Metastases in
Head and Neck Cancer

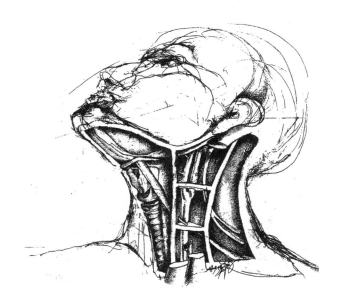

B. M. Lippert, J. A. Werner (eds.)

Proceedings of the 2nd International Symposium
January 25-27, 2001, Marburg, Germany

Tectum Verlag
Marburg 2001

Die Deutsche Bibliothek - CIP-Einheitsaufnahme

Lippert, B. M.; Werner, J. A. (Hrsg.):
Metastases in Head and Neck Cancer.
Proceedings of the 2nd International Symposium
January 25-27, 2001, Marburg, Germany.
/ herausgegeben von B. M. Lippert und J. A. Werner
- Marburg : Tectum Verlag, 2001
ISBN 3-8288-8254-4

Tectum Verlag
Marburg 2001

PREFACE

The *International Symposium on Metastases in Head and Neck Cancer* (January 25-27, 2001, Marburg, Germany) is the second conference concerning this subject organized by the editors. The first symposium took place in January 1998 in Kiel, Germany, chaired by Prof. Dr. H. M. Rudert.

The Symposium was equally focused on clinically oriented questions concerning metastases of head and neck cancer as well as on diverse theme-oriented questions out of the basic sciences. Intentionally the current meeting was structured in a way that there were no parallel sessions which should optimise the exchange of knowledge between all participants. As you can see in the contents there were several high profile representatives of the field. This fact also explains the high scientific quality of several of the contributions.

Due to the good resonance on the diversity and the quality of the presentations we intend to offer a third conference concerning the subject of metastases in head and neck cancer in a few years. The necessity of research in these fields is clear regarding the unchanged established prognostic relevance of metastatic spread.

The abstracts of the first conference were printed in the supplement of the British Journal of Cancer [77 (Suppl. 1), 1998]. A proceedings volume did not appear because of the move of the editors to Marburg, Germany. Nevertheless there were numerous inquiries concerning the publication of the presented results. Bearing this in mind it was a matter or course for us to publish this proceedings volume of the current symposium. Such a volume only makes sense when being published immediately after the meeting and including most of the contributions. Both points were achieved.

In this context we would like to thank all the authors who handed in their manuscripts before the end of the deadline. We also want to thank the publishing house Tectum that did not only make it possible to publish the volume in short terms but also to produce it at a really reasonable and for such volumes untypical price.

Burkard M. Lippert, M.D.   Jochen A. Werner, M.D.

CONTENTS

I

II

HPV AS A FACTOR IN OROPHARYNGEAL CANCER: PRESENCE, TYPE AND ROLE IN THE MALIGNANT PROCESS

Erin L. McKean[1], Ajita Narayan[1], Thomas E. Carey[1], Douglas Chepeha[1], William R. Carroll[2], Carol R. Bradford[1]

[1]The Head and Neck Oncology Laboratory, Head and Neck Oncology Division, Deparment of Otolaryngology, University of Michigan Cancer Center, Ann Arbor, MI 48109

[2]Otolaryngology-Head and Neck Surgery, University of Alabama, Birmingham, AL 35249-6889.

ABSTRACT

In order to explore the role of HPV in head and neck cancers, fresh tumors, cell lines and adjacent normal tissue were tested for the presence of HPV DNA. A subset of tumors from relatively young, nonsmoking, non-alcohol-abusing female patients with oropharyngeal cancer was the focus of this particular study. Oropharyngeal tumors from four of four female patients, ranging in age from 43 to 57 years, with lingual or tonsillar cancers were positive for HPV using PCR with L1 consensus primers. In addition, all four cases were positive for PCR signals with HPV-16-specific primers. PCR with primers specific for HPV-6, 11, 18, 31, 33, and 57 were all negative. In two cases, cell cultures from the tumors were tested. In one case, the tumor DNA showed a strongly positive result for HPV, while the culture was only weakly positive. In the other case, two separate cultures from opposite sides of the tumor were HPV-positive, whereas the DNA isolated from the tumor tissue was negative, suggesting that the cultures from this specimen might be enriched for HPV-containing cells. While our results to date support a role for high-risk HPV in the etiology of a subset of oropharyngeal cancers, there is much to be done to establish a firm linkage between HPV and head and neck squamous cell cancers. Ongoing investigations will help us to characterize the state of the viral genome, i.e. whether it is integrated or episomal; the location of the viral genome integration; the state of p53 and Rb; and the expression of viral E6, E7, and E2 genes in head and neck cancers.

INTRODUCTION

Human papillomaviruses (HPV) are associated with about 10% of cancers worldwide (mostly anogenital). Recent studies have advanced the concept that HPV plays a role in head and

1

neck squamous cell carcinogenesis. Based on polymerase chain reaction (PCR) assays, slightly one-third of head and neck squamous cell cancers (HNSCCs) contain HPV DNA[1-7]. HPV-16, a high-risk papillomavirus, has been detected in almost 90% of these positive squamous cell tumors. There appear to be no consistent significant differences in the prevalence of HPV in these tumors based on gender, age, race, lymph node status, and tobacco use. Some studies do, however, imply a strong association between HPV and an oropharyngeal tumor site[8,9]. The mode of transmission of HPV in the head and neck is unknown. No specific sexual behavior or other practices have been associated with HPV infection in the head and neck. However, prevalence of HPV in the head and neck increases with an increase in the number of sexual partners[10].

Human papillomaviruses are epitheliotropic, nonenveloped, icosahedral DNA viruses containing double-stranded, covalently closed DNA in a protein coat. The 8 kilobase HPV genome is organized into three segments: the long control region (LCR), encompassing about 10% of the genome and functioning to control gene expression; early (E) genes, comprising about 50% of the genome and encoding nonstructural proteins that regulate viral transcription and replication; and late (L) genes, making up 40% of the genome and expressing capsid proteins. Integration of HPV DNA often results in inactivation of the early E2 gene, which codes for the E2 protein, a potent downregulator of HPV E6 and E7 transcription[11]. Mechanistically, the HPV E6 and E7 oncoproteins from high-risk types not only inactivate the pRB and p53 tumor suppressor functions but also transactivate a family of cyclin-dependent kinase complexes that control eukaryotic cell division[12,13]. The HPV E6 oncoprotein complexes with the host cell p53, inducing its degradation, and may also activate telomerase[14]. E7 complexes with retinoblastoma gene products (Rb1, p107, and p130), disrupting a number of transcription factors and deregulating different check points in the cell cycle[15]. Together, E6 and E7 expression allow a cell to evade normal cell cycle control and to gain functions critical in immortalization of tumor cells.

MATERIALS AND METHODS

Samples and Primary Cultures

The tumor specimens tested were derived from the University of Michigan Department of Otolaryngology squamous cell cancer patients without the usual risk factors for head and neck cancer (July 2000 – November 2000). Established risk factors for HNSCC include alcohol and tobacco use, older age (>60 years), and male gender. The incidence of oral cancer rises with age and peaks between ages 64 and 74, though for the Black American population, this peak occurs approximately 10 years earlier. With regards to the gender factor, oral cancer is seen twice as often in men. Therefore, out of the University of Michigan HNSCC cases, four fresh tumor specimens were obtained from nonsmoking, nonalcohol-abusing, Caucasian women under the age of 60 years (Figure 1). Each tumor specimen was divided into three parts: one was cultured, one was used for DNA extraction, and one was frozen for later immunohistochemical analysis. The cultures were maintained in DMEM supplemented with nonessential amino acids, L glutamine, penicillin, streptomycin, and 10% fetal bovine serum and were grown at 37° C in 95% air/5% CO_2.

DNA extraction

Fresh tumor DNA was isolated by SDS/Proteinase K digestion. Primary culture DNA was isolated using DNAzol (Gibco BRL). DNA was extracted using phenol-chloroform-isoamyl alcohol (25:24:1), precipitated with 0.1 volume of 3 M sodium acetate and two volumes of 100% ice-cold ethanol, washed with 70% ethanol, air-dried and redissolved in 10mM Tris-0.1mM EDTA. Yield was assessed by O.D. 260 and purity by O.D. 260/O.D. 280. Aliquots were stored at -20° C.

Polymerase Chain Reaction

Specimens were analyzed by PCR for the presence of HPV DNA using the promiscuous primers MY09 and MY11, which were derived from the HPV L1 ORF and which generate a 450 base pair fragment[16]. They were further tested for HPV type using type-specific primers based on various regions of the HPV genome. Reactions used HPV-positive control cell lines (CaSki and/or HeLa) and distilled water as a reagent control. To prevent contamination, pre-PCR operations were carried out in an area physically separated from post-PCR work. A 10-µL reaction mixture was prepared consisting of 0.1-µg of sample DNA, 25mM $MgCl_2$, 0.2µL each of 10mM dNTP and both primers, and 0.25 U of recombinant Taq polymerase. Initial denaturation took place at 95° C for 5 minutes. For the promiscuous primer set, this was followed by 24 cycles of denaturation at 94° C for 2 minutes, annealing at 46° C for 2 minutes and 55° C for 1 minute, and elongation at 72° C for 1 minute. Final elongation took place at 72° C for 7 minutes. For the type-specific reactions, 30 cycles of 94° C for 30 seconds, 52° C for 1 minute, and 72° C for 1 minute were run, followed also by a 7 minute final elongation at 72° C. PCR products were run on 1.5% agarose gels, stained with ethidium bromide, and photographed.

Southern Blot

*Eco*R1 (Roche) and *Bam*H1 (Roche) were used together to digest 10µg of genomic DNA. The digested DNA was electrophoresed on a 1.2% agarose gel, transferred to a nylon ZetaProbe membrane (BioRad) and crosslinked to the membrane. The HPV DNA probe was derived from the Caski HPV-16 L1 region and was radiolabeled with 50µCi of $[\alpha^{32}P]dCTP$ using a random-primed labeling kit (Gibco BRL). Southern blots were prehybridized at 56° C in hybridization solution (5X Denhardt's, 6X SSC, 0.5% SDS, 10 µg/µL denatured salmon sperm DNA) for 2 hours. The blots were then hybridized with the HPV probe overnight at 54° C. Membranes were washed twice at 37° C in 6X SSC, 0.1%SDS and exposed to x-ray film.

RESULTS

DNA from tumor tissue and/or cell cultures from four patients were positive for HPV using L1 consensus primers (Figure 2). These results represent PCR analysis of either fresh tumor DNA or DNA extracted from primary cell culture. Fresh tumor DNA was HPV-positive in patients A, B, and D, but HPV-negative in patient C. Cultures were established successfully for patients C and D. Interestingly, in patient C, cultures from both the left and right sides of the original tumor specimen turned up positive despite a negative result using DNA extracted from the fresh tumor tissue.

3

HPV typing by PCR revealed 4 of 4 HPV-positive samples contained HPV-16 (Figure 3). Fresh tumor DNA was HPV-16-positive from patients A, B, and D. Culture DNA was positive for both patients C and D. PCR reactions for HPV 6, 11, 18, 31, 33, and 57 were all negative.

Southern blot hybridization, using both fresh and cell culture DNA, confirmed the HPV-positive results for patients C and D. There was not enough DNA available from the tumor tissue of patients A and B to perform a Southern hybridization.

DISCUSSION

HPV-16 is the most common HPV type in HNSCC. Our results are consistent with this. Additionally, we found 100% positivity in specimens from patients presumed to be at low-risk for developing HNSCC. All four were women, all had low or no tobacco exposure and none admitted to alcohol abuse. Although our sample size is low, this is quite striking. We hypothesize that HPV has a role in HNSCC, specifically in those patients without the usual head and neck cancer risk factors.

For patient C, the tumor DNA was negative, but the culture was positive. There are several explanations for this result. First, because we used fresh tissue and not microdissected material for DNA extraction, it is possible that from the original tumor specimen, DNA was extracted from tissue surrounding the cancer but not from the tumor itself. Another possibility is that oral cancers harboring HPV are composed of a heterogeneous cell population[17]. Although we did not address the question directly, literature suggests that in HPV-positive tumors, only a minority of cells harbor HPV DNA. Patient C's culture contains tumor cells in nested islands with large, pleomorphic nuclei. Enrichment of these presumed tumor cells in culture very likely led to the strong HPV-16 positive signal.

Patient D, on the other hand, had a strongly HPV-positive tumor DNA while the culture was only faintly positive. In contrast to patient C's culture, patient D's culture appears to be fibroblastic. Possibly, stromal tissue in the vicinity of the tumor focus was cultured rather than the tumor cells, causing a diminished HPV signal.

Thus, testing for HPV in culture may have clinical implications even when the original tumor specimen is negative (as seen with patient C). However, testing culture DNA alone will not necessarily give greater sensitivity (as seen with patient D). Previously in our laboratory, 22 cell lines have been screened for HPV. HPV DNA was identified in 3 of those 22 cell lines[18]. When tumor specimens were screened for HPV, 15 of 22 inverted papilloma specimens positive, as were 45 of 51 respiratory papillomas[19]. The lower prevalence of HPV in cell lines versus fresh tumors may suggest that HPV exists in an episomal state in a subset of HNSCCs. In addition, the benign papillomatous tumors actually produce viral particles making detection far more likely than in a malignant tumor where viral copy number per cell is generally low.

More tumors from "low-risk" patients (those with low carcinogen exposure) should be tested and the positive specimens that are already identified must be further characterized. We are currently using flourescence in situ hybridization (FISH) to detect HPV integration and to

4

assist in localizing the integration site. We are performing FISH on a consistently HPV-16-positive cell line established in our laboratory and also in our newly established cultures. Further, we are investigating the status of other proteins (specifically p53, Bax, and the Bcl family of proteins) in the established cell line and cultures.

Figure 1.

Patient	Age	Site	Smokes	Drinks	Stage
A	57	Tongue	No	No	T3N0
B	48	Tongue	No	No	In situ
C	43	Tongue	No	No	T1N0
D	57	Tonsil	Quit '91	No	T2N2C

Figure 2.

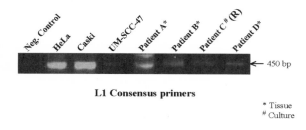

L1 Consensus primers

* Tissue
\# Culture

Figure 3.

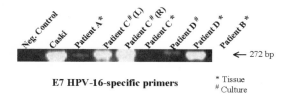

E7 HPV-16-specific primers

* Tissue
\# Culture

5

REFERENCES

1. McKaig RG, Baric RS, Olshan AF. Human Papillomavirus in Head and Neck Cancer: Epidemiology and Molecular Biology. Head and Neck May 1998;250-265.
2. Sugerman, PB, Shillitoe EJ. The high risk human papillomaviruses and oral cancer: evidence for and against a causal relationship. Oral Dis Sep 1997;3: 130-47.
3. Bouda M, Gorgoulis VG, Kastrinakis NG, Giannoudis A, Tsoli E, Danassi- Afentaki D, et al. "High-risk" HPV types are frequently detected in potentiallymalignant and malignant oral lesions, but not in normal oral mucosa. ModPathol Jun 2000;13(6):644-53.
4. Hoffman M, Kahn T, Mahnke CG, Goeroegh T, Lippert BM, Werner JA. Prevalence of human papillomavirus in squamous cell carcinoma of the head and neck determined by polymerase chain reaction and Southern blot hybridization: proposal for optimized diagnostic requirements. Acta Otolaryngol Jan 1998;118(1):138-44.
5. Sisk EA, Bradford CR, Jacob A, et al. Human papillomavirus infection in "young" versus "old" patients with squamous cell carcinoma of the head and neck. Head Neck Oct 2000:649-57.
6. Gillison ML, Koch WM, Capone RB, Spafford M, Westra WH, Wu L, et al. Evidence for a causal association between human papillomavirus and a subset of head and neck cancers. J Natl Cancer Inst May 2000;92(9):709-20.
7. Badaracco G, Venuti A, Bartolazzi A, Morello R, Marzetti F, Marcante ML. Overexpression of p53 and bcl-2 proteins and the presence of HPV infection are independent events in head and neck cancer. J Oral Pathol Med Apr 2000;29(4): 173-9.
8. Paz IB, Cook N, Odom-Maryon T, Xie Y, Wilczynski SP. Human papillomavirus (HPV) in head and neck cancer. An association of HPV 16 with squamous cell carcinoma of Waldeyer's tonsillar ring. Cancer 1997;79:595-604.
9. Snijders PJ, Cromme FV, van den Brule A, Schrijnemakers HF, Snow GB, Meijer CJ, et al. Prevalence and expression of human papillomavirus in tonsillar Carcinomas, indicating a possible viral etiology. Int J Cancer 1992;51:845-50.
10. Schwartz
11. McGlennen RC. Human papillomavirus oncogenesis. Clin Lab Med Jun 2000; 20(2):383-406.
12. Werness BA, Levine AJ, Howley PM. Association of human papillomavirus types 16 and 18 E6 proteins with p53. Science 1990;248:76-9.
13. Romanczuk H, Thierry F, Howley PM. Mutational analysis of *cis* elements involved in E2 modulation of human papillomavirus type 16 p97 and type 18 p105. J Virology 1990;64:2849-59.
14. Klingelhutz AJ, Foster SA, McDougall JK. Telomerase activation by the E6 gene product of human papillomavirus type 16. Nature 1996;168:195-9.
15. Davies R, Hicks R, Crook T, et al. Human papillomavirus type 16 E7 associated with a histone H1 kinase and with p107 through sequences necessary for transformation. J Virology 1993;67:2521-8.
16. Resnick RM, Cornelissen MTE, Wright DK, et al. Detection and typing of human papillomavirus in archival cervical cancer specimens by DNA amplification with consensus primers. J Natl Cancer Inst 1990;82:1477-84.
17. Atula S, Grenman R, Kujari H, Syrjanen S. Detection of human papillomavirus (HPV) in laryngeal carcinoma cell lines provides evidence for a heterogeneic cell population. Eur J Cancer May 1999;35(5):825-32.
18. Bradford CR, Zacks SE, Andropy EJ, et al. Human papillomavirus DNA Sequences in cell lines derived from head and neck squamous cell carcinomas. Otolaryngology- Head Neck Surg Mar 1991;104:303-10.
19. Moore CF, Wiatrak BJ, Bradford CR, Carey TE, et al. High-risk human papillomavirus types and squamous cell carcinoma in patients with respiratory papillomas. Otolaryngology- Head Neck Surg May 1999;120:698-705.

THE ROLE OF C-*ERB*B RECEPTORS IN HEAD AND NECK SQUAMOUS CELL CARCINOMAS: CORRELATION WITH MATRIX METALLOPROTEINASES AND VASCULAR ENDOTHELIAL GROWTH FACTORS

Pornchai O-charoenrat, MD[1], Peter H. Rhys-Evans, FRCS[1], Daniel J. Archer, FRCS[1], Suzanne A. Eccles, PhD[2]

[1]Head and Neck Unit, Royal Marsden Hospital, London SW3 6JJ, United Kingdom
[2]Section of Cancer Therapeutics, Institute of Cancer Research, Surrey, SM2 5NG, United Kingdom

Running title: C-*erb*B receptors in HNSCC
                    P. O-charoenrat *et al.*

Keywords: c-*erb*B receptors, epidermal growth factor receptor, head and neck cancer, matrix metalloproteinase, squamous cell carcinoma, vascular endothelial growth factor

Correspondence to: *P. O-charoenrat, Head and Neck Unit, Royal Marsden Hospital, Fulham Road, London SW3 6JJ, UK (e-mail: pornchaio@yahoo.co.uk).*

ABSTRACT

Background. We studied the profile of four c-*erb*B receptors in head and neck squamous cell carcinomas (HNSCC) and determined whether their expression was associated with clinicopathological features and key molecules involved in angiogenesis and metastasis. We also assessed the impact of expression on survival.

Methods. This prospective study included 54 cases of primary HNSCC, of which 27 cases showed lymph node metastasis. The expression of c-*erb*B receptors, matrix metalloproteinases (MMPs) and vascular endothelial growth factor (VEGF) family members was simultaneously analyzed in the tissue homogenates by semi-quantitative RT-PCR.

Results. HNSCC frequently co-expressed multiple c-*erb*B receptors and showed significant correlations amongst their levels. High expression of EGFR, c-*erb*B-2 or c-*erb*B-3 was associated with an infiltrating mode of invasion, nodal metastases and advanced pathological stages. EGFR and c-*erb*B-2 levels were strongly correlated ($P = 0.0004-0.029$)

7

with the expression of MMP-2, MMP-7, MMP-9, MMP-10, MMP-11, MMP-13, VEGF-A and VEGF-C whereas the levels of c-*erb*B-3 and B-4 showed a weaker correlation ($P = 0.049$-0.01) with some MMPs and VEGF-C. Only nodal metastasis and EGFR levels were significantly associated with poor outcome in uni- and multi-variate analysis.

Conclusions. Co-operative signaling of all four c-*erb*B receptors may play a significant role in the pathogenesis of HNSCC. Amongst these, EGFR appears to be the dominant component controlling the invasive and angio-/lymphangiogenic phenotype in HNSCC via upregulation of multiple MMPs and VEGFs.

INTRODUCTION

The c-*erb*B receptors have four homologous members in the family: the epidermal growth factor receptor (EGFR or c-*erb*B-1 or HER-1 for human EGF receptor-1), c-*erb*B-2 (*neu* or HER-2), c-*erb*B-3 (HER-3) and c-*erb*B-4 (HER-4).[1, 2] Numerous studies have suggested the potential role of the c-*erb*B receptors and their ligands in the progression of head and neck squamous cell carcinoma (HNSCC).[3-11] However, the underlying mechanisms remained unclear. Recently we demonstrated that the expression of multiple matrix metalloproteinases (MMPs) and vascular endothelial growth factors (VEGFs) is a common feature in both experimental and clinical models of HNSCC, and that the analysis of specific MMPs and VEGFs may be useful to evaluate the malignant potential in individual HNSCC.[8, 9, 12] Our *in vitro* studies also suggest a link between the c-*erb*B signaling and regulation of multiple MMPs and VEGFs in HNSCC.[6-8] The differential regulatory patterns of these key molecules by the aberration of c-*erb*B receptors may be crucial for the loss of growth regulation, angiogenesis, invasion and metastasis of the tumors expressing them. In the present study, we characterized the expression and prognostic value of four c-*erb*B receptor family members in HNSCCs and their relationship with clinicopathological characteristics. We also examined the possible roles of c-*erb*B oncogenes on expression of key molecules involved in HNSCC invasion and metastasis in particular the relationships with MMPs and VEGFs.

MATERIAL AND METHODS

Patients and Tissue Samples. The protocol for the following studies was approved by the Ethical Committee of the Royal Marsden Hospital Trust, UK. Fresh tissue samples were obtained from 54 patients undergoing major surgical resection for HNSCC at the Head and Neck Unit, the Royal Marsden Hospital, from July 1997 through October 1999. None of the patients had previously received preoperative chemotherapy or radiotherapy. All patients were treated with curative intent and adjuvant treatment was given in appropriate cases following the Hospital's protocol. In each case, the portion of tumor was resected near the advancing edge of the tumor, avoiding its necrotic center. After excision, the tissues were immediately snap-frozen and stored in liquid nitrogen until use. The adjacent tissues were submitted for histopathological study, which revealed that most of the cells were malignant. Tumors were staged according to the TNM classification 5th edition[13] and the mode of cancer invasion (MI) was histologically classified as described previously.[14] In 27 cases, tissue samples of metastatic lymph nodes (LNM) were also available for analysis. Matched histologically normal mucosae of the upper aerodigestive tract, resected 5 cm distant from the tumor area, were obtained in 32 cases.

Semi-quantitative RT-PCR. The semi-quantitative RT-PCR assay and the primer sequences have been described previously.[8,9] The following genes were assayed using specific primer pairs: EGFR, c-*erb*B-2, c-*erb*B-3, c-*erb*B-4, MMP-1, MMP-2, MMP-3, MMP-7, MMP-9, MMP-10, MMP-11, MMP-13, MMP-14 (MT1-MMP), TIMP-1, TIMP-2, VEGF-A (isoform 121, 165, 189, 206), VEGF-B, VEGF-C and VEGF-D. β-actin was used to check RNA integrity and as an internal control. In order to control gel-to-gel variability, each PCR product from SIHN-006 carcinoma cells[7-9] was also electrophoresed as a control on every gel. The level of mRNA was calculated as the ratio of tissue sample to control cell line on the same scan and was then corrected as a ratio to the corresponding β-actin level. Sequences of PCR primer sets for c-*erb*B receptors (in 5'-3' direction) were as follows: EGFR forward-AA CCGGACTGAAGGAGCTGC, backward-ACGTGGCTTCGTCTCGGAAT, product size = 392 bps; c-*erb*B-2 forward-CCTCTCTCAGATTCAAGTGG, backward-TGACAGTAGTGG AGTGATGG, product size = 852 bps; c-*erb*B-3 forward-CTGAATGGCCTGAGTGTGA, backward-TGAGGAGCACAGATGGTCTT, product size = 543 bps; and c-*erb*B-4 forward-CAGCGATTCTCAGTCAGTGT, backward-CAATGATCCTGTGCCAATGC, product size = 961 bps.

Statistical Analysis. All statistical analyses were performed on the entire patient population using the SPSS software system (SPSS for Windows, version 8.0). The association between the different clinicopathological and biological characteristics was studied by the Pearson χ^2 test. Cancer-specific survival curves and median survival times were calculated by the method of Kaplan and Meier, and differences in survivor function due to prognostic factors were calculated by the log-rank test. The joint effects of covariables that were significant at a level of 0.25 in univariate analysis were further examined via Cox multivariate regression analysis using a forward stepwise selection procedure. All *P* values were two-sided. A *P*-value of less than 0.05 was considered statistically significant and used for entering or removing a covariable from this model. Correlations between the mRNA levels of c-*erb*B receptors, MMPs and VEGFs were computed using the two-tailed Spearman nonparametric correlation.

RESULTS

Expression of c-*erb*B Receptors in HNSCC Tissues. The mRNA expression of EGFR was significantly greater in malignant tissues (primary tumors and/or LNM) in comparison with the mRNA levels in histologically normal mucosae (2.4-fold, *P* < 0.0001). Varying levels of c-*erb*B-2, c-*erb*B-3 and c-*erb*B-4 receptors were detected in tumors (primary HNSCC and LNM) and adjacent histologically normal mucosae and the expression levels between groups were not significantly different as reported previously.[3] In addition, no differences were found between expression of all c-*erb*B receptors tested in primary HNSCC *vs.* LNM (data not shown). When the patients were separated into two groups according to the cut-off values obtained from the median values of mRNA levels determined by RT-PCR in the primary tumors, 46.3 % (25/54) co-expressed high levels of EGFR and c-*erb*B-2, 37.0 % (20/54) co-expressed high levels of EGFR, c-*erb*B-2 and c-*erb*B-3, and 25.9 % (14/54) expressed high levels of all four c-*erb*B receptors.

Correlations between Clinicopathological Characteristics and Survival. As of December 31, 2000, the median follow-up period for living patients was 26 months (range, 15-41 months), 35 patients (64.8 %) were alive, whereas 15 patients (27.8 %) were dead of tumors and 4 patients (7.4 %) died from unrelated causes. The prognostic impact of clinicopathological and biological parameters on patient survival was firstly evaluated by univariate analysis. Infiltrating mode of invasion ($P = 0.027$), positive nodal status ($P = 0.0008$), and advanced pathological stage ($P = 0.0001$) were significantly associated with a worse survival. Among the c-*erb*B receptors, EGFR ($P = 0.0009$) and c-*erb*B-2 ($P = 0.0231$) were strong predictors of adverse outcome. Age, gender, tumor site, T classification, and histologic grade were not able to predict disease outcome. Cox multivariate regression analysis was performed to define the variables with independent prognostic value with respect to survival. Nodal metastasis ($P = 0.0019$, Relative Hazard = 4.13) and EGFR levels ($P = 0.0206$, Relative Hazard = 3.05) were the only characteristics to retain an independent prognostic influence on cancer-specific survival (Fig 1).

Levels of c-*erb*B Receptors in Relation to Clinicopathological Characteristics. Statistically significant correlations were demonstrated between high EGFR expression and an infiltrating mode of invasion ($P < 0.001$, Odds Ratio = 11.143), lymph node metastases ($P = 0.001$, Odds Ratio = 9.50) and advanced pathological stages ($P = 0.005$, Odds Ratio = 6.667). Enhanced expression of c-*erb*B-2 was also correlated with invasion ($P = 0.018$, Odds Ratio = 4.80) and lymph node involvement ($P = 0.003$, Odds Ratio = 7.20). High levels of c-*erb*B-3, but not c-*erb*B-4, showed significant correlations with invasion ($P = 0.007$, Odds Ratio = 5.833), lymph node involvement ($P = 0.001$, Odds Ratio = 9.917) and advanced stages ($P = 0.016$, Odds Ratio = 5.194). In contrast, there was no association between levels of the c-*erb*B family members and age, gender, size and site of primary tumors or histological grade.

Correlations between Levels of c-*erb*B Receptors, MMPs and VEGFs. We investigated the relationship between the expression levels of c-*erb*B receptors and molecules involved in the process of invasion/metastasis including MMP and VEGF family members (Table 1). The levels of EGFR were significantly correlated with those of c-*erb*B-2 ($P = 0.004$) or c-*erb*B-3 ($P = 0.006$) and the levels of c-*erb*B-2 showed good correlation with those of c-*erb*B-3 ($P = 0.002$) or c-*erb*B-4 ($P = 0.01$). In addition, the levels of c-*erb*B-3 showed strong correlation with those of c-*erb*B-4 ($P < 0.001$). EGFR levels were strongly correlated ($P = 0.0004$ - 0.029) with the expression of MMP-2, MMP-7, MMP-9, MMP-10, VEGF-A (all four isoforms), and VEGF-C. C-*erb*B-2 receptor also showed a significant correlation ($P = 0.0007$ - 0.013) with MMP-2, MMP-9, MMP-10, MMP-11, MMP-13, VEGF-A isoform 121 and 165, and VEGF-C whereas the levels of c-*erb*B-3 and B-4 receptors showed a weaker correlation ($P = 0.049$ - 0.01) with some MMPs and VEGF-C.

DISCUSSION

The present study demonstrated that a significant proportion of human HNSCC simultaneously expressed several receptors of the c-*erb*B family. Furthermore, a statistically significant direct correlation among expression of these receptors was observed in this series of patients. Enhanced expression of EGFR or c-*erb*B-2, infiltrating mode of invasion and nodal involvement were the variables found to be significantly correlated with a reduced survival by univariate analysis, but only EGFR and nodal status were shown to be independent prognostic indicators. The prognostic impact of c-*erb*B receptor aberration could relate to disordered cell growth via a variety of mechanisms, including altered growth factor production, quantitative or qualitative changes in growth factor receptors, and disturbances of intracellular signaling events following receptor binding.[2] Several experimental studies have demonstrated a causal link between c-*erb*B expression and tumor progression, for example, tumor cells overexpressing EGFR are more invasive *in vitro* and highly metastatic *in vivo*.[9,15] Although c-*erb*B-2 is an orphan receptor, the formation of heterodimer complexes between c-*erb*B-2 and ligand-occupied EGFR appears to be an important mechanism for inter-receptor activation and for synergistic signal transduction.[6,16,17] The roles of c-*erb*B-3 and c-*erb*B-4 in HNSCC progression are less clear. However, their ability to form heterodimers with other c-*erb*B family members upon stimulation by their direct ligands (i.e. heregulins) has been shown to enhance signaling via EGFR or c-*erb*B-2 and the invasive properties of HNSCC cells.[6,8]

While several MMPs have been implicated in HNSCC progression,[12, 18] the mechanism(s) which lead to their overexpression *in vivo* are largely unknown. Increasing evidence suggests a correlation between c-*erb*B signaling and some members of the MMP family, for example, major c-*erb*B ligands have been shown to upregulate the expression of several MMPs in various tumor cell lines.[6, 7, 19-21] The levels of EGFR on tumor cells, and their activation through paracrine and/or autocrine mechanisms may be an important factor affecting the production of proteolytic enzymes.[9,22] Aberrant c-*erb*B-2 activation has also been shown to increase invasive capacity by stimulating the expression of several MMPs.[23-25] In the present study, we found that the expression levels of EGFR, c-*erb*B-2 and c-*erb*B-3 have a significant association with nodal metastasis. Co-expression of all four receptors was also demonstrated in the metastatic lymph nodes as in the primary tumor samples. It is, therefore, possible that different receptor tyrosine kinases cooperate in the process of lymphatic spread.

The VEGF family of proteins including VEGF-A, VEGF-B, VEGF-C and VEGF-D are specific, highly potent angiogenic agents acting to increase vessel permeability, endothelial cell growth, proliferation, migration, and differentiation.[26] The linkage between the EGFR and c-*erb*B-2 signaling and VEGF-A regulation was firstly postulated by Petit *et al.*[27] We recently confirmed and extended this observation by showing that activation of c-*erb*B receptors by ligand binding had significant differences in the regulation of the steady-state mRNAs for VEGF-A, VEGF-B, VEGF-C and VEGF-D in HNSCC cells and suggesting that they served distinct, although perhaps complementary (VEGF-A and VEGF-C) or antagonistic (VEGF-D) functions.[8] Our unpublished observations show that the expression of VEGF family members is a common feature in both experimental and clinical models of HNSCC and enhanced expression of VEGF-A and VEGF-C is significantly correlated with the presence of lymph node metastases and highly invasive primary tumors. The present findings of significant correlation between expression of EGFR, c-*erb*B-2, or c-*erb*B-3 levels and VEGF-A or VEGF-C levels provide compelling evidence that cross-talk between the c-*erb*B family of receptors and VEGF family members exists in clinical HNSCC. The regulation of these potent angiogenic factors by c-*erb*B signals may be crucial for the promotion of HNSCC tumorigenesis and progression.

We conclude that expression of multiple c-*erb*B receptors is a characteristic of HNSCC. Co-operative signaling of all four c-*erb*B receptors may play a significant role in controlling the invasive and angio-/lymphangiogenic phenotype of HNSCC via upregulation of multiple MMPs and VEGFs. Among the c-*erb*B family receptors studied here, EGFR was the most significant factor in predicting the outcome of the patients with HNSCC, which suggests that EGFR may play the most significant role at least in these types of cancer.

Figure 1. Kaplan-Meier analysis showing the overall cancer-specific survival among 54 head and neck cancer patients according to (*A*) cervical lymph nodal status or (*B*) epidermal growth factor receptor (EGFR) levels in the primary tumor.

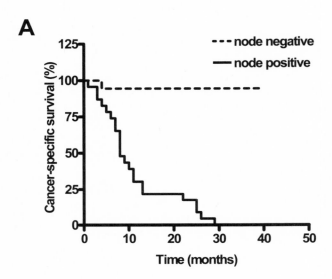

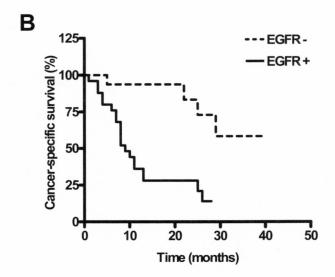

Table 1. Relationships of EGFR, c-*erb*B-2, c-*erb*B-3 and c-*erb*B-4 expression with MMPs/TIMPs and VEGFs

	EGFR	C-*erb*B-2	C-*erb*B-3	C-*erb*B-4
EGFR	N/A	$P = 0.004$	$P = 0.006$	$P = 0.387$
C-*erb*B-2	$P = 0.004$	N/A	$P = 0.002$	$P = 0.010$
C-*erb*B-3	$P = 0.006$	$P = 0.002$	N/A	$P < 0.001$
C-*erb*B-4	$P = 0.387$	$P = 0.010$	$P = 0.001$	N/A
MMP-1	$P = 0.689$	$P = 0.976$	$P = 0.857$	$P = 0.512$
MMP-2	$P = 0.019$	$P = 0.010$	$P = 0.596$	$P = 0.238$
MMP-3	$P = 0.155$	$P = 0.446$	$P = 0.875$	$P = 0.666$
MMP-7	$P = 0.029$	$P = 0.060$	$P = 0.018$	$P = 0.060$
MMP-9	$P = 0.006$	$P = 0.013$	$P = 0.010$	$P = 0.761$
MMP-10	$P = 0.014$	$P = 0.005$	$P = 0.042$	$P = 0.276$
MMP-11	$P = 0.176$	$P = 0.004$	$P = 0.087$	$P = 0.048$
MMP-13	$P = 0.140$	$P = 0.007$	$P = 0.173$	$P = 0.480$
MMP-14	$P = 0.531$	$P = 0.188$	$P = 0.372$	$P = 0.063$
TIMP-1	$P = 0.201$	$P = 0.774$	$P = 0.170$	$P = 0.740$
TIMP-2	$P = 0.474$	$P = 0.451$	$P = 0.854$	$P = 0.805$
VEGF-A isoform 121	$P = 0.002$	$P = 0.004$	$P = 0.160$	$P = 0.899$
VEGF-A isoform 165	$P = 0.0004$	$P = 0.013$	$P = 0.059$	$P = 0.827$
VEGF-A isoform 189	$P = 0.004$	$P = 0.127$	$P = 0.119$	$P = 0.063$
VEGF-A isoform 206	$P = 0.025$	$P = 0.799$	$P = 0.531$	$P = 0.612$
VEGF-B	$P = 0.537$	$P = 0.098$	$P = 0.835$	$P = 0.143$
VEGF-C	$P = 0.0006$	$P = 0.0007$	$P = 0.049$	$P = 0.186$
VEGF-D	$P = 0.729$	$P = 0.481$	$P = 0.012$	$P = 1.000$

REFERENCES

1. Eccles SA. Cell biology of lymphatic metastasis. The potential role of c-*erb* B oncogene signalling. *Recent Results Cancer Res* 2000; 157:41-54.

2. Klapper LN, Kirschbaum MH, Sela M, Yarden Y. Biochemical and clinical implications of the ErbB/HER signalling network of growth factor receptors. *Adv Cancer Res* 2000; 77:25-79.

3. Ibrahim SO, Vasstrand EN, Liavaag PG, Johannessen AC, Lillehaug JR. Expression of c-erbB proto-oncogene family members in squamous cell carcinoma of the head and neck. *Anticancer Res* 1997; 17:4539-4546.

4. Grandis JR, Melhem MF, Gooding WE, et al. Levels of TGF-alpha and EGFR protein in head and neck squamous cell carcinoma and patient survival. *J Natl Cancer Inst* 1998; 90:824-832.

5. Xia W, Lau Y-K, Zhang H-Z, et al. Combination of EGFR, HER-2/neu, and HER-3 is a stronger predictor for the outcome of oral squamous cell carcinoma than any individual family members. *Clin Cancer Res* 1999; 5:4164-4174.

6. O-charoenrat P, Rhys-Evans P, Court WJ, Box GM, Eccles SA. Differential modulation of proliferation, matrix metalloproteinase expression and invasion of human head and neck squamous carcinoma cells by c-*erb* B ligands. *Clin Exp Metastasis* 1999; 17:631-639.

7. O-charoenrat P, Modjtahedi H, Rhys-Evans P, Court WJ, Box GM, Eccles SA. Epidermal growth factor-like ligands differentially upregulate matrix metalloproteinase-9 in head and neck squamous carcinoma cells. *Cancer Res* 2000; 60:1121-1128.

8. O-charoenrat P, Rhys-Evans P, Modjtahedi H, Eccles SA. Vascular endothelial growth factor family members are differentially regulated by c-*erb* B signaling in head and neck squamous carcinoma cells. *Clin Exp Metastasis* 2000; 18:155-161.

9. O-charoenrat P, Rhys-Evans P, Modjtahedi H, Court W, Box G, Eccles S. Over-expression of epidermal growth factor receptor in human head and neck squamous carcinoma cell lines correlates with matrix metalloproteinase-9 expression and *in vitro* invasion. *Int J Cancer* 2000; 86:307-317.

10. O-charoenrat P, Rhys-Evans P, Eccles SA. Expression and regulation of c-*erb* B ligands in human head and neck squamous carcinoma cells. *Int J Cancer* 2000; 88:759-765.

11. Werkmeister R, Brandt B, Joos U. Clinical relevance of *erb* B-1 and -2 oncogenes in oral carcinomas. *Oral Oncology* 2000; 36:100-105.

12. O-charoenrat P, Rhys-Evans P, Eccles SA . Correlations between MMPs and TIMP-1 with invasion and metastasis in head and neck squamous cell carcinomas. *Clin Exp Metastasis* 1999; 17:773.

13. Sobin LH, Wittekind C, eds. UICC TNM Classification of Malignant Tumours. New York: John Wiley & Sons, Inc 1997; 5th ed.

14. Yamamoto E, Kohama G, Sunakawa H, Iwai M, Hiratsuka H. Mode of invasion: bleomycin sensitivity and clinical course in squamous cell carcinoma of the oral cavity. *Cancer* 1983; 51:2175-2180.

15. Radinsky R, Risin S, Fan D, et al. Level and function of epidermal growth factor receptor predict the metastatic potential of human colon carcinoma cells. *Clin Cancer Res* 1995; 1:19-31.

16. Yu D, Wang S, Dulski K, Tsai C, Nicolson G, Hung M. C-erb-B-2/neu overexpression enhances metastatic potential of human lung cancer cells by induction of metastasis-associated properties. *Cancer Res* 1994; 54:3260-3266.

17. Graus-Porta D, Beerli R, Duly J, Hynes N. ErbB-2, the preferred heterodimerization partner of all ErbB receptors, is a mediator of lateral signaling. *EMBO J* 1997; 16:1647-1655.

18. Thomas GT, Lewis MP, Speight PM. Matrix metalloproteinases and oral cancer. *Oral Oncology* 1999; 35:227-233.

19. Kerr LD, Holt JT, Matrisian LM. Growth factors regulate transin gene expression by c-fos-dependent and c-fos-independent pathways. *Science* 1988; 242:1424-1427.

20. Shima I, Sasaguri Y, Kusukawa J, et al. Production of matrix metalloproteinase 9 (92-kDa gelatinase) by human oesophageal squamous cell carcinoma in response to epidermal growth factor. *Br J Cancer* 1993; 67:721-727.

21. Johansson N, Airola K, Grenman R, Kariniemi AL, Saarialho Kere U, Kahari VM. Expression of collagenase-3 (matrix metalloproteinase-13) in squamous cell carcinomas of the head and neck. *Am J Pathol* 1997; 151:499-508.

22. Kusukawa J, Harada H, Shima I, Sasaguri Y, Kameyama T, Morimatsu M. The significance of epidermal growth factor receptor and matrix metalloproteinase-3 in squamous cell carcinoma of the oral cavity. *Eur J Cancer B Oral Oncol* 1996; 32B:217-221.

23.   Tan M, Yao J, Yu D. Overexpression of the c-erb-B-2 gene enhanced intrinsic metastasis potential in human breast cancer cells without increasing their transformation abilities. *Cancer Res* 1997; 57:1199-1205.
24.   Xu F-J, Stack S, Boyer C, et al. Heregulin and agonist anti-p185c-*erb* B2 antibodies inhibit proliferation but increase invasiveness of breast cancer cells that overexpression p185c-*erb* B2: increased invasiveness may contribute to poor prognosis. *Clin Cancer Res* 1997; 3:1629-1634.
25.   Watabe T, Yoshida K, Shindoh M, et al. The Ets-1 and Ets-2 transcription factors activate the promoters for invasion-associated urokinase and collagenase genes in response to epidermal growth factor. *Int J Cancer* 1998; 77:128-137.
26.   Veikkola T, Karkkainen M, Claesson-Welsh L, Alitalo K. Regulation of angiogenesis via vascular endothelial growth factor receptors. *Cancer Res* 2000; 60:203-212.
27.   Petit AMV, Rak J, Hung WC, et al. Neutralizing antibodies against epidermal growth factor and ErbB-2/neu receptor tyrosine kinases down-regulate vascular endothelial growth factor production by tumor cells *in vitro* and *in vivo*: angiogenic implications for signal transduction therapy of solid tumors. *Am J Pathol* 1997; 151:1523-1530.

mRNA-EXPRESSION OF MMP-13 IN HEAD AND NECK CANCER

Steffen Maune, MD, Roman Koch, Markus Hoffmann, MD, Tibor Goeroegh, PhD, Stefan Gottschlich, MD
Department of Otorhinolaryngology, Head and Neck Surgery, University of Kiel, Arnold Heller Str. 14, 24105 Kiel, Germany

Running title: MMP-13 expression in head and neck cancer

Key words: MMP-13; head and neck; metastasis; RT-PCR; mRNA

Correspondence to: *Steffen Maune, MD, Department of Otorhinolaryngology, Head and Neck Surgery, University of Kiel, Arnold Heller Str. 14, 24105 Kiel, Germany*

ABSTRACT

Background. Matrix metalloproteinase-13 (MMP-13), belongs to the family of matrix metalloproteinases (MMP), a group of endopeptidases, that are able to degrade extracellular matrix. The physiological inhibitors of MMP are the tissue inhibitors of matrix metalloproteinases (TIMP). It is assumed that MMPs play an important role in invasion and metastasis of malignancies. MMP-13 expression was already detected in squamous cell carcinoma of the head and neck, but the significance of MMP-13 in the process of metastasis of head and neck cancer is still unclear.

Methods. In total 40 tumor biopsies of head and neck squamous cell carcinoma were analysed with reverse transcriptase-PCR and Northern blot for their MMP-13 mRNA-expression. All tumor biopsies were also screened for TIMP-1 the physiological inhibitor of MMP-13. In 12 cases a N0-status and in 28 patients a N+-neck was present at the time of primary surgical therapy.

Results. In 32 of 40 (80%) tumor biopsies a MMP-13 mRNA-expression was detected in the head and neck carcinoma. In 10 of 12 (83.3%) cases with N0-status and 22 of 28 (78.5 %) cases with N+-neck a MMP-13 mRNA Expression could be shown. There was no correlation between MMP-13 mRNA expression in the tumor tissue and N-status of the patient. In 36 tumor biopsies (94,7%) a TIMP-1 expression was detected.

Conclusion. It seems that MMP-13 mRNA expression is not a prognostic factor for metastatic behaviour of head and neck cancer, but the high rate of MMP-13 expression in the head and neck squamous cell cancer tissue underlines the aggressive growth of this tumor entity.

INTRODUCTION

Matrix metalloproteinases (MMP) are a family of zinc-dependent endopeptidases which are all capable of degrading extracellular matrix components[1]. They play an important role in many physiological processes such as normal remodulation processes, ovulation, the implantation in the uterus, the development of the embryo, and the healing of wounds[2]. The physiological tissue inhibitors of the MMP's are the TIMP's, the tissue inhibitors of matrix metalloproteinases, of which four are known to-day[1, 3]. MMP expression can also be demonstrated in pathological processes such as arthritis, artherosclerosis, and carcinoma invasion and metastasization[1]. In many studies[4-9], the expression of different MMP's was demonstrated in both tumor and stroma cells of squamous cell carcinomas of the head and neck region.

In 1994, a new MMP, collagenase-3 or MMP-13, was described for the first time. The substrat specificity of MMP-13 seems to be different than that of other collagenases. MMP-13 degrades primarily fibrillary collagenes and especially collagen type II as compared to type I and III collagens. The physiological inhibitor of MMP-13 in the tissue is TIMP-1[3]. In the meantime, MMP-13 expression has been demonstrated in different pathological and physiological processes such as mamma- and vulva-carcinoma cells[10, 11], in osteoarthritic cartilage, and in developing fetal bones[12]. Up until now, only a few studies in the otorhinological area have explored the importance of the MMP-13 expression.

The expression of MMP-13 mRNA was able to be demonstrated both in several squamous cell carcinoma cell lines from the head and neck region[13-15] and in primary carcinomas of the larynx[16].

In this study, the question will be clarified of which connection there is between the expression of MMP-13 in primary head and neck carcinomas and their behaviour in metastasization.

PATIENTS AND METHODS

Patients
All in all, 40 tumor samples from squamous carcinomas of the head and neck (tonsils n=28, base of the tongue n=8, oral cavity n=4) were used, all shock frozen at -80°C. All patients were staged according to the TNM-classification of the UICC from the year 1987. The T-status was T-2 for 13 patients, T3 for 13, and T4 for the remaining 14 patients. Twelve patients had a N0 and 28 a N+ lymph node status. No distant metastasization was evident in any patient at the time of the first diagnosis. The T-status of the N0 patients was: T2 5 patients,T3 4 patients, and T4 3 patients. The average age of the entire group was 57.7 years

(N0: 58,5 and N+ 57.6 years). The ages of the entire group ranged from 44 to 78 years (N0: 44-79 and N+: 46-72 years). 32 patients were male and 8 were female.

Reverse transcriptase-PCR

After isolating the total-RNA, the mRNA was transcribed with oligo-(dT)-primers and the cDNA was amplified in a specific area of MMP-13 (Position 97-471) and TIMP-1 (Position 128-649) by PCR. The PCR-reaction-components and the reaction conditions were: 50 µM sense-primer, 50 µM anti-sense Primer, 5 µl 10XPCR-buffer, 1µl 10MM dNTP, 1.2 µl 50 mM $MgCl_2$, 2.5 U Taq-polymerase (all reagences Gibco, Karlsruhe) and 500 ng genomic DNA. The amplification took place in a total volume of 50 µl throughout 30 temperature cycles (94°C for 45 sec., 55°C for 30 sec. and 72°C for 1.5 min.) 10 ng of the produced PCR-product were dissolved in 16 µl Aqua dest., denatured in boiling water, and specifically labeled with the DIG High Prime Labeling and Detection Kit (Boehringer-Mannheim, Mannheim). The sample was cooled, injected with 4 µl DIG High Prime, and centrifuged. Finally, the mixture was incubated at 37°C for 20 hours.

Northern Hybridisation and Detection

For the hybridisation reaction, the total-RNA from the carcinoma sample was divided up into a 1.2% Agarosegel with 1 volume part 50-times Morpholino-Propane-Sulfone-Acid (MOPS)-buffer (1M MOPS, 250 mM Sodium acetate, 50 MM Ethylendiamintetra-vinegar-acid, pH 7.0) and 2% (v/v) 0.22 M formaldehyde. To stain the 28S and the 18S rRNS-fragments, 0.01% (v/v) of a 1% (w/v) ethidium bromide solution was added to the gel. After electrophresis, the RNA was transferred from the gel to a nylon membrane, washed in 1/10 of a 20-times-strong SSC-solution (3 M NaCl, 0.3 M sodium citrate, pH) and immobilised by 1200 µJoule UV radiation (Stratalinker, Stratagene, Heidelberg). Following that, the membrane was pre-hybridized for 1 hour at 50°C with the DIG Easy Hyb-Solution (Boehringer-Mannheim). The hybridisation followed this step. The labeled cDNA was denatured in boiling water and then cooled. The denatured sample was mixed with the DIG Easy Hyb Pre-hybridisation solution. The hybridisation reaction was carried out over 12-126 hours at 50°C.

After hybridisation, the membrane was incubated first for 2 x 15 min in double-strength SSC and 0.1% sodiumdodecylsulfate (SDS) at room-temperature, then 2 x 15 min. at 0.5-times-strong SSC and 0.1% SDS at 68°C. Then there were washings of the membrane for 5 min. in a wash-buffer and 0.3% Tween 20 (Calbiochem, Bad Soden) and for 30 min. in Blocking-solution. The membrane was then incubated for 30 minutes in antibody solution (anti-DIG-AP conjugate 1:10000 in Blocking solution (Boehringer-Mannheim) and treated 2 x 15 minutes with an equilibrations solution (Boehringer-Mannheim). After that, the membrane was placed with the RNS-side up onto a transparant sheet, layered with 1 ml CSPD-solution [Dinitrat 3- (4.Methoxyspiro) 1.2 Dioxetane-3.2- (5-chloro) tricyclodecan-4-phenylphosphate (Boehringer Mannheim)] and incubated for a few minutes. Immediately afterwards, it was sealed in an airtight transparent plastic bag and autoradiographed.

RESULTS

In 32 of the 40 (80%) tumor samples, a MMP-13 mRNA-expression was demonstrated with the help of RT-PCR in the tumor tissue. In all the tumor samples, which showed a MMP-13 mRNA-expression in the RT-PCR, this was confirmed by Northern blot hybridisation.

In 10 of the 12 cases (83.3%) with N0-status and 22 of the 28 cases (78.5%) with N+-neck, a MMP-13 mRNA Expression was demonstrated. There was no correlation between MMP-13 mRNA expression and the N-status. A connection between T-status and the MMP-13 mRNA expression was also not proved. The differences in the sexes in the MMP-13 positive group was 26 male to 6 female, and in the MMP-13 negative group 6 male to 2 female. The average age of the MMP-13 positive patient group was 57.3 years and that of the MMP-13 negative group was 57.7 years.

In 36 of the 40 tumor samples (94.7%) a TIMP-1 expression was demonstrated.

DISCUSSION

The invasion and the metastasization of a malignancy is a multi-stage process and presupposes proteolytic activity either from the tumor cells themselves or the surrounding stroma cells[1, 17]. The expression of metalloproteinases is a factor to which great importance can be attached in this process. MMP's are, in principle, capable of degrading all the components of the extra cellular matrix (ECM). Rising MMP-activity correlates to the progression of malignant tumors of the most diverse origins[3].

There are many publications about the importance of the expression of matrix metalloproteinases and the destruction of the extra cellular matrix for the invasion and the metastasization in many malignancy entities[17]. A correlation has been described between the degree of the tumor invasion and the degree of metastasization, even in head and neck carcinomas[6]. The connection between the expression of metalloproteinases in the primary tumor and the occurrence of lymph node metastases was proved in lung- and cervical carcinomas, for example[18, 19]. In oral squamous cell carcinomas, a close association was demonstrated between the reduced expression of extracellular matrix, especially the basal membrane components such as laminine, Type IV collagen and proteoglycanes, and a invasive and metastatic potential in this type of carcinoma[20]. In connection with this, an expression of MMP-1, -2, -3, and -9 was described as a possible causal factor for the reduction of ECM. In this way, a correlation was shown for the afore-mentioned MMP's between their expression and the degree of metastasization[6]. We can also assume that such an assocation might also exist between the MMP-13 expression and the metastasizing behaviour of head and neck carcinomas.

There have been only a few studies of the MMP-13 expression in malignancies and especially in squamous cell carcinomas of the head and neck region. MMP-13 was cloned for the first time in 1994 by Freije et al[10] from human mamma-carcinomas. The first study in which it was shown that MMP-13 can also be exprimed from plate epithel was published in 1997 by Johannsen et al[13]. The authors demonstrated an expression of this proteasis in the cell lines and primary tumors of the head and neck region in 76% and 88% of the cases,

20

respectively. The results of the aforementioned study show a comparable frequency of MMP-13 mRNA expression with 80% in our group of head and neck carcinomas (nearly all oropharynx), whereas Johannsen et al had a group of primary tumors located in the larynx, the oro- and hypopharynx, and in the oral cavity. From the cell lines and primary tumors that they investigated the authors draw the conclusion, that in these carcinomas there is an association between MMP-13 expression and a stronger capacity for invasion, because they either show a strong local invasion or they originated from patients with a very short time of survival. A correlation between MMP-13 mRNA-expression and lymph node status of the patients was not demonstrated in this study, so that, in accordance to this aspect, a comparison to the aforementioned results is not possible.

In a study by Cazorla et al[16] about MMP-13 expression in larynx carcinomas, a significant correlation between MMP-13 expression and local tumor invasion of the larynx carcinomas was found. If we look more closely at these results, thre seems to be a correlation between the advanced stage of a tumor and the MMP-13 expression. In this study from the year 1998[16], there are also figures indicating the N-status of the studied patients which allow comparisons to the presented study of head and neck carcinomas. In all 35 larynx carcinoma patients (N+ = n=27; N0 = n=8), 17 of the N+ patients (63%) and 3 of the N0 patients (37%) showed MMP-13 expression. From these figures, no correlation was drawn between MMP-13 expression and the lymph node metastasization. On the other hand, the results of our study of head and neck carcinomas show a much higher rate of MMP-13 expression in 83.3 % of the tumor samples examined, which might possibly underscore a more aggressive or invasive character of the head and neck carcinomas (mostly oropharynx). Additionally, the procentual distribution of the N+ and N0 patients referring to MMP-13 expression shows quite clearly the missing correlation between N+ status and MMP-13 expression.

It is conceivable that it is a modulation of the MMP-13 effect on the destruction of the ECM and therefore on the metastasizing process by the physiological inhibitor TIMP-1, which can also be exprimed from the tumor cells. The proof of a TIMP-1 expression in almost every one of the tumor samples, however, allows the conclusion that this potentially modulating effect on the MMP-13 effect does not play a role in those carcinomas which were examined.

CONCLUSION

There were no indications that MMP-13 expression in head and neck carcinomas is a significant factor as a prognosis for the metastasizing behaviour. The high rate of expression indicates aggressive growth of this carcinoma entity.

REFERENCES

1. Stetler-Stevenson WG, Aznovoorian S, Liotta L. Tumor cell interactions with the extracellular matrix during invasion and metastases. Annu Rev Cell Biol 1993;9:541-573.
2. Birkedal-Hansen H, Moore WGY, Bodden MK, Windsor LJ, Birkedal Hansen B, DeCarlo A, Engler JA. Matrix metalloproteinases: a review. Crit Rev Oral Biol Med 1991;4:197-250.
3. Curran S, Murray GI. Matrix metalloproteinases in tumor invasion and metastasis J Pathol 1999;189:300-308.
4. Balbìn M, Pendás AM, Uría JA, Jiménez MG, Freije JP, López-Otín C. Expression and regulation of collagenase-3 (MMP-13) in human malignant tumors. APMIS 1999;107:45-53.

5. Gray ST, Wilkins RJ, Tyun K. Interstitial collagenase gene expression in oral squamous cell carcinomas. Am J Pathol 1992;141:301-306.

6. Kurahara S, Shinohara M, Ikebe T, Nakamura S, Beppu M, Hiraki A, Takeuchi H, Shirasuna K. Expression of MMPs, MT-MMP, and TIMPs in squamous cell carcinoma of the oral cavity: correlation with tumor invasion and metastasis. Head Neck 1999;21:627-638.

7. Kusukawa J, Sasaguri Y, Morimatsu M, Kameyama T. Expression of metalloproteinases in stage 1 and 2 squamous cell carcinoma of the oral cavity. J Oral Maxillofac Surg 1995;53:530-534.

8. Polette M, Clavel C, Muller D, Abecassis J, Binninger I, Birembaut P. Detection of mRNAs encoding collagenase-1 and stromelysin-2 in carcinomas of the head and neck by in situ hybridization. Invasion Metastases 1991;11:76-83.

9. Répássy G, Forster-Horváth C, Juhász A, Ádány R, Tamássy R, Timár J. Expression of invasion markers CD44v6/v3, NM 23 and MMP-2 in laryngeal and hypopharyngeal carcinoma. Pathol Oncol Res 1998;4:14-21.

10. Freije JMP, Diez-Itza I, Balbin M, Sanchez LM, Blasco R, Tolivia J, Lopez-Otin C. Molecular cloning, and expression of collagenase-3, a novel human matrix metalloproteinase produced by breast carcinomas. J Biol Chem 1994;269:16766-16773.

11. Johannsson N, Vaalamo M, Grenman S, Hietanen S, Klemi P, Saarialho-Kere U, Kähäri V-M. Collagenase-3 (MMP-13) is expressed by tumor cells in invasive vulvar squamous cell carcinomas. Am J Pathol 1999;154:469-479.

12. Stahle-Bäckdahl M, Sandstedt B, Bruce K, Lindahl A, Jimenez MG, Vega JA, Lopez-Otin C. Collagenase-3 (MMP-13) is expressed during human fetal ossification and re-expressed in postnatal bone remodeling and in rheumatoid arthritis. Lab Invest 1997;76:717-728.

13. Johansson N, Airola K, Grenman R, Kariniemi, Saarialho-Kere U, Kähäri VM. Expression of collagenase-3 (matrix metalloproteinase-13) in squamous cell carcinomas of the head and neck. Am J Pathol 1997;151:499-508.

14. Koong AC, Denko AC, Hudson KM, Schindler C, Swiersz L, Koch C, Evans S, Ibrahim H, Le QT, Terris DJ, Giaccia AJ. Candidate genes for the hypoxic tumor phenotype. Cancer Res 2000;60:883-887.

15. O-Charoenrat P, Rhys-Evans P, Modjahedi H, Court W, Box G, Eccles S. Overexpression of epidermal growth factor receptor in human head and neck squamous carcinoma cell lines correlates with matrix metalloproteinase-9 expression. Int J Cancer 2000;86:307-317.

16. Cazorla M, Hernández L, Nadal A, Balbin M, López JM, Vizoso F, Fernández PL, Iwata K, Cardesa A, López-Otin, Campos E. Collagenase-3 expression is associated with advanced local invasion in human squamous cell carcinomas of the larynx. J Pathol 1998;186:144-150.

17. Chambers AF, Matrisian LM. Changing views of the role of matrix metalloproteinases in metastasis. J Natl Cancer Inst 1997;89:1260-1270.

18. Garzetti GG, Ciavattini A, Lucarini G, Goteri G, Romanini,C, Biagini G. The 72-kDa metalloproteinase immunostaining in cervical carcinoma: relationship with lymph nodal involvement. Gynecol Oncol 1996;60:271-276.

19. Tokuraku M, Sato H, Murakami S, Okada Y, Watanabe Y, Seiki M. Activation of the precursor of gelatinase A/72kDa type IV collagenase/MMP-2 in lung carcinoma correlates with the expression of membrane type matrix metalloproteinase (MT-MMP) and with lymph node metastasis. Int J Cancer 1995;64:355-359.

20. Harada T, Shinohara M, Nakamura S, Oka M. An immunohistochemical study of the extracellular matrix in oral squamous cell carcinoma and its association with invasive and metastatic potential. Virchow Archiv 1994;424:257-266.

A CYTOKERATIN EXPRESSION MODEL DETECTED BY RT PCR IN SQUAMOUS CELL CARCINOMAS OF THE HEAD AND NECK

A. Sesterhenn[1], R. Mandic[1], Anja-A. Dünne[1], R. Moll[2], J.A. Werner[1] (Marburg, Germany)
[1]Department of Otolaryngology, Head and Neck Surgery, Philipps-University of Marburg, Germany
[2]Department of Pathology, Philipps-University of Marburg, Germany

Acknowledgement: We would like to thank very much Mr T.E. Carey and Mr R.Grenman for the provided cell lines we could use in this study.

Running title: Cytokeratin Expression in Squamous Cell Carcinoma

Keywords: Cytokeratins, intermediate filaments, cell lines, RT-PCR, Squamous cell carcinoma

Correspondence to: Dr A. M. Sesterhenn, Dept. of Otorhinolaryngology, Head and Neck Surgery, University of Marburg, Deutschhausstr. 3, D-35037 Marburg, Germany, Phone: +49-6421-286-2850, Fax: +49-6421-286-2842 (e-mail: andreas.sesterhenn@med.uni-marburg.de)

ABSTRACT

Background. Cytokeratins are members of intermediate filaments which are predominantly found in epithelial cells. Different types of epithelia are characterized by a distinct composition of cytokeratin. Recent immunohistochemical investigations could demonstrate, that in contrast to some rarely expressed cytokeratins like number 8, 18 and 19, the cytokeratins 5, 6, 14, 16 and 17 are regularly expressed in benign squamous epithelia as well as in SCCHN.

Methods. We isolated total RNA from 11 primary cell lines derived from squamous cell carcinomas of the head and neck region. The expression of cytokeratins was evaluated by RT-PCR utilizing oligonuleotide primers against cytokeratins 5, 6, 14, 16 and 17.

Results. Cytokeratin 6 was detectable in all of the cases, also cytokeratin 16 with one exception. For cytokeratin 5 we could observe a frequent expression with absence just two cases. cytokeratin 14 was expressed only sporadically in 4 of 11 cell lines just as cytokeratin 17 in only one case.

Conclusion. From our results we could conclude that SCCHN, in contrast to benign squamous epithelia, exhibit a different cytokeratin expression-profil at the RNA-level.

INTRODUCTION

Cytokeratins are protein components of intermediate filaments and so responsible for the stability of the cell especially in the epithelium. Till now cytokeratins could be subclassified into 20 different subtypes. It is well established that cytokeratins are in a distinct constellation specific for different types of epithelia. Antibodies against certain cytokeratins could be utilized for histological diagnosis of epithelial tumors. It is important to know that the expression of cytokeratins is strictly conserved and maintained even in the event of malignant transformation. Recent investigations could demonstrate by immuno-histochemical and molecular biological examinations, that in contrast to some rarely expressed cytokeratins like number 8, 18 and 19, cytokeratins 5, 6, 14, 16 and 17 are usually expressed in squamous cell carcinomas of the head and neck region[1,2]. So we became particularly interested in the question, whether these immunohistochemical results could be proved on the RNA-level and whether there are potential differences in the cytokeratin expression between normal squamous epithelium and squamous cell carcinoma at the molecular level.

MATERIALS AND METHODS

We could use primary tumor cell lines derived from squamous cell carcinomas of the head and neck form the University of Michigan (UM) and from the University of Turku (UT). The primary tumors had different localizations in the head and neck area. As controls for benign tissue we used two ceratinocyte cell lines.

RNA preparation
Total cellular RNA was prepared by a Qiagen RNeasy Total RNA kit (Hilden, Germany). The cell lysates were mixed with an equal volume of 70% ethanol, transferred onto an Rneasy spin column and extracted according to the manufacturer's instructions. RNA was eluted with 40µl RNAse-free water and stored at –28°C. The Quantity of isolated RNA was determined by absorbance at 260 nm.

RT-PCR
All primers against cytokeratins used in this study have been designed by ourselfs. The required sequences were obtained form genbank. The primers were synthesized by Sigma-ARK (Darmstadt, Germany). The sequences of the primers against the different cytokeratins are as follows:
CK 5 sense: 5´CACTAGTGCCTGGTTC TCTTGCTC
CK 5 antisense: 5´GATGTACTGCTCG AACGGCTCCAG;
CK 6 sense: 5´ GACTGTGAGGCAGAA

24

CCTGGAGCCG,
CK6 antisense: 5′ GACGTGGTCGATCT CAGATCTCAG;
CK 14 sense: 5′GCAGAGCCAGGACCC ACCTGAAGACC
CK14 antisense: 5′CAGGCCTGACCTG CCGTGCTGTG C
CK 16 sense: 5′ GGATGAGCTGACCC TGGCCAGGACTGAC,
CK16 antisense: 5′CTCCAGCAGGCG GC GGTAGGTGGCAATC
CK17 sense: 5′GCACCCTCTAGCTGA CTGTAAAAC,
CK17 antisense: 5′CAGGATGTTGGCA TTGTCCACGGTGGCTGTGAG

RT-PCR was performed using the 1st Strand cDNA Synthesis Kit for RT-PCR from Boehringer (Boehringer, Mannheim). Samples containing 5μl total RNA were resuspended in a mastermix containing 2μl of 10x Reaction Buffer, 4μl of 25 mM MgCl$_2$, 2μl Deoxynucleotide Mix, 1μl of Oligo-p(dT)$_{15}$ Primer, 1 μl of Rnase Inhibitor, 0.8μl of AMV Reverse Transcriptase and 4.2μl of sterile water. Reactions in which pure water replaced the RNA template were used as RT-negative controls. The mixture was incubated at 25°C for 10 min to allow annealing of the primers to the RNA. Reverse Transcription of RNA was performed at 42°C for 60 min, stopped at 95°C for 5 min and finally placed on ice.

From this cDNA solution, 5μl was removed for a subsequent use in PCR amplification by adding each sample 95μl
of PCR Master Mix solution (10x Reaction Buffer, 25mM MgCl$_2$, deoxynuleotide mix, gelatin 0.1%, primers specific for different cytokeratins and Taq DNA polymerase. β-aktin amplification was used to demonstrate RNA integrity (not shown). The samples were briefly vortexed and covered with one drop of mineral oil. PCR was carried out under the following conditions: denaturation for 3 min at 94°C, followed by 30 cycles of 1min denaturation at 94°C, 1.5min annealing at 51°C and 1min primer extension at 72°C. The last cycle was performed for 10min at 72°C and finally stopped at 4°C. PCR products were analyzed by agarose gel electrophoresis and ethidium bromide staining against PCR size markers (Biolabs, New England).

RESULTS

Our preliminary investigations confirmed the previous immunohistochemical observations, that cytokeratins 5, 6, 14, 16 and 17 are expressed in benign squamous epithelia. In both of the ceratinocyte cell lines all cytokeratins mentioned above have been expressed. Conerning the SCCHN cell lines we could point out, that cytokeratin 6 was detectable in all of the cases, also cytokeratin 16 with just one exception in case UM11B. For Cytokeratin 5 we could observe a frequent expression with absence in just two cases (UM 11B and UT12A). To our surprise cytokeratin 14 was expressed only sporadically in 5 of 11 cell lines (UM1, UM3, UM4, UM9 and UT10) just as cytokeratin 17 in only one case (UT10).

1 2 3 4 5 6 7 8 9 10 11 M

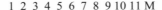

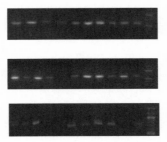

Figure 1: Results of RT-PCR. 1. Gel: CK6 at 583bp; 2. Gel: CK16 at 585 bp; 3. Gel: CK 5 at 710 bp. Lanes 1-11 SCCHN cell lines as follows: 1=UM1; 2=UM3; 3=UM4; 4=UM9; 5=UM11B; 6=UM22B; 7=UM27; 8=UT8; 9=UT10; 10=UT12A; 11=UT16A; M=Marker.

CK 6	11/11
CK 16	10/11
CK 5	9/11
CK 14	4/11
CK 17	1/11

Table 2. Cytokeratin expression in numbers of
SCCHN cell lines

DISCUSSION

From our results we could conclude that squamous cell carcinomas of the head and neck region, in contrast to benign squamous epithelia, exhibit a different cytokeratin expression-profile at the RNA-level. So we came to the hypothesis, that the absence of cytokeratins 14 and 17 as observed in head and neck squamous cell carcinomas could potentially be related to a loss of cell stability. To further investigate this hypothesis we will confirm our results at the protein level by Western blotting and subcellular fractionation. At this point it has to be mentioned that the primary tumor site of SCCHN cell lines, tumor differentiation or TNM classification has not been taken into consideration concerning the cytokeratin expression. Our data show the first results of an ongoing research project, which is going to be confirmed more detailed by further molecular biological investigations and larger numbers of cases.

REFERENCES

1. Moll R. Cytokeratine als Differenzierungsmarker: Expressionsprofile von Epithelien und epithelialen Tumoren. Stuttgart, Jena, New York: Gustav Fischer; 1993.
2. Moll R. Cytokeratins as Markers of Differentiation in the Diagnosis of Epithelial Tumors. Subcellular Biochemistry 1998; 31:205-262.

EXPRESSION AND ACTIVATION PATTERNS OF STAT3 IN SQUAMOUS CELL CARCINOMAS OF THE HEAD AND NECK REGION

R. Mandic, A. Sesterhenn, Anja-A. Dünne, B.M. Lippert, J.A. Werner (Marburg, Germany)Dept. of Otorhinolaryngology, Head and Neck Surgery, Philipps University, Marburg, Germany

Acknowledgements: We thank Nadine Eikelkamp, Roswitha Peldszus and Grazyna Sadowski for technical support.

Running title: Stat3 activation in squamous cell carcinomas

Key words: Stat3, EGF-R, SCCHN, activation, cancer

Correspondence to: *Jochen A. Werner, M.D. Dept. of Otorhinolaryngology, Head and Neck Surgery, University of Marburg, Deutschhausstr. 3, D-35037 Marburg, Germany, Phone: ++49-6421-286-6478, Fax: ++49-6421-286-6367 (e-mail: j.a.werner@mailer.uni-marburg.de*

ABSTRACT

Background. Activation of the epidermal growth factor receptor (EGF-R) is related to high activity of Stat3 proteins, which are involved in oncogene expression in squamous cell carcinomas of the head and neck region (SCCHN). In this study we investigated the Stat3 expression and activation patterns in SCCHN cell lines.

Methods. Western blotting was performed on cytosolic and nuclear extracts from nine different SCCHN cell lines with antibodies against EGF-R, Stat3, p-Stat3 and Actin utilizing standard procedures.

Results. In the cytosolic fraction we only found inactive Stat3, whereas all of the active Stat3 was present in the nuclear fraction. Interestingly, the ratio of the two Stat3 isoforms α and β differed between the cell lines.

Conclusions. Stat3 enters the nucleus upon activation. Different ratios of active Stat3 α and β were found in the nuclear extracts of the different cell lines, implicating a distinct role of these isoforms in oncogene activation of SCCHN.

INTRODUCTION

Signal transducers and activators of transcription or STATs are proteins with a dual function. They transmit signals from the cell surface to the nucleus and are directly involved in gene regulation[1].Seven mammalian STAT members are known so far, these are Stats 1-4, 5a, 5b and 6. In addition Stats1 and 3 produce 2 two different protein isoforms by the mechanism of alternative RNA splicing. These isoforms are named Stat1 (or Stat3) α and β[2-4]. It was first shown for Stat3 that STATs can be activated (phosphorylated) by oncoprotein tyrosine kinases like Src[5], resulting in a Stat3-dependent gene expression, that is linked to oncogenic transformation of the cell[6]. Stat3 was found to be highly activated in squamous cell carcinomas of the head and neck region (SCCHN)[7] and that its activation primarily depends on the phosphorylation mediated by the carboxy-terminal kinase domain of the activated epidermal growth factor receptor (EGF-R)[8], leading to dimerization, nuclear import, activation of transcription and malignant transformation of the cell due to activation and expression of oncogenes[2].

The used squamous cell carcinoma cell lines were kindly provided by T.E. Carey (University of Michigan, MI, USA) and R. Grénman (University of Turku, Finland). Cells were grown in DMEM media, supplemented with 10% fetal calf serum, containing penicillin and streptomycin. Primary antibodies, specific for EGF-R (1005), Stat3 (H-190), p-Stat3 (Tyr 705) and Actin (C-11) as well as the secondary anti-goat, anti-rabbit or anti-mouse HRP-conjugated antibodies were obtained from Santa Cruz Biotechnology (Santa Cruz, CA, USA). Cells were washed in cold PBS and the cell pellet was lysed in a buffer containing 1% NP-40, 66mM EDTA, 10 mM Tris/HCl. Protease and phosphatase inhibitors (SIGMA) were added to the buffer prior to lysis of the cells. Cell nuclei are resistant to lysis by non-ionic detergents like NP-40 and could be separated from the cytosolic fraction by high speed (13000g) centrifugation to yield the nuclear fraction. SDS-PAGE was performed under standard conditions[9]. Western blotting was performed as described earlier[10]

RESULTS

Cytosolic extracts of nine different cell lines were investigated for expression of EGF-R, Stat3, p-Stat3 and Actin. Actin was used as an internal control to verify a comparable input of the cell lysates [Fig.1A, lower panel]. EGF-R expression could be detected in all cell lines [Fig.1A, upper panel]. We also detected Stat3 expression utilizing an antibody (H-190) that can recognize but not distinguish the inactive (unphosphorylated) and active (phosphorylated) form of Stat3 [Fig.1A, second panel from the top]. However, when using an antibody that is specific for the active form of Stat3 (Tyr 705), we failed to detect any of the active form in the cytosolic fraction [Fig.1A, second panel from the bottom]. Since it was known that after phosphorylation and activation of Stat3 the protein dimerizes and enters the nucleus[2], we separated the nuclear and cytosolic fraction. We found all of the active Stat3 in the nuclear fraction (Fig.1B, upper panel; Fig. 1C). Surprisingly, the ratio of the two Stat3 isoforms α and β in the nuclear fraction varied between the different cell lines. Especially the α form was found to be dominant over the β form in two of the SCCHN cell lines (Fig.1B, upper panel, lanes 3 and 4). Interestingly, when we included the control keratinocyte cell line, which was representing healthy keratinocytes, we also found Stat3α to dominate over Stat3β (Fig.1C, K).

CONCLUSIONS

Activated Stat3 is localizing to the nucleus in cell lines derived from squamous cell carcinomas of the head and neck region (SCCHN). The amount of activated Stat3α or β present the nucleus can vary between the different cell lines. Future investigations will address potential functional differences between Stat3α and β at the molecular level. Our further studies will focus on the differences in EGF-R mediated Stat3 signaling and gene expression between the SCCHN cell lines and will include the use of microarray techniques.

REFERENCES

1. Darnell JE, Kerr IM, Stark GR. Jak-STAT pathways and transcriptional activation in response to IFNs and other extracellular signaling proteins. Science. 1994 Jun 3; 264(5164):1415-2
2. Bowman T, Jove R. STAT Proteins and Cancer. Cancer Control. 1999 Nov 6(6):615-619.
3. Schaefer TS, Sanders LK, Nathans D. Cooperative transcriptional activity of Jun and Stat3 beta, a short form of Stat3. Proc Natl Acad Sci USA. 1995 Sep 26; 92(20):9097-101.
4. Schaefer TS, Sanders LK, Park OK, Nathans D. Functional differences between Stat3alpha and Stat3beta. Mol Cell Biol. 1997 Sep; 17(9):5307-16.
5. Yu CL, Meyer DJ, Campbell GS, Larner AC, Carter-Su C, Schwartz J, Jove R. Enhanced DNA-binding activity of a Stat3-related protein in cells transformed by the Src oncoprotein. Science. 1995 Jul 7; 269(5220):81-3.
6. Bromberg JF, Wrzeszczynska MH, Devgan G, Zhao Y, Pestell RG, Albanese C, Darnell JE. Stat3 as an oncogene. Cell. 1999 Aug 6; 98(3):295-303.
7. Grandis JR, Drenning SD, Zeng Q, Watkins SC, Melhem MF, Endo S, Johnson DE, Huang L, He Y, Kim JD. Constitutive activation of Stat3 signaling abrogates apoptosis in squamous cell carcinogenesis in vivo. Proc Natl Acad Sci USA. 2000 Apr 11; 97(8):4227-32.
8. Park OK, Schaefer TS, Nathans D. In vitro activation of Stat3 by epidermal growth factor receptor kinase. Proc Natl Acad Sci USA. 1996 Nov 26; 93(24):13704-8.
9. Laemmli UK. Cleavage of structural proteins during the assembly of the head of bacteriophage T4. Nature. 1970 Aug 15; 227(259):680-5.
10. Mandic R, Lowe AW. Characterization of an alternatively spliced isoform of rat vesicle associated membrane protein-2 (VAMP-2). FEBS Lett. 1999 May 21; 451(2):209-13.

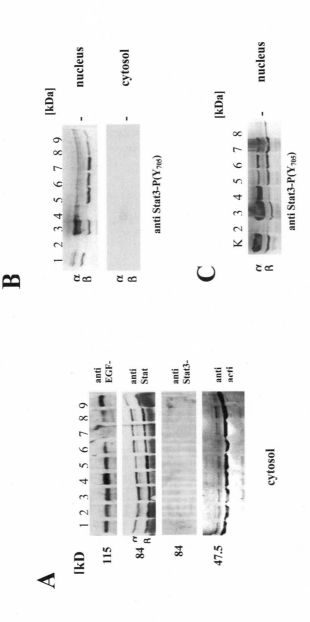

Figure 1: (*A*) Cytosolic fractions of nine different SCCHN cell lines (1-9) were tested for expression of EGF-R, Stat3 (active+inactive), Stat3-P(Y_{705})(active), and Actin. (*B*) Nuclear and cytosolic fractions of the 9 cell lines were probed for active Stat3. (*C*) Nuclear fractions of cell lines 2-8 were tested for active Stat3 and compared to a control keratinocyte cell line (K). α=Stat3α, β=Stat3β.

ABSENCE OF DCC GENE EXPRESSION IN HEAD AND NECK SQUAMOUS CELL CARCINOMA (HNSCC) CELL LINES

Ueda, Y., Jung, K-Y, Takebayashi, S., Ogawa, T., Ogawa, H., Mineta, H., Grenman, R., Bradford, C.R., Carey, T.E.
University of Michigan, Ann Arbor, MI 48109-0506, USA; Turku University, Turku, Finland, Hamamatsu University School of Medicine, Hamamatsu 431-3124, Japan.

ABSTRACT

Loss of heterozygosity (LOH) of chromosome 18q is frequent in Head and Neck squamous cell carcinomas (HNSCC). The tumor suppressor gene DCC (deleted in colorectal carcinoma) is located on the long arm of chromosome 18 in band 18q21.3. Using 42 polymorphic markers spanning all of 18q performed LOH analysis on 57 head and neck squamous cell carcinoma cell lines for which a source of normal DNA was available. DCC maps between D18S487 and D18S35. Of the 57 cell lines tested, 40 were informative for D18S487 and 39 were informative for D18S35. LOH was observed in 58% (23/40) at D18S487 and in 56% (22%) at D18S35. In contrast to these rates, we found consistent regions of loss with much higher LOH rates of 74% (D18S39 in distal 18q21), 70% (D18S61 in 18q22.2) and 75% (D18S70 in 18q23), suggesting that the important gene(s) on 18q may reside in one of these regions. Nevertheless, since DCC has been implicated as a possible tumor suppressor gene, we wished to determine the expression pattern of DCC in HNSCC lines. We tested a set of 8 cell lines (UM-SCC-11A, -11B, -17B, -22A, -22B, 74A, -74B, and –81B) established from 5 patients for which the 18q-deletion status has been determined. Six of these cell lines have LOH in the DCC region, and two cell lines, UM-SCC-74A and –74B from a primary (-74A) and recurrent (-74B) oral carcinoma in the same donor do not have LOH. We also tested normal keratinocytes and the following cell lines: HeLa (a cervical carcinoma known to have 18q loss), SJNB20 (a neuroblastoma line known to express DCC), Glio54s10 (a glioblastoma cell line transfected with a vector containing full length DCC), DCCF40 (COS1 containing full length DCC), and DCCT4 (COS1 cells containing a truncated version of DCC that encodes only the extracellular domain of DCC). RT-PCR was performed using intron-spanning primers that amplify DCC exon 1 and exon 2, as well as primers that amplify exon 27-28. In addition, antibody to the intracellular domain of DCC was used to assess DCC expression on western blots. sing RT-PCR, we could not detect DCC expression in RNA from NHK, nor from HeLa, nor from any of the HNSCC lines. However, DCC was detected in SJNB20, Glio54s10, and DCCF40 using primers for both exons 1-2 and exons 27-28. For

DCCT4, DCC was detected using only the exon 1-2 primers set. This is as expected since this cell line lacks the intracellular domain encoding exons 27-28. Similarly, in western blots using antibody to the DCC intracellular domain, DCC protein could be detected only in extracts from SJNB20, Glio54s10 and DCCF40. From these results we conclude that either DCC is not expressed in NHK and the HNSCC cells we tested, or that our methods are too insensitive to detect low levels of expression of this gene product. Thus, we can neither implicate nor exclude DCC as a tumor suppressor gene in HNSCC at this time.

INTRODUCTION

LOH (loss of heterozygosity) and chromosome deletions are the most common genetic events observed in cancers. These allelic losses are generally thought to reflect the existence of tumor suppressor genes[1,2]. In our previous study, loss of heterozygosity was frequent in long arm of chromosome 18 in HNSCC. We confirmed the study of LOH using 42 polymorphic markers in 57 HNSCC cell lines. As much as 75% LOH occurs in these regions. These results suggest that there might be important genes on 18q in HNSCC[3,4].

The DCC (Deleted in Colorectal Carcinoma) gene, located in the chromosome 18q21.3 band, was originally identified as a possible tumor suppressor gene that is frequently subject to LOH in colorectal carcinomas[5]. DCC mRNA is made from 29 exons and the coding sequence of DCC predicts a trans-membrane polypeptide with an extracellular domain and a cytoplasmic domain. The DCC is located on 18q21.3 between the D18S487 locus and the D18S35 locus. In our previous study, D18s487 marker has 58% LOH and D18S35 has 56% LOH in HNSCC cell lines. That is indicating DCC might be acting as a tumor suppressor gene in HNSCC. There are many reports of LOH and Loss of expression of DCC being very common in other types of tumors, prostate[6], gastric[7], esophageal[8], oral[9], pancreatic[10], breast[11], renal[12] and glial[13] malignancies. And Expression of full length wild type DCC was actually shown to inhibit tumor growth in one study.

DCC is highly homologous to N-CAM (neural cell adhesion molecule), which is an adhesion molecule abundantly expressed in neural tissue[5]. So it might play an important role in cell-cell, or cell-extracellular matrix interaction during development or differentiation. A reverse correlation between DCC protein level and frequency of liver metastasis in colon cancer was suggested by a quantitative analysis of the protein[14]. Therefore, inactivation of DCC function may be associated with decreases in cell-cell interactions and attachment, thereby, increasing the potential for metastasis.

In this study, we determine the expression pattern of DCC between primary and recurrent or metastatic HNSCC cell lines.

MATERIAL AND METHODS

Cell lines (Table1)
8 HNSCC cell lines that were established from the University of Michigan (UM) patients with HNSCC were tested. A indicates primary site and B indicates recurrence or metastatic site from same patient. UMSCC 11A was derived from larynx SCC and UMSCC 11B from

32

recurrence of the same patient, UMSCC-22A from hypopharynx SCC and UMSCC-22B from neck lymph node metastasis, UMSCC-74A from larynx SCC and B from recurrence, UMSCC-17B from neck lymph node metastasis of larynx SCC and UMSCC-81B from reccurence of hypopharynx SCC. We also tested HeLa cell, which is a cervivcal carcinoma cell lines, and NHK is derived from normal human keratinocytes. As positive controls, SJNB20, Glio54s10, DCC F40 and DCC-T4 were used. SJNB20 is a neuroblastoma cell line known to express DCC protein. Glio54S10 is the glioblastoma cell line transfected with the DCC gene and expresses full length DCC. DCC F40 is COS1 cells transfected with and express the full length DCC and DCC-T4 is also COS1 cell transfected with the truncated version of DCC and hence, expresses only the extracellular domain of DCC. DCC F40, DCC T4 and Glio54s10 were gift from Dr. Fearon.

RT-PCR

Total RNA was extracted from each cell lines using Rneasy Midi kit (Qiagen) in accordance with the manufacture's instructions. cDNA was synthesized from 2ug of total RNA using Moloney murine leukaemia virus reverse transcriptase (GIBCO-BRL) with the random hexamer that was used as the template for the polymerase chain reaction (PCR). The 2 sets of primers for PCR to amplify the DCC gene-coding region were used. They are intron-spanning primers, one set amplifying DCC exon 1 to 2, sense and anti-sense primers used were 5'cccaagctggcttttgtact3' and 5'tgcttcctttcatccattcc3', corresponding to nucleotides 31-50 and 269-250, and the other set amplifying DCC exon 27 to 28, sense and anti-sense primers used were 5'gttcgaccaactcacccct3' and 5'atcctctgttggtttgtggc3', corresponding to nucleotides 2424-2433 and 2712-2731. The former primer amplifies part of the extracellular domain of DCC and the latter, part of the cytoplasmic domain. The PCR procedure was performed with 30cycles of denaturation at 94C for 1min, annealing at 60C for 1min and extension at 72C for 1min in a thermal cycler (Gene Amp PCR System 9700, PE). RT-PCR products were electrophoresed on 1.5% agarose gels and visualized with UV light following ethidium bromide staining. Their identities were confirmed by Southern transfer and hybridization with a 32P-labeled DCC cDNA probe.

Western Blotting

Proteins were extracted by Lysis buffer from approximately 80% confluent cells in T75 flasks. Usually, 100ug of protein determined using the Bradford method was resolved by SDS-PAGE and transferred to a PVDF membrane (Immobilon-PSQ, Millipore) for 3 h at 100V in blotting buffer consisting of 0.025M Tris, 0.192M glycine and 20% methanol. For blocking, the protein blots were incubated in TBS with 5% non-fat dry milk and 5% tween. The membranes were incubated with monoclonal antibody targeted to the cytoplasmic domain of DCC (clone G97-449, Pharmingen) at room temperature for 1 h. Visualization of antibody complexes was carried out with a ECL detection kit (Amasham) and subsequent exposure to reflection film.

RESULTS

RT-PCR

We could not detect DCC gene expression in Normal Human Keratinocyte, or in HeLa, or in any of the HNSCC cell lines both on primary site and on reccurence or metastasis site. However, DCC was detected in positive controls, SJNB20, Glio54s10 and DCC-F40, on both cytoplasmic domain and extracellular domain. DCC-T4 only expresses the extracellular domain of DCC, as expected, has a band corresponding to the extracellular domain. (Figure 1, Table 2)

Western blotting

Additionally, we assessed DCC protein expression by western blot using an anti-human monoclonal antibody targeted to the cytoplasmic domain of DCC. A 185kDa protein can be detected in SJNB20, Glio54s10 and DCC-F40, but not in Normal Human Keratinocytes, DCC-T4 or in any of HNSCC cell lines, both primary tumors and recurrent or metastatic tumor. These results are similar to those seen in the RT-PCR analysis. (Table 2)

DISCUSSION

Several reports have suggested that the inactivation of DCC is relatively late event in the carcinogenesis of colorectal cancer, especially metastasis. There is a homology to the neural cell adhesion molecule (N-CAM) family proteins. Inactivation of DCC function is correlate with decreases in cell to cell attachment there it may increase the potential of metastasis. In recent report, DCC induces apoptosis in the absence of ligand binding, but blocks apoptosis when engaged by netrin-1[15]. Therefore DCC may function as a tumor suppressor protein by inducing apoptosis in settings in which ligand is unavailable, for example, during metastasis.

In this report, we tested the DCC expression of primary site and metastasis or reccurence site on HNSCC cell lines, but we cannot detect the DCC expression on neither HNSCC cell lines we tested both of primary site and metastasis site nor normal human keratinocyte. From these results we conclude that either DCC is not expressed in NHK and the HNSCC cells we tested, or that our methods are too insensitive to detect low levels of expression of this gene product. Thus, we can neither implicate nor exclude DCC as a tumor suppressor gene in HNSCC at this time.

UM-SCC 11A	Larynx cancer
UM-SCC 11B	Recurrence of UM-SCC 11A
UM-SCC 22A	Hypopharynx cancer
UM-SCC 22B	Neck lymph node metastasis from UM-SCC 22A
UM-SCC 74A	Larynx cancer
UM-SCC 74B	Recurrence of UM-SCC 74A
UM-SCC 17B	Neck lymphnode metastasis from larynx cancer
UM-SCC 81B	Recurrence of hypopharynx cancer
HeLa	Cervical carcinoma
NHK	Normal human keratinocyte
SJNB20	Neuroblastoma
Glio54s10	Glioblastoma transfeted DCC expression vector
DCC F40	Cos1 expressing full length DCC
DCC T4	Cos1 expressing extracellular domain of DCC

Table 1. Tested cell lines.

34

	Extracellular domain	Cytoplasmic domain	
	mRNA	mRNA	protein
UM-SCC 11A	-	-	-
UM-SCC 11B	-	-	-
UM-SCC 22A	-	-	-
UM-SCC 22B	-	-	-
UM-SCC 74A	-	-	-
UM-SCC74B	-	-	-
UM-SCC 17B	-	-	-
UM-SCC 81B	-	-	-
HeLa	-	-	-
NHK	-	-	-
SJNB20	+	+	+
Glio54s10	+	+	+
DCC F40	+	+	+
DCC T4	+	-	-

Table 2. Result of DCC expression on each cell lines

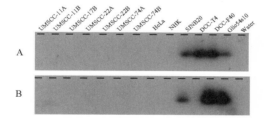

Figure 1. RT-PCR of DCC gene. A: DCC exon 1-2 region (extracellular domain). B: DCC exon27-28 region (cytoplasmic domain).

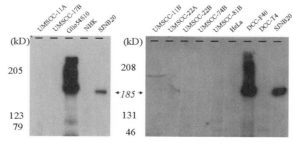

Figure 2. Expression of DCC protein using a monoclonal antibody targeted to the cytoplasmic domain of DCC.

REFERENCES

1. Cavenee WK, Dryja TP, Phillips RA, Benedict WF, Godbout R, Gallie BL, Murphree AL, Strong LC,White RL. Expression of recessive alleles by chromosomal mechanisms in retinoblastoma. Nature. 1983 Oct 27-Nov 2;305(5937):779-84.

2. Vogelstein B, Fearon ER, Kern SE, Hamilton SR, Preisinger AC, Nakamura Y, White RAllelotype of colorectal carcinomas. Science 1989 Apr 14;244(4901):207-11

3. Takebayashi S, Ogawa T, Jung KY, Muallem A, Mineta H, Fisher SG, Grenman R, Carey TE. Identification of new minimally lost regions on 18q in head and neck squamous cell carcinoma. Cancer Res. 2000 Jul 1;60(13):3397-403.

4. Frank CJ, McClatchey KD, Devaney KO, Carey TE. Evidence that loss of chromosome 18q is associated with tumor progression. Cancer Res. 1997 Mar 1;57(5):824-7.

5. Fearon ER, Cho KR, Nigro JM, Kern SE, Simons JW, Ruppert JM, Hamilton SR, Preisinger AC, Thomas G, Kinzler KW, et al. Identification of a chromosome 18q gene that is altered in colorectal cancers. Science. 1990 Jan 5;247(4938):49-56.

6. Gao X, Honn KV, Grignon D, Sakr W, Chen YQ. Frequent loss of expression and loss of heterozygosity of the putative tumor suppressor gene DCC in prostatic carcinomas. Cancer Res. 1993 Jun 15;53(12):2723-7.

7. Uchino S, Tsuda H, Noguchi M, Yokota J, Terada M, Saito T, Kobayashi M, Sugimura T, Hirohashi S. Frequent loss of heterozygosity at the DCC locus in gastric cancer.Cancer Res. 1992 Jun 1;52(11):3099-102.

8. Huang Y, Boynton RF, Blount PL, Silverstein RJ, Yin J, Tong Y, McDaniel TK, Newkirk C, Resau JH, Sridhara R, et al. Loss of heterozygosity involves multiple tumor suppressor genes in human esophageal cancers. Cancer Res. 1992 Dec 1;52(23):6525-30.

9. Kim MS, Li SL, Bertolami CN, Cherrick HM, Park NH. State of p53, Rb and DCC tumor suppressor genes in human oral cancer cell lines. Anticancer Res. 1993 Sep-Oct;13(5A):1405-13.

10. Hohne MW, Halatsch ME, Kahl GF, Weinel RJ. Frequent loss of expression of the potential tumor suppressor gene DCC in ductal pancreatic adenocarcinoma. Cancer Res. 1992 May 1;52(9):2616-9.

11. Thompson AM, Morris RG, Wallace M, Wyllie AH, Steel CM, Carter DC. Allele loss from 5q21 (APC/MCC) and 18q21 (DCC) and DCC mRNA expression in breast cancer. Br J Cancer. 1993 Jul;68(1):64-8.

12. Brooks JD, Bova GS, Marshall FF, Isaacs WB. Tumor suppressor gene allelic loss in human renal cancers. J Urol. 1993 Oct;150(4):1278-83.

13. Scheck AC, Coons SW. Expression of the tumor suppressor gene DCC in human gliomas. Cancer Res. 1993 Dec 1;53(23):5605-9.

14. Goi T, Yamaguchi A, Nakagawara G, Urano T, Shiku H, Furukawa K. Reduced expression of deleted colorectal carcinoma (DCC) protein in established colon cancers. Br J Cancer. 1998;77(3):466-71.

15. Mehlen P, Rabizadeh S, Snipas SJ, Assa-Munt N, Salvesen GS, Bredesen DE. The DCC gene product induces apoptosis by a mechanism requiring receptor proteolysis. Nature. 1998 Oct 22;395(6704):801-4.

ASSESSMENT OF P53 MUTATIONS IN SQUAMOUS CELL CARCINOMAS OF THE HEAD AND NECK: THE CRITICAL IMPACT OF APPLIED METHODS.

Henning Bier[1], Ulrich Hauser[1], Thomas Carey[2], Reidar Grénman[3], and Vera Balz[1]
[1]Department of Otorhinolaryngology, Head & Neck Surgery, Heinrich-Heine-University, Düsseldorf, Germany
[2]Laboratory of Head & Neck Cancer Biology, University of Michigan, Ann Arbor, MI, USA
[3]Department of Otorhinolaryngology, Head & Neck Surgery, University of Turku, Turku, Finland

Running title: p53 mutations

Key words: cell lines, mutation frequency, sequence analysis, protein detection

Correspondence to: Henning Bier, M.D., Department of Otorhinolaryngology, Head & Neck Surgery, Heinrich-Heine-University, Moorenstrasse 5, D-40225 Düsseldorf, Germany, Phone: +49 211 811 7570, Fax: +49 211 811 8880 (e-mail: bierh@uni-duesseldorf.de)

ABSTRACT

Background. Mutations of the p53 tumorsuppressor gene are a common genetic alteration in squamous cell carcinomas of the head and neck (SCCHN). However, numerous papers have reported a remarkable range of mutation frequencies, and the predictive value of mutant p53 is continuing to be an issue of controversy.

Methods. We determined the p53 status in a panel of 23 established SCCHN cell lines by direct analysis of the entire coding region of both genomic DNA and transcript as well as immunohistochemistry and Western blotting.

Results. 21 of the 23 tumor lines have mutated p53 (92%), and expression of wild type transscript occurs in 4 of these 21 cell lines. Four of the p53 mutations are located outside exons 5-9 (20%). Protein detection recognized only 12 of the 21 mutations (57%).

Conclusions. Depending on the applied methodical approach, a considerable number of p53 mutations may remain unidentified.

INTRODUCTION

The huge p53 literature provides a highly interactive and complex picture of how this transcription factor is produced, activated, modified, localised, and, finally, degraded. However, despite these manifold and, so far, poorly understood protein-protein interactions, an unanimously accepted concept about p53 is that it serves as a molecular stress response device[1,2]. This activity is characterized by the integration of signals emanating from a wide range of cellular insults and the response to these insults by activating a set of genes to induce protective and adaptive measures – for example cell cycle arrest, DNA repair and apoptosis.

There have been many attempts to establish p53 as a marker for the development, progression, response to antineoplastic treatment, and prognosis of cancer. In general, these investigations have focused on mutations of the p53 gene. In squamous cell carcinomas of the head and neck (SCCHN), employing immunohistochemical detection of mutated and therefore accumulated protein, or partial sequence analysis, numerous papers have reported a considerable range of mutation frequencies. Discussions on the predictive value of p53 mutations are dominated by more or less contradictory results[3, 4, 5, 6, 7].

In the past, we have created an autologous multicellular in vitro model of squamous cell carcinomas of the head and neck[8]. For the characterization of these tumors, we also performed a detailed p53 analysis and were surprised by some of the results obtained, such as the high proportion of mutations and the number of mutations located outside exons 5-9. Therefore, we decided to extend these investigations and determined the p53 status in a panel of 23 established cell lines of SCCHN.

MATERIALS AND METHODS

Cell lines
The cell line panel included: UM (University of Michigan) -SCC 10A/B, 11B, 14A/B/C, 17A/B, and 22B, UT (University of Turku) -SCC 7, 9, 14, 15, 22, 23, 24A/B, 33, 34, and 50, and UD (University of Düsseldorf) -SCC 1, 2, 3, 4, 5, 6, 7A/B/C, and 8. In these tumor lines, immunhistochemistry and Western blotting as well as direct analysis of the whole coding region for both genomic DNA and transcript was performed.

Cell culture
Tumor cell monolayers were cultured in plastic flasks (Greiner, Solingen, Germany) under standard conditions (37°C, 5% CO_2, fully humidified atmosphere) in MEM medium (Gibco, Eggenstein, Germany) supplemented with 10% (v/v) heat inactivated fetal calf serum (Sigma, St. Louis, USA), 2mM l-glutamine, 50 IU/ml penicillin, and 50µg/ml streptomycin (all ICN, Amsterdam, The Netherlands). To transfer or passage cell cultures, confluent monolayers were detached with 0.05% trypsin/0.02% EDTA solution (Boehringer, Mannheim, Germany). Subsequently, cells were washed twice in medium or cold PBS and resuspended or processed as required.

p53 protein detection

For p53 protein detection the antibody DO-1 was used (Immunotech, Krefeld, Germany). This clone recognizes an epitope in the N terminal region (AA 37-45) and has been described to identify wild type and mutant forms of p53. For immunohistochemistry, tumor cell monolayers cultered, washed (PBS), fixed (acetone), and air dried on microscope slides were exposed to primary antibody, biotinylated secondary antibody, Vectastain ABC complex (Vector Lab., Burlingame, USA), DAB for visualization, and Mayer's hemalaun for counterstaining. In controls, the primary antibody was omitted. Western blotting was performed according to a routine protocol, employing protein separation by SDS-PAGE and transfer by electroblotting on nitrocellulose membranes. Blocking was obtained with Tween 20, and for visualization a secondary detection system was employed, including biotinylated secondary antibody, streptavidin coupled alkaline phosphatase, and NBT/BCIP.

p53 sequence analysis

For p53 sequence analysis, RNA was prepared with the QIAshredder and RNeasy-kit (Qiagen, Hilden, Germany). Tumor cells were obtained from frozen tumor specimens (UD-SCC 1-8) or harvested from culture falsks, and lysed. RNA was reverse transcribed using random-hexanucleotides and Superscript (Gibco) according to the manufacturers protocol. Aliquots of the conversion mixture were amplified by PCR in a Perkin Elmer thermal cycler as described previously[8]. RT-PCR products were checked by electrophoresis on a 1% agarose gel and staining with ethidium bromide. Genomic DNA was processed similarly. After purification (QIAquick, Qiagen), RT-PCR products were mixed with PRISM AmpliTaq FS Ready Reaction Dye Terminator sequencing kit (Applied Biosystems, Weiterstadt, Germany) and specific oligo-nucleotide primers. After the sequencing reaction (25 cycles of denaturing for 15 sec at 96°C, and annealing and extension for 4 min at 60°C), the reaction products were ethanol-precipitated and analysed with an automated sequencer (Applied Biosystems). Identified p53 mutations underwent confirmation by repeated RT-PCR analysis.

RESULTS

The p53 status of all UD cell lines was confirmed in preparations obtained from frozen tissue sections of the respective tumor specimens (UD-SCC 1, 2, 3, 4, 5, 6, 7, 8). Furthermore, all subpopulations of a particular tumor, for example cell lines that were established from recurrent or metastatic disease (UM-SCC 10A/B, 14A/B/C, 17A/B, and UT-SCC 24A/B) or outgrown from seperately cultured tissue explants (UD-SCC 7A/B/C), always showed the same p53 mutation.

All but two cell lines (UD-SCC 2, UM-SCC 17 A/B), 21 of 23 (92%), harbor mutated p53 transcript. Besides point mutations we found deletions, splice mutations and one insertion. In addition to the mutated allele a wild type allele is present in 9 of these 21 lines. However, expression of wild type transcript occurs only in 4 cases (UD-SCC 1, UT-SCC 14, 24, and 50).

Four of the 21 p53 mutations (20%) are located outside exons 5-9, and17 within exons 5-9. Accordingly, restriction to the widely employed analysis of these exons only would have yielded a mutation frequency of 74%, leaving a notable proportion of p53 mutations unidentified.

Immunohistochemistry and Western blotting with the antibody DO-1 led to identical results. Both methods recognized 12 of the 21 mutations only (57%). In all cases, the mutation caused major alterations of the protein, such as truncation (UD-SCC 1, 3, and 4) deletion (UT-SCC 9, 15, 23, 34, and 50), and insertion (UT-SCC 24) which may give rise to rapid degradation thus preventing protein accumulation.

DISCUSSION

These findings clearly indicate that a considerable number of mutations of the p53 tumor suppressor will be missed when the methodical approach is confined to immuno-histochemistry/western blotting (43%) or partial sequencing of the core domain (20%). Since our investigations were performed in established cell lines of head and neck carcinomas, this result may reflect a selection of tumors which are able to grow under in vitro conditions. However, in a recent paper from Kropveld et al., a very similar observation was reported for a limited number of specimens from consecutive patients with squamous cell carcinomas of the head and neck[4]. Determination of the p53 status in a larger series of unselected head and neck cancers should allow a more validated and probably final statement.

Furthermore, two other aspects deserve consideration. Besides mutations other mechanisms do exist to interfere with the regular function of p53, and we still do not know if and to what extent recently identified members of the p53 family are capable to substitute p53 functions. For example, in our panel of cell lines we have found two tumors without p53 mutation. In one of these tumors (UD-SCC 2), however, considerable amounts of HPV 16 DNA were detected, suggesting an accelerated inactivation of p53 protein through complex formation with the virus protein E6[9]. Consequently, the percentage of cell lines supposed to lack normal p53 function rises to 96% (22 of 23). Hence, suitable test systems are required to obtain meaningful data on the presence or absence of functional p53.

Comming back to the predictive value of p53 mutations, we should like to conclude that, of course, particular mutations like contact or structural mutations in the core domain may have an impact on the course of disease[10], for example because of a gain of function. And, of course, overexpression of p53 as detected by immunohistochemistry may be of clinical importance, for example in generating an immune responses against inadequately expressed protein[11]. However, if we want to look for the significance of p53 inactivation, more sophisticated methods as currently employed are needed.

REFERENCES

1.   Levine AJ. p53, the cellular gatekeeper for growth and division. Cell 1998;88:323-331
2.   Prives C, Hall PA. The p53 pathway. J Pathol 1999;187:112-126
3.   Calzolari A, Chiarelli I, Bianchi S, et al. Immunohistochemical vs. molecular biology methods. Complementary techniques for effective screening of p53 gene alterations in head and neck cancer. Am J Clin Pathol 1997;107: 7-11
4.   Kropveld A, Rozemuller EH, Leppers FGJ, et al. Sequencing analysis of RNA and DNA of exons 1 Through 11 shows p53 gene alterations to be present in almost 100% of head and neck squamous cell cancers. Lab Invest 1999;79:347-353
5.   Raybaud-Diogène H, Tétu B, Morency R, Fortin A, Monteil RA.

p53 overexpression in head and neck squamous cell carcinoma: review of the literature. Oral Oncol 1996;32:143-149

6. Saunders ME, Mac Kenzie R, Shipman R, Fransen E, Gilbert R, Jordan RCK.
    Patterns of p53 mutations in head and neck cancer: full-length gene sequencing and results of primary radiotherapy. Clin Cancer Res 1999;5: 2455-2463

7. Taylor D, Koch WM, Zahurak M, Shah K, Sidransky D, Westra WH. Immunohistochemical detection of p53 protein accumulation in head and neck cancer: correlation with p53 gene alterations. Hum Pathol 1997;30:1221-1225

8. Balló H, Koldovsky P, Hoffmann T, et al. Establishment and characterization of four cell lines derived from human head and neck squamous cell carcinomas for an autologous tumor-fibroblast in vitro model. Anticancer Res 1999;19:3827-3836 ()

9. Scheffner M, Wernes BA, Huibregtse JM, Levine AJ, Howley PM. The E6 oncoprotein encoded by human papillomavirus types 16 and 18 promotes the degradation of p53. Cell 1990;63:1129-1136

10. Erber R, Conradt C, Homann N, et al. TP53 DNA contact mutations are selectively associated with allelic loss and have strong clinical impact in head and neck cancer. Oncogene 1998;16:1671-1679

11. Hoffmann TK, Nakano K, Elder E, Dworacki G, Finkelstein SD, Apella E, Whiteside TL, DeLeo AB. Generation of T cells specific for the wild-type sequence p53$_{264-272}$ peptide in cancer patients – implications for immunoselection of epitope-loss variants. J Immunol 2000;165:5938-5944

DISSIMILAR CELL CYCLE RESPONSES AFTER γ-IRRADIATION AND CISPLATIN TREATMENT ARE INDUCED BY *P53* IN HEAD AND NECK SQUAMOUS CELL CARCINOMAS

A. Narayan[1], E. Stein[1], M. Johnson[1], K. Dornfeld[1], M. Kukuruga[1], S. Fisher[2], T. Carey[1], C. Bradford[1]

[1]University of Michigan, Ann Arbor, MI 48109-0506
[2]Loyola University, Chicago, IL

ABSTRACT

Until recently, surgery and postoperative radiation was the mainstay of conventional therapy for squamous cell carcinomas of the head and neck region (HNSCC). The combined use of chemotherapy and radiation has since become a novel approach in the search for more effective treatment regimens. Though the mechanisms of action of individual anticancer agents are well understood, there is still speculation as to how the resulting DNA damage can induce specific and different cellular responses. To verify whether the *p53* tumor suppressor gene has a role in determining the response of HNSCC cell lines to cisplatin, a chemotherapeutic drug, our laboratory had previously investigated its growth inhibitory effects on HNSCC cell lines. The study suggested that there was a direct correlation between mutant *p53* and sensitivity to cisplatin. The UM-SCC-5 laryngeal cell line contains a mixed population of cells with wild-type and mutant *p53*. After successive cycles of exposure to increasing doses of cisplatin, a population of cells resistant to this drug was selected. Analysis of *p53* in the newly-emerged resistant cells (UM-SCC-5PT) showed that the cells now had only wild-type *p53*. To further characterize the correlation between chemo- or radiosensitivity and *p53*, both parental and resistant cells were analyzed by flow cytometry after exposure to cisplatin or γ-radiation. UM-SCC-5PT cells with wild-type *p53* exhibited a dramatic decrease in the percentage of cells in the G1-phase of the cell cycle 20 hours following γ–radiation with 6 or 10 Gy respectively. This was accompanied by considerable increase in the percentage of irradiated cells in the G2/M fraction. However, when this cell line was exposed to 100 µM of cisplatin, there was only a modest decrease in the percentage of cells in the G1-phase but a large increase in the percentage of cells in the S-phase. Furthermore, there was no observable accumulation of cisplatin-treated cells in the G2/M fraction. In contrast, the parental UM-SCC-5 cell line, with a large population of mutant p53 containing-cells, irradiated with 6 Gy or 10 Gy exhibited an almost negligible decrease of G1-phase cells when compared to the unirradiated set. Moreover, cells in the G2/M fraction increased only slightly. After exposure to cisplatin, the percentage of cells in the S-phase decreased by about 26-38%. These data suggest that p53 is important in inducing G2/M arrest of HNSCC cells with DNA damage induced by γ-radiation. Cisplatin appears to induce a different set of responses in the cells. Furthermore, it appears that G2/M arrest in these cells may be more important than G1/S arrest in resistance to radiation-induced damage. The dissimilar mechanisms of repair of the damage induced by these two therapeutic agents may, in part, be responsible for the diverse set of biological responses. This could explain the effectiveness of combined use of chemotherapy and radiation in the treatment of HNSCC.

INTRODUCTION

Head and neck squamous cell carcinoma (HNSCC) is the 6th most common malignant disease in the world and about 2-6% of all deaths in the United States are due to cancer of the upper aerodigestive tract (oral cavity, pharynx, larynx, esophagus)[1]. In advanced HNSCC, the 5-year survival rates are dismal (ranging from 0-40% depending on the tumor site). Conventional treatment of the advanced disease is through a combination of surgery and radiation therapy[2-4]. For advanced laryngeal cancer, laryngectomy is the surgical treatment and is followed by post-operative radiation. The considerable morbidity associated with such an approach encompasses speech, taste, smell, swallowing and more importantly, quality of life[5]. An approach involving organ-preservation has been fraught with difficulties due to the prolonged treatment course, lack of major impact on distant tumor relapse and patient survival and requirement for salvage surgery in a number of patients with recurrence or persistent local or regional disease. However, there is evidence that concomitant chemotherapy and radiation can achieve high rates of functional larynx (organ) preservation[6]. The cure rates achieved by this modality of therapy are also comparable to those seen after the usual treatment (surgery and post-operative radiation).

Cisplatin is a chemotherapeutic drug used in the treatment of HNSCC. The cytotoxic properties of this drug were reported many years ago[7]. It diffuses into the cell and upon activation, reacts with cellular DNA to form inter- and intra-strand links. DNA replication and transcription are subsequently affected leading to DNA double stranded breaks (DSBs) and miscoding that have lethal or mutagenic effects on the cell. Ionizing radiation can be either particulate or electromagnetic in nature[8, 9]. X-rays and γ-rays exemplify electro-magnetic ionizing radiation. Radiation-induced lesions in the cell include DNA-protein and DNA-DNA cross links, single-strand breaks (SSBs), DSBs, base alterations and base detachments, sugar alterations and bulky lesions (defined as clusters of base damage involving at last 3 unpaired bases and not necessarily combined with a strand break[9]). Repair of breaks and adducts formed by these genotoxins involves non-homologous end rejoining (NHEJ), nucleotide-excison repair and to lesser extents, mismatch-repair, homologous recombination and single-strand annealing[10-12].

The *p53* tumor suppressor gene product plays a crucial role in sensing DNA damage and mediating the appropriate repair (cell cycle arrest) or apoptotic responses[13, 14]. Especially in the case of HNSCC, status of the *p53* gene is a significant predictive factor for successful organ preservation[15]. When overexpression of p53 was studied in tumors of patients with advanced laryngeal carcinoma, the outcome of larynx preservation was significantly associated with p53 overexpression[15]. Tumors that lacked *p53* mutations as detected by single

44

strand conformational polymorphism (SSCP) and sequencing, tended not to overexpress p53[16]. Preliminary *p53*-mutation data from tumors of patients that did not respond to the chemoradiation arm of the Department of Veterans Affairs Laryngeal Cancer Cooperative Study, demonstrated that the most tumor specimens of this non-responding group lacked p53 mutations (unpublished). This and *in vitro* experiments suggested that there is a direct correlation between the presence of mutant *p53* and sensitivity to cisplatin. To characterize a similar association, if it existed, between the status of the *p53* gene in HNSCCs and radiation sensitivity, we assessed the functional performance of p53 in its ability to induce cell cycle arrest after DNA damage. Wild-type p53 is known to mediate a G1/S and G2/M cell cycle arrest after ionizing radiation[17, 18]. However, there are also p53-independent pathways of arrest at the G2/M checkpoint[19-21]. Furthermore, if mutations in *p53* correlated with radiation sensitivity, then it could be used as a possible predictive marker in treatment of HNSCC.

MATERIALS AND METHODS

Cell lines
Cell lines established at the University of Michigan (UM) were used in these experiments. UM-SCC-5 is a laryngeal carcinoma cell line that is very sensitive to cisplatin. This heterogeneous population of cells predominantly harbors cells that have a mutation in exon 5 of the *p53* gene. There is also a small percentage of cells that are wild-type for that same exon. UM-SCC-5 PT is a subline derived from UM-SCC-5 by passing it through successive cycles of increasing concentrations of cisplatin *in vitro*[22]. The resistant cells were found to have wild-type *p53* after completion of selection. Cells were grown in T-75 flasks (Falcon) at 37°C in a humidified atmosphere with 5% CO_2. Medium for growth was Dulbecco's modified Minimum Essential Medium (Life Technologies) supplemented with 10% fetal bovine serum (Hyclone), penicillin (100 units/ml; Life Technologies), streptomycin (100 µg/ml; Life Technologies) and non-essential amino acids (1%; Life Technologies).

γ-Irradiation of cells
Rapidly growing cells were passaged the day before irradiation to ensure a logarithmically growing population. They were irradiated in T-75 flasks at 6 or 10 Gy using a ^{60}Co-irradiator at a dose of approximately 1 Gy/min. Flasks were then incubated in the incubator until cells were harvested at 20 hours post-irradiation.

Cisplatin treatment of cells
Cisplatin (Sigma-Aldrich) was dissolved in 0.9% saline (Sigma-Aldrich) at a concentration of 1 mg/ml. Exponentially growing cells were treated with 50 or 100 µM of cisplatin, which was left in the medium until harvesting.

Flow Cytometry
Supernatant medium in the flasks with cells was collected at the beginning of the procedure. Then the cells were rinsed in phosphate-buffered saline (PBS; Fisher) and the wash was collected in the same set of tubes. The cells were trypsinized in trypsin-EDTA (Life Technologies) and centrifuged at 1000 rpm for 10 minutes at 4°C. Supernatant was discarded and cell pellet was resuspended in PBS and centrifuged again at 1800 rpm for 15 minutes. Supernatant was discarded and cell pellet was resuspended in a PBS solution containing 0.1% sodium citrate (Sigma-Aldrich), 0.1% Triton-X (Sigma-Aldrich), propidium iodide (100

μg/ml; Sigma-Aldrich) and RNase T1 (2 units/ml; Promega) at an approximate concentration of 10^6 cells /ml of PI solution. The cells were cytometrically analyzed on an Epics Elite Cell Sorter (Beckman-Coulter). 20,000 events were assessed and the scattergrams were evaluated on a multicycle software (Phoenix Flow Systems) program that gave the best "fit" for the cells in the various phases.

RESULTS

Twenty hours post-irradiation, UM-SCC-5 PT cells (wild-type *p53*) irradiated with 6 or 10 Gy accumulate to a large extent in the G2/M fraction of the cell cycle compared to the unirradiated cells. The magnitude of accumulation (50-60%) of cells at G2/M is impressive and striking in that the expected result would have been arrest of the cells at the G1/S boundary[17]. However, there are reports about the strong and considerable arrest of cells at the G2/M phase of the cell cycle after exposure to ionizing radiation[18]. Additionally, our results show absence of any debris or fragmentation of cells in the sub-G1 area. In the case of the cells with predominantly mutant *p53* (UM-SCC-5), a much reduced proportion of the cells exhibit arrest in the G2/M phase of the cell cycle compared to the unirradiated cells as observed by flow-cytometric analysis. Additionally, cells are still cycling and there are many cells in the S-phase. Presence of debris in the sub-G1 area of the cell cycle indicates that cells are dying and fragmenting, a feature that was not seen in UM-SCC-5 PT, the population of cells with wild-type *p53*.

Exposure of cells with wild-type *p53* (UM-SCC-5 PT) to 100 μg/ml of cisplatin induces considerable decrease in the proportion of cells in the synthetic phase of the cell cycle 20 hours after treatment. This is in stark contrast to the radiation response of these cells in which the cells piled up in the G2/M phase. This difference in response suggests a different mechanism of sensing the DNA damage. The UM-SCC-5 cell line with mutant p53-containing cells exhibits very little increase in the proportion of cells in the S-phase compared to the untreated controls. However, in the UM-SCC-5 cell line, a large fraction of cells are dying, as evidenced by the amount of debris in the sub-G1 area of the cell cycle. This is presumably because they are suffering subsatntial damage to their DNA and are unable to repair the damage.

DISCUSSION

Our results indicate that wild-type p53 appears to mediate a G2/M arrest in HNSCC cells after exposure to ionizing radiation. This arrest is quite impressive in that more than half of the cycling cells accumulate in that region. Although a G1/S arrest would be a more likely result in normal cells post-irradiation[17, 23], a G2/M arrest is not unexpected. p53-dependent mechanisms of G2/M arrest through the 14-3-3 and Chk2 proteins have recently been elucidated[24, 25] and there is increasing acceptance of the idea that p53 has an important role in the G2/M arrest of cells post-radiation[18]. However, the observation that UM-SCC-5 PT cells displayed a G1/S slow-down after exposure to cisplatin suggests that the mechanism of response to damage induced by cisplatin and γ-radiation is different. Incidentally, it is not clear whether the cells are arrested in mitosis *per se* or whether they have been held up at the G2/M boundary. Nocadozole trapping experiments[18] could be used to monitor escape from

G2 into mitosis and help clarify the situation. Additionally, it is interesting that exposure to neither cisplatin nor γ-radiation resulted in the fragmentation of the 5 PT cells which would contribute to signal in the sub-G1 area. This might be due to the chemo- and radiation-resistant properties of the cells, which in turn could be due to the acquisition of a wild-type *p53* status during the course of selection from the parental cell line, UM-SCC-5. Wild-type *p53* would allow a cell to arrest, repair the damage that it has suffered and contribute to emergence of resistance to the agent in question.

The parental cell line is known to have a mutation in exon 5 of *p53*. Preliminary results from our laboratory favors the hypothesis that HNSCC cells with mutant *p53* are chemosensitive (to cisplatin) in comparison to cells with wild-type *p53*. This is because cells that are unable to arrest, continue cycling and accumulate damage which ultimately leads to cell death (thrugh apoptosis or non-apoptotic means).

γ-irradiation of UM-SCC-5 cells results in a much less striking arrest of cells at the G2/M boundary and furthermore, the cells continue cycling through the various phases of the cell cycle. The S-phase cell-depletion seen in the derived subline UM-SCC-5 PT, is not observed in UM-SCC-5. Genotoxins, especially cisplatin, appear to induce lethal damage in these cells which results in observable cell debris (sub-G1 signal) 20 hours after treatment. Therefore, there is definitely cell death post-treatment with these agents. That UM-SCC-5 is a heterogenous population and has both, wild-type *p53*- and mutant *p53*-containing cells, might explain the small G2/M arrest post-irradiation. Cell death in the mutant fraction of cells might lead to an inflated contribution of the wild-type p53-containing cells to the arrest in the G2/M phase after exposure to ionizing radiation.

Therapeutic implications of such data are wide-ranging. Treatment protocols for HNSCC, combining chemotherapy concomitantly with radiation therapy, could be justified by the following: 1) Different genotoxins have different mechanisms of causing DNA damage and inducing repair. This might enable the overwhelming of a tumor cell's defense pathways. 2) Use of different agents simultaneously (with care to not increase side-effects) might prevent the emergence of resistance through faithful repair of damage. 3) An individually-tailored, logical approach to the treatment of such tumors should be based on appreciation of the molecular events in tumor cells post-treatment.

REFERENCES

1.   Lansford, CD., *et al*., 1999 Human Cell culture Vol II; 185-255 (JRW Masters and B Palsson (Eds)), Head and Neck Cancers.
2.   Wolf GT, *et al*., NEJM, 1988 324:1685-1690, Induction chemotherapy plus radiation compared with surgery plus radiation in patients with advanced laryngeal cancer.
3.   Wolf GT, Hong WK, Head Neck, 1995 17 (4): 279-83, Induction chemotherapy for organ preservation in advanced laryngeal cancer: is there a role?
4.   Sharma VM, Wilson WR, Eur Arch Otorhinolaryngol, 1999;256 (9):462-5, Radiosensitization of advanced squamous cell carcinoma of the head and neck with cisplatin during concomitant radiation therapy.
5.   Bradford, CR, Carey, TE, 1999 Comprehensive Management of Head and Neck tumors Vol I; 321-342 (SE Thawley, WR Panje, JG Batsakis, RD Lindberg (Eds)) Molecular Biology of Head and Neck Tumors.
6.   Jacobs C, *et al*., Cancer, 1987; 60 (6): 1178-83, Chemotherapy as a subsititute for surgery in the treatment of advanced resectable head and neck cancer.

7.   Rosenberg B, *et al.,* Nature, 1969; 222 (191): 385-6, Platinum compounds: a new class of potent antitumor agents.

8.   Ward, JF, Prog Nucleic Acid Res Mol Biol, 1988; 35:95-125, DNA damage produced by ionizing radiation in mammalian cells: identities, mechanisms of formation, and reparability.

9.   Frankenberg-Schwager, M, Radiat Environ Biophys., 1990; 29 (4): 273-92, Induction, repair and biological relevance of radiation-induced DNA lesions in eukaryotic cells.

10.   Corda Y, *et al.,* Biochemistry, 1993; 32 (33): 8582-8, Spectrum of DNA--platinum adduct recognition by prokaryotic and eukaryotic DNA-dependent RNA polymerases.

11.   Mello JA, *et al.,* Biochemistry, 1995; 34 (45): 14783-91, DNA adducts of cis-diamminedichloroplatinum(II) and its trans isomer inhibit RNA polymerase II differentially *in vivo.*

12.   Karran, P, Curr Opin Genet Dev. 2000; 10 (2): 144-50, DNA double strand break repair in mammalian cells.

13.   Levine, AJ, Cell, 1997; 88 (3): 323-31, p53, the cellular gatekeeper for growth and division.

14.   Ljungman, M, Neoplasia, 2000; 2 (3): 208-25, Dial 9-1-1 for p53: Mechanisms of p53 activation by cellular stress

15.   Bradford, CR, *et al.,* Otolaryngol Head Neck Surg., 1995; 113 (4): 408-12, Overexpression of p53 predicts organ preservation using induction chemotherapy and radiation in patients with advanced laryngeal cancer.

16.   Bradford, CR, *et al.,* Arch Otolaryngol Head Neck Surg., 1997; 123 (6): 605-9, p53 mutation as a prognostic marker in advanced laryngeal carcinoma

17.   Kastan, MB *et al.,* Cancer Res., 1991; 51 (23 Pt 1): 6304-11, Participation of p53 protein in the cellular response to DNA damage.

18.   Bunz, F, *et al.,* Science, 1998; 282 (5393): 1497-501, Requirement for p53 and p21 to sustain G2 arrest after DNA damage

19.   Waldman, T, *et al.,* Cancer Res., 1995; 55 (22): 5187-90, p21 is necessary for the p53-mediated G1 arrest in human cancer cells

20.   Deng, C, *et al.,* Cell, 1995; 82 (4): 675-84, Mice lacking p21CIP1/WAF1 undergo normal development, but are defective in G1 checkpoint control.

21.   Brown JP, *et al.,* Science, 1997; 277 (5327): 831-4, Bypass of senescence after disruption of p21CIP1/WAF1 gene in normal diploid human fibroblasts.

22.   Oldenburg, J, *et al.,* Cancer Res. 1994; 54 (2): 487-93, Characterization of resistance mechanisms to cis diamine dichloroplatinum (II) in 3 sublines of CC5331 colon adenocarcinoma cell line *in vitro.*

23.   Agami R, Bernards R, Cell, 2000; 102 (1): 55-66, Distinct initiation and maintenance mechanisms cooperate to induce G1 cell cycle arrest in response to DNA damage.

24.   Hermeking H *et al.,* Mol Cell, 1997; 1 (1): 3-11, 14-3-3 sigma is a p53-regulated inhibitor of G2/M progression.

25.   Hirao A, *et al.,* Science, 2000; 287 (5459): 1824-1827, DNA damage-induced activation of p53 by the checkpoint kinase Chk2.

p53 GENE ANALYSIS CANCER OF UNKNOWN PRIMARY IN THE HEAD AND NECK

Stefan Gottschlich, MD, Oliver Schumacher, Markus Hoffmann, MD, Tibor Goeroegh, PhD, Steffen Maune, MD
Department of Otorhinolaryngology, Head and Neck Surgery, University of Kiel, Arnold Heller Str. 14, 24105 Kiel, Germany

Running title: p53 mutations in CUP

Key words: CUP; p53; mutation; head and neck

***Correspondence to**: Stefan Gottschlich, MD, Department of Otorhinolaryngology, Head and Neck Surgery, University of Kiel, Arnold Heller Str. 14, 24105 Kiel, Germany*

ABSTRACT

Background. Lymphnode metastasis in the head and neck region with an occult primary carcinoma are a rare tumor entity in head and neck cancer. Tumorbiological parameters as well as mechanism and cause for the development of this so called „cancer of unknown primary" (CUP) are not well understood and examined. Mutations of the p53 tumorsuppressor gene are the most prevalent genetic changes of human malignancies and an incidence of up to 50% is described in head and neck cancer. For tumorbiological characterization of CUP the p53 status was determined.

Methods. Twenty-nine archival formalinfixed paraffined CUP of an occult squamous cell carcinoma of the head and neck region were examined. In all cases a primary cancer was never diagnosed. The DNA extracted from the tumor material was amplified with specific primers for exon 4-9 of the p53 gene and then sequenced.

Results. None of the 29 CUP cases showed a mutation in exon 4-9 of the p53 gene.

Conclusion. The total absence of p53 mutations in the so called mutational „hot spots" shows a significant difference to the frequency of primary tumors of the head and neck region. May be this tumorbiological characterisation helps to further elucidate the growth behaviour of CUP in the head and neck region and the reason for their development.

INTRODUCTION

Squamous cell carcinoma metastases in cervical lymph nodes from a cancer of unknown primary in the head and neck region make up about 3-5% of all diagnosed malignancies in the upper aerodigestive tract[1, 2] and therefore form a rather rare entity. There are multiple studies of the clinical behaviour, the diagnostic, and the prognosis of the cancer, and a combination of surgical and radiation treatments has proved to be the optimal therapeutical concept for this tumor entity[5]. It is surprising that there have been so few studies on the tumorbiological characterisation of this so-called „cancer of unknown primary" (CUP). A closer definition of the tumorbiological growth phenomenon of the CUP could help us better understand the carcinogenesis. There are different model conceptions for the emergence of the CUP. One of them assumes that a primary developed tumor shows spontaneous regression, so that there is no primary tumor at the diagnosis of the neck lymph node metastasis. This regression model seems to be accepted for the CUP of the malignant melanoma[6]. In a second hypothesis, it is assumed that early metastases of a small primary tumor are revealed before the primary tumor by rapid growth with tumorbiological or immunological modulations of the growth in the lymph nodes, so that there is only a very small tumor focus at the time of the clinical diagnosis of the CUP[1].

Mutations of the p53 gene are among the most frequent genetical changes observed in human malignancies[7-9] and mutations of the p53 gene are also the most frequent alteration of the genome in squamous cell carcinomas of the head and neck region[10-13]. The product of the p53 gene is a nuclear protein which plays an important role in the regulation of the growth of the cell[9, 14]. It is assumed that more than 95% of these mutations of the p53 gene are in the exons 5-8[7, 8].

In the following study, the status of the tumor suppressor gene p53 was therefore examined in the exons 4-9 of the CUP of the head and neck region in order to characterize this carcinoma entity and possibly to define factors for the genesis of this exceptional form of cancerogenesis.

MATERIAL AND METHODS

All in all, 29 histologically-secured squamous cell carcinoma metastasis in cervical lymph nodes with CUP were used for this study. We are referring to paraffined, formalin-fixed archival material from patients who were diagnosed and treated between 1989 and 1995 at the Kiel University Otorhinolaryngology Clinic. All patients underwent a combined treatment of surgery and radiation. In none of the cases were we able to diagnose a primary tumor. HE-stains were prepared, and then the tumormaterial was identified and removed. The DNA was extracted from the tumor material by using a DNA Extraction Kit (Qiagen, Hilden) and then amplified using the PCR with the help of primers specific to exons 4-9. The PCR was prepared in a thermocycler (9600; Perkin Elmer, Norwalk, USA) under the following conditions for 100 μl reactions mixture: 10 μl 10x PCR buffer, 2,4 μl of 50 mM MgCl$_2$, 0.5 μl of 5U/μl 100 μM Sense and Antisense Primer and 300 ng Template DNA in 83.1 μl H$_2$O (all PCR Reagences from Gibco BRL, Karlsruhe). The high stringency PCR went through 35 cycles at 96° (10 s), 59° (5 s) and 60° (4 min). The PCR-product was then purfied with a GFX Purification Kit (Pharmacia, Freiburg) and then sequenced with the „Dideoxy-chain-termination" method while using the „Big Dye Terminator Cycle Sequencing Ready Reaction kit" (Applied Biosystems, Weiterstadt). All amplified exons were sequenced upstream and downstream with the DNA Sequencer ABI Prism 310 (Applied Biosystems).

RESULTS

After the DNA extraction there was a sufficient amount of DNA from 20 to 50 µg in all 29 cases. After the primer specific amplification with the help of the PCR, sufficient amounts of DNA for up- and downstream sequencing were able to be demonstrated in all 23 amplicons. The evaluation of the sequencing showed no proof of any mutation in any of the 29 CUP cases in the exons 4-9 which were examined.

DISCUSSION

„Cancer of unknown primary" in lymph nodes of the head and neck region have an incidence rate of 3-5%[1, 2]. Strangely, this tumorbiological phenomenon has not been the subject of many molecular studies. The scientific studies of the CUP concentrate more on the possibilities of diagnosis[3, 4, 15], clinical classification[16] and potential schemes of treatment[5]. Because of these missing molecularbiological characterizations, in 29 cases of a CUP in which a primary tumor was not able to be identified, the tumor-DNA was examined for p53 mutations, the most frequent genetical alteration of head and neck carcinomas

The tumor suppressor gene p53 plays a central role in the cell cycle regulation. Normally, p53-protein prevents those cells with DNA damage from progressing from the G1-phase to the S-phase during the cell cycle, and therefore permits the damaged DNA to be repaired[9, 14]. If the damage that has already occurred is irreparable, then p53 is also involved in the introduction of the apoptosis[14]. The expression of cDNA or genomic clones of wild-type p53 suppresses the transformation of cells in culture by other oncogenes, the growth of transformed cells in culture, and the tumorigenic potential of cells in animals[9, 14]. These examples underline the importance of the tumor suppressor gene p53 for the carcinogenesis.

Nowadays, two main hypotheses about the formation of the CUP are being discussed[1]. On the one hand, we assume that a tumor involution takes place after the initial growth of the tumor and the beginning of the metastasization, and that the primary source no longer exists at the time of diagnosis. This assumption seems to be guaranteed for malignant melanomas[6, 9, 17, 18]. For the other hypothesis, we assume that the true primary tumor focus is too small to be identified by to-day's diagnostic. That means it is a well-known clinical phenomenon of the ear nose and throat medicine, which is that the primary tumor mass is distinctly smaller than the volume of the metastases. In both cases, the growth of the primary tumor is very slow, which could result in the case of a CUP with the tumor not being identified, and in both cases, it results in a metastasization, which shows more rapid growth in the different surroundings of the neck lymph nodes.

As far as we know, there are no results of studies of the p53 status in CUP cases from the head and neck region in larger groups. Within the framework of studies on heterogenous groups of patients with head and neck carcinomas, there have been isolated tests for p53 mutations in CUP. Koch et al[10] had one patient with a CUP in a group of 110 patients, and there was a mutation of the p53 gene in this CUP. Boyle et al[13] also reported a patient with a CUP in their group. This one also showed a mutation of the p53 gene, in this case in the codon 237. Mutations in the p53 gene were detected in two patients with CUP in the study of Ma et al[19]. Wood et al were also able to identify a mutation in exon 9 in the single patient with a CUP of 38 patients in all. There are no further clinical data available for these patients with CUP, so that it remains unclear if they were „genuine" CUP cases in which a primary tumor was never diagnosed, as in the group of patients of this study. Comparative numbers of a larger group of CUP patients are not available. The frequency of the p53 mutations in primary head and neck carcinomas is distinctly higher in comparison. Studies of different groups[10-13, 20, 21] even reach a frequency of mutations in the so-called hot-spot regions of exons 5-9 which ranges from 18%-45% for primary tumors in the head and neck region. A study by Kropveld et al[22] which is investigated all 11 exons of the p53 gene even reaches a frequency of almost 100% in a mixed group of patients with head and neck carcinomas.

In conclusion, it can be recorded that the frequency of p53 mutations in lymph node metastases in the head and neck region with occult primary tumors seems to be lower than with primary tumors, which seems to allow the conclusion that a functioning p53 mechanism enables tumor involution or a slower tumor growth, respectively. But in the multifactoral carcinogenesis, one factor alone cannot be responsible for a tumorbiological phenomenon such as the CUP. It is possible, however, that the p53-suppressor gene does play an important role here.

REFERENCES

1. Jungehülsing M, Eckel HE, Staar S, Ebeling O. Diagnostik und Therapie des okkulten Primärtumors mit Lymphknotenmetastasen im Kopf-, Halsbereich. HNO 1997; 45: 573-583.
2. Coker DE, Casterline PF, Chambers RG, Jaques DA. Metastases to the lymph nodes of the head and neck from an unknown primary site. Am J Surg 1977; 134: 517-522.
3. Schipper JH, Schrader M, Arweiler D, Müller S, Sciuk J. Die Positronenemissions-tumographie zur Primärtumorsuche bei Halslymphknotenmetastasen mit unbekanntem Primärtumor. HNO 1996; 44: 254-257.
4. Califano J, Westra WH, Koch W, Meininger G, Reed A, Yip L, Boyle JO, Lonardo F, Sidransky D. Unknown primary head and neck squamous cell carcinoma: molecular identification of the site of origin. J Natl Cancer Inst 1999; 91: 599-604.
5. Lefebvre JL, Coche-Dequeant B, Ton Van J, Buisset E, Adenis A. Cervical lymphnodes from an unknown primary in 190 patients. Am J Surg 1990; 160: 443-446.
6. Schultz-Coulon HJ, Peter HH. Melanommetastasen im Halsbereich bei unbekanntem Primärtumor. Laryngo-Rhino-Otol 1984; 63: 17-20.
7. Nigro JM, Baker SJ, Preisinger AC, Jessup JM, Hostetter R, Cleary K, Bigner SH, Davidson N, Baylin S, Devilee P, Glover T, Collins FS, Weston A, Modali R, Harris CC, Vogelstein B. Mutations in the p53 gene occur in diverse human tumor types. Nature 1989; 342: 705-708.
8. Hollstein M, Sidranski D, Vogelstein B, Harris CC. p53 mutations in human cancers. Science 1991; 253: 49-53.
9. Levine AJ, Momand J, Finlay CA. The p53 tumour suppressor gene. Nature 1991; 351: 453-455.
10. Koch WA, Brennan JA, Zahurak M, Goodman SN, Westra WH, Schwab D, Yoo GH, Lee DJ, Forastiere AA, Sidransky D. p53 mutation and locoregional treatment failure in head and neck squamous cell carcinoma. J Natl Cancer Inst 1996; 88: 1580-1586.
11. Nylander K, Nilsson P, Mehle C, Roos G. p53 mutations, protein expression and cell proliferation in squamous cell carcinomas of the head and neck. Br J Cancer 1995; 71: 826-830.
12. Somers KD, Merrick MA, Lopez ME, Incognito LS, Schechter GL, Casey G. Frequent p53 mutations in head and neck cancer. Cancer Res 1992; 52: 5997-6000.

13. Boyle JO, Hakim J, Koch W, van der Riet P, Hruban RH, Roa RA, Carreo R, Eby YJ, Rupert JM, Sidransky D. The incidence of p53 mutations increases with progression of head and neck cancer. Cancer Res 1993; 53: 4477-4480.
14. Vogelstein B, Kinzler KW. p53 function and dysfunction. Cell 1992; 70: 523-526.
15. Lang FJW, Grosjean P, Monnier P. Aktueller Stand der Broncho-Ösophagoskopie in der Hals-Nasen-Ohrenheilkunde. 1997; 76:704-708.
16. Fernandez JA, Suarez C, Martinez JA, Llorente JL, Rodrigo JP, Alvarez JC. Metastatic squamous cell carcinoma in cervical lymph nodes from an unknown primary tumour: prognostic factors. Clin Otolaryngol 1998; 23: 158-163.
17. Balm AJ, Kroon BB, Hilgers FJ, Jonk A, Mooi WJ. Lymph node metastases in the neck and parotid gland from an unknown primary melanoma. Clin Otolaryngol 1994; 19:161-165
18. Serna MJ, Vazquez-Doval J, Sola MA, Ruiz de Erenchun F, Quintanilla E. Metastatic melanoma of unknown primary tumor. Cutis 1994; 53: 305-308.
19. Ma L, Ronai A, Riede UN, Köhler G. Clinical implication of screening p53 gene mutations in head and neck squamous cell carcinomas. J Cancer Res Clin Oncol 1998; 124: 389-396.
20. Wood NB, Kotelnikov V, Caldarelli DD, Hutchinson J, Panje WR, Hegde P, Leurgans S, LaFollette S, Taylor SG, Preisler HD, Coon JS. Mutation of p53 in squamous cell cancer of the head and neck: Relationship to tumor cell proliferation. Laryngoscope 1997; 107: 827-833
21. Mineta H, Borg A, Dictor M, Wahlberg P, Akervall J, Wennerberg J. p53 mutation but not p53 overexpression, correlates with survival in head and neck squamous cell carcinoma. Br J Cancer 1998; 78: 1084-1090.
22. Kropveld A, Rozemuller EH, Leppers FGJ, Scheidel KC, de Weger RA, Koole R, Hordijk GJ, Slootweg PJ, Tilanus MGJ. Sequencing analysis of RNA and DNA of exons 1 through 11 shows p53 gene alterations to be present in almost 100% of head and neck squamous cell carcinomas. Lab Invest 1999; 79: 347-353.

QUANTIFICATION OF MICRONUCLEI IN ORAL EPITHELIAL CELLS AND PERIPHERAL LYMPHOCYTES IN ORAL CANCER PATIENTS

Enno-Ludwig Barth, MD, DDS, Andre Eckardt, MD, DDS, PhD
Department of Oral- and Maxillofacial Surgery, Medical School, Hanover, Germany

Keywords: Micronucleus, oral cancer, biomarker, buccal mucosa cells, human lymphocytes

Correspondence to: *E.-L. Barth, Department of Oral- and Maxillofacial Surgery, Medical School, Carl-Neuberg-Str. 1, 30625 Hanover, Germany (e-mail: ELBarth@gmx.de)*

ABSTRACT

Cancers of oral cavity and pharynx belong to the most frequent cancers world wide. Apart from exogenous risk factors like tobacco smoke the individual-determined endogenous susceptibility plays an important role for developing a cancerous disease. In about 10 – 30 % of the oral cancer patients synchronous or metachronous second primary tumors occurred. This may be due to a process called field cancerisation. One possible reason for tumorgenesis is damage to the DNA caused by different chemical or physical carcinogens. Quantification of genomic damage can be done by measuring micronuclei, which result from chromosome breakage or alteration of the mitotic fuse during cellular division. Aim of this study was to evaluate the use of the MN-assay as a biomarker to predict the indivi-dual risk of oral cancer patients for developing secondary tumors. Concerning this intention it was found, that only the MN-assay on peripheral blood lymphocytes could be a useful instrument.

INTRODUCTION

Oral cancer constitutes 2 – 3 % of all cancers in Europe and about 4 % of neoplasms in the United States. The majority of oral cancers is caused by tobacco smoke, and there is a marked synergistic effect between smoking and drinking alcohol. Besides, the individual-determined endogenous susceptibility plays an important role for developing a cancerous disease.

Moreover, in about 10 – 30 % of the oral cancer patients second primary tumors are found. The development of second primary cancer in the upper aerodigestive tract may be due to the diffuse mucosal initiation and promotion by exogenous carcinogen exposure such as tobacco

55

and alcohol placing the entire epithelial tissue at risk of tumor genesis by a process called field cancerisation.

Today cancer is known as the result of a multi-step process of genetic mistakes and changes, which proceeds to dysregulation of cell growth, proliferation and differentiation. Cumulative genetic damage during multistage carcinogenesis can be assessed by several genomic markers.

One of these biological markers – namely the micronucleus-assay – we used in our examinations as a tool to estimate the individual risk of tumor diseases in the oral cavity, especially for developing second primaries.

Micronuclei (MN) are defined as microscopically visible, round or oval cytoplasmic chromatin masses next to the nucleus (Fig. 1 and 2). They are formed after a mitotic division when whole chromosomes or parts of chromosomes lag behind the other chromosomes, and become incorporated into a small body adjacent to the main nucleus. Thus, the micronucleus analysis indirectly reflects chromosome breakages or impairment of the mitotic spindle. Chromosome breakages again represent a form of DNA damage, caused by different chemical carcinogens or radiation, which depends on the amount of ultimate carcinogen available to react with DNA as well as on the efficacy of the enzymatic repair process. Therefore micronuclei can be used as indicators of cytogenetic damage.

In all, five criteria were established to identify micronuclei[1]
1. the Diameter is less than 1/5 of the nucleus,
2. its intensity is equal to that of the nucleus
3. it is round or oval with no intended margins
4. it is completely separated from the nucleus
5. the number of micronuclei must not be more than 2 per cell (otherwise the nucleus is considered fragmented)

MATERIAL AND METHODS

Within the scope of our study we carried out a MN-assay in 149 patients with squamous cell carcinoma of the head and neck, in 27 of these patients we found a second primary tumor (18.1 %), 19 persons showed a local relapse (12.8 %), at 10 patients we found a nodal relapse (6.7 %). 64 patients without any tumor in their medical history were used as healthy controls. Further characteristics of the study participants are listed in Table 1.

The MN-Assay was carried out on both non-stimulated peripheral blood lymphocytes and on oral epithelial cells. The peripheral blood lymphocytes were isolated from whole blood by density centrifugation over Ficoll-Hypaque, cells from the buccal mucosa were sampled with a premoistened wooden spatula.

After purification of the cell solution slides were prepared, fixed with methano-acetic acid solution (3:1) and stained for micronuclei analysis with *Acriflavin*, a variation on the *Feulgen*-technique for fluorescence microscopy specific for DNA. For each slide, micronucleated cells were scored by examining 1.000 lymphocytes and epithelial cells respectively.

The evaluation of the smears was done by fluorescence microscopy using a high-power objec-tive in 1000fold magnification; the statistical analysis was done by the t-test for independent groups. P values less than 0.05 were considered significant.

RESULTS

We could confirm some well-established results from other studies: There was no significant difference in micronucleus frequency in peripheral blood lymphocytes as well as in epithelial cells between men and women[2]. Generally in exfoliated cells the frequency of micronuclei tends to be lower than in human blood cells of the same individuals.

Moreover there are signs of an effect of age on micronucleus formation in lymphocytes but not in epithelial cells[3-5].The age effect on micronucleus formation may be caused either by accumulated mutagenic damage or by true ageing processes such as altered cell metabolism or decreased repair capacity. On the other hand the lack of such a correlation between age and MN in epithelial cells could be evidence, that the cytogenetic damage in oral epithelium is local and acute.

Besides there is an influence of smoking on the frequency of micronuclei in both epithelial cells and lymphocytes, but only in heavy smokers with at least 10 pack-years this trend is significant[6-9].

Furthermore we found a higher MN rate in both peripheral blood lymphocytes and epithelial cells in individuals with malignant tumors in comparison with healthy probands[9-11].

Comparing the number of micronucleated cells in patients with a local relapse or a nodal relapse to patients without relapse we did not find any significant difference neither in lymphocytes nor in epithelial cells.

Only in patients with second primary tumor we found a significant higher frequency of micro-nuclei in peripheral blood lymphocytes, in epithelial cells however this high significance was not so clear. Further some patients showing high frequencies of micronuclei in lymphocytes without having second malignancies at the time of the MN-assay later developed a second primary tumor.

Before drawing any conclusions from these results, it is necessary to understand the kinetics of the production of MN in epithelial tissue. Epithelial tissues are comprised of basal, intermediate and superficial cells. The basal layer contains the stem cells, which are capable of self-renewal. These cells also divide to produce daughter cells that undergo maturation to the other cell types and migrate to the surface to replace cells, which are lost.

Micronuclei are formed by chromosomal damage in the basal cells of the epithelium. When these cells divide, chromosomal fragments lag behind and are excluded from the main nuclei in the daughter cells. These fragments form – as already explained – micronuclei in the cell cyto-plasm. It is these cells that later mature and are exfoliated.

The pattern of micronucleus formation in an individual will be strongly dependent on the type of carcinogen exposure he is receiving and on the individual efficacy of the DNA-repairing systems.

In our studies we found the known fact as well, that patients undergoing radiotherapy to head and neck region showed an increase in micronucleated mucosal cells during the treatment, after radiotherapy micronuclei in oral epithelial cells decline to values observed before treatment[12, 13]. So MN frequencies in epithelial cells change in response to carcinogen exposures. Therefore patients who received radiotherapy were removed from the analysis

The micronucleus test in epithelial cells is a marker of the extent of chromosome breakage a few weeks previously, when the cells currently exfoliated were dividing in the basal layer of buccal mucosa. So this test can only reflect the current risk in buccal mucosal cells, but not the cumulative risk over the years.

On the other hand in some studies it is demonstrated, that chromosomal damage, measured by the frequency of MN, persists in peripheral blood lymphocytes of patients up to nine years after polychemotherapy[14]. Since estimates of the mean lifetime of human peripheral blood T-lymphocytes (PBTL) range from 1.5 to 10 years[15], in these cells the MN-assay may reflect the accumulation of cytogenetic damage over the years.

DISCUSSION

The main aim of our study was to evaluate the use of MN-assay as a biomarker in tumor patients indicating an increased risk for developing second primary tumors.

Because there is a differing individual susceptibility, which influences the degree of cytogenetic damage, on the one hand people with similar lifestyle could develop cancer and on the other, there are people, who never develop a malignant tumor until a later date. It is the same with second malignancies.

So there are advices of a higher genetic instability in patients with increased tumor risk. The amount of genomic change in a cell is dependent not only on exposure to external carcinogenic or genotoxic agents but also on the capacity of internal protective mechanisms to prevent or repair damage to the cell's genome, or both.

Consequently individuals with both inborn chromosomal instability and an elevated incidence of cancer, such as patients with *Bloom*-syndrome, ataxia-teleangiectasia, *Fanconi's* anemia, and xeroderma pigmentosum[16, 17] can be found.

It is possible, that "normal" individuals belonging to the general population could acquire genomic instability in individual cells of a tissue by mutation in genetic loci responsible for

58

the maintenance of genomic integrity. Such mutation could result from exposure to a carcinogenic agent or, alternatively, from spontaneous processes like endogenous sources of DNA damage. An elevation in genetic instability in a premalignant cell would lead to an accelerated process of genetic change in a tissue, thereby increasing the probability of the cell's accumulation the multiple changes required for tumor genesis.

Micronuclei as DNA fragments may thus provide a marker of cytogenetic damage either caused by inborn or acquired chromosomal instability or by carcinogenic agents.

Because of longevity of lymphocytes in comparison to epithelial cells these cells could be used to predict the individual risk for developing a second primary cancer.

Table 1: Characteristics of the study participants

		Tumor patients	Healthy controls
Number		149	64
Gender	Male	122	43
	Female	27	21
Smoking habit	Smokers	113	33
	Non-smokers	41	31

Table 2: Results: Frequencies of micronuclei ($p < 0.05$, n.s.: not significant, sig.: significant)

	Frequency of MN in 1000 cells (±SE/Significance)	
	Epithelial cells	Lymphocytes
Tumor patients (all)	2.58 (± 1.42)	3.51 (± 1.39)
Local relapse	2.71 (± 1.66 / n.s.)	3.57 (± 1.70 / n.s.)
Nodal relapse	2.66 (± 0.98 / n.s.)	3.58 (± 1.21 / n.s.)
Second primary	3.01 (± 1.66 / n.s.)	5.18 (± 1.81 / sig.)
Health control	1.31 (± 0.61 / sig.)	2.05 (± 0.60 / sig.)

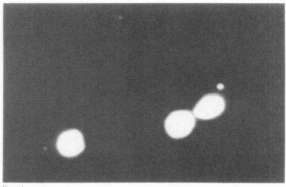

Figure 1

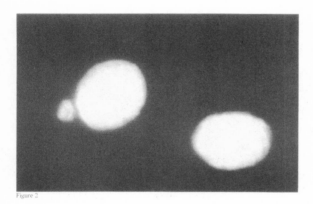

Figure 2

Figure 1. Micronucleus in PBL (Acriflavin, 1000x)
Figure 2. Micronucleus in oral mucosa epithelial cell (Acriflavin, 1000x

REFERENCES

1.   Countryman PI, Heddle JA. The production of micronuclei from chromosome aberrations in irradiated cultures of human lymphocytes. Mutation Res 1976; 41: 321 - 332
2.   Di Giorgio C, De Méo MP, Laget M, Guiraud H, Botta A, Duménil. The micronucleus assay in human lymphocytes: screening for inter-individual variability and application to biomonitoring. Carcinogenesis 1994; 15: 313 - 317
3.   Högstedt B. Micronuclei in lymphocytes with preserved cytoplasm. A method for assessment of cytogenetic damage in man. Mutation Res 1984; 130: 63 – 72
4.   Nair U, Obe G, Nair J et al. Evaluation of frequency of micronucleated oral mucosa cells as a marker for genotoxic damage in chewers of betel quid with or without tobacco. Mutation Res 1991; 261: 163 – 168
5.   Xue KX, Ma GJ, Wang S, Zhou P. The in vivo micronucleus test in human capillary blood lymphocytes: methodological studies and effect of ageing. Mutation Res 1992 ; 278: 259 – 264
6.   Xue KX, Wang S, Ma GJ et al. Micronucleus formation in peripheral blood lymphocytes from smokers and the influence of alcohol- and tea-drinking habits. Int. J. Cancer 1992; 50: 702 – 705

60

7. Carstensen U, Alexandrie AK, Högstedt B, Runnug A, Bratt I, Hagmar L. B- and T- lymphocytes in chimney sweeps with respect to genetic polymorphism for CYP1A1 and GST1 (class Mu). Mutation Res 1993; 289: 187 – 195

8. Trivedi AH, Dave BJ, Adhvaryu SG. Monitoring of smokeless tobacco consumers using cytogenetic endpoints. Anticancer Res 1993; 13: 2245 – 2250

9. Bloching M, Hofmann A, Lautenschläger C, Berghaus A, Grummt T. Exfoliative cytology of normal buccal mucosa to predict the relative risk of cancer in the upper aerodigestive tract using the MN-assay. Oral Oncology 2000; 36: 550 – 555

10. Scala M, Comandini D, Monteghirfo S et al. Micronucleus test on exfoliated oral cavity cells in patients with head and neck neoplastic and preneoplastic lesions. In: Werner JA, Lippert BM, Rudert HH, editors. Head and Neck Cancer – Advances in Basic Research, Elsevier Science B.V.; 1996. p 587 – 592

11. Venkatachalam P, Paul SFD, Mohankumar MN et al. Higher frequency of dicentrics and micronuclei in peripheral blood lymphocytes of cancer patients. Mutation Res 1999; 425: 1- 8

12. Rosin MP. Micronuclei as intermediate end points in Intervention. In: Newell GR, Hong WK, editors. The Biology and Prevention of Aerodigestive Tract Cancers, Plenum Press, New York; 1992. p 95 - 104

13. Belien JAM, Copper MP, Braakhuis BJM, Snow GB, Baak JPA. Standardization of counting micronuclei: definition of a protocol to measure genotoxic damage in human exfoliated cells. Carcinogenesis 1995; 16: 2395 - 2400

14. Osanto S, Thijssen JCP, Woldering VM, van Rijn JLS, Natarajan AT, Tates AD. Increased frequency of chromosomal damage in peripheral blood lymphocytes up to nine years following curative chemotherapy of patients with testicular carcinoma. Environmental and Molecular Mutagenesis 1991; 17: 71 – 78

15. Bogen KT. Reassessment of human peripheral T-lymphocyte lifespan deduced from cytogenetic and cytotoxic effects of radiation. Int J Radiat Biol 1993 ; 64 : 195 – 204

16. Rosin MP, German J. Evidence for chromosome instability in vivo in Bloom syndrome: increased numbers of micronuclei in exfoliated cells. Hum Genet 1985; 71: 187 - 191

17. Rosin MP, Ochs HD, Gatti RA, Boder E. Heterogeneity of chromosomal breakage levels in epithelial tissue of ataxia-telangiectasia homozygotes and heterozygotes. Hum Genet 1989; 83: 133 – 138

MOLECULAR DIAGNOSIS OF HEAD AND NECK CANCER

Ulrike Bockmühl, M.D. Ph.D.
Dept. of Otorhinolaryngology, Charité-Hospital, Humboldt-Univ., Augustenburger Platz 1, 13353 Berlin, e-mail: ulrike.bockmuehl@charite.de

INTRODUCTION

Histopathological tumor classification is still considered the gold standard for the classification of solid tumors and for the decision which treatment modality should be used. But it is well known that the established TNM parameters do not satisfactorily predict the clinical outcome in individual cases or the response to radiochemotherapy. This is primarily due to the different biological behaviour of the tumors which partially escape conventional biological analysis. To overcome these limits there is an increased demand for a refined initial characterization of the tumor by genetic alterations. In an idial setting, by a small biopsy of the primary tumor the pathologist should not only set up the diagnosis but also answer the question whether or not the tumor carries the potential for metastatic spread or if it is resistent to radiation and/or chemotherapy and he should provide a statement on the patients prognosis. In this regard we have focussed on the characterization of head and neck squamous cell carcinomas (HNSCC) by chromosomal alterations classifying the tumors concerning their biological behaviour.

MATERIAL AND METHODS

Tumor samples. Tumor specimens were obtained from surgical resections of 113 HNSCC treated at the Department of Otorhinolaryngology of the Charité Hospital at the Humboldt-University Berlin during the period, 1994 through 1996. None of the patients had previous malignancies or received treatment before initial tumor biopsy. They were all treated for cure by surgical removal of the primary carcinoma along with a neck dissection being complemented by adjuvant postoperative radiation in advanced stages. Operation specimens were transferred to the Institute of Pathology within 1 hour after surgical removal. One aliquot was frozen in liquid nitrogen and kept at -80°C until DNA extraction. DNA was extracted from several 30 μm cryostat tissue sections by proteinase K and phenol-chloroform extraction which was verified to consist of a minimum of 70% tumour cells in each case. A second aliquot was submitted to formalin fixation and paraffin embedding. The

63

histopathological diagnosis was established in every case according to the WHO guidelines on H&E stained tissue sections.

One group comprised 44 non-metastatic (pN0) tumors with no evidence for recurrence or metastasis formation in the mean follow up period of 4 years. In the second group, 69 primary metastasizing (pN+) HNSCC were analyzed and the third group consisted of 38 corresponding metastatic lesions (36 synchronous lymph node metastases, 2 metachronous lymph node metastasis).

CGH preparation. Chromosome metaphase spreads, DNA labeling, hybridization and detection were performed essentially as described previously.[1,2] Detailed protocols are available at the Web site http://amba.charite.de/cgh. The digital image analysis was performed by a custom made CGH software in all cases. Details are published [3,4] and are also available at the Web site http://amba.charite.de/cgh/. The alterations were determined by a statistical procedure as described.[4] The individual ratio profiles and their confidence intervals of all tumors are available at http://amba.charite.de/cgh/.

Analysis of CGH results. The chromosomal imbalances of a large tumor collective were visualized by a histogram as discribed.[5] Similarly the calculation of the difference histogram for the comparison of tumor subgroups has already been reported.[2,6] The case-by-case histogram is a recently introduced tool for the comparison of tumor pairs.[6] It visualizes those changes that differ most frequently between the primary tumors and their corresponding metastases. To examine the similarity between tumor pairs a percent concordance measure was applied to CGH changes on the level of chromosome arms, chromosomal loci and alteration based.[6]

RESULTS

Summarizing the genetic data of all 113 tumors it turned out that HNSCC are characterized by a pattern of chromosomal alterations consisting of deletions of chromosomes 3p, 4, 5q, 6q, 8p, 9p, 11, 13q, 18q, 21q and overrepresentations of 3q, 11q13, 8q, 9q, 16p, 17q, 19, 22q.

To examine the similarity between tumor pairs the percent concordance measure was used and the mean concordance ranged from 64 – 68% whether the CGH changes were calculated on the level of chromosome arms or chromosomal loci or alteration based. To identify the metastasis belonging to a primary tumor within the pool of all metastatic lesions similarity scores were calculated on the different resolutions, i.e. chromosome arms, bands and loci. Thereby, between 23 and 30 tumor pairs were correctly identified. Including those cases in which the corresponding metastasis reached at least the 3rd best match, the numbers ranged between 26 and 34 of the 38 tumor pairs. Visualizing those changes that differ most frequently between related tumor pairs we used the case-by-case histogram comparison. It shows that the common changes between the pairs are dominating refelecting the clonal nature of the tumors. Interestingly, there are chromosomal regions in which additional changes are mainly seen in the primary tumors, e.g. deletions of chromosomes 4, 11 and 13q and gains of 1q implicating their occurence early during tumor development in contrast to gains of 7, 8q23-24 and chromosome 10 and 14q deletions which accumulate in the metastatic lesions.

Since chromosomal alterations with relevance for the metastatic process should be enriched in tissue samples from metastases we compared the CGH pattern of 38 lymph node metastases with 44 non metastasizing primary carcinomas by a difference histogram. In particular, the analysis showed that the deletions of chromosomes 10, 11 and 14q as well as gains of 3q are statistically significant associated with the metastatic phenotyp in HNSCC.

By our custom made software we are able to assess individual chromosomal loci and to correlate them with patients survival. Follow up of our patients was performed on an ambulant basis after completed therapy and lasted 44 month in duration. 33 patients died because of their cancer during this period. The survival analysis was done using the Kaplan-Meier method. For every single chromosomal alteration as well as the clinicopathological data (TNM status, UICC stage, Grading, tumor site) survival was evaluated with respect to disease-free interval (dfi) as well as disease-specific survival (dss). The difference of the survival curves was tested for significance with the Logrank test. Relative to the clinicopathological parameters only the lymph node status showed significance in correlation with the disease-free interval. Among the chromosomal alterations there were 5 locations, i.e. gains of 3q21-29, 11q13 and losses of 8p21-22, 11q23-25 and 18q21 being statistically significant concerning the disease-free intervall as well as the disease-specific survival. To examine the relative impact of these variables we used Cox proportional hazards models. The presence or absence of lymph node metastases was included as the only clinical parameter in the multivariate analysis resulting totally in 6 binary variables. For the disease-free interval the Cox model determined the nodal status, gains of 3q21-29 and 11q13 as well as deletions of 8p21-22 as remaining variables. The regression analysis for the disease-specific survival however reduced the variables to the gains of 3q21-29 and 11q13. To test the influence of the genetic markers in conventionally defined tumor subgroups we performed Kaplan-Meier analysis for each of the 3 imbalances that were assessed in the multivariate analysis in patients with defined pT and pN stages. In particular for the pN0 subgroup, the analysis confirmed the validity of the three independent markers, i.e. 3q21-29 gain, 11q13 gain and 8p21-22 loss, yielding significant p values of the Logrank test both for the disease-specific survival and the disease-free interval. Other significant p values were observed for the combinations: pT2 – 3q21-29 gain (dss and dfi), pT2 - 11q13 gain (dfi) and pN1 – 3q21-29 gain (dfi).

CONCLUSION

Taken together, our CGH studies supplement the genetic data on HNSCC pathogenesis and provide criteria predicting metastatic spread and prognosis and criteria for multiple tumor analysis. The molecular dissection of tumor groups by specific chromosomal alterations, e.g. 3q and 11q13 gain or the deletions of chromosome 10 and 14q, and the classification by the TNM system apparently identify different features of the patients tumors that influence their clinical outcome. Thus, it clearly points to the necessity and feasibility of a genetic classification of HNSCC.

REFERENCES

1. Bockmühl U, Schwendel A, Dietel M, Petersen I. Distinct patterns of chromosomal alterations in high and low grade head and neck squamous cell carcinomas. Cancer Res 1996;56:5325-5329.
2. Bockmühl U, Petersen S, Schmidt S, et al. Patterns of chromosomal imbalances in metastasizing and non metastasizing head and neck cancer. Cancer Res 1997;57:5213-5216.
3. Petersen I, Langreck H, Wolf G, et al. Small cell lung cancer is characterized by a high incidence of deletions on chromosomes 3p, 4q, 5q, 10q, 13q and 17p. Br J Cancer 1997;75:79-86.

4.   Roth K, Wolf G, Dietel M, Petersen I. Image analysis for comparative genomic hybridization (CGH) by a windows-based karyotyping program. Anal Quant Cytol Histol 1997;19:461-474.
5.   Bockmühl U, Schlüns K, Küchler I, Petersen S, Petersen I. Genetic imbalances with impact on survival in head and neck cancer patients. Am J Pathol 2000;157:369-375.
6.   Bockmühl U, Schlüns K, Schmidt S, Matthias S, Petersen I. Chromosomal alterations during metastasis formation of head and neck squamous cell carcinoma. Am J Pathol 2001;158:in press.

66

WHAT DO HEAD AND NECK CARCINOMAS HAVE IN COMMON WITH ADENOIDS ON THE LEVEL OF GENE EXPRESSION?

Tibor Görögh, PhD,[1] Stefan Gottschlich, MD,[1] Markus Hoffmann, MD,[1] Claudia Holtmeier,[1] Sun H. Hu, MD,[2] Jens E. Meyer, MD,[1] Stefan Naumann,[1] Jan Maass, MD,[1] Heinrich Rudert, MD,[1] Steffen Maune, MD[1]

[1] Department of Otorhinolaryngology Head and Neck Surgery, University of Kiel, Germany
[2] Department of Otorhinolaryngology, University of Zhejiang, China

Running title: Gene Expression in Head and Neck Carcinomas and Adenoids

Keywords: carcinoma; adenoid, gene expression; amplification; hybridization,

Acknowledgement: This work was supported by grands of the IZKF of the University of Kiel, Germany

Correspondence to: Dr. T. Görögh, Department of Otorhinolaryngology, Head and Neck Surgery, University of Kiel, Arnold-Heller-Str. 14, 24105 Kiel, Germany, Phone: +49-431-597-2240, Fax.: 2272 (e-mail: gorogh@hno.uni-kiel.de)

ABSTRACT

Background. Recently we reported remarkable repression of fibronectin (FN) mRNA expression and protein production in head and neck squamous cell carcinomas (HNSSC) versus benign phenotypes and that the repression was correlated with different alterations of the gene sequence preceding the transcriptional initiation codon. To prove whether the FN expression could be one of the molecular mechanisms involved only in the carcinogenesis additional experiments with this gene were performed.

Methods. Total RNA was isolated from frozen specimens of 15 larynx-, 20 oropharynx-, and 5 hypopharynx carcinomas with metastases, 15 adenoides and 10 benign mucosa biopsies following reverse transcription. Resulting cDNA was amplified using FN gene specific oligonucleotides. RT-PCR results were verified by Northern hybridization using a 790 bp digoxigenin-labeled FN-cDNA as probe.

Results. A strong reduction in 30% of the head and neck carcinoma biopsies analyzed, an absence in 45% and the normal expression level in only 25% was detected for FN-mRNA and protein in contrast to benign adjacent mucosal biopsies. Surprisingly the FN-mRNA expression was quite absent in all 15 adenoides.

Conclusion. These results suggest that both transcriptional and translational regulation of the FN is differentially controlled between HNSSC and their benign phenotypes. If the loss of FN in malignant metastasizing cells contributes to decrease of cell adhesion and to contact inhibition, as it is often reported, the question arises, whether the loss of FN in adenoides affects similar effect with regard to the amoebic migration of the reticulo-endothelial cells which is additionally supported by different cytokines.

INRODUCTION

Squamous cell carcinoma (SCC) of the head and neck is one of the most aggressive growing tumors among the malignancies, yet relatively little is known about the genes that are important in both the genesis and the progression of this disease. Alterations in the tumor suppressor gene p53,[1,2] and oncogenes, such as ras, myc, and erb-B2,[3-5] activity of matrix metalloproteinase,[6] or the incidence of human papilloma virus[7] (HPV) appear to affect only a subset of this carcinoma. To obtain more information on genes that are involved in this neoplastic disorder compared with benign phenotype, the PCR based differential display was applied. Using this technique, we found and recently reported a gene that was present in benign counterpart, but absent or strong repressed in SCC[8] . Comparatively, we analyzed the expression of this gene in some benign tumors.

MATERIALS AND METHODS

For the in-vitro analysis two well-characterized laryngeal SCC cell-lines, UMSCC-10A,[9] and UTSCC-19A,[10] and two keratinocyte cultures, derived from adjacent normal mucosa of the larynx were used and routinely cultured. For rapid and reproducible preparation of total RNA, the Rneasy Kit (Qiagen, Hilden, Germany) was used in accordance with the manufacturer's instructions. After measurement of the RNA concentration, samples of total RNA were adjusted to 3.5 µg for subsequent first-strand cDNA synthesis. Quantitative analysis of the mRNA content was done by RT-PCR using glyceraldehyde 3-phosphate dehydrogenase (GAPDH) as a control.

mRNA Differential Display. After heat denaturation, the cDNA was incubated with 0.5 µM of one of the H-AP arbitrary primer set (GenHunter, Nashville, TN), 2.5 µM of the corresponding anchored oligo (dT) primer, 2.5 µM dNTPs, 1.5 µM $MgCl_2$, 2µCi [α^{33}P]dATP (Amersham, Braunschweig, Germany), and 2.5 U *Taq* polymerase in a final volume of 50 µl. Low-stringency PCR was carried out for 40 cycles at 95°C for 60 sec, 40°C for 120 sec, 72°C for 30 sec, with a final extension step at 72°C for 10 min (Thermocycler 9600; Perkin-Elmer, Norwalk, CT). After thermocycling 3.5 µl of the amplicon plus 2µl loading dye [97% deionized formamid, 10 mM EDTA, 0.1% xylen cyanole, 0.1% bromphenol blue] were mixed, incubated at 80 °C for 2 min, and loaded onto a 6% denaturing polyarcylamide sequencing gel. After electrophoresis the gel was dried and autoradiographed.

After developing the film, bands of interest were isolated and reamplified under the same conditions as mentioned above, except that the concentration of dNTP was 20 µM and no isotopes were added. Routinely, 5 µl of the 40 µl reamplified products were separated in 1% agarose gel and stained with 0.01% ethidium bromide. Purified double-stranded cDNA fragments were ligated into the pGEM-T-cloning vector (Promega, Heidelberg, Germany), cloned, and sequenced on a DNA-sequencing apparatus Abi Prism 310 (Applied Biosystems, Weiterstadt, Germany).

Northern hybridization. A 790 bp probe was designed for Northern hybridization using the sense primer 5'-CTCAACAGACAACCAAACT-3' and the anti-sense primer 5'-CCTTGTCAT CCTTGACAGTG-3'which was labeled by chemoluminescence (Boehringer Mannheim, Germany). Total RNA was isolated from the in-vitro cultures used for the gene expression analysis as well as from frozen specimens of 15 larynx-, 20 oropharynx-, and 5 hypopharynx carcinomas with metastases, 15 adenoides and 10 benign mucosa biopsies. After agarose electrophoresis, blotting the membranes, hybridization, and chemiluminescence detection with disodium 3-(4-methoxyspiro 1,2-dioxetane-3,2'-(5'-chloro)tricyclodecan-4-yl)phenyl phosphate (Boehringer Mannheim) were carried out according to the manufacturer's instructions. A GAPDH probe was used to verify that the lanes were equally loaded. Finally, the blots were exposed to X-ray film (2-20 min) using an intensifier screen. Quantitation of the Northern results was performed using the gel documentation system E.A.S.Y. Win-32 (Herolab, Wiesloch, Germany).

RESULTS

A part of the comparative analysis of mRNA fingerprints is shown in Fig.1. Among the amplified products a gene fragment was detected the expression of which was considerably repressed in SCC cells compared to benign keratinocytes. DNA sequencing of this PCR product designated FN encompassing the region from 4357 to 4547 of the coding sequence. To verify the differential expression of FN Northern hybridization was performed using total RNA extracted from frozen specimens of 40 metastasizing SCC, of 10 adjoining benign mucosa and of 15 adenoids. As shown in Tab.1 an absence of the FN gene expression in 18 (=45%), strong reduction in 12 (=30%), and normal expression level in only 10 (=25%) SCC biopsies could be detected in contrast to adjoining benign mucosa samples. Alteration of the FN gene expression was also found in benign biopsies. In 2 out of the 15 adenoids strong reduction and in the remaining 13 the absence of the expression of this gene was detectable.

DISCUSSION

In head and neck SCCs investigated in this study, the gene expression pattern was comparatively analyzed with benign phenotyp and alteration of the FN gene expression was found. The loss of FN is a hallmark of many tumors and might reflect cell-growth and adhesion properties that mainly differ from those of the wildtyp, however, the factors contributing to the development of the malignant phenotyp is not sufficient investigated. Studying the mechanisms of the down-regulation, nuclear factors binding to different elements of the 5'-flanking region of the FN gene have been found.[11,12,13] Yet, it is not known whether the FN gene expression is only a carcinoma-specific feature or does this gene repress in benign tumors too. To determine this, poly(A)RNA from adenoids were subjected to Northern hybridization. Interestingly, in all adenoids used strong down-regulation or absence of FN expression could be found.

SCCs account for the majority of head and neck tumors, have the propensity for invasion into the extracellular matrix (ECM). It is know from a variety of experimental systems that the ability of tumor cells to migrate and metastasize is strongly affected by the adjacent normal tissue and cells, particularly mesenchymally derived stromal cells.[14]

In case of adenoid, the reactive area is very rich on B-or T-cells which are capable of migrating in tissue even through-breaking the basement membrane, however, from inside to outside unlike tumor cells. Their amoebic migration and interaction with follicular dentritic cells (FDC) are critically depending on integrin-mediated adhesion.[15] Beside the expression of integrin the extracellular matrix proteins (EMP) laminin and FN promote this process as well.[16,17] Comparing tumor cells with B-and T-cells a similarity exists at following point: These cells have the potential to migrate in tissue without producing FN. Therefore, in both SCC and adenoid the stromal cells should provide FN as a ligand for integrin necessary for promotion of cell-migration.

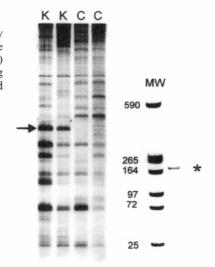

Figure 1. Messenger RNA fingerprint generated by differential display and visualized by autoradiography. The arrow indicates a gene fragment in benign keratinocytes (K) which is strongly repressed in SCC cells (C). After cloning and sequencing the fragment reamplification was performed indicated by the star (MW: molecular weight).

REFERENCES

1. Dolcetti R, Doglioni C, Maestro R, et al. p53 over-expression in an early event in the development of human squamous cell carcinoma of the larynx: genetic and prognostic implications. Int J Cancer 1992;52:178-182.
2. Tamas L, Kraxner H, Mechtler L, et al. Prognostic significance of p53 histochemistry and DNA histogram parameters in head and neck malignancies. Anticancer Res 2000;20:4031-4038.
3. Saranath D, Chang SE, Bhoite LT, et al. High frequency mutation in codons 12 and 61 of Ha-ras oncogene in chewing tobacco-related human oral carcinoma in India. Br J Cancer 1991;63:573-578.
4. Fan CS, Wong N, Leung SF, et al. Frequent c-myc and Int-2 overrepresentations in nasopharyngeal carcinoma. Hum Pathol 2000;31:169-178

5.   Xla W, Lau YK, Zhang HZ, et al. Strong correlation between c-erbB-2 overexression and overall survival of patients with oral squamous cell carcinoma. Clin Cancer Res 1997;3:3-9.

6.   Repassy G, Forster-Horvath C, Juhasz A, et al. Expression of invasion markers CD44v6/v3, NM 23 and MMP-2 in laryngeal and hypopharyngeal carcinoma. Pathol Oncol Res 1998;4:14-21.

7.   Mellin II, Freisland S, Lewensohn R, et al. Human papillomavirus (HPV) DNA in tonsillar cancer: clinical correlates of relapse, and survival. Int J Cancer 2000;20:300-304.

8.   Görögh T, Maune S, Lippert BM, et al. Transcriptional repression of the human fibronectin gene in laryngeal squamous cell carcinoma cells. Cancer Res Clin Oncol (in press)

9.   Carey TE. Head and neck tumor cell lines. In: Hay RJ, Park JG, Gazdar A, editors. Atlas of human tumor cell lines. San Diego: Academic Press; 1994. p 79-117.

10.   Liisa E, Joensuu H, Kulmala J, et al. Squamous cell carcinoma is highly sensitive to taxol, a possible new radiation sensitizer. Acta Otolaryngol 1995;115:340-344.

11.   Nakamura T, Nakajima T, Tsunoda S, et al. Induction of E1A-responsive negative factors for transcription of the fibronectin gene in adenovirus E1-transformed rat cells. J Virol 1992;66:6436-6450.

12.   Oda E, Shirasuna K, Suzuki M, et al. Cloning and characterization of a GC-box binding protein, G10BP-1, responsible for repression of the rat fibronectin gene. Mol Cell Biol 1998;18:4772-4782.

13.   Bowlus CL, McQuillan J, Dean DC. Characterization of three different elements in the 5'-flanking region of the fibronectin gene which mediate a transcriptional response to cAMP. J Biol Chem 1991;266:1122-1127.

14.   Ramos DM, Chen B, Regezi J, et al. Tenascin-C matrix assembly in oral squamous cell carcinoma. Int J Cancer 1998;75:680-687.

15.   Pals ST, Taher TE, van der Voort R, et al. Regulation of adhesion and migration in the germinal center microenvironment. Cell Adhes Commun 1998;6:111-116.

16.   Shibayama H, Tagawa S, Hattori H, et al. Laminin and fibronectin promote the chemotaxis of human malignant plasma cell lines. Blood 1995;86:719-725.

17.   Shibayama H, Tagawa S, Hattori H, et al. Interleukin-6 inhibits the chemotaxis of human malignant plasma cell lines. Br. J Haematol 1996;93:534-541.

ANALYSIS OF CHROMOSOMES IN METASTASING TUMOUR CELLS OF LARYNX BY MOLECULAR AND CONVENTIONAL CYTOGENETICS

K.Szyfter[1,2], M.Kujawski[1], M.Jarmuż[1], R.Grenman[3], K.Szukała[1], W.Golusinski[3], W.Szyfter[3]
[1]Institute of Human Genetics, Polish Academy of Sciences, Poznań, Poland
[2]Chair and Clinic of Otolaryngology, K.Marcinkowski University of Medical Sciences, Poznań, Poland
[3]Otolaryngology Clinic - Head and Neck Surgery, University of Turku, Finland

Key words: laryngeal cancer - metastasis - chromosome aberrations - 13q loss

Correspondence to: *K.Szyfter, Institute of Human Genetics, Polish Academy of Sciences, ul. Strzeszyńska 32, 60-479 Poznań, Poland, Phone: (48 61) 8233011, Fax: (48 61) 8233235 (e-mail: szyfkris@rose.man.poznan.pl)*

Acknowledgements: The studies were supported by the grants KBN PO5C 016 19 and 4 PO5A 095 18 from the State Committee of Scientific Investigations. M. Kujawski was awarded with The Annual Stipend for Young Scientists founded by The Foundation for Polish Science.

ABSTRACT

A genetic progression model for HNSCC provides an accumulation of chromosome alterations in relation to disease evolution. Chromosomes 1q, 3, 5p, 9p, 11q and 13q were found to be the most frequent abnormalities in laryngeal cancer. Further, using comparative genomic hybridization (CGH) and FISH technique losses of 13q were studied in detail in primary tumour v. corresponding lymph node metastases (20 cases).

A pattern of 13q chromosome abnormalities seems to indicate that the common region lost is different than 13q14 coding for *RB1* gene whose function in metastasis of head and neck cancer were already risen. Furthermore, 9 cell lines derived from subjects with various stages of HNSCC were taken under conventional cytogenetic for karyotyping. Monosomy of 13 chromosome was detected in 8 of 9 cell lines. Besides of a variety of numerical and structural aberrations a large number of marker chromosomes were found.

Altogether, the analysis of chromosomes in clinical material and in cell lines imply an involvement of a new putative locus at 13q in metastasis in laryngeal cancer.

In search for useful prognostic markers of progression of head and neck cancer attention was paid for chromosome abnormalities. It has been already hypothesised that chromosome alterations are a subject of changes accompanying disease progression [1]. The investigation attempts were focused mostly on early events and on metastasis [2-6]. Using the technique of comparative genomic hybridization we have studied differences between patterns of chromosome abnormalities in two groups of samples. First, we described chromosome aberrations in primary locations of laryngeal tumours divided according to metastatic phenotype [7]. Next, we analysed material derived from laryngeal cancer subjects with local metastasis to compare chromosome abnormalities in primary location and its corresponding metastasis to the adjacent lymph nodes [8]. The main conclusions of these studies were as follows: (i) there is an accumulation of imbalances of genetic material towards cancer progression, (ii) deletions of genetic material considerably exceed amplifications, (iii) a pattern of the most frequent re-arrangements seem to be similar in primary tumours and their corresponding metastasis. However, in some regions (e.g. 13q) the deletions of genetic material were found far more often. The present study was aiming for further analysis assuming a role of chromosome 13 losses in expansion of tumour cells from larynx to the adjacent lymph nodes. The clinical material studied before obtained after surgical treatment was supplemented by cytogenetic studies of cell lines derived from tumours of variable characteristics concerning primary location inside larynx, staging and histologic aggressiveness. A preliminary report on karyotyping of 8 cell lines was already published [9].

MATERIAL AND METHODS

All the subjects (males, cigarette smokers) were diagnosed as squamous cell carcinoma of larynx. 13 paired samples derived from primary tumour location and corresponding metastases to adjacent lymph nodes were taken for cells and DNA isolation; next 7 paired samples is under analysis. Patients were not subjected to radiotherapy before surgery. The clinical material was examined by histopathologist. Cell lines were derived from primary tumours at the University of Turku, Finland.

The following methodologies were applied: comparative genomic hybridization as published [7,8] and molecular cytogenetic analysis by interphase fluorescence *in situ* hybridization (FISH). To analyse locus of *RB1* the probe LSI 13 (labeled with Spectrum Orange, Vysis) was hybridized with CEP6 (Vysis) as a control of hybridization. Karyotypes of cell lines were established by conventional cytogenetic technique with Giemsa staining to obtain a GTG banding pattern.

RESULTS

Looking at losses of the region containing *RB1* gene it was established that a vast majority of metastases and primary tumours (12 of 13) were lacking both or one signal as shown by FISH technique (Table 1). However, the detected losses could be recognised mostly as "soft" (present in 10% of cells or less); "solid" aberrations (present in at least 20% of cells) occurred only in 6/13 metastases and 2/13 primary tumours. There was only one case of *RB1* loss in tumour cells with no apparent changes detected in the same material by CGH. In contrast, in two samples there were found two signals derived from two alleles where CGH analysis has proven a loss of genetic material in chromosome 13. The latter observation may indicate for an involvement of another locus (different from *RB1*) in metastasis to the neck lymph nodes in laryngeal cancer. The losses of 13q shown by FISH technique were mostly consistent with the findings using CGH technique.

In the separate experiments the karyotypes of the cell lines derived from laryngeal cancer were analysed. As an example the karyotype of the cell line UT-SCC-22 derived from a male with an early laryngeal cancer of G2 histologic aggressiveness is shown (Fig.1). The final results of cell lines karyotyping are still under analysis. At present al least some common features are to be mentioned. The total number of chromosomes is higher than 46 because of triploidy (chromosomes 3, 8, 12, 14, 15 and 16 - examples refer to the karyotype shown) and tetraploidy (chromosomes 5, 9, 10 and 20). Concerning aberrations of chromosome 13 in 6 of 7 cell lines a monosomy of chromosome 13 was found. Monosomy of chromosome 13 was seen at all the cells analysed. In the remaining cell line (UT-SCC-19A) a trisomy of chromosome 13 was established.

A number of marker chromosomes are observed. The experiments designed to explain their origin are in progress and at the moment we cannot exclude that a lost part of chromosome 13 could be translocated to one of the marker chromosomes.

DISCUSSION

Recently in tumour biology there is a considerable shift of interest from molecular markers to subcellular ones that includes studies on chromosomes. Molecular markers appear to be more restricted to pre-malignant carcinogenesis or an early tumourigenesis [10-12]. Another reason of a growing interest in cytogenetic studies is connected with expanding of research area following introducing such techniques as fluorescent *in situ* hybridization (FISH) and comparative genomic hybridization (CGH) known as molecular cytogenetics to put a difference with a conventional cytogenetics. On this way, many projects were undertaken aiming for a correlation of specific chromosome abnormalities with head and neck cancer and its staging, aggressiveness and prognosis.

The chromosomes with frequent structural abnormalities found by us previously [7,8] were already described by other authors dealing with head and neck cancer [2,3,5]. It must be stressed in this point that the material used here is very compact and restricted to squamous cell carcinoma of the larynx contrary to other head & neck cancer projects.

Hence, we decided to join the current interest in some "tiny" abnormalities as 18q [4], 11q13 [3] or 3p21.3 [13] and their predictive significance. Our attention was paid on the region 13q containing a locus of oncosuppressor *RB* gene. The preferential losses at 13q14 and 13q32-ter were documented in head and neck carcinomas [14]. The studies on esophageal squamous cell carcinoma established only allelic loss of 13q12-13 [15]. On the other hand, a well-documented study on hereditary breast cancer has proven frequent deletions in 13q21 region that could implicate another cancer susceptibility locus different from *RB*. Our preliminary results could be interpreted as an extention of the latter supposition into head and neck cancer. Hence, a role of *RB* gene in laryngeal cancer does not seem to be significant.

The results established by molecular and conventional cytogenetics are often divergent, at least for two reasons. CGH is applicable to non-balanced chromosome alterations leaving the other non-detected. On the other hand, classical cytogenetics deals with the same resolution but with that method analysis of balanced aberrations (translocations, inversions etc.) is possible. A number of marker chromosomes have to be taken also into account. Because of their small size they could be lost in analysis by CGH that in turn can cause an overestimation of losses. Nevertheless, in our opinion a combination of CGH, FISH and conventional cytogenetics should contribute well to get complementary results.

Table 1. Aberrations of chromosome 13q in primary site and lymph node metastasis of laryngeal cancer cells studied by FISH and CGH techniques

case	occurrence of RB1 gene in cells (%)									
	primary tumour					metastasis				
	FISH signal				CA	FISH signal				CA
	loss	1^0	2^0	3^0		loss	1^0	2^0	3^0	
1	0.5	7.5	91.5	0.5		1.5	6.5	92.0	0	-13q21-31
2	2.0	6.5	91.5	0		**16.5**	**33.5**	49.5	0.5	-13
3	2.5	7.5	90.o	0		3.5	10.0	86.5	0	
4	3.0	10.5	86.5	0	-13	2.5	18.0	79.0	0.5	-13
5	1.5	11.5	87.o	0		0.5	23.5	76.0	0	-13q21-ter
7										-13q14-31
8	2.5	12.0	86.5	0		**8.0**	**20.5**	71.5	0	
9	0	1.0	99.0	0		0.5	6.0	93.0	0.5	13q14-q31
10	0	6.5	92.5	1.0		0	0.5	39.5	60.0	+13q14-31
11	3.0	8.0	89.0	0		1.5	6.5	89.5	2.5	
12	0	9.5	90.5	0		3.0	7.o	89.5	0	
13										-13q21-31
14	**16.0**	**28.5**	55.5	0	-13	**90.0**	**6.5**	3.5	0	-13
15					-13					-13
17	**74.5**	**20.0**	5.5	0	-13	**91.5**	**7.0**	1.5	0	-13
20					-13					-13
21					-13q21-ter					-13q21-ter
26					-13					-13
27					-13q14-21					-13q14q21
28	1.5	10.0	88.5	0		5.0	9.5	85.5	0	

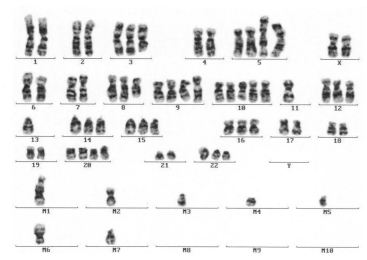

Fig. 1. Karyotype of UT-SCC-22 cell line

REFERENCES

1. Califano J, van der Riet P, Westra W, Nawroz H, Clayman G, Piantadosi S, Corio R, Lee D, Greenberg B, Koch W, Sidransky D. Genetic progression model for head and neck cancer: Implication for field cancerization. *Cancer Res* 1996; 56:2488-2492

2. Bockmühl U, Schwendel A, Dietel M, Petersen. Distinct patterns of chromosomal alterations in high- and low-grade head and neck squamous cell carcinoma. *Cancer Res* 1996; 56:5325-5329

3. Bockmühl U, Petersen S, Schmidt S, Wolf G, Jahnke V, Dietel M, Petersen I. Patterns of chromosomal alterations in metastazing and nonmetastazing primary head and neck carcinomas. *Cancer Res* 1997; 57:5213-5316

4. Frank JF, McClathey KD, Devaney KO, Carey TE. Evidence that loss of chromosome 18q is associated with tumor progression. *Cancer Res* 1997; 57:824-827

5. Jin Ch, Jin Y, Wennerberg J, Dictor M, Mertens F. Nonrandom pattern of cytogenetic abnormalities in squamous cell carcinoma of the larynx. *Genes Chrom Cancer* 2000; 28:66-76

6. Nawroz H, van dr Riet P, Hruban RH, Koch W, Ruppert JM, Sidransky D. Allelotype of head and neck squamous cell carcinoma. *Cancer Res* 1994; 54:1152-1155

7. Kujawski M, Alto Y, Jaskuła-Sztul R, Szyfter W, Szmeja Z, Szyfter K, Knuutila S. DNA copy number losses are more frequent in primary larynx tumors with lymph node metastasis than in tumors without metastases. *Cancer Gen Cytogenet* 1999;114:31-34

8. Kujawski M, Sarlomo-Rikala M, Gabriel A, Szyfter K, Knuutila S. Recurrent DNA copy number losses associated with metastasis of larynx carcinoma. Genes Chrom Cancer 1999; 26:253-257

9. Jarmuż M, Szyfter K, Grenman R, Golusinski W, Szyfter W. Analysis of chromosome alterations in cell lines derived from laryngeal tumours as a tool for estimation of larynx cancer. Otolaryng Pol 2000; 54:567-572

10. Sidransky D. Molecular genetics of head and neck cancer. *Current Opinion Oncol* 1995; 7:229-233

11. Szyfter K, Szmeja Z, .Szyfter W, Hemminki H, Banaszewski J, Jaskuła-Sztul R, Louhelainen J. Molecular and cellular alterations in tobacco smoke-associated larynx cancer. *Mutat Res* 1999, 445:259-274

12. Gray JW, Collins C. Genome changes and gene expression in human solid tumors. *Carcinogenesis* 2000; 21:443-452

13. Wu X, Zhao Y, Honn SE, Tomlinson GE, Minna JD, Hong WK, Spitz MR. Benzo(a)pyrene dio epoxide-induced 3p21.3.aberrations and genetic predisposition to lung cancer. *Cancer Res* 1998; 58:1605-1608

14. Maestro R, Piccinin S, Doglioni C, Gasparatto D, Vukosavljevic T, Sulfaro S, Barzan L, Boiocchi M. Chromosome 13q deletion mapping in head and neck squamous cell scarcinomas: Identification of two distinct regions of preferential loss. *Cancer Res* 1996; 56:1146-1150

15. Harada H, Tanaka H, Shimada Y, Shinoda M, Imamura M, Ishizaki K. Lymph node metastasis is associated with allelic loss on chromosome 13q12-13 in esophageal squamous cell carcinoma. Cancer Res 1999; 59:3724-3729

16. Kainu T, Juo SHH, Desper R, Schäffer AA, Gillander E, Rozenblum E, Freas-Lutz D, Weaver D, Stephan D, Bailey-Wilson J, Kallioniemi OP, Tirkkonen M, Sirjäkoski T, Koivisto P, Karhu R, Hollo K, Arason A, Johannesdottir G, BergthorsonJT, Johannsdottir H, Egilsson V, Barkardottir RB, Johannsson O, Haraldsson K, Sandberg T, Holmberg E, Grönberg H, Olsson K, Borg A, Vehmanen P, Eerola H, Heikkilä P, Pyrhönen S, Nevanlinna H. Somatic deletions in hereditary breast cancers implicate 13q21 as a putative novel breast cancer susceptibility locus. *Proc.Nat.Acad.Sci* 2000; 97:9603-9608

ON THE ROLE OF CELL-CELL ADHESION IN METASTASIS FORMATION IN HEAD AND NECK CANCER

Franz X. Bosch[1], Antje Schuhmann[1], Jürgen Kartenbeck[2]
[1]Department of Otolaryngology, Head and Neck Surgery, University of Heidelberg, INF 400, D-69120 Heidelberg, Germany
[2]Division of Cell Biology, German Cancer Research Center, INF 280, D-69120 Heidelberg, Germany

ABSTRACT

We challenge the dogma of downregulated expression of cell-cell contact components as a prerequisite of metastasis formation. 187 tumors was analyzed for changes in expression of E-Cadherin, desmoplakin and desmogleins by immunohistochemistry (IHC), and the patterns observed were compared with clinical parameters. Selected cases were further studied by mRNA-in situ-hybridization (ISH), Western Blotting and electron microscopy (EM).

Partially reduced protein expression of cell adhesion components was common in invasive tumors. However, downregulation of gene expression of E-Cadherin as well as of the desmosomal components occurred only in a minority of cases. Various defects in the adhesive structures were seen in EM, but expression and formation of some intact desmosomes and of E-Cadherin persisted in the metastasizing primary tumors and in the lymph node metastases. Of interest, the extent of reduction of E-Cadherin but not of the desmosomal components, as seen in IHC, had predictive and prognostic power. This was independent of tumor site, tumor size and stage. Expression and assembly of desmosomes did not correlate with tumor progression.

We propose that metastasis involves only a temporarily reduced expression of E-Cadherin and desmosomes. Expression of E-Cadherin but not of the desmosomes is of predictive and prognostic value.

INTRODUCTION

Stability and maintenance of epithelial tissue depends on the integrity of junctional structures. Key elements in intercellular adhesion are transmembrane glycoproteins of the cadherin

79

family.[1,2] Best investigated in this respect are E-cadherin and its cytoplasmatically associated proteins α- and β-catenin.[3] The desmosomes with their main constituents desmoplakins and desmogleins also represent an important adhesive structure.[4] There is evidence that malfunction of these adherens junctions, mainly caused by reduced expression of the above-mentioned adhesion molecules, results in loss of adhesion, dedifferentiation, tumorigenesis and metastasis.[5-7] Statistical results from a number of different tumors seem to point to a correlation between reduced expression and poor prognosis.[8,9]

While the published data demonstrate that tumor differentiation and invasiveness correlate with a changed expression pattern of junctional proteins, the correlation to survival rates of the affected patients is less strong. A reliable association of abnormal expression patterns of adhesive or attached junctional proteins with the clinical outcome requires registration of multitude factors like, e.g. tumor size and stage at initial diagnosis, exact tumor site, choice of treatment, age and performance status of the patients, and, depending on the impact of the molecular factor analyzed, a sufficient number of cases included in the study.

In the current study we analyzed untreated primary head and neck SSC (HNSCC) for the expression of the desmosomal proteins desmoplakin and desmoglein and for the adherens junction protein E-cadherin by immunohistochemistry (IHC). We also compared the expression patterns of the above-mentioned proteins from the primary tumors with metastases derived therefrom. In a part of this cohort, immunofluorescence microscopy and electron microscopy was performed. The patterns of changes seen in IHC were compared with the clinical course of the disease and the survival rates during a median follow-up of over three years (ranging from 2 to 9 years).

MATERIALS AND METHODS

Patients and tissues
187 cases of primary SCC and 60 metastases were selected from patients attending the Department of Head and Neck Surgery (University of Heidelberg, Germany) between 1990 and 1998. Clincial and histologial diagnosis of SCC and no prior treatment of the tumor were criteria for the selection in this study. Tumor biopsies were taken during surgical dissection under general anaesthesia and after the signed consent of the patients. The specimens to be used in immunohistochemistry and immunofluorescence microscopy were snap-frozen in isopentane precooled with liquid nitrogen and stored at -80°C. Tissue sections (3 to 5 μm) were prepared with a cryotome. For electron microscopcal analysis, small tissue pieces were fixed with 2.5% glutaraldehyde in 50 mM cacodylate buffer (pH 7.2, 50 mM KCl, 1.25 mM $CaCl_2$) for 30 to 45 min.

Indirect Immunofluorescence (IIF), Immunohistochemistry (IHC), Electron Microscopy (EM).
These were performed according to standard protocols. For EM, tissues were embedded in Epon. Epon blocks were cut using a Reichert-Jung microtome (Ultracut). Electron micrographs were taken with a Zeiss EM 910 (Carl Zeiss, Oberkochen, Germany).

Antibodies.

The following primary antibodies were used: anti-E-cadherin 1: HECD-1, Transduction Laboratories, and L-CAM/Uvomorulin, clone 6F9; Progen Biotechnik, Heidelberg, Germany; anti-desmoglein I&II: DSG 3.10; anti-desmoplakin I&II (cocktail); anti-desmoglein III: DSG 194, all Progen Biotechnik, Heidelberg, Germany.

Evaluation of IHC staining results with E-Cadherin, Desmoglein and Desmoplakin.

The expression levels of these proteins in normal squamous epithelium were examined by staining mucosal biopsies derived from non-tumor patients. All three antigens revealed a strong and uniform membraneous staining in all living cell layers. For each antigen, staining in the tumors was graded in the following manner: indistinguishable from normal mucosa, score 0; some cytoplasmic staining in addition to membraneous staining, score 1; weakly reduced membraneous staining, score 2; weakly reduced membraneous staining plus some cytoplasmic staining, score 3; moderately reduced membraneous staining, score 4; moderately reduced membraneous staining plus some cytoplasmic staining, score 5; strongly reduced membraneous staining, score 6; strongly reduced or absent membraneous staining with weak cytoplasmic staining left, score 7; total absence of staining, score 8.

Statistical Analysis

Survival rate was estimated using the Kaplan-Meier method. All endpoints, i.e. local recurrences, regional recurrences to lymph nodes and second primary carcinomas, were measured from the first day of treatment. If patients died for reasons not related to cancer, they were censored at the time of their death or at their last follow up. Patients who have not experienced any of the endpoints were censored at the time of their last follow up. Survival was defined as the time to death (related to cancer). Significance testing between groups was performed using a two-sided log-rank test. Only the immunohistochemical/immuno-fluorescence patterns were evaluated in relation to follow-up events.

RESULTS

IHC of primary tumors for the desmosomal components desmoglein I&II and desmoplakin I&II

For desmoplakin (DP) staining, a single monoclonal antibody, DP-2.15, was used for all tumors. The validity of this antibody was confirmed by staining part of the cohort with a cocktail of monoclonal antibodies against DP, and the staining results were very similar.

IHC of primary tumors for E-Cadherin, the prototype component of Adherens Junctions

There were two well established monoclonal abtibodies against E-cadherin available, HECD-1 and L-CAM clone 6F9. The sensitivity and specificity in Western Blots of these two antibodies were similar, so we initially decided to use L-CAM clone 6F9, for historical reasons. However, during the course of this study we noted discrepancies between the staining results and results of Western Blot analyses of a subset of the tumors, and also discrepancies between the staining results and analyses of mRNA expression by in situ-hybridization (data not shown). This suggested that masking of the epitope recognized by the 6F9 antibody occurred in a substantial fraction of the tumors. All tumors in which epitope masking might have occurred, were stained again with HECD-1. Indeed, in many cases much stronger staining was observed with HECD-1, and the staining scores were corrected accordingly.

Summary of the IHC and IIF results

After grouping the primary tumors according to the tumor site, tumor stage, histological grading and lymph node involvement, it became clear that virtually all invasive squamous cell carcinomas examined in this study (n=187) revealed at least slight reductions in the expression and localization patterns both of the desmosomal components, as well as of E-Cadherin, as seen by IHC or IIF. The mean scores of the individual components as well as the sumscores of the three components did not vary significantly between the different tumor sites larynx, oral cavity, oropharynx and hypopharynx, between the tumor stages, and the histological grades. The extent of changes observed was highly variable among the tumors, and we also observed in many cases a marked intra-tumoral heterogeneity. Fig. 1 illustrates typical changes observed by IIF after staining of tumors representing different stages from early invasive (a) to late stage highly metastatic primary tumors (c, e).

In many cases, the changes observed in staining of the desmosomes and E-cadherin were independent from each other. Surprisingly, most metastasizing primary tumors and most metastases showed at least partially retained expression of these adhesive structures, and only a minority of the tumors showed reduced mRNA expression of desmogleins and E-cadherin (data not shown).

Comparison of Indirect Immunofluorescence (IIF) and Electron Microscopy (EM)

In a subset of primary tumors and lymph node metastases, the immunostaining patterns were directly compared with the ultrastructural appearance of the adhesion structure, which at the EM level was restricted to the desmosomes. We noted three main tumor categories at the EM level.

Tumors of category 1 (T_1) appeared to be typical for early invasive but non-metastasizing primary tumors, with strong staining for desmoplakin I&II glycoprotein (Fig. 1a), desmoglein I&II and E-cadherin (not shown). At EM, T_1 showed densely packed desmosomes, evenly distributed at the periphery of the cells (Fig. 1b). The general appearance was comparable with a normal squamous epithelium. Tumors of category 2 (T_2) showed at the light microscopic level heterogenous staining for all three adhesion proteins (both strongly and weakly stained areas present; Fig. 1c), and at the EM level a strikinlgy reduced number and size of desmosomal structures. Single closed membrane vesicles in the cytoplasm, closely resembling internalized desmosomes, were seen (Fig. 1d, arrow head). The lymph node metastasis derived from T_2 also showed such internalized desmosomes (not shown). The desmosomal staining of category 3 tumors (T_3) was further reduced when compared with T_2 (Fig. 1e). In EM of T_3, the desmosomes connecting cellular extensions or cell bodies were much less frequent, they were smaller in diameter and many showed signs of degeneration (Fig. 1f, arrow heads). Occasionally, cytokeratin filaments were still attached to these rudimentary desmosomes (left of the two arrow heads in Fig. 1f).

Clinical relevance of the IHC expression patterns of E-cadherin, desmoplakin and desmoglein 1,2 assessed by statistical analysis

The changes seen in the primary tumors were independent of the tumor site and stage (TNM) at time of diagnosis, and they only weakly correlated with tumor differentiation and with relapse events during follow-up. However, E-cadherin, but not the desmosomal proteins analyzed, strongly correlated with survival. The Kaplan Meier analysis of the relationship between the E-cadherin staining scores above and below the median and overall survival is presented in Fig. 2, which demonstrates that patients with E-cadherin scores above median (i.e. score 2) had a significantly poorer prognosis as compared to those with a score up to median. In contrast to E-Cadherin, desmoplakin I&II and desmoglein I&II as well as the sumscore of the desmosomal components failed to show prognostic and pedictive relevance. When the scores of all three adhesion molecules were added up, the predictive and prognostic power of E-cadherin was strongly diminished, confirmimg the selective association of prognosis with E-cadherin. The prognostic impact of reduced E-cadherin expression on shortened overall survival was as strong as that of the tumor stage, the nodal status and the tumor site (not shown).

DISCUSSION

Changed expression patterns of molecules present in adherens junctions which are responsible for epithelial cell-cell adhesion, especially E-cadherin and the associated catenins, have been shown to cause abnormal organization and dedifferentiation of the tissue and to result in the initiation of invasive and metastatic behavior. However, in squamous epithelia, adhesion and tissue stability also depend on the adhesive properties of the multiple desmosomal complexes. It has been reported that the desmosomes are affected in a parallel manner as adherens junctions during dedifferentiation and in metastasis of various tumor types.[5,7,10-12] Whether reduced or absent expression of desmosomal components is actually governed by changes in E-cadherin expression or may occur independently of E-cadherin, and whether changes in desmosomes are of diagnostic and prognostic value, has not been rigorously analysed.

In this study, we have addressed these questions. The desmosomes in SCC of the head and neck of 187 patients were examined for the relationship between expression and clinical parameters including patient survival. In turn, the data were then compared with the results from the parallel assessment of E-cadherin. Desmoplakin staining served as a reliable indicator of the number and state of the desmosomes. In addition, the desmosomal cadherins desmoglein I&II were also analysed. The expression of these appear to be differentiation dependent in squamous epithelia.[13,14]

In accordance to the above-mentioned earlier studies, we also noticed an enhanced reduction of junctional complexes, i.e. desmosomes and adherens junctions with increasing tendency to metastasize. However, we never detected tumor cells or metastatic cells, positively identified as of epithelial origin with cytokeratin antibodies, which were devoid of adhesive structures. Even tumor cells invading the connective tissue always revealed dotted immunosignals, indicating ongoing synthesis of desmosomal components, despite apparent reduction in adhesive properties.

Furthermore, although in many cases there seemed to be a coordinate change in E-cadherin and in the desmosomes, there was also a sizable portion of the tumors in which this was not the case. Statistical analysis showed that there was no significant correlation between the two adhesive structures. Most importantly, our data have revealed a strong prognostic impact of reduced E-Cadherin expression on the survival of the patients. In fact, E-cadherin turned out to be equal to or even superior to the known clinical prognostic factors tumor site, tumor stage and lymph nodal status at the time of first diagnosis (Fig. 2). No such relationship existed between changes in the desmosomes and the clinical course of the disease in our patient cohort. The latter finding confirmed that the changes we have documented were not strictly coupled.

Finally, since we did not detect tumor cells devoid of adhesive structures, neither in the primary metastasizing tumors nor in the matched lymph node metastases, we conclude that there are as yet unidentified factors involved in cellular detachment and metastatic outgrowth. Besides the partial but not complete downregulation of expression and assembly of the adhesive structures which we have described, there may be temporarily active signals inhibiting intercellular adhesion despite the presence of adhesive structures. This would allow metastasizing cells to reassociate to cell clusters in suitable environments at possible sites of implantation.

Figure 1. Desmoplakin staining by Indirect Immunofluorescence (IIF) and Electron Microscopy (EM) of different tumor stages of HNSCC. In a, c and e, IIF staining for desmoplakin I&II is shown, in b, d, and f, EM pictures of the same tumors are presented. Tumor in a and b, T3N0M0 of supraglottic larynx; tumor in c, and d, T3N2M0 of oropharynx; tumor in e and f, T4N2M0 of hypopharynx. Note that in a, b, the tumor shows largely normal desmoplakin staining in IIF and normal desmosome morphology in EM. In contrast, the tumor in c, d shows diminishion of desmoplakin staining and ultrastructural alterations; the arrow head points to an internalized desmosome. These changes in IIF and EM are further increased in the tumor depicted in e and f; the arrow heads point to damaged desmosomes.

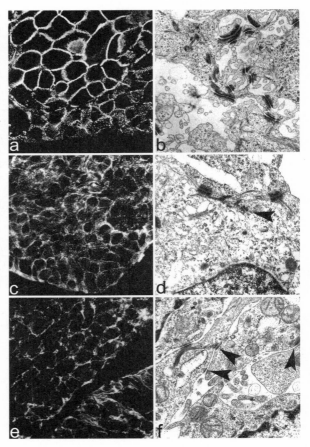

Figure 2. Correlation of reduced E-Cadherin expression with shortened overall survival. The median score of E-cadherin staining was 2 (see Materials and Methods). Patients with a score >2 had a significantly reduced survival (n=87), as compared with the patients with a score </=2 (n=100), as assessed by Kaplan Meier analysis and log rank test (p=0.0203).

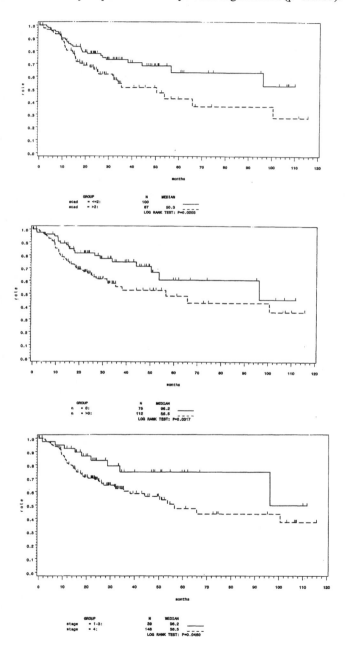

REFERENCES

1.   Takeichi M. Cadherins in cancer: Implications for invasion and metastasis. Curr Opin Cell Biol 1993;5:806-811.
2.   Gumbiner BM. Cell adhesion: the molecular basis of tissue architecture and morphogenesis. Cell 1996;84:345-357.
3.   Wheelock MJ, Knudsen KA, Johnson KR. Membrane-cytoskeleton interactions with cadherin cell adhesion proteins: Roles of catenins as linker proteins. Curr Top Membr 1996;43:169-185.
4.   Garrod DR. Desmosomes and hemidesmosomes. Curr Opin Cell Biol 1993;5:30-40.
5.   Alroy J, Pauli BU, Weinstein RS. Correlation between numbers of desmosomes and the aggressiveness of transitional cell carcinoma in human urinary bladder. Cancer 1981;47:104-112.
6.   Schipper JH, Frixen UH, Behrens J, Unger A, Jahuke K, Birchmeier W. E-cadherin expression in squamous cell carcinoma of the head and neck: inverse correlation with tumour differentiation and lymph node metastasis. Cancer Res 1990;51:6328-6337.
7.   Hiraki A, Shinohara M, Ikebe T, Nakamura S, Kurahara S, Garrod DR. Immunhistochemical staining of desmosomal components in oral squamous cell carcinomas and ist association with tumpour behaviour. Br J Cancer 1996;73:1491-1497.
8.   Mattijssen V, Peters HM, Schalkwijk L, Manni JJ, van't Hof-Grootenboer B, de Mulder PH, Ruiter DJ. E-cadherin expression in head and neck squamous –cell carcinoma is associated with clinical outcome. Int J Cancer 1993;55:580-585.
9.   Behrens J. Cell contacts, differentiation, and invasiveness of epithelial cells. Invasion Metastasis 1994;14:61-70.
10. Krunic ALJ, Garrod DR, Smith NP, Orchard GS, Svcijetic OB. Differential expression of desmosomal glycoproteins in keratoacanthoma and squamous cell carcinoma of the skin: an immunohistochemical aid to diagnosis. Acta Derm Venerol (Stockholm) 1996;76:394-398.
11. Shinohara M; Hiraki A, Ikebe T, Nakamura S, Kurahara S-I, Shirasuna K, Garrod DR. Immunohistochemical study of desmosomes in oral squamous cell carcinoma: Correlation with cytokeratin and E-cadherin staining, and with tumour behaviour. J Pathol 1998;184:369-381.
12. Garrod DR, Chidgey MAJ, North AJ. Desmosomes: differentiation, development and disease. Curr Opin Cell Biol 1996;8:670-678.
13. Schäfer S, Koch PJ, Franke WW. Identification of the ubiquitous human desmoglein, Dsg2, and the expression catalogue of the desmoglein subfamily of desmosomal cadherins. Exp Cell Res 1994;211:391-399.
14. Schmidt A, Heid HW, Schäfer S, Nuber UA, Zimbelmann R, Franke WW. Desmosomes and cytoskeletal architecture in epithelial differentiation: cell-type specific plaque components and intermediate filament anchorage. Eur J Cell Biol 1994;65:229-245.

ASSESSING GENETIC CHANGES IN PRIMARY AND METASTATIC TUMORS

Thomas E. Carey, Ph.D., Satoru Takebayashi, MD, Tetsuya Ogawa, MD, PhD, Yo Ueda, MD.
University of Michigan Department of Otolaryngology/Head and Neck Surgery, Head and Neck Cancer Research Laboratory, 1301 East Ann Street, Ann Arbor, MI 48019-0506

ABSTRACT

It has become clear that genetic changes play a major role in the development and progression of tumors. Furthermore, the biology of individual tumors is controlled by the alterations in protein expression that are secondary to these genetic changes. Thus, analysis of genetic changes is a valuable approach to understanding the biology of individual tumors and provides a means to identify new targets for therapy. Two of the principal concerns are those early factors associated with tumor genesis and those later genetic events that are associated with tumor progression. The former provide us with clues as to how tumors arise and are useful markers of clonality which have helped to clarify our understanding of how some tumors spread. In the case of head and neck cancer this is particularly important since so-called "second primary" cancers are the leading cause of death in patients with early stage tumors. The important question for us to understand is whether these second primary cancers are really new cancers, or clones that spread from the earlier lesion. Clonal genetic markers are useful for addressing this issue. For those genetic changes associated with progression we can learn how these changes affect tumor biology and why they provide a selective advantage to clones that acquire them. In this brief discussion we will use some examples to illustrate how analysis of genetic change in primary and secondary tumors can guide our understanding of tumor biology and tumor progression. The first example illustrates that apparent second primary tumors are, in at least some cases, actually derived from the same clone and therefore are primary and metastatic tumors. By the same token tumors that are obviously primary and metastatic tumors each contain independent events that arise in both clones once they become separate populations. Thus, clonal markers must be early events that are shared by all progeny of the original tumor population. Genetic events that arise late in tumor progression may be present in only the primary tumor, which continues to evolve after separation of metastatic clones, or only in the metastatic tumor cells as they progress. Either way, such late events may indicate the presence of genes whose function is altered with progression. To illustrate this we will outline our recent investigation of a common chromosome deletion and the discovery of a target gene. From this we present our analysis of how the alteration may be involved in changes tumor behavior.

INTRODUCTION

Head and neck squamous cell cancer is a difficult neoplastic disease to manage. Despite improvements in diagnostic tools, surgical techniques and improved radiotherapy and combinations with chemotherapy there has not yet been a significant improvement in survival in thirty years. Thus it is necessary to improve our understanding of the biology of this cancer type and to learn to develop better methods of treatment. Our laboratory has focused on identifying genetic changes that arise in the development and progression of head and neck cancer to use these changes to better understand tumor origin and dissemination. In this paper we will discuss clonal markers and the implications of these markers to better understand mechanisms of tumor spread. We will also outline the search for a putative tumor suppressor gene on chromosome 18q that appears to be an event associated with tumor progression.

Early events as clonal markers

Second primary tumors arise at an annual rate of 4-7% in patients with early stage head and neck cancers[1]. These secondary tumors, which can arise at some distance from the primary tumor and 1-5 years or more after the primary tumor has been treated, were originally postulated to be the result of field cancerization[2]. Field cancerization was described as areas of "condemned" mucosa at high risk for new carcinogenic events because of prolonged exposure to carcinogens. This concept has been further interpreted to mean that each second primary tumor represents the development of a new malignant clone arising de novo. Thus, a new tumor could arise anywhere in the upper aerodigestive tract. This perception is unfortunate since it suggests that nothing can be done to prevent the development of new tumors. New data supports a different perspective that suggests that many of the so-called second primary tumors are actually progeny of the original tumor clone. The significance of this observation is that if we understand the mechanisms of spread and the process that leads to progression at secondary sites then therapy can be designed to control this type of tumor progression.

Worsham et al.[3] described a patient with a primary tumor of the floor of mouth who on careful examination was also found to have a second tumor in the pyriform sinus. This was initially thought to be an example of a second primary tumor arising contemporaneously at a distant site. However, when specimens were obtained from both sites and examined for genetic changes a dicentric marker chromosome that arose from an unbalanced translocation of Yp to 14p with loss of the long arm of Y was discovered in the floor of mouth tumor. When tissue from the pyriform sinus tumor was examined by fluorescence in situ hybridization with probes for the long and short arms of the Y chromosome the same rearrangement was present. Furthermore when centromeric probes for chromosomes known to be present in multiple copies or in only two copies in the floor of mouth tumor, the same numerical changes were also present in the pyriform sinus tumor. Thus, it became very clear that the second tumor was genetically derived from the tumor in the floor of mouth. It is impossible to know with certainty the mechanism of spread that allowed the secondary focus to develop where it did. However, the location of the second tumor suggests that tumor cells floated away from the primary locus and lodged in the pyriform sinus and eventually invaded into the mucosa. In vitro experiments with cultured head and neck tumor cells[4] support this idea since tumor cells can grow easily on the surface of epithelial tissue plugs and can invade at locations of a thinned or excoriated epithelial layer. If the patient also had gastroesophageal reflux then the mucosa of the pyriform sinus may have been inflamed and predisposed to such a mechanism.

Other studies[5,6] also support the idea that the primary tumors give rise to secondary mucosal tumors that may develop several centimeters away from the primary tumor locus. In these cases, molecular markers have shown that the same clone of cells spread laterally within the mucosa away from the primary tumor. One particularly instructive example used immunohistochemistry to demonstrate clonal expansion of cells that over express cyclin D1 in an early oral cavity lesion[7]. In this case arborization from a single site of origin spread laterally over a wide area, illustrating one mechanism by which foci of cells might later begin to grow leading to a second nidus of tumor growth. Such a mechanism in a subset of head and neck cancers could explain the origin of some second primary tumors. Several studies have argued that second primary cancers are unique because different molecular markers were detected in the primary and secondary tumors. Unfortunately, although the presence of an identical marker is strong support for clonal origin, the presence of different markers does not support unique origin, only that clonal evolution may have occurred. In fact when known primary and metastatic tumors are compared numerous genetic differences can be identified. However, if careful comparisons are made several common clonal genetic changes are also readily identifiable in both the primary and metastatic tumors[8]. Thus, for determining clonal relationships it is necessary to identify the early genetic events.

Clonal evolution and progression
In the course of examining the chromosome changes in primary and metastatic tumors in the same patients we observed that loss of chromosome 18q often was present in only one of the tumors[9]. This indicated that the loss of 18q is not an early event in tumor development, but rather this event occurred with tumor progression. Consistent loss of a chromosome segment in specific tumor types has been linked to loss of function of tumor suppressor genes. Therefore, we hypothesized that loss of function of a gene on 18q may be associated with tumor progression in head and cancer. To test this hypothesis we examined 57 primary tumor cell lines with 42 microsatellite markers to determine the common minimal region of loss. Three regions of loss were identified. One was a discrete region centered on D18S70 in band 18q23 that was lost in 30/40 (75%) informative cases. In contrast, the nearest centromeric and telomeric markers were lost in only 53% and 63% respectively, indicating that the lost gene is likely to be close to D18S70[10]. Review of the genetic databases at the time of this analysis revealed that only three known genes and 5 expressed sequence tags (ESTs) were mapped to this region of 18q. Of the three known genes, one was a G-protein coupled receptor (GPCR). Such receptors and their ligand hormones are implicated in multiple signaling mechanisms and specific examples such as gastrin releasing peptide and neuromedin B that bind to the bombesin GPCR are known to affect tumor cell proliferation. Thus we focused on the galanin receptor 1 (GALNR1) gene as a possible target of loss and inactivation within 18q23.

Galanin receptor 1, Galanin and Galanin receptor 2.
The galanin receptors are typical of GPCRs, which are expressed as seven transmembrane spanning integral membrane proteins. In general when an agonist (hormones and

neuropeptides) binds to the receptor conformational changes expose binding sites for trimeric G-proteins that then initiate a signaling cascade that can alter gene expression. Galanin is a neuropeptide hormone of 30 amino acids. It is involved in numerous functions including regulation of appetite, blood pressure and sexual activity[11]. Galanin has also been implicated in growth stimulation in small cell lung cancer[12,13]. Furthermore, the galanin gene maps to 11q13 a region of frequent gene amplification in HNSCC, suggesting that it might be over expressed in tumors with this common genetic change. To understand how galanin and its receptors might be involved in progression of HNSCC we examined the expression and mutational status of GALNR1 and GALNR2 and the expression of galanin using western blotting, SSCP analysis, and RT-PCR in tumor cells with and without 18q LOH and in normal keratinocytes.

We first examined expression of GALNR1. Among tumor cell lines with 18q loss at *D18S70* expression of GALNR1 was weak or undetectable. In contrast, in normal keratinocytes and cell lines that retained both copies of 18q GALNR1 was expressed. Furthermore, two examples of mutations in the transmembrane domain known to affect signaling of other GPCRs were found in cell lines from two different patients, suggesting that the mutations may have affected the ability of the receptor to function. When reverse transcriptase (RT)-PCR was carried out to examine expression of galanin nearly all of the tumor lines and normal keratinocyte cultures were positive. Since it appeared that GALNR1 was either not expressed and/or mutated in tumors with 18q LOH we suspected that another galanin receptor might be expressed. GALNR2 had been implicated in small cell lung cancer as a factor involved in multiple signaling pathways[14]. Therefore we investigated the mutational status and expression of this protein in the same cells we had studied for GALNR1 and galanin expression. In contrast to the GALNR1 results, GALNR2 was strongly expressed in several of the cell lines with 18q LOH, but not in the cell lines that retained both copies of 18. Furthermore, we found a mutation of the GALNR2 gene that resulted in a stop codon and probable loss of at least one transmembrane domain. Surprisingly this tumor cell line strongly expressed the GALNR2 protein and experiments are now underway to discover if this is the truncated form that is expressed. When all of our findings are considered together it appears that loss of 18q is frequently associated with loss of expression of GALNR1. Similarly, it appears that galanin is commonly expressed by squamous carcinomas and immortalized keratinocytes. However, GALNR2 is apparently not expressed at high levels in normal cells or even tumor cells that retain 18q and express GALNR1. Thus we hypothesize that inactivation of both copies of GALNR1 disrupts the normal signaling pathway of galanin and GALNR1. Furthermore, when GALNR1 is not expressed, GALNR2 expression comes on and in the presence of constitutive galanin expression initiates an alternate signaling cascade that supports tumor progression. Clearly much more work is required to understand how these changes do in fact affect signaling and tumor behavior since we have only just discovered this explanation for how loss of 18q might be linked to tumor progression.

REFERENCES

1. Khuri, FR, Lippman, SM, Spitz, MR, Lotan, R, Hong, WK. Molecular epidemiology and retinoid chemoprevention of head and neck cancer. J Natl Cancer Inst 89:199-211, 1997.
2. Slaughter, DP, Southwick, HW, Smejkal, W. "Field cancerization" in oral stratified squamous epithelium: Clinical implications of multicentric origin. Cancer 6:963-968, 1953.

3. Worsham, MJ, Wolman, SR, Carey, TE, Zarbo, RJ, Benninger, MS, Van Dyke, DL: Common clonal origin of synchronous primary head and neck squamous cell carcinomas: Analysis by tumor karyotypes and fluorescence in situ hybridization. Human Path 26:251-261, 1995

4. Varani, J, Zeigler, ME, Perone, P, Carey, TE, Datta, SC. Human squamous carcinoma cell invasion in organ-cultured skin. Cancer Lett 111:51-7, 1997.

5. Bedi, GC, Westra, WH, Gabrielson, E, Koch, W, Sidransky, D. Multiple head and neck tumors: Evidence for common clonal origin. Cancer Res 56:2484-2487, 1996.

6. Califano, J., van der Riet, P., Westra, W., Nawroz, H., Clayman, G., Piantadosi, S., Corio, R., Lee, D., Greenberg, B., Koch, W. Sidransky, D. Genetic progression model for head and neck cancer: Implications for field cancerization. Cancer Research, 56, 2488-2492, 1996.

7. Izzo, JG, Papadimitrakopoulou, VA, Li, XQ, Ibarguen, H, Lee, JS, Ro, JY, El-Naggar, A, Hong, WK, Hittelman, WN. Dysregulated cyclin D1 expression early in head and neck tumorigenesis: in vivo evidence for an association with subsequent gene amplification. Oncogene 17:2313-2322, 1998.

8. Carey TE, Worsham MJ and Van Dyke DL. Chromosomal biomarkers in the clonal evolution of head and neck squamous neoplasia. J Cell Biochem Suppl 17F:213-222, 1993.

9. Frank CJ, McClatchey KD, Devaney KO, and Carey TE. Evidence that loss of chromosome 18q is associated with tumor progression. Cancer Res 57:824-827, 1997.

10. Takebayashi, S, Ogawa, T, Jung, K-Y, Muallem, A, Mineta, H, Fisher, S.G., Grenman, R, Carey, TE. Identification of New Minimally Lost Regions on 18q in Head and Neck Squamous Cell Carcinoma. Cancer Res 60:3397-3403, 2000.

11. Crawley, J. N. Biological actions of galanin. Reg. Peptides., *59:* 1-16, 1995.

12. Sethi, T., and Rosengurt, E. Galanin stimulated Ca^{2+} mobilization, inositol phosphate accumulation, and clonal growth in small cell lung cancer cells. Cancer Res., *51:* 1674-1679, 1991.

13. Sethi, T., and Rozengurt, E. Multiple neuropeptides stimulate clonal growth of small cell lung cancer: effects of bradykinin, vasopressin, cholecystokinin, galanin, and neurotensin. Cancer Res., *51:* 3621-3623, 1991.

14. Wittau, N, Grosse, R, Kalkbrenner, F, Gohla, A, Schultz, G, Gudermann. The galanin receptor type 2 intitiates multiple signaling pathways in small cell lung cancer cells by coupling to Gq, Gi, and G12 pathways. Oncogene 19:4199-4209, 2000.

MOLECULAR AND CELLULAR MECHANISMS
OF LYMPHOGENIC METASTATIC SPREAD:
UNDERLYING CHANGES IN GENE EXPRESSION PATTERNS

Jonathan P. Sleeman[1], Natasha Novac, Wolf-Gerolf Thies, Andrea Nestl[2], Oliver von Stein and Martin Hofmann[3]

[1]Forschungszentrum Karlsruhe, Institut für Toxikologie und Genetik, Postfach 3640, D-76021 Karlsruhe, Germany
[2]LYNX Therapeutics GmbH, Im Neuenheimer Feld 515, D-69120 Heidelberg, Germany
[3]Lion bioscience AG, Im Neuenheimer feld 515, D-69120 Heidelberg, Germany

Correspondence to: J. P. Sleeman, Forschungszentrum Karlsruhe, Institut für Toxikologie und Genetik, Postfach 3640, D-76021 Karlsruhe, Germany, Tel. (+49) 7247 826089, Fax. (+49) 7247 823354 (*e-mail: sleeman@igen.fzk.de*)

ABSTRACT

Metastasis is the lethal component of cancer. Tumor cells have to possess many cellular and molecular properties in order to successfully metastasize, and many of these properties are common for different types of metastatic cancers. The properties which a cell possesses are determined by the profile of genes it expresses. Thus, to fully define and understand the cellular and molecular events which lead to metastasis, and to gain an insight into how to intervene in metastatic disease, one needs to know which genes are responsible for providing tumor cells with metastatic properties. We have therefore undertaken a study to compare the gene expression profiles of genetically matched pairs of metastatic and non-metastatic cell lines from rat carcinoma models using the technique of Suppression Subtractive Hybridisation (SSH). Thereby we identified a panel of 268 genes, many of which have not been previously described. Analysis of these genes and their expression patterns in tumors has and will further illuminate cellular and molecular processes which lead to metastasis, in addition to providing possible avenues for therapeutic intervention.

For the vast majority of carcinomas, including squamous cell carcinoma, tumor metastasis follows the sequence of local invasion, entry into vessels of the circulatory system and subsequent depostion and growth at distant sites[1]. Another feature of virtually all carcinomas is their predilection to metastasize initially into regional lymph nodes[2]. These and other similarities suggest that common processes are operating during the metastatic dissemination of carcinomas. Characterization of these processes holds the promise of identifying ways in which of intervene in the course of metastatic disease.

It has long been recognized that the process of tumor metastasis is dependent on changes in the cellular and molecular properties of the tumor cell. For local invasiveness, at least three properties are required (reviewed in 2). Tumor cells need to change their adhesive properties, thereby loosing contact with other cells in the primary tumor and making new contacts with the extracellular matrix and host cells they encounter as they invade. They also need to be able to penetrate into the surrounding host tissue, and here the modulation of protease activity in the vicinity of the tumor cells plays a critical role. Tumor cells also need to be able to migrate away from the primary tumor and so may need to gain motility functions. These same three properties, changes in adhesive properties, modulation of protease activity and motility are also thought to be important when tumor cells extravasate, for example, out of the blood stream and into the surrounding tissue. Here, the tumor cells need to bind to the endothelium at the site where a metastasis will form, and invade through the endothelial layer and into the underlying host tissue. Other properties are also required. For example, metastatic deposits need to be able to survive and grow at sites distant to the primary tumor. Here, factors such as the ability to respond to local growth factors or to grow in an autocrine fashion, to overcome apoptosis-inducing signals and to induce angiogenesis are important. Although we know many details about the process of metastasis, we still do not have a complete picture. New concepts are continuing to emerge[3]. For example, recent work shows that local invasion in critically dependent on the induction of angiogenesis by tumors[4].

The properties of a cell are determined by the genes they express, and thus one would predict that the expression of many genes must change quantitatively or qualitatively to endow tumor cells with the properties required for the complex process of metastasis. It is therefore not surprising that during the study of metastasis, the differential expression of a plethora of genes has been associated with the metastatic phenotype. These include cell adhesion molecules such as E-cadherin, selectins, integrins and members of the immunoglobulin superfamily[5, 6], enzymes such as matrix metalloproteinases, serine proteases and members of the cathepsin family[7], and motility factors such as epitaxin and autocrine motility factor[8, 9]. However, what has remained unclear is exactly how many genes change in their expression pattern as tumor cells develop the capability to metastasize. Moreover, are any of these genes absolutely required for metastasis formation, or can the same property required for metastasis be provided by several different genes or groups of genes? To what extent are genes which do not play a role in the metastatic process upregulated during progression to the metastatic phenotype? To begin to find answers to these important questions, it would be necessary to describe and compare the repertoire of genes specifically expressed in metastasizing cells but not in their non-metastasizing counterparts.

Differential screening methods have been used to screen for genes up and down regulated during progression to metastatic competence, and each of these studies has identified one or several such genes[10-16]. However, none of these studies was able to analyse efficiently or exhaustively differences in the gene expression profiles of metastatic compared to non-metastatic cells. We set out to address this issue by using Suppression Subtractive Hybridisation in an attempt to describe more fully the global changes in gene expression which occur as tumors develop metastatic properties[17]. Specifically, we compared the gene expression profiles of related metastatic and non-metastatic tumor cells. As source material we used cells from rat pancreatic and mammary carcinoma models which metastasize agressively via the lymphatic system.

Our SSH screens suggest that the genetic background to tumor metastasis is rather complex (Figure 1). We isolated 268 independent differentially expressed genes, approximately half of which were already known genes (full information about these genes will be available on the following web site: http://igtmv1.fzk.de/www/itg/sleeman/sleeman.html). The expression of some of these known genes has already been associated with metastasis. The remaining genes we isolated were novel, previously unpublished sequences. Only 11 of the genes were isolated in both of the SSH screens, and thus the majority of genes were isolated in one of the screens but not the other. However, when we randomly checked expression of genes which were isolated in only one of the SSH screens, a high proportion of them were observed to be differentially expressed in a metastasis-related manner in both the mammary and pancreatic carcinoma models[17]. This suggests two things. Firstly, the pool of genes differentially expressed in both the mammary and the pancreatic carcinoma models is much bigger than the 11 genes which were isolated in both of the SSH screens. Secondly, the number of genes differentially expressed between the metastasizing and non-metastasizing cells we used must be considerably higher than the 268 independent sequences we obtained.

Our data show that many genes change in their expression patterns during metastatic progression. Genomic instability is the likely genetic driving force behind these changes. The genomes of tumors cells are unstable due to mutation or deletion of genes such as p53 which are crucially involved in the cell's response to DNA damage[2, 18, 19]. This has the consequence that cells with damaged DNA may survive and proliferate, with the danger that mutations persist and/or genes are amplified. The mutations and chromosomal aberrations so generated will be cell specific, leading to diversification within a developing tumor. During tumor dissemination, only those tumor cells that have acquired changes in gene expression which endow them with the properties required for metastasis will overcome the selection pressures they encounter and will go on to form progressively growing secondary tumors. However, many changes in gene expression resulting from genomic instability may have no functional relevance for metastasis, as the consequences of genomic instability will not only change the expression patterns of genes which are metastatically relevant, but also of genes which are neutral or even deleterious for metastasis. Hence not all genes differentially expressed in metastasizing cells are necessarily required for the metastatic process.

To identify those genes in our panel of strongest relevance to metastasis, we have used a variety of screening methods. For example, we have used Northern blots to identify genes whose expression is associated with metastasis in multiple tumor models. Such genes include CD24 and the ribosomal protein S7[17]. We have shown that CD24 and S7 are also upregulated in human metastatic tumors. Their functional relevance to metastasis is currently being tested by ectopic expression and gene inactivation studies. It is also of interest that many of the genes so far tested by Northern blot are only upregulated in one tumor model, suggesting these may be tumor type-specific, that they are not absolutely required for metastasis, or that their upregulation is coincident with but does not contribute to metastasis. As enhanced motility is often a feature of metastatic cells, we have also screened for genes in our panel which are also expressed in activated lymphocytes and macrophages. Thereby we identified the immediate early gene Pip92 and a novel as yet undescribed gene. Again, these genes are upregulated in certain human tumors, and we are currently determining if their expression is functionally important for metastasis. Continued study of our panel of metastasis-associated genes will provide further important insights into the genetic basis of tumor metastasis, and may identify targets for therapeutic intervention in metastatic disease.

Figure 1. Summary of genes identified by SSH which are differentially expressed in metastasizing cells compared to related non-metastasizing ones. In the mammary carcinoma SSH screen, MTPa cells (non-metastatic) were compared with MTLy (metastatic cells). In the pancreatic carcinoma SSH screen, 1AS cells (non-metastatic) were compared with ASML (metastatic cells). Together, a total of 268 differentially expressed genes were identified, of which 11 were found in both the mammary and pancreatic carcinoma SSH screens. See reference 17 for details.

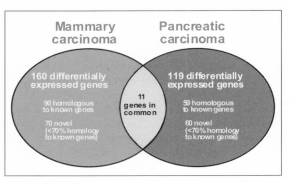

REFERENCES

1. Liotta L, Stetler-Stevenson W In: DeVita, Hellman, Rosenberg (eds) Cancer, Principles and Practice of Oncology, Fourth Edition. J. B. Lippincott Co., Philadelphia, 1993. p134-149
2. Sleeman JP. The lymph node as a bridgehead in the metastatic dissemination of tumors. Recent Results Cancer Res 2000; 157: 55-81
3. Sleeman JP, Thies WG, Nestl A, von Stein O, Hofmann M. Fact and Fiction: changing concepts in tumor metastasis. In The Sentinel Lymph Node Concept in Oncology - Facts and Fiction (Ed. Munz, D.). W. Zuckswerdt Verlag, Berlin, 2001. In press
4. Birchmeier W, Behrens J. Cadherin expression in carcinomas: role in the formation of cell junctions and the prevention of invasiveness. Biochim Biophys Acta 1994; 1198:11-26.
5. Duffy MJ. The role of proteolytic enzymes in cancer invasion and metastasis. Clin Exp Metastasis 1992; 10:145-155.
6. Honn KV, Tang DG. Adhesion molecules and tumor cell interaction with endothelium and subendothelial matrix. Cancer Metastasis Rev 1992; 11:353-375.
7. Liotta LA, Mandler R, Murano G, Katz DA, Gordon RK, Chiang PK, Schiffmann E. Tumor cell autocrine motility factor. Proc Natl Acad Sci U S A. 1986; 83:3302-3306.
8. Shimonaka M, Yamaguchi, Y. Purification and biological characterization of epitaxin, a fibroblast-derived motility factor for epithelial cells. J Biol Chem 1994; 269:14284-14289.
9. Skobe M, Rockwell P, Goldstein N, Vosseler S, Fusenig NE. Halting angiogenesis suppresses carcinoma cell invasion. Nat Med 1997; 3:1222-1227.
10. Pencil SD, Toh Y, Nicolson GL. Candidate metastasis-associated genes of the rat 13762NF mammary adenocarcinoma. Breast Cancer Res Treat 1993; 25: 165-174
11. Daigneault L, Beaulieu R, Filion M, Gaboury L, Royal A, Babai F. Cloning and identification of genes differentially expressed in metastatic and non-metastatic rat rhabdomyosarcoma cell lines. Clin Exp Metastasis 1995; 13: 345-356
12. Salesiotis AN, Wang CK, Wang CD, Burger A, Li H, Seth, A. Identification of novel genes from stomach cancer cell lines by differential display. Cancer Lett 1995; 91: 47-54
13. van Groningen JJ, Bloemers, HP, Swart GW. Identification of melanoma inhibitory activity and other differentially expressed messenger RNAs in human melanoma cell lines with different metastatic capacity by messenger RNA differential display. Cancer Res 1995; 55: 6237-6243
14. Ishiguro T, Nakajima M, Naito M, Muto T, Tsuruo T. Identification of genes differentially expressed in B16 murine melanoma sublines with different metastatic potentials. Cancer Res 1996; 56: 875-879
15. Hashimoto Y, Shindo-Okada N, Tani M, Takeuchi K, Toma H, Yokota J. Identification of genes differentially expressed in association with metastatic potential of K-1735 murine melanoma by messenger RNA differential display. Cancer Res 1996; 56: 5266-5271

16.   Clark EA, Golub TR, Lander ES, Hynes RO. Genomic analysis of metastasis reveals an essential role for RhoC. Nature 2000; 406: 532-535
17.   Nestl A, von Stein OD, Zatloukal K, Thies W-G, Herrlich P, Hofmann M, Sleeman JP. Gene expression patterns associated with the metastatic phenotype in rodent and human tumors. Cancer Res 2001; in press
18.   Kinzler KW, Vogelstein B. Lessons from hereditary colorectal cancer. Cell 1996; 87: 159-170
19.   Cahill DP, Kinzler KW, Vogelstein B, Lengauer C. Genetic instability and darwinian selection in tumours. Trends Cell Biol 1999; 9: M57-M60

MECHANISMS OF METASTASIS
WITH SPECIAL REFERENCE TO SQUAMOUS CELL CARCINOMA

Suzanne A. Eccles[1] Ph.D and Pornchai O-charoenrat[2] M.D.
[1]CRC Centre for Cancer Therapeutics, Institute of Cancer Research, McElwain Laboratories, Cotswold Rd., Belmont, Sutton, Surrey SM2 5NG UK
[2]Head and Neck Unit, Royal Marsden Hospital, London SW3 6JJ UK

Running title: Mechanisms of metastasis

Key words: metastasis, angiogenesis, c-erbB oncogenes, VEGF, metalloproteinases

Correspondence to: Dr S. A. Eccles, CRC Centre for Cancer Therapeutics, Institute of Cancer Research, McElwain Laboratories, Cotswold Rd., Belmont, Sutton, Surrey SM2 5NG, UK, Tel: +44 (0)20 8722 4210; Fax: +44 (0)20 8643 0223; (*email suzan@icr.ac.uk*)

ABSTRACT

While the management of HNSCC has improved, there is no evidence to suggest that therapeutic advances have resulted in better survival rates[1], indeed there has been an increase in presentation of distant metastases. Clearly, a more sophisticated understanding of the pathogenesis of these tumours could provide information for predicting outcome and for developing novel therapies. Our work focusses on the c-erbB family of oncogenes which are frequently upregulated in HNSCC, with the aim of determining the molecular mechanisms underlying their association with poor prognosis. Metastasis is known to require changes in cell-cell and cell-matrix adhesion, neoangiogenesis, imbalances in proteolytic enzymes and the ability of tumour cells to survive and proliferate in "ectopic" sites. This minireview shows how tumour cells with activated EGFR and c-erbB receptors specifically upregulate key angiogenic growth factors and matrix metalloproteinases, leading to enhanced invasion and the opportunity for lymphatic and haematogenous spread.

THE C-ERBB RECEPTOR FAMILY AND LIGANDS

C-erbB receptors of the transmembrane type I receptor tyrosine kinase family, have four members: the epidermal growth factor receptor (EGFR/c-erbB-1/HER-1) c-erbB-2/neu/ HER-2), c-erbB-3/HER-3 and c-erbB-4/HER-4. EGFR over-expression in several studies has been associated with poor prognosis in squamous cell carcinoma of the oral mucosa (e.g. Kusukawa et al)[2]. The c-erbB-2 receptor is a 185 kDa receptor-like phosphoglycoprotein with constitutive tyrosine kinase activity in the absence of ligand. So far, no ligands have been identified which bind directly to the c-erbB-2 receptor. Experimental studies suggest that c-erbB-2 serves as a fundamental signalling component that that co-operates with other c-erbB receptor family members in the formation of heterodimers. The c-erbB-3 protein distribution is distinctly different from that of EGFR and c-erbB-2. C-erbB-3 does not have an intrinsic tyrosine kinase activity but it can be transphosphorylated by both the EGFR and c-erbB-2[3-5] C-erbB-4 protein and mRNA have been shown to distribute widely in both adult and foetal tissues[6]. Xia et al[7] have recently indicated that expression of all four receptors is associated with shortened survival in patients with oral SCC, with the combination of EGFR, c-erbB-2 and c-erbB-3 (but not c-erbB-4) giving the greatest prognostic information.

The c-erbB ligand family consists of more than 30 members. We have utilised three ligands with distinct receptor binding profiles: transforming growth factor (TGF) α, betacellulin (BTC) and heregulin (HRG) β1, to study the effects of activation of different signalling pathways. Ligand binding induces receptor homo- or heterodimerization and subsequent auto- or cross-phosphorylation. This initiates a complex series of molecular events causing a spectrum of biological activities via simultaneous stimulation of multiple signal transduction pathways.

TGFα binds specifically to the EGFR receptor with an affinity similar to EGF. HNSCC has been reported to express TGF-α mRNA and protein, and TGF-α activity has been detected in the urine of patients with disseminated HNSCC. The overexpression of TGF-α in HNSCC is frequently accompanied by elevated levels of EGFR[8], suggesting the possibility of autocrine stimulation. Issing et al[9] observed that patients with HNSCC overexpressing EGFR and TGFα had a significantly shorter survival than patients overexpressing EGFR only, whereas Grandis et al[10] reported that both TGF-α and EGFR protein levels in primary HNSCC were each independently associated with adverse outcomes. BTC has the ability to efficiently activate all four members of the c-erbB receptor family. The third class of ligands (HRGs) do not bind to EGFR, but bind directly to c-erbB-3 and c-erbB-4 and activate c-erbB-2 through formation of complexes with c-erbB-3 or c-erbB-4[11]. HRG-β1 has been shown to be the most potent in terms of receptor tyrosine phosphorylation and activation of downstream signal elements such as mitogen-activated protein kinase (MAPK)[12]

Activation of the c-erbB receptors is recognized as being important in the progression of many human cancers including HNSCC[13-16] and recent studies have shown that this is due not simply to mitogenic stimulation, but also to their involvement in many aspects of malignancy including invasion and angiogenesis.

Molecular Biology of Invasion and Metastasis in HNSCC

HNSCC are characterised by local invasiveness and a propensity for dissemination to cervical lymph nodes. Cancer cell invasion and metastasis is a complex, multistep process involving active interactions between the invading cell, the extracellular matrix (ECM) and other stromal elements[17] (Figure 1). Normal epithelial cells exist in close association with a basement membranes, with which they dynamically interact via integrins and other cell-matrix connections. Detachment of normal cells from this substratum results in death by anoikis; tumour cells are frequently resistant to this form of programmed cell death due to loss of p53 and other cell cycle control elements. In addition, epithelial cells are firmly attached to one another via a multiplicity of adhesion molecules including cadherins and desmosomal proteins which also maintain the architecture and integrity of the epithelia.

The first step in the formation of a malignant focus is loss of the normal growth control processes, which leads to hyperplasia. Cells then frequently show loss or aberrant localisation of E-cadherin and desmosomal proteins, changes in integrin expression, acquisition of a motile phenotype and enhanced proteolytic activity leading to invasion. This can be due to upregulation of various proteases (either by the cancer cells themselves or neighbouring host cells) and/or by downregulation of natural inhibitors such as TIMPs. Proteolysis of the extracellular matrix (ECM) is also involved in the neoangiogenesis necessary for the continued growth of solid tumours[18]. Invasion can be considered, at its simplest, to be motility coupled to localised proteolysis. We and others have shown that activation of c-erbB receptors can induce many of the phenotypic traits associated with invasion, including loss of E-cadherin, acquisition of a fibroblastoid, motile phenotype and upregulation of a variety of proteases.

Matrix Metalloproteinases (MMPs) in HNSCC
Accumulating evidence indicates that MMPs may play a causal role in tumour progression[17]. The MMPs are a family of zinc- and calcium-dependent endopeptidases that can collectively degrade virtually all protein components of the ECM. Most MMPs can be divided into four subclasses. The first group (collagenases) which degrade types I, II, and III fibrillar collagens comprises MMP-1, MMP-8 and MMP-13. Stromelysins include MMP-7, MMP-3 MMP-10 and MMP-11. Gelatinases MMP-2 and MMP-9 are able to cleave both the denatured forms of collagen and type IV collagen, a key component of endothelial basal laminae. The final group of MMPs are the membrane-type matrix metalloproteinases (MT-MMPs 1-5) which have the unique property of binding to the cell membrane, where at least some members co-operate in the activation of other MMPs such as MMP-2. The net activity of MMPs is determined by the amount of proenzyme expressed, the extent to which it is activated and the local concentration of specific inhibitors, i.e. the tissue inhibitors of metalloproteinases (TIMPs). The local balance of these enzymes and inhibitors appears to be a crucial factor in tumour invasion and metastasis.

The first study of MMPs in HNSCC in vivo was reported by Polette et al[19]. Using in situ hybridisation, they showed that tumour cells and adjacent stromal cells (fibroblasts, macrophages) frequently expressed MMP-1 and MMP-10 along disrupted basement membrane. MMP-11 expression was detected in stromal cells immediately surrounding invasive cancer cells[20] and MMP-7 was observed both in normal and malignant tissues. MMP-3 was detected primarily in the advancing front of cancers and was found to correlate with invasion and metastasis in oral SCCs[2]. MMP-2 and MMP-9 have been shown to be highly expressed and strongly correlated with the malignant phenotype and lymph node metastasis in HNSCC[21]. Several studies have shown that the MMP-2 may be derived not from the tumour cell, but from the surrounding stroma; in contrast, MMP-9 is expressed by malignant keratinocytes and localized at the tumour/stroma interface[22]. Recently, MMP-13 was detected in the majority of HNSCC tissues but not in normal skin or oral mucosa[23]. MT1-MMP is produced by stromal cells and, like MMP-2, taken up by adjacent epithelial cells. Expression of other MT-MMPs in HNSCC has not yet been reported. The finding that expression of some MMPs is higher in stromal cells suggests that tumour cells are capable of inducing and utilizing host tissue MMPs and support an active role of the stroma in HNSCC invasion.

We and others have found that activation of c-erbB oncogenes by all major ligands selectively induces MMP expression in vitro. The highest upregulation we found was that of MMP-9 induced by betacellulin, and we speculate that the potency of this ligand is due to its ability to activate all four c-erbB receptors and hence multiple downstream signaling pathways. Heregulin β1 also induced MMP-9 expression, but much higher concentrations were needed (10-100nM versus 1-10 nM)[24]. Anti-EGFR monoclonal antibodies reversed the effects of the ligands, indicating that this receptor was a key component of the response. EGFR activation also (to a lesser extent) upregulated MMP-3 and MMP-7. Their induction was an early event, suggesting that they may initiate a proteolytic cascade, since both are capable of activating other MMPs including MMP-9. The levels of expression of EGFR on a panel of cell lines correlated with their MMP-9 enzyme activity and invasive potential. Invasion was inhibited completely by anti-EGFR antibodies, and partially by anti-MMP-9 antibodies, suggesting that other proteases also contribute[25]. In addition, we have recently shown significant correlations between EGFR, c-erbB-2 and c-erbB3 levels in clinical samples of HNSCC with infiltrating mode of invasion and nodal metastases. Cancers with high EGFR or c-erbB-2 also expressed high levels of multiple MMPs with the strongest statistical correlation being found with MMP-9 (O-charoenrat- this Conference)

We also checked the effects of a broad spectrum hydroxamate MMP inhibitor on HNSCC invasion and found that, in addition to inhibiting invasion as expected, there was an anti-proliferative effect in some cell lines. These inhibitors are generally considered to be non-toxic, and we had not observed these cytostatic effects in breast carcinoma cell lines. The effects were reversible, and we found that they could be prevented by the addition of exogenous ligand such as EGF or TGFα, but much less efficiently by HRG (unpublished observations). It is well known that all EGFR ligands are synthesised as transmembrane precursors which are subjected to proteolytic cleavage of the ectodomain to yield a soluble growth factor which is then available to activate the receptor. The enzymes responsible have not been fully identified, although metalloproteinases including ADAMs[26] and MMPs have been implicated; for example, MMP-3 has been shown to release active HB-EGF[27]. We found that addition of MMP inhibitors to HNSCC in vitro inhibited the release of autocrine TGFα into the supernantant (unpublished observations). Thus MMPs induced by EGFR activation (and to a lesser extent c-erbB-3 and c-erbB-4) may promote cell invasion through ECM and basement membranes, and may also contribute to a positive feedback loop via release of active ligands. It has been shown in some experimental systems that intravasation is not a rate-limiting step, and also lymphatic vessels may prevent less of a physical barrier than capillaries since they have a discontinuous basement membrane. Therefore, the classical role defined for MMPs as molecular "wire-cutters" assisting tumour cell escape and dissemination through lysis of structural proteins may be only one aspect of their role(s) in invasion[28] and angiogenesis (discussed below).

102

Neoangiogenesis in HNSCC

Neoangiogenesis is of particular significance in the processes of tumour growth, invasion and metastasis because it is not only supplies the nutritional requirements of the developing neoplasm, but also increases the opportunity for tumour cells to enter the circulation and disseminate. Tumour angiogenesis is an active process involving multiple distinct steps. Initially, the basal lamina surrounding the ECM and endothelial cell layer is broken down by proteolytic enzymes such as MMPs and plasminogen activators secreted from tumour or host cells. The ability of HNSCC to induce an angiogenic response has been demonstrated in in vitro and in xenograft models[29]. In addition, histological examination of human HNSCC specimens has confirmed that increased microvascularity is a common feature of HNSCC. However, the results of studies associating microvessel density and various clinicopathological parameters and/or outcome are inconclusive[30].

The major inducers of neoangiogenesis are the vascular endothelial growth factors (VEGFs) although fibroblast growth factors, angiopoetin 1, interleukins and other growth factors also contribute. VEGFs are highly potent angiogenic agents acting to increase blood vessel permeability, endothelial cell growth, proliferation, migration, and differentiation. The VEGF-A gene gives rise to four isoforms as a result of alternative splicing. These differ in their molecular masses (121, 165, 189 and 206 amino acids) and possess different biological activities. VEGF-B is transcribed as a mature protein with 167 (VEGF-B$_{167}$) and 186 (VEGF-B$_{186}$) amino acid residues. VEGF-C is suggested to be a selective lymphangiogenic factor, which induces proliferation of lymphatic endothelial cells and lymphatic vessels[31]. VEGF-C and VEGF-D can bind to and induce tyrosine autophosphorylation of the same receptors namely VEGFR-2 (KDR/ Flk1) and VEGFR-3 (Flt-4). VEGFR-1 (Flt-1) and VEGFR-2 are receptor tyrosine kinases for VEGF-A whereas VEGF-B binds only to VEGFR-1. VEGFR-1 and VEGFR-2 are expressed on vascular endothelium whereas VEGFR-3 is exclusively confined to the lymphatic endothelium in normal adult tissues. However, interestingly, VEGFR-3 can also be found in tumour endothelia[32], possibly due to the re-expression of a more undifferentiated phenotype.

Increased expression of VEGF-A has been demonstrated in both HNSCC cell lines [29] and clinical specimens[33]. However, the clinical relevance of VEGF-A expression is not clear, and it may be that receptor levels are also important. Few studies have examined VEGF B, C and D in HNSCC, although Saaristo et al[34] reported that VEGF-C was evident in nasopharyngeal tumour cell islands with VEGFR-3 on adjacent angiogenic vessels. Our own studies[35] have shown that enhanced expression of VEGF-A (isoforms 121 and 165) and VEGF-C in HNSCC had predictive value for the presence of cervical nodal metastases.

Of the many known inducers of VEGF-A, besides hypoxia, two of the most potent are EGF and TGF-α[36]. This may be due to signals involving the AP-1 and AP-2 transcription binding sites which are found in the promoters of the VEGF-A and VEGF-C genes (and also many MMP genes). Treatment of A431 cell line with the blocking mAb against EGFR (C225) has been shown to down-regulate VEGF-A expression both in vitro and in vivo[37]. We have found that stimulation of HNSCC in vitro with EGFR and c-erbB ligands leads to significant upregulation of all isoforms of VEGF-A and VEGF-C with the same relative potency as induction of MMPs (BTC> EGF> HRG). VEGF-B was unaffected, and VEGF-D was simultaneously down-regulated. These effects were reversed by anti-EGFR and anti-c-erbB-2 monoclonal antibodies[38]. These data suggest that signalling through these receptors may be critically important in stimulating angiogenesis of capillary and lymphatic vessels in HNSCC (perhaps preferentially the tumour vessels which express both VEGFR-2 and VEGFR-3) and may also increase vessel permeability and tumour cell escape.

Most angiogenic factors (including VEGFs and bFGFs), like the EGFR ligands require proteolytic processing to develop their full activity. This may include release from sequestration in ECM and/or stepwise cleavage to produce forms with enhanced binding capacity to receptors. For instance, only fully-processed VEGF-C can bind to VEGFR-3 and VEGFR-2; this is accomplished by as yet unidentified cellular protease(s)[39]. Another example is the release of active HB-EGF and TGF-β (which are angiogenic) by MMP-3, and more importantly MMP-9 has recently been implicated as the key mediator of the "angiogenic switch" in transgenic tumour models. It seems that MMP-9 is able to mobilise VEGF from extracellular reservoirs in lesions undergoing malignant transformation, inducing ingrowth of new vessels and sustained tumour growth[40].

Positive feedback mechanisms in c-erbB signalling, angiogenesis and invasion.

Taken together, the evidence suggests that co-operative signalling via c-erbB receptors can regulate many key processes of angiogenesis and invasion in HNSCC, and this is illustrated in Figure 2. Ligands binding to EGFR and c-erbB-3 and c-erbB-4 affect cell-cell adhesion via downregulation of E-cadherin and desmosomal proteins, and alter the tumour cell's relationship with the matrix microenvironment via changes in integrin expression (eg MMP-7 disrupts adhesion mediated by β-4 integrins). Cell motility is enhanced, and again MMPs upregulated by c-erbB signalling can release tumour cell and endothelial cell growth factors and chemotactic fragments from matrix components, and potentiate invasion by proteolysis of matrix and basement membrane components. C-erbB activation also upregulates VEGF-A and VEGF-C expression, further stimulating proliferation of vascular and lymphatic endothelial cells, and increasing vessel permeability. The enhanced angiogenic activity sustains growth of the primary tumour, potentiates dissemination and also supports the establishment of micrometastases. Although most of these relationships have been established in vitro, correlations observed in clinical material suggest that they may also be operative in patients. These key contributors to invasion, angiogenesis and metastasis would therefore provide ideal targets for therapeutic intervention, and by aiming at the "master switches" of the c-erbB oncogene proteins (which are accessible at the cell membrane) it may be possible to simultaneously inhibit many different aspects of the malignant phenotype.

Figure 1: Changes in epithelial organisation during carcinoma invasion.
Epithelial cells become less adherent, transiently acquire a motile, mesenchymal morphology, invade through stroma and basement membranes and gain access to blood and lymphatic vessels

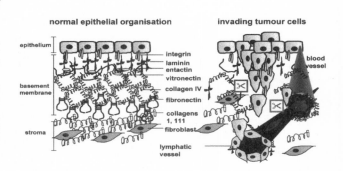

Figure 2: Some putative positive feedback loops in invasion and angiogenesis induced by c-erbB receptor activation

1. Autocrine or paracrine ligands activate receptors by either direct binding or transphosphorylation
2. EGFR (and c-erbB-2) activation leads to enhanced production of VEGF-A isoforms and VEGF-C
3. Capillary and lymphatic endothelial cells respond to VEGFs (< cell proliferation, migration, permeability)
4. Tumour growth and dissemination are potentiated by neoangiogenesis
5. EGFR activation also leads to upregulation of specific MMPs (predominantly MMP-9; also MMP-3 and MMP-7)
6. MMPs activate proteolytic cascade and potentiate tumour cell invasion and angiogenesis
7. MMPs release sequestered growth factors and process ligands

The cycle continues

REFERENCES

1.   Mork J. Forty years of monitoring head and neck cancer in Norway- no good news. Anticancer Res 1998; 18:3705-8.
2.   Kusukawa J, Harada H, Shima I, Sasaguri Y, Kameyama T, Morimatsu M. The significance of epidermal growth factor receptor and matrix metalloproteinase 3 in squamous cell carcinoma of the oral cavity. Oral. Oncol. 1996; 32B:217-221
3.   Graus-Porta D, Beerly R, Daly JM, Hynes NE. ErbB2, the preferred heterodimerization partner of all ErbB receptors is a mediator of lateral signalling. EMBO J. 1997; 16:1647-55
4.   Riese DJ and Stern DF. Specificity within the EGF family/erbB receptor family network. Bioessays 1998; 20:41-48
5.   Slikowski MX, Schaefer G, Akita RW et al . Coexpression of erbB2 and erbB3 proteins reconstitutes a high affinity receptor for heregulin. J. Biol. Chem. 1994 269: 14661-5
6.   Srinivasan R, Poulsom R, Hurst HC and Gullick WJ. Expression of the c-erbB4/HER4 protein in normal human fetal and adult tissues and in a survey of nine solid tumor types. J. Pathol. 1998; 185:236-45
7.   Xia W, Lau Y-K, Zhang H-Z, et al. Combination of EGFR, HER-2/neu and HER-3 is a stronger predictor for the outcome of oral squamous cell carcinoma than any individual family members. Clin Cancer Res. 1999; 5:4164-74
8.   Ibrahim, S. O., Vasstrand, E. N., Liavaag, P. G., Johannessen, A.C and Lillehaug, J R. Expression of c-erbB proto-oncogene family members in squamous cell carcinoma of the head and neck. Anticancer Res. 1997; 17:4539-46,.
9.   Issing, WJ, Liebich C Wustrow, TP and Ullrich A. Coexpression of epidermal growth factor receptor and TGF-alpha and survival in upper aerodigestive tract cancer. Anticancer Res. 1996, 16:283-8,.
10.   Grandis JR, Melhem MF, Gooding WE, Day R, Holst VA, Wagener MM, Drenning SD, Tweardy DJ. Levels of TGFα and EGFR protein in head and neck squamous cell carcinoma and patient survival. J. Natl. Cancer Inst. 1998; 90:824-832
11.   Karunagaran D, Tzahar E, Beerli RR et al. ErbB2 is a common auxiliary subunit of NDF and EGF receptors: implications for breast cancer. EMBO J. 1996; 15:254-64
12.   Weiss FU, Wallasch C, Campiglio M, Issing W, Ullrich A. Distinct characteristics of heregulin signals mediated by HER3 or HER4. J. Cell Physiol. 1997; 173:187-95
13.   Gullick WJ. Type 1 growth factor receptors: current status and future work. Biochem. Soc. Symp. 1998; 63:193-8

14. Eccles SA Cell biology of lymphatic metastasis: the potential role of c-erbB signalling. Recent Results Cancer Res 2000; 157: 41-54.

15. Eccles SA c-erbB-2 as a target for immunotherapy. Exp. Opin. Invest. Drugs 1998; 7: 1879-96

16. Klapper LN, Kirschbaum MH, Sela M, Yarden Y. Biochemical and clinical implications of the ErbB/HER signalling network of growth factor receptors. Adv Cancer Res 2000; 77:25-79.

17. Mignatti P, Rifkin DB. Nonenzymatic interactions between proteinases and the cell surface: novel roles in normal and malignant cell physiology. Adv Cancer Res 2000:103-157.

18. Hahnfeldt P, Panigrahy D, Folkman J, Hlatky L. Tumor development under angiogenic signaling: a dynamical theory of tumor growth, treatment response and postvascular dormancy. Cancer Res. 1999; 59:4770-5

19. Polette M, Clavel C, Muller D, Abecassis J, Binninger I, Birembaut P. Detection of mRNAs encoding collagenase 1 and stromelysin 2 in carcinomas of the head and neck by in situ hybridisation. Invasion Metastasis 1991; 11:76-83

20. Muller D, Wolf C, Abecassis J et al. Increased stromelysin 3 gene expression is associated with increased local invasiveness in head and neck squamous cell carcinomas. Cancer Res. 1993; 53:165-9

21. Kawamata H, Nakashiro K, Uchida D, Harada K, Yoshida H, Sato M. Possible contribution of active MMP-2 to lymph node metastasis and secreted cathepsin L to bone invasion of newly established human oral-squamous-cancer cell lines. Int. J. Cancer 1997; 70:120-7

22. Pyke C, Ralfkiaer E, Huhtala P, Hurskainen T, Dano K and Tryggvason K. Localization of messenger RNA for Mr 72,000 and 92,000 type IV collagenases in human skin cancer by in situ hybridization. Cancer Res.1992; 52:1336-1341

23. Johansson N, Airola K, Grenman R et al. VM. Expression of collagenase-3 (matrix metalloproteinase-13) in squamous cell carcinomas of the head and neck. Am J Pathol 1997;151:499-508.

24. O-charoenrat P, Modjtahedi H, Rhys-Evans P, Court W, Box G and Eccles S. Epidermal Growth factor-like ligands differentially upregulate matrix metalloproteinase-9 in head and neck squamous carcinoma cells. Cancer Res. 2000; 60: 1121-1128

25. O-charoenrat P, Rhys-Evans P, Modjtahedi H, Court W, Box G, Eccles S.A. Over-expression of epidermal growth factor receptor in human head and neck squamous carcinoma cell lines correlates with matrix metalloproteinase-9 expression and in vitro invasion. Int. J. Cancer 2000; 86:307-317

26. Dong J, Opresko LK, Dempsey PJ, Lauffenberger DA, Coffey RJ, Wiley HS. Metalloprotease-mediated ligand release regulates autocrine signaling through the epidermal growth factor receptor Proc. Natl. Acad. Sci USA 1999; 96: 6235-40.

27. Suzuki M, Raab G, Moses MA, Fernandez CA, Klagsbrun M. Matrix metalloproteinase-3 releases active heparin-binding EGF-like growth factor by cleavage at a specific juxtamembrane site. J. Biol. Chem 1997; 272:31730-37.

28. McCawley LJ and Matrisian LM. Matrix metalloproteinases: multifunctional contributors to tumor progression. Molec. Med. Today 2000; 6:149-156

29. Petruzzelli GJ, Benefield J, Taitz AD, Fowler S, Kalkanis J, Scobercea S, et al. Heparin-binding growth factor(s) derived from head and neck squamous cell carcinomas induce endothelial cell proliferation. Head Neck 1997; 19: 576-82.

30. omer JJ, Greenman J, Stafford ND. Angiogenesis in head and neck squamous cell carcinoma. Clin. Otolaryngol. 2000; 25: 169-80

31. Joukov V, Pajusola K, Kaipainen A, Chilov D, Lahtinen I, Kukk E, et al. A novel vascular endothelial growth factor, VEGF-C, is a ligand for the Flt4 (VEGFR-3) and KDR (VEGFR-2) receptor tyrosine kinases. EMBO J 1996; 15: 290-8.

32. Partanen TA, Alitalo K, Miettinen M. Lack of lymphatic vascular specificity of endothelial growth factor receptor 3 in 185 vascular tumors. Cancer 1999; 86:2406-12

33. Smith BD, Smith GL, Carter D, Sasaki CT, Haffty BG. Prognostic significance of vascular endothelial growth factor protein levels in oral and oropharyngeal squamous cell carcinoma. J Clin Oncology 2000; 18: 2046-52.

34. Saaristo A, Partanen TA, Arola J et al. Vascular endothelial growth factor-C and its receptor VEGFR-3 in the nasal mucosa and in nasopharyngeal tumors. Am J Pathol. 2000; 157:7-14

35. O-charoenrat, P Rhys-Evans P, Eccles, SA . Expression of vascular endothelial growth factor family members in head and neck squamous cell carcinoma correlates with lymph node metastasis Cancer In press 2001

36. Gille J, Swerlick RA, Caughman SW. Transforming growth factor-alpha-induced transcriptional activation of the vascular permeability factor (VPF/VEGF) gene requires AP-2-dependent DNA binding and transactivation. EMBO J 1997; 16: 750-9.

106

37. Petit AMV, Rak J, Hung WC, et al. Neutralizing antibodies against epidermal growth factor and ErbB-2/neu receptor tyrosine kinases down-regulate vascular endothelial growth factor production by tumor cells in vitro and in vivo : angiogenic implications for signal transduction therapy of solid tumors. Am.J. Pathol. 1997;151:1523-1530.

38. O-charoenrat P, Rhys-Evans P, Modjtahedi H, and Eccles SA. Vascular endothelial growth factor family members are differentially regulated by c-erbB signaling in head and neck squamous carcinoma cells. Clin. Exp.Metastasis 2000; 18:155-161

39. Joukov V, Sorsa T. Kumar V et al. Proteolytic processing regulates receptor specificity and activity of VEGF-C. EMBO J. 1997; 16:3898-911.

40. Bergers G, Brekken R, McMahon G et al. Matrix metalloproteinase-9 triggers the angiogenic switch during carcinogenesis. Nature Cell Biol 2000; 2: 737-44

PLK (POLO-LIKE-KINASE), A NEW PROGNOSTIC MARKER FOR PPHARYNGEAL CARCINOMAS

Rainal Knecht[1], Christine Oberhauser[1], Klaus Strebhardt[2]
[1]Departmment of Otorhinolarynngology
[2]Departmment of Obstetrics and Gynecology, School of Medicine, J.W. Goethe-Universitiy, Theodor-Stern-Kai 7, 60590 Frankfurt, Germany

Running title: Prognostic value of PLK in oropharyngeal carcinomas

Correspondence to: *PD Dr. R. Knecht, Department of Otolaryngology, School of Medicine, J.W. Goethe-University, Theodor-Stern-Kai 7, 60590 Frankfurt, Germany, Tel.: +49-69-6301-4471, Fax.: +49-69-6301-7710 (e-mail.: Knecht@uni-frankfurt.de)*

The worldwide annual incidence of squamous cell carcinomas of the head and neck (HNSCC) is about 500.000. The prognosis of these patients is mainly based on the clinicophatological tumor stage in particular the lymph node status pN, even though it is generally accepted that despite the sam stage patient´s outcome can be different. Therefore, this study focuses on the identification of molecular parameters for the improvement of the daily clinical diagnosis which contribute to further prognostic differentiation.

Polo-like-kinase (PLKs) are implicated in the regulation of the eukaryotic cell cycle[1]. The expression of PLK-mRNA, a novel marker for cellular proliferation correlates with the prognosis of patients suffering from different types of tumors[2-4]. Here, we have examined for the first time the prognostic role of PLK-protein expression in human cancer. Primary tumors from 157 patients with HNSCC, which were collected over a period of one year, were evaluated for their PLK-immunoreactivity. Therapy and posttherapeutical investigations (5 years) of the patients (115 male, 42 female) suffering from oropharyngeal carcinomas (stage I=14, stage II=30, stage III=34, stage IV=79) were performed as follows: Patients in tumor stages I and II underwent surgery whereas patients in stage III and IV were subjected to surgery and postoperative radiotherapy (2 Gy fractions given as once-a-day treatment to a total dose of 700 Gy applied to the primary region and the neck). Chemotherapy was given non concomitantly, applying thhree cycles of cisplatin (20 mg/qm/day) and 5-flourourascil (1000 mg/qm/day) acc ording to a standard schedule[5]. Tumor recurrences were treated chemotherapeutically with the same regimen until no response or progressive disease was measured in two dimensions by computed tomography scan. The length of follow-up was between 5 and 132 months.

Paraffin-embedded tumor sections were immunolabeled with an affinity purified PLK-specific, polyclonal rabbit serum. The primary antibody, which was used in a dilution of 1:80, was visualized with the APAAP technique, sections were counterstained with hematoxylin. For comparative purposes sections were labeled with antibodies for Ki67 (Dako, Hamburg, 1:50) and PCNA (Dako, Hamburg, 1:1000) using the same technique. Three independent investigators calculated the number of tumor cells (stained nuclei) positive for PLK, Ki67 or PCNA respectively per 5000 counted tumor cells. Thereby a minimum of 15 fields (400x) per tumor was investigated. Prognostic evaluations were based on the observer´s mean PLK-index (positive cells/5000 cells x 100).

Levels of PLK-protein in microscopically normal oropharyngeal mucosa (median=12.0%, minimum=0,1%, maximum=41.0%) surrounding the tumor of the same patient were low. In 10% of the investigated cases we observed in the surrounding tissue (in a distance of 3-5 cm to the tumor) dysplasia (grade I/II). Under these conditions levels of PLK-protein expression were slightly clevated. Compared to the periphery PLK-protein was overexpressed (median=59,4%, minium=22,3%, maximum=74,8%) in oropharyngeal carcinomas (Wilcoxon test: p=0.016). A correlation of PLK-expression with clinicopathological parameters revealed a siignificant correlation with the pathological tumor stage (p=0.007) and the pN stage (p=0.012) but not with the N stage (p=0.09,Kruskal-Wallis-Test) A Kaplan-Meier-analysis based on a median cut-off showed that patients exhibiting moderate PLK-expression (<59,4%) had longer survival times than those with high expression tumors (>59,4% figure, log rank: p=0.013). The median survival times were 52 months (95% CI, 36-67 months) and 26 months (95% CI, 14-37 months) respectively. To test the selectivity of PLK prognostic information, we performed a Cox regression analysis. During stepwise backward selection from entered variables (age, sex, pT, pN, PLK-expression, therapy) only pN (e^B =1,87, 95% CI: 1.14-2.89; p=0-007) and PLK (e^B=2.31,95%CI: 96-5.56; p=0.039) were significant predictors of survival. In contrast, the proliferation marker, Ki67 and PCNA, which are frequently discussed as prognostic parameters for HNSCC, were not associated with tumor stage, pN or survival in our study, which is in line with recent reports[6].

Based on immunohistochemical methods PLK sems to be a new prognostic marker for the daily routine diagnosis judging the risk of dying for patients with oropharyngeal carcinomas in additation to the pN stage more precisely. Moreovoer, if the pN stage is unkonwn and the prognostic information relies only on clinical investigations, determination of PLK-expression in tumor-derived specimens could improve the prediction of survival.

Figure 1: Kaplan-Meier curve of survival of patiients with HNSCC (n=157). Adjusted survival rate is given in percent. The PLK-expression indices are grouped according to the median of 59,4% into moderate (<59,4%; n=78) and high (>59.4%; n=79). (log rank test p=0.013)

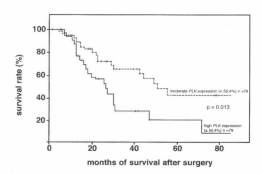

110

REFERENCES

1.   Lane H.A., and Nigge E. A., Cell-cycle control: polo-like kinases join the outer circle. Cell Biol, 7, 63-68, (1997)

2.   Holtrich, U., Wolf, G., Bbräuninger,A, Kern,T., Böhme,B.; Rübsamen-Waigman, H. and Strebhardt, K., Induction and downregulation of PLK, a human serine/threonine kinase expressed in proliferating cells and tumors. Proc. Natl. Acad. Sci USA, 91, 1736-40 (1994).

3.   Wolf G., Elez R., Doermer A., Holtrich U., Ackermann H., Stutte H.J., Altmannsberger H.-J., Rübsamen-Waigmann H. and Strebhardt K., Prognostic significatnce of polo-like kinase (PLK) expression in non-small-cell lung cancer. Oncogene, 14, 543-49 (1997)

4.   Knecht R., Elez R., Oechler M., Solbach C., von Ilberg C., Strebhardt K., Prognostic significance of polo-like kinase (PLK) expression in squamous cell carcinomas of the head and neck. Cancer Res., 59:2794-97, 1999

5.   Forastiere, A.A., Metch,B., Schuller,D.E., Ensley, J.F., Hutchins, L.F., Triozzi, P., Kish, J.A., Mc Clure, S., Von Feldt E., Williamson SK., et al. Randomized comparision of cisplatin plus flourourracil and carboplatin plus flourouracil versus methotrexate in advanced squamous-cell carcinoma of the head and neck: a Southwest Oncology Group Study. J. Clin. Oncol., 10, 1245-1251 (1992)

6.   Sommer T. and Olofsson J., Significance of p53, PCNA and Ki67 in the prognosis of squamous cell carcinomas of the oral cavity. Laryngo-Rhino-Otol 76, 89-96 (1997)

S100A2 CA2+ BINDING PROTEIN IN PRIMARY LARYNGEAL SCC: A PROGNOSTIC FACTOR OF NECK NODE RELAPSE.

M. Maurizi[1], G. Almadori[1], G. Cadoni[1], J. Galli[1], F. Michetti[2], C. Heizmann[3], L. Lauriola[4], F.O.Ranelletti[4].

[1]Institute of Otolaryngology,Università Cattolica S. Cuore, 00168 Roma, Italy
[2] Institute of Anatomy,Università Cattolica S. Cuore, 00168 Roma, Italy
[3]Division of Clinical Chemistry and Biochemistry, Department of Pediatrics, University of Zurich, Zurich, Switzerland.
[4]Institute of Pathology,Università Cattolica S. Cuore, 00168 Roma, Italy.

Running title: S100A2 in laryngeal cancer.

Correspondence to*: Almadori Giovanni, Institute of Otolaryngology, Catholic University of the Sacred Heart, Largo A: Gemelli, 8, Rome 00168. Italy.*

SUMMARY

Background. S100A2 belongs to a family of calcium-binding proteins implicated in the regulation of cell proliferation, differentiation, motility and extracellular signal transduction as well as apoptosis and cancer metastasis.

Material and methods. We investigated by immunocytochemistry the expression of the Ca^{2+} binding protein S100A2 in 62 cases of laryngeal squamous cell carcinoma (SCC).

Results. S100A2 was detected in 18/19 (95%) low-grade tumors and in 22/43 (51%) high-grade tumors, which were partially keratinizing. The remaining 21/43 (49%) high-grade tumors were all non-keratinizing, anaplastic tumors and clearly S100A2 negative. A correlation was found between S100A2 tumor positivity and longer relapse-free (p=0.0005), metastasis free survival (p=0.0232) and overall survival (p=0.0095).

Conclusion. The evaluation of the expression of the Ca^{2+} binding protein S100A2 may allow the identification of a subset S100A2 negative laryngeal SCC patients who are more susceptible to loco-regional relapse and then require that therapy should be adapted accordingly.

INTRODUCTION

In laryngeal SCC, conflicting results have been reported between survival and tumor cell differentiation[1]. The identification of factors related to tumor cell differentiation may be useful for a better understanding of the relationship between histological grading and tumor behavior. The S100 family of calcium-binding proteins has been implicated in regulation of cell proliferation, differentiation, motility and extracellular signal transduction as well as apoptosis and cancer metastasis[2, 3]. It has recently been reported that S100A2 is a member of the S100 protein family that appears expressed specifically in the basal-parabasal layer of normal skin and in well-differentiated skin tumors[4]. The vast majority of laryngeal cancers are of the squamous cell type with a variable degree of differentiation ranging between well-differentiated, keratinizing and anaplastic, non-keratinizing tumors[1]. Preliminary immunohistochemical experiments showed that both normal squamous laryngeal epithelium and laryngeal squamous cell cancer (SCC) express S100A2 protein. Since S100A2 protein expression seems to be positively associated with squamous cell differentiation[4], we studied the clinical significance of S100A2 expression in laryngeal SCC.

MATERIALS AND METHODS

Patients. Our study included 62 untreated consecutive primary laryngeal SCC patients. Histological grading and TNM classification were performed on conventional paraffin sections according to the recommendations of the International Union Against Cancer. Thirty-eight patients underwent total laryngectomy, 17 supraglottic laryngectomy, 2 hemilaryngectomy and 5 cordectomy. At surgery, 8 patients with clinically positive neck nodes underwent a therapeutic neck dissection. The median follow-up period was 44 months (range = 2-90 months).

Immunohistochemical analysis. Tumor tissues obtained at surgery and two autoptic specimens of normal larynx were fixed in formalin and paraffin-embedded according to standard procedures. Tissue sections were treated with 0.3% H_2O_2 in methanol for 10 min to block endogenous peroxidase activity. For the immunolocalization of S100A2, sections were incubated with normal rabbit serum for 15 min, then with rabbit antiserum against S100A2, diluted 1:200, for 1 h. The specificity of rabbit antiserum against human recombinant S100A2 was assessed by Western blot analysis as described elsewhere[5]. Indirect immunostaining was achieved using the ABC (Vector Laboratories, Burlingame, CA) technique. Endogenous biotin was saturated by a biotin blocking kit (Vector Laboratories). The peroxidase was developed with a DAB substrate kit (Vector Laboratories). Negative controls were performed using normal rabbit or mouse serum, omitting the primary antibodies. For statistical evaluation, cut-off points were chosen to categorize tumors as positive or negative relative to S100A2 expression. Arbitrarily, a cut-off point of $\leq$ 5% immunostained tumor cells was chosen based on an initial overview of the cases in order to determine the range of positive cells in the study slides. Cut-offs were chosen before any attempt of correlating histology with expression. In S100A2+ tumors, the percentages of stained cells were: up to 25% in 6 cases; up to 50% in 9 cases, and > 50% in 25 cases.

Statistical analysis. Fisher's exact test for proportions was used to analyze the distribution of S100A2 status according to various clinico-pathological parameters. Survival data were available for all 62 patients. All medians and life tables were computed using the product-limit estimate by Kaplan and Meier, and the curves were examined by means of the log-rank test. Univariate and multivariate analysis was performed by Cox's proportional hazards model. Relapse-Free Survival (RFS) and Metastasis-Free Survival (MFS) was calculated, respectively, from the date of first surgery to that of clinical or pathological loco-regional and regional neck-node recurrence. Overall survival was calculated from the date of first surgery to that of death.

RESULTS

According to the cut-off criteria (see Materials and Methods), the number of S100A2 positive (S100A2+) and negative (S100A2-) tumors was 40 and 22, respectively. A significant correlation was observed between S100A2 + and low grade differentiation (G1-G2 vs G3-G4, p=0.001) The percentage of S100A2+ tumors was 18/19 (95%) and 22/43 (51%) in low grade (G1+G2) and high grade (G3+G4) tumors, respectively. During the follow-up period, loco-regional recurrences were observed in 31/62 (50%) cases and only 14/62 (22.6%) patients had only a regional neck-node recurrence. At the end of the study, 25/62 (40%) patients had died of cancer. A significant relationship was found between S100A2 tumor negativity and short overall survival. The 5-year survival rate was 68% (95% C.I.: 53% - 84%) for patients with S100A2+ tumors compared with 32% (95% C.I.: 8% - 56%) for patients with S100A2- tumors (p = 0.0095). Similarly, the relapse-free survival (RFS) and metastasis-free survival (MFS) curves have indicated that patients with positive tumors have respectively a longer RFS and MFS than those with negative tumors. The 5-year RFS was 61% (95% C.I.: 45% - 77%) for patients with positive tumors compared with 23% (95% C.I.: 4% - 41%) for those with negative tumors (p = 0.0005). The 5-year MFS was 81% (95% C.I.: 67%-95%) for patients with positive tumors compared with 55% for those with negative tumors (p=0.0232). Table I shows the univariate analysis of prognostic variables for overall, metastasis and relapse-free survival.

DISCUSSION

The results of this study indicate that the expression of S100A2 in laryngeal SCC could be of some potential in predicting prognosis. The highly significant association between S100A2+ and tumor keratinizing status suggests that, in laryngeal SCC, the prognostic effectiveness of S100A2 expression is probably due to the fact that this Ca^{2+}-binding protein is related to cell commitment to differentiation. in the direction of keratinization. Controversy exists as to whether very simple methods of histological grading of squamous cell carcinoma bear a direct relationship to a patient's survival or to loco-regional recurrence rates. For larynx SCC the very simple and rapidly assessed histopathological grading into keratinizing and non-keratinizing anaplastic tumors has been demonstrated to provide an independent significant contribution to the prediction of prognosis[1].

The management of laryngeal cancer has improved greatly in recent years, particularly for initial disease control as well as quality of life related to the function and/or organ preservation of the larynx[6]. What is more, the prognostic significance of S100A2 protein expression might identify more chemio-radiosensitive tumors candidates to the novel clinical trials of induction chemotherapy or definitive irradiation. Although the application of experimental results to clinical practice is generally slow, we suggest that the evaluation of the expression of the Ca^{2+} binding protein S100A2 may allow the identification of a subset S100A2 negative laryngeal SCC patients who are more susceptible to loco-regional relapse and then require that therapy should be adapted accordingly. An aggressive initial management of these S100A2 negative tumors may be considered to avoid undertreatment. On the other hand, a much less aggressive treatment could be considered in S100A2+ tumors.

Table 1. Univariate analysis of prognostic variables for relapse-free, metastases-free and overall survival in 62 LSCC patients.

	RFS	MFS	OS
Variable	RR[1] (CI 95%)[2] p	RR (CI 95%) p	RR (CI 95%) p
Histopath. Grading			
G1-G2	1	1	1
G3-G4	1.22 (0.6-2.7) 0.48	1.24 (0.5-3.0) 0.63	1.04 (0.4-2.5) 0.93
Stage			
I-II	1	1	1
III-IV	1.30 (0.6-3.0) 0.54	1.6 (0.6-4.2) 0.33	1.93 (0.7-5.2) 0.19
Lymph-node involvement			
No	1	1	1
Yes	2.99 (1.3-6.7) 0.008	2.1 (0.7-6.2) 0.20	5.43 (2.3-12.8) 0.0001
T-classification			
1-2	1	1	1
3-4	1.35 (0.6-2.8) 0.43	1.8 (0.7-4.4) 0.19	1.6 (0.7-3.6) 0.26
S100A2 immunostaining			
Positive	1	1	1
Negative	3.26 (1.6-6.7) 0.001	3.2 (1.1-9.3) 0.032	2.72 (1.2-6.0) 0.013

[1]unadjusted relative risk; [2]95% confidence intervals

REFERENCES

1. Wiernik, G., Millard, P.R., Haybittle, J.L., The predictive value of histological classification into degrees of differentiation of squamous cell carcinoma of the larynx and hypopharynx compared with the survival of patients. Histopathology 1991; 19: 411-417.
2. Schäfer, B.W., Wicki, R., Hengelkamp, D., Mattei, M.C., Heizmann, C.W., Isolation of a YAC clone covering a cluster of nine S100 genes of human chromosome 1q21. Rationale for a new nomenclature of the S100 protein family. Genomics 1995; 25: 638-643.
3. Heizmann, C.W. and Cox, J., New perspectives on S100 proteins: a multifunctional Ca^{2+}-, Zn^{2+}- and Cu^{2+}-binding protein family. Biometals 1998; 11: 383-397.
4. Shrestha, P., Muramatsu, Y., Kudeken, W., Mori, M., Takai, Y., Ilg, E.C., Schafer, B.W., Heizmann, C.W., Localization of Ca^{2+}-binding S100 proteins in epithelial tumours of the skin. Virchows Arch. 1998; 432: 53-59.
5. Ilg, E.C., Schäfer, B.W., Heizmann, C.W., Expression pattern of S100 calcium-binding proteins in human tumors. Int. J. Cancer 1996; 68: 325-332.
6. Magnano, M., Bussi, M., De Stefani, A., Milan, F., Lerda, W., Ferrero, V., Gervasio, C., Ragona, R., Gabriele, P., Cortesina, G., Prognostic factors for head and neck tumor recurrence. Acta Otolaryngol. (Stockh), 1995; 115: 833-838.

RELEVANCE OF OCCULT TUMOR CELLS IN THE BONE MARROW OF HEAD AND NECK CANCER PATIENTS

Barbara Wollenberg MD, PhD, Stephan H. Lang, MD, Michaela Andratschke, MD, Cristof Pauli, MD, Reinhard Zeidler, PhD
Department of Otorhinolaryngology, Head and Neck Surgery; Grosshadern Medical Center, Ludwig-Maximilians-University Munich, Germany

Running title: Occult tumor cells in SCCHN

Key words: SCCHN, occult tumor cells, micrometastasis, bone marrow

Acknowledgement: This work was supported by the Deutsche Forschungsgemeinschaft DFG WO 483 / 1-2 donated to B. Wollenberg

Correspondence to: *Priv.-Doz. Dr. B. Wollenberg, MD, Dep.of Otorhinolaryngology, HNS, LMU Munich, Grosshadern Medical Center, Marchioninistr. 15, 81377 Munich, Germany, Phone: +49/ 89/ 7095-1, Fax: +49/ 89/ 7095 5874 (e-mail: bwollen@hno.med.uni-muenchen.de)*

ABSTRACT

Background. The presence of tumor cells in the bone marrow is associated with a poor prognosis in malignoma patients.

Methods. In the present paper we investigate bone marrow samples from 176 patients suffering from head and neck squamous cell carcinoma (SCCHN) for the presence of disseminated tumor cells using anti-cytokeratin 19 (CK 19) antibody to immuno-histochemically detect disseminated tumor cells in the bone marrow.

Results. CK19-positive cells could be detected in the bone marrow from 54 out of 176 SCCHN patients. All healthy control donors tested (n=52) revealed a complete absence of CK 19-positive cells in this compartment. The presence of disseminated tumor cells was associated with a significantly higher incidence of loco-regional or distant tumor recurrence and a significantly reduced survival rate.

117

Conclusion. The early detection of micrometastases could help to identify those patients who are likely to benefit from adjuvant therapeutic strategies.

INTRODUCTION

Patients suffering from squamous cell carcinoma of the head and neck (SCCHN) are at high risk to develop loco-regional recurrence or distant metastases. Therefore, the early detection of disseminated tumor cells could be helpful in defining new therapeutic or diagnostic strategies resulting in the improvement of the poor survival rate.

The cytoskeleton of epithelial cells contains intermediate sized filaments which are composed of characteristic cytokeratins. Since neoplastic cells retain the main cytoskeletal properties of their progenitors, cytokeratins are found in normal as well as in malignant epithelia. In the present study we used an antibody directed against cytokeratin 19 (CK 19). This CK 19 cytokeratin is expressed in cultured keratinocytes and in normal as well as malignantly transformed squamous epithelia and was used for the detection of disseminated tumor cells in bone marrow of patients. Expression of CK 19 is restricted to epithelial cells that are usually absent from the peripheral blood or bone marrow of healthy persons. The detection of CK 19-positive cells in the peripheral blood and bone marrow of patients, suffering from epithelial malignoma, therefore indicates the unphysiological presence of epithelial cells, i.e. systemic spread of the cancer.

In the present study, CK 19-positive cells could be detected in the bone marrow from 54 out of 176 SCCHN patients. All healthy control donors tested revealed a complete absence of CK 19-positive cells in this compartment. The presence of disseminated tumor cells was associated with a significantly higher incidence of loco-regional tumor recurrence or distant metastases and a significantly reduced survival rate.

PATIENTS AND METHODS

The study comprised 176 patients with histologically proven SCCHN classified in accordance to the TNM-staging system. During the 5-year follow-up, patients were clinically examined at regular intervals and 5-year-survival rates were analyzed for all patients.

Bone marrow aspirates and immunohistochemistry. Bone marrow aspirates were taken intraoperatively through a small skin incision from both iliac crests in heparin-coated syringes. Bone marrow samples of healthy donors (n=52) served as negative controls, whereas FaDu cells (pharyngeal squamous cell carcinoma, ATCC, Rockville/USA) served as positive controls. After a Ficoll/Hypaque density centrifugation cytospin-preparations were prepared.

CK 19-expression was investigated immunohistochemically by the APAAP-method, using the monoclonal KS 19.1 antibody (5 µg/ml; Progen, Germany) against CK 19. Binding of the antibody was visualised using newfuchsin (5% in 2N HCl) and cell-nuclei were counter-stained with hemalaun (Merck, Germany). Bone marrow samples were classified CK 19-positive if one or more clearly red stained cells could be identified.

Statistical analysis. The Kaplan-Meier method was used for the calculation of survival-rates and the chi-square-test in order to evaluate differences between clinicopathological parameters and CK 19-positivity. Differences were found to be statistically significant if p<0.05.

RESULTS

CK 19 in patients bone marrow. CK 19-expressing cells were detected in 54 out of 176 SCCHN patients (= 30.68%). In contrast, bone marrow samples of all healthy volunteers (n=52) stained negative for CK 19.

CK 19 and recurrent tumor disease. As depicted in table 1, the presence of CK 19-expressing cells in the bone marrow was associated with a significantly higher incidence of loco-regional tumor recurrence or distant metastasis as compared to patients with CK 19-negative bone marrow aspirates.

	total	loco-regional recurrence	metastasis
CK19+ patients	54	27 (=50%)	13 (=24.07%)
CK19- patients	122	33 (=27.05%)	14 (=11.48%)
p value		0.003	0.032

Table 1: Association between loco-regional recurrence, metastasis and CK 19-positive or -negative cells in the bone marrow.

Kaplan-Meier Analysis for the survival. The survival in all of the 176 patients assessed for the presence of CK 19-positive cells in the bone marrow were calculated using the Kaplan-Meier method during a 5-year follow-up period: Presence of disseminated tumor cells in the bone marrow was associated with a significantly lower survival (p< 0.001) as compared to patients showing no signs for CK 19-positive cells in this compartment (Figure 1).

Figure 1. The Kaplan-Meier analysis demonstrates a significantly reduced survival rate for SCCHN patients yielding disseminated tumor cells, i.e. CK 19-positive cells, in the bone marrow in contrast to patients showing no CK 19-positive bone marrow aspirates.

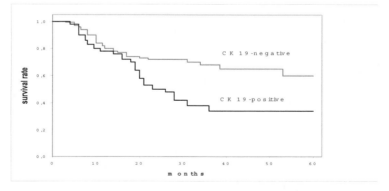

DISCUSSION

SCCHN has to be considered as a systemic disease and more than 50% of the patients develop recurrent disease. This strongly indicates that (i) small histologically undetectable tumor deposits remain at the primary site of the tumor close to the draining lymph vessels or (ii) that the formation of distant metastases is due to the systemic dissemination of tumor cells. Tumor cells present in the bone marrow are considered to be a clinically relevant prognostic factor.[1,2] Various markers have been used for the detection of these disseminated tumor cells, predominantly antibodies to cytokeratins.[3] Characterization of those cells revealed a loss of MHC class I and an expression of proliferation markers such as Ki 67.[4,5]

The objective of the present study was the detection of tumor cells present in the bone marrow of SCCHN patients and the impact on tumor recurrence and survival.

Using an anti-cytokeratin 19 antibody we could detect CK 19-positive cells in the bone marrow of 30.68% of the patients by means of immunohistochemistry. The presence of disseminated tumor cells was associated with a significantly higher incidence of loco-regional or distant tumor recurrence and a significantly reduced survival rate.

In the future, the early detection of micrometastases could be helpful in defining new therapeutic or diagnostic strategies thus resulting in the improvement of the poor survival rate of SCCHN patients.

REFERENCES:

1.   Wollenberg B, Ollesch A, Maag K, Funke I, Wilmes E: [Micrometastases in bone marrow of patients with cancers in the head and neck area]. Laryngorhinootologie 1994; 73:88-93.
2.   Pantel K, Gath H, Heissler E. Staging of head and neck cancer [letter; comment]. N Engl J Med 1995; 332:1788; discussion 1789-1790.
3.   Chaubal S, Wollenberg B, Kastenbauer E, Zeidler R. Specific detection of minimal residual disease in head and neck cancer by EpCAM RT-PCR. Anticancer Research 1999; 19:2237-2242.
4.   Wollenberg B, Chaubal S, Andratschke M, Pauli C, Stein M, Kastenbauer E. Loss of MHC Class I Antigens on epithelial cells in bone marrow of patients with undifferentiated squamous cell cancer of the head and neck. (submitted)
5.   Wollenberg B, Wilmes E. The relevance of the Ki 67-antigen expression on tumor cells in the bone marrow of patients with head and neck-cancer. 3rd International Head and Neck Cancer Congress, San Francisco, USA, 1992.

HISTOLOGICAL DIAGNOSIS OF LYMPH NODE METASTASES – INCLUDING MICROMETASTASES – IN HEAD AND NECK CANCER

Roland Moll, Annette Ramaswamy, Philipps University of Marburg, Institute of Pathology, D-35033 Marburg, Germany

Correspondence to: *Roland Moll, M.D., Philipps University of Marburg, Institute of Pathology, Baldingerstrasse, D-35033 Marburg, Germany, Phone: (+49) 6421-28 62270, Fax: (+49) 6421-28 65640*

The histopathological examination of cervical lymph nodes is an important part of the medical care of patients with head and neck cancer. Based on the information which the head and neck surgeon expects to receive from the pathologists, there are two main tasks for the latter regarding cervical lymph nodes: on the one hand the histological typing, defining the kind of tumor present, and on the other hand the histological staging, describing the extension of the malignant disease. This paper will give an overview of the current state of histopathological diagnosis of cervical lymph node metastases, with a particular focus on micrometastases.

Histopathology of squamous cell carcinoma of the upper aerodigestive tract

In cervical lymph node metastases, the most common histopathologic finding is metastatic squamous cell carcinoma derived from a primary tumor which has arisen in the mucosal tissues of the upper aerodigestive tract. Establishing the tumor entity, i.e. typing, usually poses little problems with conventional squamous cell carcinoma, which is composed of either keratinizing or nonkeratinizing, atypical squamous epithelium. Exceptions are very poorly differentiated squamous cell carcinomas, the squamous nature of which may be difficult to ascertain; in such cases the immunohistochemical demonstration of stratified squamous epithelial markers such as cytokeratins CK5/6 may be helpful.[1] After typing, histopathological grading is performed, i.e., determination of the grade of differentiation (G1 to G3). Relevant parameters include features of differentiation (including intercellular bridges and keratinization) as well as features of cytological malignancy (nuclear pleomorphism, frequency of mitoses, presence of atypical mitoses) and histological malignancy (infiltration). Thus, well differentiated squamous cell carcinomas (G1) exhibit well-developed features of differentiation and few features of malignancy, whereas the reverse is the case with poorly differentiated tumors (G3). These grading parameters (for definition by the WHO see [2]) all form a continuous spectrum and are not clearly defined at distinct quantitative levels.

Therefore, the grading procedure is rather subjective and shows relatively poor interobserver agreement.[2] The problems are enhanced by histological tumor heterogeneity which is a feature of many squamous cell carcinomas. In view of such problems, modifications of the grading procedure have been proposed, such as considering the mode of invasion and the lymphoplasmacytic infiltrate[3] and applying selective tumor front grading.[4] Altogether, despite being generally used, the grading of squamous cell carcinomas is not fully satisfactory. When primary tumor and lymph node metastases are compared, the differentiation grade is often identical, but there may also be differences in the one or the other direction of differentiation.

There are several histological variants of squamous cell carcinoma, some of which are clinically important.[2,5,6] *Basaloid squamous cell carcinoma* exhibits basal cell-like tumor cells with little cytoplasm, numerous mitoses, often peripheral palisading and central necrosis. Keratinization is absent. There may be interstitial hyalinosis and deposition of mucinous material. These tumors mainly arise in the hypopharynx, base of tongue and supraglottic larynx. Clinically, they behave similarly to poorly differentiated conventional squamous cell carcinoma.

Undifferentiated (lymphoepithelial) carcinoma (lymphoepithelioma, tumor of Schmincke) is a particular clinico-pathologic entity which should be correctly recognized. These tumors typically arise in the nasopharynx. They show a broad age distribution, also including children. Most cases are associated with Epstein-Barr virus (EBV). Undifferentiated lymphoepithelial carcinomas typically produce early lymph node metastases, often as the presenting sign, whereas the primary tumor may initially remain occult. Histopathologically, the tumor is composed of undifferentiated cells with vesicular nuclei and high mitotic index. Cell borders are inapparent, often suggesting the presence of a syncytium. Very typical is the presence of a diffuse lymphoplasmacytic infiltrate which may create a high dispersion of tumor cells, which then may resemble immunoblasts or Hodgkin cells. Therefore, malignant lymphoma of Hodgkin or non-Hodgkin type is important in the differential diagnosis of undifferentiated lymphoepithelial carcinoma. In lymph node metastases of lymphoepithelial carcinomas, the lymphoplasmacytic infiltrate may be present or absent.

Spindle cell carcinomas, which mainly arise in the larynx and frequently are exophytic, are a biphasic variant of squamous cell carcinoma. Per definition they must include a squamous cell carcinoma component which, however, may be minor. The predominant component usually is a malignant spindle cell component reminiscent of a sarcoma. This tumor portion may be undifferentiated, reminiscent of malignant fibrous histiocytoma, or show osteoid or cartilage production, reminiscent of osteosarcoma or chondrosarcoma. The epithelial origin is, however, often made evident by at least focal cytokeratin expression. The differential diagnosis includes squamous cell carcinoma with prominent stroma proliferation, various types of sarcomas (including rhabdomyosarcoma) as well as the spindle cell type of malignant melanoma.[5]

Further variants include *adenoid squamous cell carcinoma* and *adenosquamous carcinoma.*

Squamous cell carcinomas and their variants need to be discriminated from other types of carcinomas which also may present as cervical lymph node metastases such as salivary gland carcinomas, various kinds of adenocarcinomas, and malignant melanomas. In some instances, immunohistochemistry may be required for differential diagnosis.

Micrometastases of head and neck cancer in lymph nodes

Histological staging of cervical lymph node metastases describes the extent of tumor involvement of the lymph nodes and cervical tissues (in the following, only conventional squamous cell carcinoma is considered). In the initial process of lymphatic metastasis, a subpopulation of cells of the primary tumor invades lymphatic vessels, which may be visible in histologic specimens as lymphangiosis carcinomatosa. Tumor cells washed into the regional lymph node become visible as tumor cell emboli in the subcapsular sinus or in a capsular lymphatic vessel.[7] When such tumor cells survive and start to proliferate, a micrometastasis develops (Fig. 1).

Regarding the incidence of cervical micrometastases, among histologically tumor-positive neck dissection specimens 10% to 20% have been reported to exhibit only micrometastases.[8,9] Histologically, micrometastases are defined as small tumor cell nodules measuring up to 3 mm in diameter. The majority are localized in the subcapsular sinus, the minority in medullary sinuses.[8,9] Notably, there is only minimal disturbance of the lymph node architecture; any stroma formation or angiogenesis have not yet started. Usually, lymph nodes containing micrometastases are normal in size or only slightly enlarged, and micrometastases may be present even in lymph nodes smaller than 5 mm. Commonly, there is one micrometastatic focus per lymph node; occasionally, two to three foci may be found. In a careful study of micrometastases of oral squamous cell carcinoma,[10] the size distribution of 29 micrometastatic foci present in 23 cervical lymph nodes revealed a range between 0.3 mm and 3.0 mm, with a mean of 1.36 mm. Notably, only a single micrometastatic focus was smaller than 0.3 mm. In contrast, micrometastases of breast cancer, which have been more extensively studied, are on average considerably smaller; in some studies the majority are smaller than 0.2 mm.[11] Micrometastases of squamous cell carcinomas thus usually show little degree of cellular dispersion and rarely singly cell dissolution but rather tend to form larger, more compact foci with an apparently higher degree of intercellular adhesion which in part is mediated by relatively abundant desmosomes.

Is the routine histopathological technique of analysis of neck dissection specimens[12] sufficient to detect such small tumor structures such as micrometastases? Several authors have performed extensive serial and semiserial sectioning of cervical lymph nodes which in conventional histology were tumor-free.[10,13,14] In one of these studies, only very few micrometastases were detected (2 in 716 lymph nodes, corresponding to 0.3%) using 5 μm serial section intervals. Higher rates were reported by Ambrosch et al.[14] and in particular Hamakawa et al.[10] who detected micrometastases in 23 out of 554 lymph nodes (4.2%) using semiserial sectioning at 200 μm intervals. In the last two studies, as a consequence 10% to 12% of the patients needed to be upstaged in their pN stage. Concerning routine diagnosis, Hamakawa et al.[10] consequently recommended to prepare, from the paraffin blocks, step sections at 1 mm intervals to obtain acceptable sensitivity for detection of micrometastases. On the other hand, the majority of authors including those of the first study mentioned [9,12,13] currently believe that it is of no great value to prepare multiple sections. Rather, attention should be directed to careful embedding of the lymph node specimens, which, if large, should be sliced at 3 to 4 mm thickness; then one section of each of these slices stained by hematoxylin and eosin (H & E) would be sufficient for routine staging. It should also be considered that the diagnostic sensitivity depends to a large extent on careful macroscopic preparation, during which all recognizable lymph nodes, including the small ones, should be identified and sampled.

Immunohistochemical staining for epithelial markers such as cytokeratins, which has proven to be useful in the detection of micrometastases of breast cancer, appears to lack improved diagnostic sensitivity in head and neck cancer metastases.[8,10,14] Instead, H & E staining is usually sufficient, which is probably due to the relatively large size of head and neck cancer micrometastases (see above). Of course, analysis of a single histological section from a 3 to 4 mm thick slice must fail to detect some small micrometastases. In situations in which highest diagnostic sensitivity with more or less complete detection of micrometastases is desired, such as in the histological analysis of sentinel lymph nodes,[15] a more extensive technique with higher numbers of sections is appropriate. However, a clinically relevant prognostic significance of micrometastases, justifying routine application of multiple sectioning, has not yet been unequivocally proven for head and neck cancer. Hamakawa et al.[10] suggested a prognostic relevance of micrometastases but their series studied was small. In contrast, Woolgar[9] was not able to find an influence on the prognosis (although her study was limited to the short-term outcome); in her series, the prognosis of patients with only micrometastases was similar to that of patients without any lymph node metastases. Prospective studies with sufficient numbers of cases and longer follow-up would be required to establish the biological and clinical significance of cervical micrometastases.

Extracapsular spread in lymph node metastases
Mostly at an advanced stage of lymphatic metastasis, the tumor breaks through the lymph node capsule and proceeds in extracapsular spread. The initial stage of this process is characterized by invasion of the connective tissue layer of the lymph node capsule. Then microscopic and subsequently macroscopic extracapsular spread develop. The latter may result in fusion of neighbouring nodes. Eventually, the tumor may invade other tissue structures such as the internal jugular vein, skeletal muscle and skin. The occurrence of extracapsular spread is correlated with the size of the lymph node, but approximately 20 % of lymph nodes with extracapsular spread measure less than 1 cm in diameter.[16] The main importance of extracapsular spreads lies in its prognostic significance.[16] Recently, it has been suggested that only macroscopic extracapsular spread (present in 55% of N^+ patients) is, in multivariate analysis, an independent prognostic parameter of high significance.[17] If this would be confirmed, it would seem necessary from the histological point of view to define a clear-cut border for the distinction between microscopic and macroscopic extracapsular spread (such as the depth of invasion into the perinodal tissue in mm).

In conclusion, one function of histopathological analysis of lymph node metastases is the diagnosis of the tumor type, in particular the recognition of special variants of squamous cell carcinoma such as undifferentiated lymphoepithelial carcinoma and spindle cell carcinoma. In some cases, particularly when the primary tumor is occult, sophisticated differential diagnosis (which may require immunohistochemistry) should be able to identify different tumors such as adenocarcinomas, salivary gland carcinomas and malignant melanoma. Regarding the staging of cervical lymph node metastases, a currently disputed item is the presence of micrometastases, the sensitive detection of which clearly is relevant for sentinel lymph node biopsies, requiring more extensive sectioning than usual. The prognostic significance of micrometastases remains, however, to be established. In routine diagnosis of neck dissection specimens, conventional histologic technique is currently recommended. Regarding macrometastases, their extracapsular spread has particular prognostic relevance and therefore should be carefully documented in histopathology reports. The results of the histological lymph node staging are summarized in the pN classification.[18] Unfortunately, important pathologic features discussed above, i.e. micrometastases (with possible prognostic significance) and extracapsular spread (with proven prognostic significance) are not considered in the present pN classification of head and neck cancer (in contrast to breast cancer), although proposals for improved classification schemes have repeatedly been made (e.g.[19]). Clearly, a high standard in the quality of histopathological analysis of cervical lymph node metastases is a prerequisite for an adequate stage-optimized care of head and neck cancer patients.

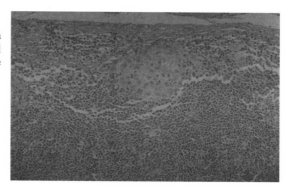

Figure 1. Micrometastasis (0.25 mm diameter) of a pharyngeal squamous cell carcinoma in a cervical lymph node. Note the typical subcapsular localization (H & E).

REFERENCES

1. Moll R. Cytokeratins as markers of differentiation in the diagnosis of epithelial tumors. In: Intermediate Filaments, Herrmann H, Harris JR, eds. Subcellular Biochemistry, Vol. 31. 1998; Plenum Press, New York, pp 205-262.
2. Pindborg JJ, Reichart PA, Smith CJ, van der Waal I: International Histological Classification of Tumours / World Health Organization: Histological typing of cancer and precancer of the oral mucosa. 2nd ed. 1997; Springer, Berlin, pp 1-87.
3. Jakobsson PA, Eneroth CM, Killander D, Moberger G, Martensson B. Histologic classification and grading of malignancy in carcinoma of the larynx. Acta Radiol Ther Phys Biol 1973;12:1-8.
4. Bryne M, Koppang HS, Lilleng R, Stene T, Bang G, Dabelsteen E. Ney malignancy grading is a better prognostic indicator than Broders´ grading in oral squamous cell carcinomas. J Oral Pathol Med 1989;18:432-437.
5. Mills SE, Gaffey MJ, Frierson HF: Atlas of Tumor Pathology, Third Series, Fascicle 26: Tumors of the upper aerodigestive tract and ear. 2000; Armed Forces Institute of Pathology, Washington, D.C., pp 1-455.
6. Seifert G: Orale Karzinome. In: Seifert G (ed) Oralpathologie III: Mundhöhle, angrenzende Weichteil- und Knochengewebe. 2000; Springer, Berlin, pp 291-378.
7. Toker C: Some observations on the deposition of metastatic carcinoma within cervical lymph nodes. Cancer 1963;16:364-374.
8. van den Brekel MW, Stel HV, van der Valk P, van der Waal I, Meyer CJ, Snow GB. Micrometastases from squamous cell carcinoma in neck dissection specimens. Eur Arch Otorhinolaryngol 1992;249:349-353.
9. Woolgar JA. Micrometastasis in oral/oropharyngeal squamous cell carcinoma: incidence, histopathological features and clinical implications. Br J Oral Maxillofac Surg 1999;37:181-186.
10. Hamakawa H, Takemura K, Sumida T, Kayahara H, Tanioka H, Sogawa K. Histological study on pN upgrading of oral cancer. Virchows Arch 2000;437:116-121.

11. Nasser IA, Lee AK, Bosari S, Saganich R, Heatley G, Silverman ML. Occult acillary lymph node metastases in „node-negative" breast carcinoma. Hum Pathol 1993;24:950-957.
12. Devaney SL, Ferlito A, Rinaldo A, Devaney KO. The pathology of neck dissection in cancer of the larynx. ORL J Otorhinolaryngol Relat Spec 2000;62:204-211.
13. Shingaki S, Ohtake K, Nomura T, Nakajima T. The value of single versus multiple sections for detection of lymph node metastasis. J Oral Maxillofac Surg 1991;49:461-463.
14. Ambrosch P, Kron M, Fischer G, Brinck U. Micrometastases in carcinoma of the upper aerodigestive tract: detection, risk of metastasizing, and prognostic value of depth of invasion. Head Neck 1995;17:473-479.
15. Werner JA, Dünne AA, Brandt D, Ramaswamy A, Kuelkens C, Lippert BM, Folz BJ, Joseph K, Moll R. Studies on significance of sentinel lymphadenectomy in pharyngeal and laryngeal carcinoma. Laryngorhinootologie 1999;78:663-670.
16. Snyderman NL, Johnson JT, Schramm VL, Myers EN, Bedetti CD, Thearle P. Extracapsular spread of carcinoma in cervical lymph nodes: impact upon survival in patients with carcinoma of the supraglottic larynx. Cancer 1985;56:1597-1599.
17. de Carvalho MB. Quantitative analysis of the extent of extracapsular invasion and its prognostic significance: a prospective study of 170 cases of carcinoma of the larynx and hypopharynx. Head Neck 1998;20:16-21.
18. Sobin LH, Wittekind C (eds): TNM classification of malignant tumours. 5th ed. 1997; Wiley & Sons, New York.
19. Glanz H, Hermanek P, Kleinsasser O, Popella C. Further development in TNM classification of laryngeal cancers. Laryngorhinootologie 1993; 72:568-573.

PREOPERATIVE DETECTION OF HEAD AND NECK METASTASIS: INFLUENCE ON THERAPEUTIC DECISION MAKING

Nils-Claudius Gellrich PhD MD DMD [1], Alexander Schramm MD DMD [1], M. Nilius MD DMD[1], Carola Runer DMD[1], Andreas Warzecha MD[1], Martin Zerfowski, PhD MD DMD [2]

[1]Dept. of Oral&Maxillofacial Surgery, Albert-Ludwigs-University Freiburg i. Br., Germany (Chairman: Prof. Dr. Dr. R. Schmelzeisen)

[2]Dept. of Oral&Maxillofacial Surgery, Eberhard-Karls-University Tübingen, Germany (Chairman: Prof. Dr. Dr. S. Reinert)

Running title: Preoperative detection of head and neck metastasis

Key words: oral cancer, staging, metastasis, simultaneous tumor

Acknowledgements: We thank Professor E. Machtens, former head of the bochum unit of oral and maxillofacial surgery, where 3 of the authors (NC, AW, MZ) were affiliated, for his generous support of this study.

Correspondence to: Priv.-Doz. Dr. Dr. Nils-Claudius Gellrich, Dept. of Oral&Maxillofacial Surgery, Albert-Ludwigs-University Freiburg, Hugstetterstr. 55, D-79106 Freiburg i.Br., Germany, Phone: 0049-761-270-4919, Fax.: 0049-761-270-4800 (e-mail: gellrich@zmk2.ukl.uni-freiburg.de)

ABSTRACT

Background. Preoperative staging is an important prerequisite for therapeutic decision making in head and neck cancer.

Methods. This comparative retrospective study was aimed to evaluate the efficacy of a specific pretherapeutic staging schedule to detect therapy relevant findings, metastases and synchronous primary malignancy. In-patients of 2 maxillofacial units (Freiburg: n=152 [A]; Bochum: n=139 [B]) with primary squamous cell carcinoma of the oral cavity without prior treatment were included.

Results. 8.6 % (group A) and 9.9 % (group B) resp. of patients had to be excluded from surgical tumor therapy due to pertinent staging results. 86.0 % (group A) and. 83.2 %

(group B) resp. of the patients underwent surgery alone or combined surgical therapy. Simultaneous tumors were found in 7 % in group A and in 12 % in group B. Pathohistologic investigation of neck specimens showed significant clinical overstaging of neck node involvement.

Conclusions. A careful and distinct preoperative staging schedule in oral cancer patients is important to define the adequate treatment in respect of radicality and quality of life.

INTRODUCTION

Staging means determination of tumor size by surgical exploration or biopsy and classification to the individual TNM-stage[1]. However, the therapeutic decision and the prognosis in oral SCC patients depends not only on the TNM-related stages but on all health related findings pertinent for tumor therapy[2,3]. Over- or understaging as to tumor size and nodal involvement can lead to a wrong therapeutic concept[4]. Although staging mainly addresses pretherapeutic findings it has to be updated according to possible findings during therapy or even following therapy[1]. However, the frequency of second primary tumors [10-30%] e.g. is a reflection of the diligence with which they are sought[5,6]. No universally accepted pretherapeutic staging protocol exists yet and likewise surgical therapy of the neck, especially the N_0 neck, is under debate in view of oncologic soundness and morbidity of neck dissection.

This study investigated the efficacy of pre- and intraoperative staging procedures as far as diagnostic findings influenced therapeutic decision making.

PATIENTS AND METHODS

291 patients with histologically proven squamous cell carcinoma (SCC) of the oral cavity participated in this comparative retrospective study. They were consecutively seen in the departments of oral and maxillofacial surgery of Freiburg (n= 152; group A) and Bochum (n=139; group B) university. Patients underwent the following staging procedures: clinical investigation; biopsy; imaging, including plain x-rays (orthopantomograms, Water's view, chest), ultrasonography (head and neck, abdomen), bone scintigraphy, CT-scan (head and neck); endoscopic investigations, comprising flexible esophago-gastro-duodenoscopy and bronchoscopy (group B) or ENT rigid panendoscopy (group A). The extended staging protocol was variable and included MRI, CT scan of the brain, chest or abdomen, colour coded ultrasound, PET. Group A patients routinely were consulted in both the ENT and radiotherapy department. 66 % of group B patients received neoadjuvant hyperfractionated radiotherapy (20 Gy) over 5 days.

Further preoperative investigations included ECG, pulmonary function testing, routine lab screening and in selected cases if required echocardiography, myocardial scintigraphy.
Synchronous malignancies and other non-malignant, therapy-relevant findings were registered as pathologic.

Surgical treatment included radical local tumor resection with an intended safety margin of 1.5 cm three-dimensionally and uni- or bilateral neck-dissection of different extent, mostly modified radical neck dissection with of without preservation of the sternocleidomastoid muscle or selective (supraomohyoid) neck dissection (level I-III).

Group A and B were compared concerning the preoperative N- and the pN-stage.

RESULTS

Group A and B are specified in table I. The 2 most frequent primary sites of the intraoral SCC were floor of the mouth and tongue: 66 % and 11 % of cases in group A; 35 % and 29 % of cases in group B. 14 % of group A patients had no surgical tumor therapy and likewise could not be classified as to pTN-stage. In group B 17 % of patients could not be scheduled for surgery. The clinical N-stage was overestimated in both groups compared to the pN-stages. There was a tendency to higher pN-stages in group B patients (fig. 1).

The number of pathologic findings due to radiological investigation is given in table II. Pathologic findings in case of orthopantomograms include osseous lesions (e.g. osteolysis), loss of teeth, remaining dental roots; in case of chest x-rays pulmonary masses, cardial insufficiency, and costal osteolysis were found. In Table III pathologic findings of CT-scans are specified. There is a considerably higher tumor involvement of bone, lymph nodes and vessels in group B as compared to group A. In accordance with the CT findings are the ultrasound findings in the head and neck area (table IV). The majority of abdominal ultrasound findings (table IV) were hepatic steatosis, cystic renal changes, prostatic hyperplasia, masses in abdominal organs, ascites. Bone scintigraphy (table IV) typically revealed degenerative spots as the most frequent pathologic feature followed by tumor infiltration at the primary site, arthroses, fractures and osteomyelitis or ostitis. In certain cases plain x-rays were ordered to confirm the scintigraphic finding.

In most cases of endoscopy chronic bronchitis was diagnosed followed by tumor, inflammation. Endoscopy from the esophagous to the duodenum showed most often inflammation (esophagitis, gastritis, duodenitis) or varicosis, ulcers of the stomach or duodenum. The frequency of each of the endoscopic investigation differed strongly (table V); although the number of positive biopsies was low for bronchoscopies and esophago-gastro-duodenoscopies in both groups. 8 patients in group B with second primary cancer could be detected. Among the number of pathologic findings in rigid panendoscopies the percentage of malignancies was high. In decreasing frequency they were followed by leucoplakia, vocal polyps, retention cysts. Due to the preoperative investigations in group A 11 patients (7 %) and in group B 17 patients (12 %) with simultaneous second primary cancer could be detected.

DISCUSSION AND CONCLUSIONS

Although there are several publications on the value of screening parameters in preoperative tumor staging in oral cancer patients, there is no guideline as to number and extent of pre- and intraoperative investigations[7,8,9,10,11,12,13,14]. The two patient groups in this study match other publications as to epidemiologic data[10,15]. Due to advanced age and aggravated by the known risk factors for oral cancer patients there is a high prevalence of associated diseases, i.e. vascular and cardial disorders, lung diseases, metabolic diorders, all affecting possible radical surgical tumor treatment. However, the majority of patients is denying their general illness and their tumor specific problems, at least as long as pain does not force them to seek medical help. Despite modern techniques to provide more radical surgical treatment - due to improved reconstructive strategies - more sophisticated planning and realization of radiotherapy and better chemotherapy options it is mainly a thorough preoperative check-up and staging that allows for adequate decision making for the individual patient[16]. 7 % and. 12 % resp. of patients with SCC of the oral cavity, who present with a synchronous second malignancy, justify the energy and expense of a comprehensive staging schedule[17,18]. Depending on the severity of accompanying diseases preoperative treatment is possible - e.g. in helicobacter pylori infections by eradication therapy – or leads to different treatment strategies. This is an important contribution to a quality-of-life-oriented treatment policy i.e. to avoid a type of therapy, which cannot be regarded as adequate to the individual patient[19].

In both participating tumor centers the first choice of treatment is radical resection of the intraoral tumor combined with ipsilateral selective neck dissection (level I-III) or modified radical neck dissection Type III. The contralateral neck treatment is performed in N+-staged tumors; in these cases selective neck dissection (level I-III) is performed and extended to modified radical neck dissection Type III if positive lymph nodes of the middle parajugular chain are histologically proven. This strategy implies a high chance to add an pathohistologically based intraoperative staging result to the preoperative tumor staging[20]. Thus a distinct definition of the pN-stage is possible, which allows as well intraoperative limitation to a low morbidity surgery like the SND I-III is with removal of lymph nodes at highest risk for metastases.

Table I: Description of group A and B

	Group A	Group B
Total number of patients	152	139
Sex ratio m : f [%]	77:23	76:24
Age (mean ± 1 SD) [yrs]	59 ± 9	58 ± 10
pT-classification [%]		
pT1	38	41
pT2	36	37
pT3	6	6
pT4	14	15
pN-classification [%]		
pN0	68	63
pN1	14	13
pN2a	-	1
pN2b	6	16
pN2c	2	5
pN3	-	1
pNx	8	2
no operation feasible	14	17

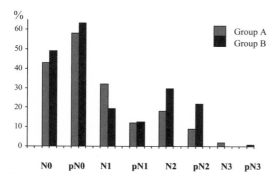

Figure 1. Clinical and pathohistological neck stages

Table II: Imaging investigations

	Group A		Group B	
	n	pathologic [%]	n	pathologic [%]
Orthopantomogram	113	86	107	90
Chest x-ray	148	29	139	22
CT head and neck	133	62	131	81
MRI head and neck	12	75	31	13

Table III: Pathologic findings in CT scans

	Group A (n = 133) [%]	Group B (n = 131) [%]
Bony arrosion	4	22
positive cervical nodes	45	65
Infiltration of jugular vein	1	6
Infiltration of carotid	0	5

Table IV: US investigations and bone scintigraphy

	Group A		Group B	
	n	pathol. [%]	n	pathol. [%]
US head & neck	145	38	130	73
US abdomen	125	49	129	54
bone scintigraphy	129	30	87	47

Table V: Endoscopic investigations

	Group A				Group B			
	n	pathol. [%]	biopsy	Tu*	n	pathol. [%]	biopsy	Tu*
Bronchoscopy	11	27	0	0	127	49	32	4
Esophago-gastro-duodenoscopy	28	36	16	0	138	64	134	4
Panendoscopy	70	37	23	3	40	37	6	3

*number of patients with histologically proven malignancy

REFERENCES

1. Gellrich N-C, Bremerich A, Akuama-Boatenge E, Brechtelsbauer D. Die Bedeutung des Lymphknotenstagings im Trigonum caroticum bei der suprahyoidalen Ausräumung. Fortschr Kiefer Gesichts Chir 1992; 37:115-117.

2. Werner JA, Gottschlich S, Folz BJ, Goeroegh T, Lippert BM, Maass JD, Rudert H. p53 serum antibodies as prognostic indicator in head and neck cancer. Cancer Immunol Immunother 1997; 44(2):112-116.

3. Klutmann S, Bohuslavizki KH, Brenner W, Hoft S, Kroger S, Werner JA, Henze E, Clausen M. Lymphoscintigraphy in tumors of the head and neck using double tracer technique. J Nucl Med. 1999; 40(5):776-782.

4. Beyers RM, El-Naggar AK, Lee Y-Y et al. Can we detect or predict the presence of occult nodal metastases in patients with squamous carcinoma of the oral tongue? Head Neck 1998; 20:138-144.

5. Bohuslavizki KH, Klutmann S, Sonnemann U, Thoms J, Kroger S, Werner JA, Mester J, Clausen M. F-18 FDG PET for detection of occult primary tumor in patients with lymphatic metastases of the neck region. Laryngo- Rhino- Otol 1999; 78(8):445-449.

6. Curtin HD, Ishwaran H, Mancuso AA, Dalley RW, Caudry DJ, McNeil BJ. Comparison of CT and MR imaging in staging of neck metastases. Radiology 1998; 207:123-130.

7. Yoshida H, Yusa H, Ueno E, Tohno E, Tsunoda-Shimizu H. Ultrasonographic evaluation of small cervical lymph nodes in head and neck cancer. Ultrasound Med Biol 1998; 24:621-629.

8. Dhooge IJ, De Vos M, Alberts FWJ, van Cauwenberge PB. Panendoscopy as a screening procedure for simultaneous primary tumors in head and neck cancer. Eur Arch Otorhinolaryngol 1996; 253:319-324.

9. Singh B, Bhaya M, Zimbler M, Stern J, Roland JT, Rosenfeld RM, Har-El G, Lucente FE. Impact of comorbidity on outcome of young patients with head and neck squamous cell carcinoma. Head Neck 1998; 20:1-7.

10. Hicks WL, Loree TR, Garcia RI et al. Squamous cell carcinoma of the floor of mouth: a 20-year review. Head Neck 1997; 19:400-405.

11. Hiratsuka H, Miyakawa A, Nakamori K, Kido Y, Sunakawa H, Kohama G-I. Multivariate analysis of occult lymph node metastasis as a prognosis indicator for patients with squamous cell carcinoma of the oral cavity. Cancer 1997; 80:351-356.

12. Houghton DJ, Hughes ML, Garvey C et al. Role of chest CT scanning in the management of patients presenting with head and neck cancer. Head and Neck 1998; 20:614-618.

13. Fukano H, Matsuura H, Hasegawa Y, Nakamura S.Depth of invasion as a predictive factor for cervical lymph node metastasis in tongue carcinoma. Head Neck 1997; 19:205-210.

14. Kowalski LP, Medina JE. Nodal metastasis. Predictive Factors. Otolaryngol Clin North Am 1998; 31:621-637.

15. Fröhlich M, Bernstein P, Metelmann H-R, Möhner M. Zur Epidemiologie der Lippen- und Mundhöhlenmalignome. Fortschr Kiefer Gesichtschir 1992; 37:1-3.

16. Mohr C, Bohndorf W, Carstens J et al. Preoperative radiochemotherapy and radical surgery in comparison with radical surgery alone. A prospective, multicentric, randomized DOSAK study of advanced squamous cell carcinoma of the oral cavity and the oropharynx (a 3-year follow-up). Int J Oral Maxillofac Surg 1994; 23:140-148.

17. Barbone F, Franceschi S, Talamini R et al. A follow-up study of determinants of second tumor and metastasis among subjects with cancer of the oral cavity, pharynx and larynx. J Clin Epidemiol 1996; 49:367-372.

18. Cohn AM , Peppard SB. Multiple primary malignant tumors of the head and neck. Am J Otolaryngol 1980; 1:411-417.

19. Gellrich N-C, Bremerich A, Kugler J, Welzel-Ruhrmann C, Ruhrmann S. Rehabilitation in der Mund-, Kiefer- und Gesichtschirurgie – eine patientengestützte Studie beim Mundhöhlenkarzinom. Dtsch Z Mund Kiefer Gesichts Chir 1993; 17:215-217.

20. Pellitteri PK, Robbins KT, Neumann T. Expanded application of selective neck dissections with regard to nodal status. Head Neck 1997; 19:260-265.

132

COLOR DUPLEX SONOGRAPHY IN THE POSTTHERAPEUTIC NECK: PRELIMINARY RESULTS

E. Di Martino[1], G. Krombach[2], B. Nowak[3], M. Zimny[3], R. Hausman[1], B. Sellhaus[4], J. Haensel[1], M. Westhofen[1]

[1]Dept. of ENT Diseases and Plastic Head and Neck Surgery, Univ. of Aachen
[2]Dept. of Radiology, Univ. of Aachen
[3]Dept. of Nuclear Medicine , Univ. of Aachen
[4]Institute of Pathology, Univ. of Aacchen

Correspondence to: Ercole Di Martino M.D., Dept. of ENT Diseases and Plastic Head and Neck Surgery, Univ. of Aachen, Pauwelsstr. 30, D-52074 Aachen, Germany

INTRODUCTION

Advanced head and neck carcinomas have a high incidence of local recurrences and metastases. A regular posttherapeutic control of these patients is obligatory since the early detection of a recurrence is crucial for the further therapeutic strategy. Neck evaluation can be sometimes difficult because of scarrification and the lack or destruction of typical anatomic landmarks. Clinical examination is often inconlusive. The imaging procedures most frequently applied during the postoperative course are sonography and computed tomography.

As it was shown functional imaging by positron emission tomography can be of value in the detection of unknown primary tumor localisation and for the diagnosis of primary and recurrent head and neck disease .[1,2,3]

Sonography has gained a widespread acceptance due to the easy application, repeatability and high sensitivity. The diagnostic value of this method can be enhanced by the use of color duplex scanning. Vascularisation patterns can provide additional diagnostic information with regard to the dignity of a tumor. This study focuses on the value of color duplex sonography in posttherapeutic neck evaluation.

PATIENTS AND METHODS

In a non-randomized prospective study the necks of 40 patients with head and neck cancer were monitored posttherapeutically for a follow-up period up to 32 months by color duplex sonography, computed tomography, positron emission tomography and clinical examination.

The patients were seen monthly in the first year, every three months in the second and three times a year in the third year of follow-up. Sixty of eighty neck sides to be evaluated had previously undergone a neck dissection with subsequent radiotherapy. In the remaining necks a neck dissection only (n=14) or a radiochemotherapy was performed.

Color duplex sonography was performed with a variable transducer (5.2-9.0 MHz). The type of vascularisation detected in lymph nodes was decisive for the evaluation.[4] Computed tomography scans were obtained with a reconstruction thickness of 5 mm. In all patients an ionated contrast medium was applied. Scans were assessed along routine criteria such as diameter, signs of necrosis and irregular margins. Positron emission tomography was performed using F-18 fluoridedeoxyglucose. Regions with increased glucose metabolism were suspective for a recurrent disease. Histopathology was the golden standard for the evaluation of the diagnostic information obtained by the various procedures applied.

RESULTS

In 6/40 patients a recurrent disease was found in the neck. A total of 21 neck nodes were dissected. 76% showed histopathologically a recurrent disease. Seven of eighty neck sides were affected. The largest diameter of the malignant lymp nodes detected was 8-28 mm.

In the detection of these recurrences clinical neck examination had a sensitivity of 14%, specifity was 95%. Positive predictive value was 25% and negative predictive value was 92%. Sensitivity of CT and PET was 85% each. Specifity was found to be 97% for both procedures. PPV and NPV were 75% and 98% for these modalities. Color duplex sonography was able to detect all neck recurrences. The sensitivity was 100%. Specifity of this procedure was 95%. PPV and NPV were found to be 70% and 100% respectively.

DISCUSSION

The diagnosis of a recurrence can be significantly impaired by posttherapeutic tissue alterations. As palpation is not a reliable procedure, imaging techniques play an important role. Motion artifacts, dental fillings and superficial tumor spread impair the validity of Computed tomography and MRI. MRI has advantages in differentiation of tumor and scar but edema formation as often found after therapy can spoil diagnosis. The application of PET can be of value in these cases as a number of studies demonstrated. [5,6]

Color duplex sonographic imaging is a highly sensitive procedure that allows a differentiation of malignant and benign lymph nodes with a good specifity. The device used in this study was able to demonstrate the occurence of nodes with a size of 3 mm. The depiction of vascularisation patterns can be impaired in these nodes. Due to to the small size of vessels and the problem of finding the appropriate plane it was sometimes difficult to sufficiently evaluate the dignity of nodes with a diameter of 6mm and below. The malignant nodes found in our patients all had a size of at least 8 mm. In a number of patients nodes of a diameter of 10-14 mm showed normal vascularisation pattern. In all these cases the lymph nodes became smaller or dissapeared during the further course of the disease so they could be assumed to be benign lesions. The sonographic evaluation of the vascularisation was decisive not to perform a surgical intervention although size criteria alone would have justified an excision.

Due to the high sensitivity duplex sonography can detected lymph nodes earlier that other methods. So it is a valuable procedure in the postoperative follow-up. However sonography is as other methods unable to identify micrometastasis. It has to be assumed that some early lesions are overlooked, whatever method applied.

CONCLUSION

Anatomic imaging with vascular depiction by color duplex sonography was the most reliable diagnostic procedure for the detection of recurrence in the posttherapeutic neck. The excellent short term result has yet to be confirmed by a prolonged follow-up. In lymph nodes with a diameter of 6mm and below the specifity of the method can be impaired.

REFERENCES

1. Steinkamp HJ, Mäurer J, Cornehl M et al: Recurrent cervical lymphadenopathy: differential diagnosis with color-duplex sonography. Eur Arch Otorhinolaryngol 1994;251:404-409
2. Lell M, Baum U, Greess H et al.: Head and Neck tumors: imaging recurrent tumor and posttherapeutic changes with CT and MRI. Eur J Radiol 2000;33:239-247
3. Hanasono MM, Kunda LD, Segall GM et al: Uses and limitations of FDG positron emission tomography in patients with head and neck cancer Laryngoscope 1999;109:880-885
4. Leuwer RM, Westhofen M, Schade G: Color duplex echography in Head and Neck cancer. Am J Otolaryngol 1997;18:254-257
5. Sercarz JA, Bailet JW, Abermayor E et al: Computer coregistration of positron emission tomography and magnetic resonance imaging in head and neck cancer. Am J Otolaryngol 1998;19:130-135
6. Lonneux M, Lawson G, Die C et al: Positron Emission Tomography with Fluorodeoxyglucose for suspected Head and Neck Tumor recurrence in the symptomatic patient. Laryngoscope 2000;110:1493-1497

IS B-SONOGRAPHY A THERAPEUTIC GUIDELINE
IN THE „N0 NECK"?

C. Arens, H. Glanz, C. Popella Department of Otorhinolaryngology, University of Giessen, Germany

Keywords: ultrasound, N0 neck, micrometastasis

ABSTRACT

Background: Management of the suspected N0 neck in squamous cell carcinoma of the head and neck remains difficult and controversial. Precautionary neck dissection versus a conservative wait-and-see policy taking into account the risk of missing micrometastases have been discussed.

Methods. In a retrospective study we analyzed the pretherapeutic ultrasound (7.5MHz) examinations of 190 patients with histologically proven pN0 and pN1 neck dissection specimens.

Results. Out of 190 examined necks, 88% were correctly staged by B-sonography. Sensitivity amounted to 82% and specificity to 91%. The positive predictive value to correctly diagnose a metastasis by ultrasound was 80 %. The negative predicted value amounted to 91%.

Conclusion. As our results demonstrate, B-sonography in comparison to other imaging techniques can be considered an economical and reliable tool in the evaluation of the N0 neck but cannot be the therapeutic guideline in the N0 neck on ist own. Other parameters like differentiation, site and size of the primary cancer as well as lymph angiosis carcinomatosa of the primary have to be taken into account.

INTRODUCTION

The management of the suspected N0 neck in squamous cell carcinoma of the upper aerodigestive tract remains difficult and controversial. For many years, the aggressive but proven precautionary neck dissection versus a conservative wait-and-see policy taking into account the risk of missing micrometastases have been discussed. A frequency of occult metastases exceeding 15 – 20 % is considered to justify elective treatment of neck nodes in patients with squamous cell carcinoma of the upper aerodigestive tract.

Over the last two decades, ultrasound has become a very important and widely used tool for many clinicians in approaching this problem and has proven to be a valuable tool in detecting lymph nodes of the neck. On that basis, ultrasound has achieved an important function in the diagnostic work-up of patients with head and neck cancer. Despite the ability to detect lymph nodes down to 2 mm in diameter however, ultrasound misses micrometastasis. Mere detection of enlarged lymph nodes alone does not imply the presence of metastasis. This difficulty of differentiating between reactively enlarged and metastatic lymph nodes may lead to an increase in the number of false-positive results. Several authors published different relevant sonomorphological criteria for the detection of metastatically altered lymph nodes by B-sonography alone[1,2]. According to these criteria, sensitivity as well as specificity came close to 90%. At the same time, other techniques for the depiction and therapy of metastatic lymph nodes have been examined, e.g. sonographically guided cytology by van den Brekel et al[3] or color-coded duplex sonography by Rickert et al[4]. Werner et al[5] were more concerned about removing only sentinal lymph nodes in order to avoid more advanced neck dissection because of its side effects.

MATERIAL AND METHODS

In a retrospective study we analyzed the pretherapeutic ultrasound examinations of 190 patients with histologically proven pN0 and pN1 neck dissection specimens treated at our university hospital during the last 5 years in order to assess the value of B-sonography in the N0 neck. pN2 and pN3 neck were excluded. Sonographical results were compared to histopathological findings. All examinations were carried out with a frequency of 7.5 MHz. During ultrasound examinations, five different sonomorphological criteria for metastatic neck disease were applied: borders, echo pattern, hilus structure, shape and size. According to these criteria lymph nodes were diagnosed as being malignant when they presented a loss of the hilus structure, had a homogenous echo pattern and showed a more spheroid like shape. Increasing size and undefined borders of lymph nodes in the drainage of the primary were also considered as signs of metastatic settlement.

RESULTS

The distribution of primary cancer sites is shown in Table 1. Already 15% of pT1 carcinomas showed metastasis. 27% pT2 primaries were diagnosed with positive regional lymph nodes to the neck. The decreasing number of metastasis in pT4 tumors is due to the high number of laryngeal carcinomas in this group (Table 2).

Out of 190 neck dissection specimens analyzed, 88% were correctly staged by B-sonography. Sensitivity amounted to 82% and specificity to 91%. The positive predictive value to correctly diagnose a metastasis by ultrasound was 80 %. The negative predicted value amounted to 91% (Table 3). All 11 false negative cases showed lymph nodes smaller than 1 cm in diameter during ultrasound examination. Micrometastases were found in 3 of these cases with undifferentiated primaries. Six of these 11 false negative results were examined by

138

more or less experienced examiners. Nevertheless ultrasound depicted 82% of metastatic neck nodes. Furthermore, 83% of false positive ultrasound examinations presented lymph nodes larger 1 cm.

DISCUSSION

Until today, metastatic neck disease presents one of the most challenging problems in oncology of head and neck cancer. Cervical lymph node evaluation is an important part of the pretherapeutic staging procedure in patients with tumors of the upper aerodigestive tract. In addition to localization, size and spread of the primary tumor, the existence and the extent of lymph node metastases determine the prognosis of affected patients and influence treatment modalities. Therefore, an accurate pretherapeutic staging in patients with squamous cell carcinoma of the head and neck is necessary especially in the suspected N0 neck. Beside the use of fine needle aspiration biopsy or color-coded duplex sonography, B-sonography remains the most important imaging technique in the pretherapeutic assessment of the neck.

In the pretherapeutic assessment of head and neck cancer, sonomorphological criteria like borders, echo pattern, hilus structure, shape and size have been developed to be applied in the lymphatic drainage of suspected or known primaries. They may also be helpful in the detection of metastasis during post-therapeutic follow-up in cancer patients by a wait-and-watch strategy. The key criteria are loss of hilus structure, shape and echo pattern. The size of a lymph node alone may only indicate the probability of metastasis and therefore seems to be of minor importance. By taking only a 1 cm size limit into acount many lymph nodes are diagnosed as false positive and many metastases remain undiagnosed.

In 251 neck dissection Eichhorn[6] found 5747 lymph nodes. A positive predictive value of only 44% was obtained. By the use of 1 cm as a size criterion, as many as 42% of histologically diagnosed lymph node metastases were smaller than 1 cm. The evaluation of these lymph nodes even with the application of the above mentioned sonomorphological criteria as well as the application of duplex sonography or ultrasoundguided fine needle aspiration biopsy, is extremely difficult. Our smallest sonographically detected lymph node metastasis was 0.6 cm in maximum diameter.

Sonomorphological criteria may not be used in every routine examination of the neck. In applying these criteria to any pathologically enlarged lymph nodes, pit falls must be considered. During routine neck sonography, we observed four patients without cancer history presenting sonomorphological criteria of lymph node metastasis. Upon histological examination of the excised lymph nodes, evidence of follicular hyperplasia and sinus histiocytosis but no histological evidence of metastatic involvement was reported.

The criteria described should primarily be applied to lymph nodes between 5 and 15 mm in maximum diameter. Smaller lymph nodes are hard to classify. Larger lymph nodes develop central necrosis and become more inhomogenous. Furthermore, larger nodes tend to conglomerate with other reactive or metastatic nodes.

Our results clearly characterize the dilemma of the pretherapeutic assessment of the suspected N0 neck. 118 patients (62%) were treated electively without histologically proven lymph node metastasis. On the other hand, ultrasound led to a false diagnosis in 23 cases (12%). False negative results were related to histologically proven micrometastasis in three cases with sonographically diagnosed N0 necks in the drainage of a cancer. On primary ultrasound, there were no detectable lymph nodes at all. Micrometastasis however, remains a key problem. Even routine histopathological examination of neck dissection specimens like the gold standard fails to detect micrometastases. Ambrosch et al[7] found 7.9% micrometastasis in primarily staged pN0 neck dissection specimens. Six of these 8 micrometastases were located in lymph nodes 3 to 6 mm in diameter. Additionally, van den Breckel[8] found micrometastasis in elective neck dissection specimens for clinically N0 neck in 22%. On the other hand, elective neck treatment in histologically staged pN0 neck dissection specimens may show relapses in 2-4%. If ultrasound according to our results produces false negative results in 6% and histology misses micrometastasis by 8%, we will have to presume a development of metastasis in a not precautionarily treated neck of 14%. Therefore, a wait-and-see policy in suspected N0 necks will consequently lead to the development of metastases in some patients therefore requiring a close sonographic examination in 4-6 weeks intervals. Schipper et al[9] found that a wait-and-see strategy will not necessarily alter the prognosis when patients get a close follow-up by B-sonography.

CONCLUSION

Our results demonstrate, that B-sonography, in comparison to other imaging techniques, remains a cost-effective and reliable tool in the evaluation of the N0 neck. But B-sonography alone cannot be the only therapeutic guideline in the N0 neck. Other parameters like differentiation, site and size of the primary cancer as well as lymph angiosis carcinomatosa have to be taken into account. B-sonography is a diagnostic tool suitable for close follow-up in selected patients undergoing a wait-and-see concept. Whether precautionary neck dissection or a wait-and-see policy will be performed remains an individualized process. New sonographical technologies, e.g. high-frequency ultrasound or chirp-coded excitation, will improve B-sonography and decrease the risk of missing micrometastasis.

Table 1

Site of the primary	%
Floor of the mouth	16
Tongue	9
Oropharynx	27
Larynx	24
Hypopharynx	20
Other locations	4

Table 2

T-stage of the primary	n / %	% of metastases
pT1	36 / 19	15
pT2	67 / 35	27
pT3	42 / 22	48
pT4	45 / 24	33

140

Table 3

Histology N=190 B-Sonography	Positive n = 60	Negative n = 130
Positive n = 61	49(26%)	12(6%)
Negative n = 129	11(6%)	118(62%)

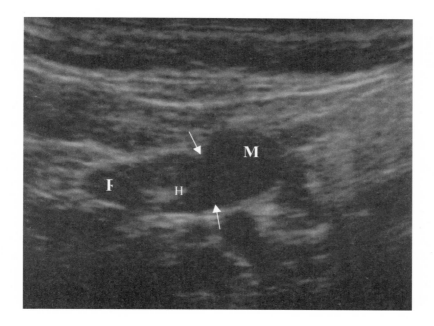

M - Metastatic lymph node
R - Reactive enlarged lymph node
H - Hilus strcture

B-sonography (7.5 MHz) of two lymph nodes in the drainage of an oropharyngeal cancer demonstrating the different sonomorphological criteria. In contrast to the reactive enlarged lymph node, metastasis presents a homogenous dark echo pattern, loss of the hilus structure and a spheroid shape. Arrows point out the border between both lymph nodes.

REFERENCES

1. Arens C, Popella C, Klimek T, Glanz H.: Sonomorphologic pattern of lymph node metastasis in head and neck cancer. Br J Cancer (77) Supplement1:14
2. Yusa H, Yoshida H, Ueno E.: Ultrasonographic criteria for diagnosis of cervical lymph node metastasis of squamous cell carcinoma in the oral and maxillofacial region. J Oral Maxillofac Surg. 1999 Jan;57(1):4
3. Van den Brekel MW, Reitsma LC, Quak JJ, Smeele LE, van der Linden JC, Snow GB, Castelijns JA.: Sonographically guided aspiration cytology of neck nodes for selection of treatment and follow-up in patients with N0 head and neck cancer. AJNR Am J Neuroradiol. 1999 Oct;20(9):1727-31.
4. Rickert D, Jecker P, Metzler V, Lehmann T, Ernst E, Westhofen M.: Color-coded duplex sonography of the cervical lymph nodes: improved differential diagnostic assessment after administration of the signal enhancer SH U 508A (Levovist) Eur Arch Otorhinolaryngol. 2000;257(8):453-8.
5. Werner JA, Dünne AA, Brandt D, Ramaswamy A, Kulkens C, Lippert BM, Folz BJ, Joseph K, Moll R.: Studies on significance of sentinel lymphadenectomy in pharyngeal and laryngeal carcinoma. Laryngorhinootologie. 1999 Dec;78(12):663-70.
6. Eichhorn T, Schroeder HG.: Ultrasound in metastatic neck disease. ORL J Otorhinolaryngol Relat Spec. 1993 Sep-Oct;55(5):258-62.
7. Ambrosch P, Kron M, Fischer G, Brinck U.: Micrometastases in carcinomas of the upper aerodigestive tract: detection, risk of metastasizing, and prognostic value of depth of invasion. Head Neck. 1995 Nov-Dec;17(6):473-9.
8. van den Brekel MW, van der Waal I, Meijer CJ, Freeman JL, Castelijns JA, Snow GB.: The incidence of micrometastases in neck dissection specimens obtained from elective neck dissections. Laryngoscope. 1996 Aug;106(8):987-91.
9. Schipper J, Gellrich NC, Marangos N, Maier W.: Value of B-image ultrasound in patients with carcinomas of the upper aerodigestive tract and N0 lymph node stage. Laryngorhinootologie. 1999 Oct;78(10):561-5.

99mTc-SESTAMIBI SPET VALUE IN DETECTING LYMPH NODES METASTASES IN HEAD AND NECK TUMORS: COMPARISON WITH CT AND SURGICAL RESULTS.

G. Almadori[1], J. Galli[1], G. Cadoni[1], L. Corina[1], M. L. Calcagni[2], A. Giordano[2]
[1]Institute of Otolaryngology, Università cattolica del Sacro Cuore, Rome, Italy
[2]Institute of Nuclear Medicine, Università cattolica del Sacro Cuore, Rome, Italy

Correspondence to: Prof. Giovanni Al madori, Ist. Clinica Otorinolaringoiatria, Università Cattolica del Sacro Cuore, Largo A. Gemelli, 8, 00168 Roma, Phone: 039630154439, Fax 03963051194

ABSTRACT

Background. CT is the diagnostic technique most frequently employed in the preoperative staging of head and neck tumors. It has some limitations especially in the differential diagnosis between reactive and metastatic lymph nodes. Recently oncotropic capacity of some radiotracers currently used in clinical practice, i.e. perfusion tracers , has been reported. The aim of this study was to verify the diagnostic accuracy of 99mTc-sestamibi SPET in assessing neck nodes metastases.

Methods. 24 patients (age range 40-75, 22 males, 2 females) with head and neck tumors underwent 99mTc-sestamibi SPET and CT before surgery . The sites of primary lesions were as follows: oral cavity (n=6), nasopharynx (n=1), oropharynx (n=4), hypopharynx (n=3), larynx (n=10). Scintigraphy procedure required: injection of 740 MBq of 99mTc-Sestamibi, dynamic acquisition during the injection, planar scintigraphy at 5 minutes and 2-3 hours post-injection (in order to evaluate tracer wash-out), SPET scintigraphy at 15 minutes post-injection evaluation of the images to detect the primary tumors and lymph-nodes metastases.

Results. Detailed results of SPET and CT in detecting lymph-nodes metastases has been examined. Sensibility, specificity and accuracy were 80%, 82%, 82%, respectively, for SPET and 80%, 58% 65%, respectively, for CT. In most cases SPET diagnosis was achieved by analysing the coronal slices only. Planar scintigraphic images were negative in 85% of primary tumors and in 100% of lymph nodes metastases.

Conclusions. Our data show that 99mTc-sestamibi SPET is more accurate than CT in detecting lymph nodes metastases, thus SPET seems better suited than CT to identify at the time of diagnosis a subset of patients to submit to neck dissection. This preliminary study suggests that this scintigraphic procedure can have a possible role in the preoperative staging and treatment of head and neck cancer patients and in the follow-up, as a complementary technique to CT scan and its possible widespread clinical application in a near future is envisaged.

INTRODUCTION

In recent years, together with the clinical and endoscopic evaluation, diagnostic imaging (CT,MRI, sonography, color-Doppler US) has been commonly used in the study of head and neck tumors[1].

In fact, these procedures enable the noninvasive assessment of the local extent and volume of primary tumor, its regional infiltration, the in-depth invasion and the tumor relationship with adjacent structures for a more careful clinical staging in support of therapeutic decision-making[1,2].

Even if these procedures are increasingly sophisticated and of high definition, some diagnostic problems are still to be solved. Among them, the most important are the characterization between reactive or metastatic laterocervical adenopathies, the search for occult metastases in N0 cases and the identification of postoperative and/or post-radiochemotherapy recurrence, occult primary tumors and distant metastases, the latter simultaneously to the study of primary tumor[3,4].

Recently, the advanced technology has allowed the use of diagnostic nuclear medicine in oncology. The methods applied in still limited series have been [18]FDG PET, 11c-methionine, L-tyrosine immunoscintigraphy with radiolabeled monoclonal antibodies and very recently SPET with positive indicators (^{201}Tl, ^{99m}Tc-sestamibi or [99m]Tetrofosmin). Among these procedures, PET is the most sophisticated as for the image quality, definition, sensitivity and specificity of results[5-10], but its widespread use is prevented by high costs, complex management and poor availability on the national territory of adequate machines and relative cyclotrons. Immunoscintigraphy already suggested in literature with the use of aspecific monoclonal ^{111}In labeled anti-CEA[11-13] and subsequently with specific monoclonal antibodies (E48, U36) against squamous cell head and neck carcinomas, even if interesting in perspective and of high diagnostic specificity, seems useful in therapy as radioimmunotherapy with encouraging preliminary results on minimal residual tumors[14].

Recently oncotropic capacity of some radiodrugs currently used in clinical practice, i.e. perfusion tracers (^{99m}Tc-sestamibi, ^{201}Tl), has been detected[15].

The aim of this study was to verify the diagnostic accuracy of 99mTc-sestamibi SPET in assessing neck nodes metastases and to pinpoint the pattern of identification in SPET images through their comparative evaluation with specifically morphologic procedures as spiral CT.

144

MATERIAL AND METHODS

24 patients (age range 40-75, 22 males, 2 females) with head and neck tumors underwent 99mTc-sestamibi SPET before surgery. The sites of primary lesions were as follows: oral cavity (n=6), nasopharynx (n=1), oropharynx (n=4), hypopharynx (n=3), larynx (n=10). The nodal conditions (benign or malignant involvement) was known in 22 patients thanks to a neck dissection (in 14/22 patients) or to a follow-up lasting at least one year (8/22 patients). CT results were available in 17 of these patients. Overall 5 patients showed a malignant involvement at histopathological examination of surgical specimen. Scintigraphic procedure required: injection of 740 MBq of 99mTc SestaMIBI, dynamic acquisition during the injection, planar scintigraphy in anterior view at 5 minutes and 2-3 hours post-injection (in order to evaluate tracer wash-out), SPET scintigraphy at 15 minutes post-injection, evaluation of the images to detect the primary tumors and lymph-nodes metastases. Transverse, coronal and sagittal tomographic sections were reconstructed by filtered back-projection. The images were read by two experts (A.G and M.L.C.) who were not informed of the clinical conditions of the patients. Discrepancies in evaluation were solved by joint re-evaluation.

RESULTS

Detailed results of SPET and CT in detecting lymph-nodes metastases has been examined. Significant uptake of 99mTc-Sestamibi was observed in 4 out of 5 patients with malignant limphnodal involvement. Overall SPET results are reported in Table 1 as compare to CT data. Sensibility, specificity and accuracy for detection of lymph nodes metastases were 80%, 82%, 82%, respectively, for SPET and 80%, 58% 65%, respectively, for CT. In most cases SPET diagnosis was achieved by analysing the coronal slices only. Planar scintigraphic images were negative in 85% of primary tumors and in 100% of lymph nodes metastases.

DISCUSSION

At present a major problem in the prognosis of head and neck tumours is the assessment of lymph node status. Clinical examination and computerized tomography (CT), the diagnostic technique most frequently employed in the preoperative staging of head and neck tumors, do not readily discriminate between reactively enlarged and early infiltrated lymph nodes. SPET is an interesting procedure in the diagnosis of tumors of head and neck region both for its technical ability to rapidly acquire planar images with their 3D reconstruction according to axial, coronal and sagittal planes and the availability in the clinical practice of perfusion tracers as ^{201}Tl, ^{99m}Tc-sestamibi, ^{99m}Tc-tetrofosmin recently shown to be endowed of good tropism for tumors of numerous organs and apparatus[16,17].

These radiopharmaceuticals were originally used as indicators of blood flow in myocardial scintigraphy, whose peculiar ability to be electively taken up by various tumors in time, was evidenced. Their uptake and subsequent cellular retention seems to be proportional to the amount of blood flow and cell metabolism, phenomena which occur during tumor growth in relation with the frequent neoangiogenesis and high metabolism of rapid cellular duplication. This involves the activation of mitochondrial functions, which, in case of sestamibi, seem responsible for its retention[16].

Valdes Olmos et al. have recently reported the results achieved in a large series of 79 patients with head and neck tumors, and stressed the validity of ^{201}Tl SPET, in the diagnosis, preoperative staging and post chemoradiotherapy and/or surgery restaging and its possible use together with conventional morphological procedures (CT, MRI) to gather additional clinicodiagnostic and therapeutic information. The authors also stressed the high ^{201}Tl affinity for neoplastic cells as indicator of active tumor proliferation.

As for head and neck tumors, there are no homogeneous data on the efficacy of ^{99m}Tc-sestamibi except for those reported by Pui et al.[10] and Kostakoglu et al.[18] concerning the diagnosis and response to radiochemotherapy respectively in patients with rhinopharyngeal carcinoma.

The preliminary results of our still small series seem encouraging.

As for primary tumors, we observed a good affinity of the method and tracer for all head and neck regions under study and the role of SPET in the differentiation of neoplastic tissue from the physiologic high uptake of salivary glands, thyroid and nasal region thanks to the tomographic features of the technique here employed. The rather poor diagnostic performance of dynamic and planar scintigraphic imaging are not surprising due to the inherent 2D characteristics of these types of imaging.

Most of metastatic adenopathies were also correctly diagnosed by sestamibi SPET as confirmed by histology and showing the potentials of the procedure in the differentiation of reactive and metastatic lymphadenopathies. The single false positive case is an evidence of the possible main limitation of the procedure, namely the presence of similar functional aspects also in non neoplastic pathologic conditions. In fact, active inflammatory lesions or repair or regeneration processes may also show increased blood flow and increased cell metabolism with consequent high uptake of tracer[16].

Furthermore, concerning the follow-up of patients after radiochemotherapy or surgery, this procedure might improve the still non optimal specificity of conventional morphological exams (CT and MRI) (Paulus, Valdes) together with the possible simultaneous diagnosis of multiple synchronous tumors, distant metastases and micrometastasis in N0 cases to optimize N treatment (over or under treatment)[19].

The advantages of ^{99m}Tc-sestamibi SPET are represented by its low invasiveness, optimum tolerance and very promising specificity and diagnostic accuracy.

Whether its limitations (poor anatomic detail, inadequate information on the relationships with adjacent structures, depth invasion and number of involved lymph nodes, still non optimum spatial resolution) rule out a generalized diagnostic application, is still to be assessed.

CONCLUSIONS

Our data show that 99mTc-sestamibi SPET is more accurate than CT in detecting lymph nodes metastases, thus SPET seems superior to identify at the time of diagnosis a subset of patients to submit to neck dissection. This preliminary study suggests that this scintigraphic procedure seems to afford a valid contribution in the preoperative staging of head and neck cancer patients as a complementary technique to CT scan. Additional studies on larger series are necessary for a careful comparison betwen SPET, histopathology findngs, CT and MRI and the analysis of involved lymph node location. The improvement in spatial resolution and a better knowledge of how tracer uptake and wash-out occur and their possible diagnostic role (different uptake, tracer retention and wash-out between neoplastic and non neoplastic lesions, possible correlation with tumor angiogenesis) will probably confirm the role of the method in the clinical practice.

Table 1. Results of SPET and CT in detecting lynph nodes metastases

	TRUE POSITIVES	TRUE NEGATIVES	FALSE POSITIVES	FALSE NEGATIVES
SPET (in 22 pts)	4	14	3	1
CT (in 17 cases)	4	7	5	1

REFERENCES

1. Dillon W.P., Harnsberger H.R. The impact of radiologic imaging on staging of cancer of the head and neck. Semin Oncol 1991; 18: 64-79.
2. Madison M.T., Remley K.B., Latchaw R.E., Mitchell S.L. Radiologic diagnosis and staging of head and neck squamous cell carcinoma. Radiol Clin North Am 1994; 32: 163-181.
3. Cole I., Chu J., Kos S., et al. Metastatic carcinoma in the neck: a clinical, computerized tomography scan and ultrasound study. Aust N Z J Surg 1993; 63: 468-474.
4. Valdes Olmos R.A., Balm A.J.M., Hilgers F.J.M., Koops W., Loftus B.M., Tan I.B., Muller S.H., Hoefnagel C.A., Gregor R.T. Thallium-201 SPECT in the diagnosis of head and neck cancer. J Nucl Med 1997; 38: 873-879.
5. Bailet J.W., Abemayor E., Jabour B.A., et al.: Positron emission tomography: a new, precise imaging modality for detection of primary head and neck tumors and assessment of cervical adenopathy. Laryngoscope 1992; 102: 281-288.
6. Casani A., Vannucci G., Fattori B., Ursino F., Sellari-Franceschini S., Neri E., Piragine F. Indicazioni e limiti della diagnostica endoscopica e per immagini nella patologia del rinofaringe e loro correlazioni. In: Piragine F.: Endoscopia e diagnostica per immagini in otorinolaringoiatria. REL. UFFIC. LXXXVI Congr. Naz. S.I.O., Venezia 26-29 Maggio 1999, ed. Pacini, 235-267.
7. Anzai Y., Carroll W.R., Quint D.J., et al.: Recurrence of head andneck cancer after surgery or irradiation: prospective comparision of 2-deoxy-2(^{18}F)fluoro-D-glucose PET and MR imaging diagnoses. Radiology 1996; 200: 135-141.
8. Davis J.P., Maisey N.M., Chevreton E.B. Positron emission tomography: a useful imaging technique for otolaryngology, head and neck surgery? J Laryngol Otol 1998; 112: 125-127.
9. Paulus P., Sambon A., Vivegnis D., Hustinx R., Moreau P., Collignon J., Deneufbourg J.M., Rigo P. 18FDG-PETfor the assessment of primary head and neck tumors: clinical, computed tomography, and histopathological correlation in 38 patients. Laryngoscope 1998; 108: 1578-1583.
10. Pui M.H., Du J.Q., Yuch T.C., Zeng S.Q. Imaging of nasopharyngeal carcinoma with Tc-99m MIBI. Clin Nucl Med 1998; 23: 29-32.
11. Galli J., Almadori G., Paludetti G., Giordano A., De Rossi G., Maurizi M. Immunoscintigrafia nella diagnosi e nel follow-up delle neoplasie della testa e del collo. In: Attualità nella ricerca sperimentale in otorinolaringoiatria. XII Congreso Nazionale Soc. Ital. Ped., S. Tecla 1992; 281-284.
9. Maurizi M., De Rossi G., Giordano A., Almadori G., Galli J., Cadoni G., Rosignoli M., Paludetti G. Immunoscintigraphy in head and neck tumors: preliminary results.Acta Med Rom 1993; 31: 354-360.

10. De Rossi G., Maurizi M., Almadori G., Di Giuda D., Paludetti G., Cadoni G., Ottaviani F., Galli J. The contribution of immunoscintigraphy to the diagnosis of head and neck tumors. Nucl Med Commun 1997; 18: 10-16.

11. De Bree R., Kuik D.J., Quak J.J., Roos J.C., van den Brekel M.W.M., Castelijns J.A., van Wagtendonk F.W., Greuter H., Snow G.B., van Dongen G.A.M.S. The impact of tumour volume and other characteristics on uptake of radiolabeled monoclonal antibodies in tumour tissue of head and neck cancer patients. Eur J Nucl Med 1998; 25: 1562-1565.

12. Maublant J., de-Latour M., Mestas D., et al. Technetuium-99m—SestaMIBI uptake in breast tumor and associated lymph nodes. J Nucl Med 1996; 37: 922-925.

13. Chisin R. Nuclear medicine in head and neck oncology: reality and perspectives. J Nucl Med 1999; 40: 91-95.

14. Leitha T., Galser C., Pruckmayer M., Rasse M., Millesi W., Lang S., Nasel C., Backfrieder W., Kainberger F. Technetium-99m-MIBI in primary and recurrent head and neck tumors: contribution of bone SPECT image fusion. The Journal of Nuclear Medicine 1998; Vol. 39 (7): 1166-1171.

15. Kostakoglu L., Uysal U:, Ozyar E., Hayran M., Uzal D., Demirkazik F.B., Kars A., Atahan L., Bekdik C.F. Monotoring response to therapy with Thallium-201 and Technetium-99m-SestaMIBI SPECT in nasopharyngeal carcinoma. J Nucl Med 1997; 38: 1009-1014.

16. Myers L.L., Wax M.K., Nabi H., Simpson G.T., Lamonica D. Positron emission tomography in the evaluation of the N0 neck. Laryngoscope 1998; 108: 232-236.

148

F18-FDG DETECTION OF LYMPH NODE METASTASES IN HEAD AND NECK CANCER WITH A DUAL-HEAD COINCIDENCE CAMERA: ABSENCE OF BENEFIT IN A ROUTINE CLINICAL SETTING

Robert J.J. van Es MD, DMD[1]; Sem Gonesh MD, DMD[1]; Peter P. van Rijk MA, MD, PhD[2]; Pieter J. Slootweg MD, DMD, PhD[3]; Ron Koole MD, DMD, PhD[1]

[1]Department of Oral and Maxillofacial Surgery, University Medical Center Utrecht the Netherlands
[2]Department of Nuclear Medicine, University Medical Center Utrecht the Netherlands
[3]Department of Pathology, University Medical Center Utrecht the Netherlands

Running title: Dual-head F18-FDG lymph node detection

Keywords: oral cancer; oropharyngeal cancer, FDG-PET, cervical lymph node detection; dual-head coincidence camera

Correspondence to: *R. J. J. van Es, MD, DMD, Department of Oral and Maxillofacial Surgery, University Medical Center Utrecht the Netherlands, PO box 85.500, 3508 GA Utrecht, the Netherlands, Phone: ++33 30-2507751, Fax: ++31 30-2541922 (e-mail: omfsurg@kmb.azu.nl)*

ABSTRACT

Background. Accurate detection of lymph node metastases in patients with head and neck cancer is important for both prognosis and treatment planning. The application of F18-FDG detection with dedicated PET scanners is limited to specialized centers and not applicable in a routine clinical setting. In a previous pilot study the use of a dual-head coincidence camera proved to be superior to conventional imaging and was cost effective. The current investigation assesses the clinical value of routine dual-head PET scanning using F18-FDG, in the staging of head and neck cancer.

Methods. This prospective study included 117 patients who had received surgery as primary therapy for oral or oropharyngeal squamous cell carcinomas. Group I: 19 patients with resection of the primary tumor only and follow-up of the neck >1 year. Group II: 98 patients in whom 130 neck dissections had been performed. Histological assessment of the size and number of cervical lymph node metastases was carried out. Preoperative staging

149

with CT scan, ultrasound and F18-FDG imaging with a dual-head coincidence gamma camera in a routine clinical setting was undertaken.

Results. Group I:1 patient died postoperatively and 2 (11%) patients developed nodal metastases 0.5-1.0 years postoperatively, despite a PET-negative neck. Group II: 19 false positive and 18 false negative necks, with sensitivity: 55%, specificity: 79%, positive predictive value: 54%, negative predictive value: 80% and accuracy: 72%. Diameters of missed metastases ranged from 0.5-20 mm (average 7.7 ± 4.9 mm), of which 39% ≤5 mm and 69% ≤10 mm.

Conclusion. F18-FDG imaging with a dual-head coincidence camera does not improve neck staging when CT-scanning and ultrasound are applied, and therefore the problem of accurate assessment of the N0 neck in a routine clinical setting remains to be solved.

INTRODUCTION

The development of the first dedicated Positron Emission Tomography (PET) scanner by Phelps et al. in 1976, marked a new era in the application of positron emitting radionuclides for use in medical imaging.[1] In 1991, Strauss and Conti demonstrated that F18-fluoro-deoxy-glucose (FDG) is metabolically trapped in the intracellular space, and can be used to identify tumors using PET based on accelerated glycolytic rates.[2]

In the 1990s, several studies demonstrated a possible value of the application of FDG-detection with dedicated PET scanners in head and neck oncology with respect to:
1. Initial diagnosis and treatment planning.
2. Treatment monitoring and detection of recurrent disease.

Accurate identification of neck node metastases plays a crucial role in prognosis and choice of therapy for the patient with a head and neck squamous cell carcinoma (HNSCC). Several studies applying F18-FDG detection in HNSCC in recent years have been successful in imaging cervical lymph node metastasis.[3-8] Sensitivities varied from 70-90%, specificities varied from 85-100% and the accuracy proved 80-95%. However, the costs of a complete PET-center including the dedicated PET scanner, the cyclotron and laboratory facilities are high. Therefore, since it is not practicable in a routine clinical setting, PET scanning for HNSCC is at present limited to specialized medical centers and is not part of the standard diagnostic program.[8, 9]

In 1994, Drane et al. reported the construction of a detection system using two modified standard gamma cameras, which could be used for both positron and normal gamma imaging.[10] This system became known as a "dual-head coincidence camera". To improve detection efficiency of the camera which is about 10% compared to the dedicated PET-scanners, ultra high-energy collimators, increased sodium iodide crystal thickness and new high-count rate digital electronics were applied.[11] In a pilot study by Stokkel et al., the preoperative assessment of neck node metastasis with this dual head coincidence camera yielded a sensitivity of 96% and specificity of 90%, which seemed comparable to the diagnostic quality of the dedicated PET scanners.[12] The question remained as to whether this

150

would be a technique of choice, accurate enough for routine practice in the preoperative staging of the neck. The following prospective study was carried out in order to provide an answer to this problem.

PATIENTS AND METHODS

Patients. From September 1997 to December 1999, 117 patients with oral or oropharyngeal SCC's (56 male and 62 female; age 36-85 years) who received surgery as primary therapy, were included in this study. Nineteen patients received only resection of the primary tumor (Group I). The other 98 patients (Group II) also underwent a neck dissection, which was bilateral in 32 cases. This made a total of 130 neck dissections.

PET-imaging. All patients underwent morphologic imaging 2-4 weeks before surgery with a dual-head coincidence PET scanner, using 130-185 MBq (3.5-5 mCi) F18-FDG. Patients fastened for 6 hours before scanning and serum glucose levels were tested. A serum glucose level between 4.0 and 10.0 mmol/l was required. For PET imaging a dual-head coincidence camera (Vertex-MCD ADAC, Milpitas, USA) was used. Acquisition involved rotation of each detector 180° with 32 stops at 45 sec per stop. Images were visually analyzed by experienced nuclear physicians unaware of the patient's history and of the findings of other imaging results.

Histology. In group II, histopathological specimens were routinely assessed. At pathology examination, the size and number of lymph node metastases were recorded in each individual neck.

Analysis. The necks of all 19 patients with only local tumor treatment (Group I) were followed up for at least 1 year to check for the development of lymph node metastases (i.e. conversions). The results of the preoperative FDG-PET scans were compared with the results of histopathological findings. Effectiveness of detection was expressed in terms of sensitivity, specificity, positive predictive value, negative predictive value and accuracy. Statistical significance was defined as $p \leq 0.05$.

RESULTS

In group I, 1 patient died postoperatively, leaving 18 patients for analysis. There were 13 T1, 2 T2 and 3 T4 tumors (Table 1.). During follow-up 3 necks developed nodal metastases in 3 patients: One patient with a SCC of the buccal mucosa had a positive PET scan preoperatively but the other 2(11%) patients with pT1 SCC's of the maxilla and soft palate respectively, had initial negative PET-scans.

In group II, there were 31 T1, 22 T2, 10 T3 and 35 T4 tumors (Table 1.). Of the 130 neck dissections in group II, 22 were true positive 19 false positive, 18 false negative and 71 true negative. This resulted in a sensitivity of 55%, a specificity of 79%, a positive predictive value of 54%, a negative predictive value of 80% and an accuracy of 72% (Table 2.). There was no significant difference in plasma glucose levels between these subgroups.

Of the 18 false negative necks, 6 (33%) contained only nodal metastases ≤5 mm in diameter. Three FDG-negative necks contained necrotic rest suggesting remnants of lymph node metastases. In all, 36 lymph node metastases were missed with dual-head PET, ranging in diameter from 0.5 to 20.0 mm, with an average of 7.7 ± 4.9 mm. Of the missed nodes, 39% proved ≤5 mm and 69% were ≤10 mm.

DISCUSSION

After initial optimism in applying PET detection for neck node metastases, we now have to weigh up the value of implementing this imaging modality in routine clinical practice. Considering its relatively low costs, the dual-head coincidence camera would seem an attractive option. However, its sensitivity and accuracy prove less satisfactory in this prospective study, when compared to earlier pilot studies.[12] This may be related to the routine of every day practice in this prospective investigation versus optimal study conditions, high alertness of PET-dedicated nuclear physicians or bias due to patient selection during a pilot study. When compared to studies with dedicated PET scanners, the less favorable results of the dual-head coincidence camera may also be due to the inferior detection capacity, the lower count-rate capability and a longer acquisition time leading to movement artifacts.[11, 13]

However, even dedicated PET scanning has its limitations: Paulus et al.[14] obtained a sensitivity of only 50% in assessing lymph node metastases of pharyngeal SCC and Lerut et al.[15] obtained a sensitivity of 22% with an accuracy of only 48% in lymph node staging of oesophageal SCC. Problems of accurate imaging are related to:
1. Overshadowing of metastases by the primary tumor. Intense tracer accumulation and ill-defined anatomical boundaries of the primary tumor which interfere with accurate discrimination of lymph node metastases nearby.[15]
2. Insufficient accumulation of activity in small metastases or extensive tumor necrosis, resulting in a reduced glucose metabolism and uptake of F18-FDG with a negative PET imaging result.[7] Others also report difficulties in detection of unknown primaries and lymph node metastases smaller than 5-10 mm, in spite of the use of dedicated PET scanners.[13, 14, 16] In our material, 40% of the missed metastases was smaller than 5 mm and almost 70% was smaller than 10 mm. Owing to the limits in resolution of the dual-head coincidence camera, this would theoretically result in a sensitivity of 85% at most, when all metastases larger than 5 mm indeed were detected.
3. Background FDG activity due to swallowing or contraction of neck muscles.
4. A substantial inter-observer variation in interpretation of the images, probably related to the experience of the nuclear physician.[15] Indeed, revision of all dual-head coincidence PET scans in this study by a PET-dedicated nuclear physician improved the accuracy of the images substantially.

Although imaging of neck node metastases with the dual-head coincidence camera is less appropriate, this camera does seem to play a role in head and neck cancer with respect to treatment monitoring following chemo-radiotherapy[17] and in detection of unknown primaries.[18] In the future, fusion of PET and CT-scan images may prove to be a valuable technique.[19]

CONCLUSION

Considering the relatively marginal improvement of neck staging when already applying routine CT-scan and ultrasound as well as the significant costs of F18-FDG PET scanning even using dual-head cameras, it is concluded that dual-head FDG-PET has not yet solved the problem of accurate staging of the N0 neck in a routine clinical setting

Table 1. Tumor sites and stages

Tumor stage	Group I	Group II
T1	13	31
T2	2	22
T3	0	10
T4	4	35
N0	19	58
PN1	-	16
PN2	-	24
Sites		
Tongue	7	21
Floor of mouth	3	35
Mandible	0	22
Maxilla	5	2
Oropharynx	2	10
Other	2	8
Total	19	98

Table 2. Group II, Comparison of PET and histology

		HISTOLOGY		
		+	–	
PET	+	22	19	41
	–	18	71	89
Total		40	90	130

Sensitivity	55%	
Specificity	79%	
	PPV	54%
	NPV	80%
Accuracy	72%	

REFERENCES

1. Phelps ME, Hoffman EJ, Mullani N, Higgins CS, Ter-Poggosian MM. Design considerations for a positron emission transaxial tomograph (PET III). IEE Trans Biomed Eng 1976;23:516-22.
2. StrausLG, Conti PS. The applications of PET in clinical oncology. J Nucl Med 1991;32:623-48.
3. Braams JW, Pruim J, Freling NJM, Nikkels PGJ, Roodenburg JLN, Boering G et al. Detection of lymph node metastases of squamous cell cancer of the head and neck with FDG-PET and MRI. J Nucl Med 1995;36:211-216.
4. Laubenbacher C, Saumweber D, Wagner-Manslau C, Kau RJ, Herz M, Avril N, Ziegler S, Kruschke C, Arnold W, Schwaiger M. Comparison of fluorine-18-fluorodeoxyglucose PET, MRI and endoscopy for staging head and neck squamous-cell carcinomas. J Nucl Med 1995;36:1747-1757.
5. Myers LL, Wax MK, Nabi H, Simpson GT, Lamonica D. Positron emission tomography in the evaluation of the N0 neck. Laryngoscope 1998;108:232-226.

6. Adams S, Baum RP, Stuckensen T, Bitter K, Hor G. Prospective comparison of 18F-FDG PET with conventional imaging modalities (CT, MRI, US) in lymph node staging of head and neck cancer. Eur J Nucl Med 1998;25:1255-1260.

7. Kau RJ, Alexiou C, Laubenbacher C, Werner M, Schwaiger M, Arnold W. Lymph node detection of head squamous cell carcinomas by positron emission tomography with fluorodeoxyglucose F 18 in a routine clinical setting. Arch Otolaryngol Head Neck Surg 1999;125:1322-1328.

8. Di Martino E, Nowak B, Krombach GA, Selhaus B, Hausmann R, Cremerius U, Bull U, Westhofen M. Results of pretherapeutic lymph node diagnosis in head and neck tumors. Clinical value of 18 18-FDG positron emission tomography. Laryngorhinootologie 2000;79:201-206.

9. Kau RJ, Alexiou C. Stimmer H, Arnold W. Diagnostic procedures for detection of lymph node metastases in cancer of the larynx. ORL J Otorhinolaryngol Relat Spec 2000;64:199-203.

10. Drane WE, Abbott FD, Nicole MW, Mastin CNMTST, Kuperus JH. Technology for FDG SPECT with a relatively inexpensive gamma camera. Radiology 1994;191:461-465.

11. Jarrit PH, Acton PD. PET imaging using gamma camera systems: a review. Nucl Med Commun 1996;17:758-766.

12. Stokkel MT, ten Broek FW, van Rijk PP. Preoperative assessment of cervical lymph nodes in head and neck cancer with fluorine-18 fluorodeoxyglucose using a dual-head coincidence camera: a pilot study. Eur J Nucl Med 1999;26:499-503.

13. Budinger TF. PET instrumentation: what are the limits? Semin Nucl Med 1998;28:247-267.

14. Paulus P, Sambon A, Vivegnis D, Hustinx R, Moreau P, Collignon J, Deneufbourg JM, Rigo P. 18FDG-PET for the assessment of primary head and neck tumors: clinical, computed tomography, and histopathological correlation in 38 patients. Laryngoscope 1998;108:1578-1583.

15. Lerut T, Flamen P, Ectors N, Van Cutsem E, Peeters M, Hiele M, De Wever W, Coosemans W, Decker G, De Leyn P, Deneffe G, Van Raemdonck D, Mortelmans L. Histopathologic validation of lymph node staging with FDG-PET scan in cancer of the esophagus and gastroesophageal junction: a prospective study based on primary surgery with extensive lymadenectomy. Ann Surg 2000;232:743-752.

16. Greven KM, Keyes JW, Williams DW, McGuirt WF, William TJ. Occult primary tumors of the head and neck. Lack of benefit from positron emission tomography imaging with 2-[F-18]fluor-2-deoxy-D-glucose. Cancer 1999;86:115-118.

17. Kostakoglu L, Uysal U, Ozyar E, Hayran M, Uzal D, Demirkazik FB, Kars A, Atahan L, Bekdik CF. Monitoring response to therapy with thallium-201 and technetium-99m-sestamibi SPECT in nasopharyngeal carcinoma. Nucl Med 1997;38:1009-1014.

18. Stokkel MP, Terhaard CH, Hordijk GJ, van Rijk PP.The detection of unknown primary tumors in patients with cervical metastases by dual-head positron emission tomography. Oral Oncol 1999;35B:390-394.

19. Faulhaber P, Nelson A, Mehta L, O'Donnell J The fusion of anatomic and physiologic tomographic images to enhance accurate interpretation. Clin Positron Imaging 2000;3:178.

THE PRELIMINARY RESULTS OF FDG-PET IN SCREENING FOR DISTANT METASTASES AND SYNCHRONOUS PRIMARY TUMORS BELOW THE CLAVICLES IN PATIENTS WITH HEAD AND NECK CANCER AT INITIAL EVALUATION.

Remco de Bree, MD [1], Jolijn Brouwer, MD [1], Emile F.I. Comans, MD [2], Otto S. Hoekstra, MD [2], Gordon B. Snow, MD [1], Charles R. Leemans, MD[1]
Departments of [1] Otolaryngology / Head and Neck Surgery and [2] Nuclear Medicine / PET center, VU Medical Center, Amsterdam, The Netherlands

Correspondence to*: R. De Bree, MD, Department of Otolaryngology / Head and neck surgery, VU Medical Center, P.O. Box 7057, 1007 MB, Amsterdam, The Netherlands, Phone: +31 20 4443690, Fax: +31 20 4443688*

The detection of distant metastases at the time of initial evaluation influences the prognosis and the selection of treatment modality in patients with head and neck squamous cell carcinoma (HNSCC). Distant metastases usually occur late during the course of disease. The lungs, bone and liver are the most frequent sites of distant metastases. Patients with distant metastases are generally not considered curable and often receive only palliative treatment. No effective systemic treatment for disseminated HNSCC is currently available.

The overall incidence of clinically detected distant metastases in HNSCC is 4% to 26%, while the incidence found at presentation in HNSCC patients with advanced stage disease is 7% to 12%.[1,2] Comparison of the incidence found at initial evaluation and the incidence found during follow up indicate that a lot of distant metastases are missed at initial evaluation. It is considered that distant metastases in HNSCC patients who achieved loco-regional control develop because of distant spreading that is already present when treatment of locoregional tumor is carried out.

In a previous study[2] we evaluated the value of screening for distant metastases retrospectively in 101 patients with advanced stage HNSCC, scheduled for major surgery, who underwent chest X-ray, CT scan of the thorax, ultrasound or CT scan of the liver and bone scintigraphy. We identified several risk factors for development of distant metastases: three or more lymph node metastases, bilateral lymph node metastases, lymph node metastases of 6 cm or larger, low jugular lymph node metastases, locoregional recurrence and second primary tumors.

155

Because almost all (94%) of the patients with distant metastases had metastases in the thorax, we concluded that CT scan of the thorax was the single most important technique that was available at that time for screening for distant metastases in HNSCC patients. Besides lung metastases, a CT scan of the thorax can also detect primary lung cancer, mediastinal lymph node metastases, bone metastases in vertebrae and ribs, and can also be extended to the liver. Therefore, our policy in HNSCC patients with aforementioned risk factors was CT scan of the thorax only.

Recently we analyzed the follow up results of the 84 patients with initially negative screening (unpublished data). Forty-nine patients died of disease (median 11 months, range 1 to 46 months) and 15 patients died due to other causes (median 10 months, range 2 to 41 months). The median follow up of the other 20 patients was 56 months (range 2 to 82 months). Eighteen patients developed distant metastases. In 15 patients these distant metastases were found within 12 months. The sites of the distant metastases were lungs (n=11), bone (n=6), liver (n=2), brain (n=2) and mediastinum (n=1). Of these 18 patients 12 developed locoregional recurrence. Nine of those patients had locoregional recurrence at the time of detection of distant metastases. Of the 6 patients without locoregional recurrence at the time of detection of distant metastases 4 were diagnosed within 12 months after screening. If it is considered that major surgery with curative intent is senseless when distant metastases become manifest within 12 months at least 4 patients underwent unnecessary extensive treatment.

Also second primary tumors have impact on survival and may alter the selection of therapy in HNSCC patients. Second primary tumors occur in about 13 % of all HNSCC patients. Synchronous second primary tumors are diagnosed in about 4% of the HNSCC patients. Although the head and neck is the most frequent site, synchronous second primary tumors also occur below the clavicles: lungs, esophagus and other sites.[3]

Because of the amount of missed distant metastases by CT scan of the thorax and the incidence of synchronous primary tumors below the clavicles, in screening for distant metastases and synchronous second primary tumors at initial evaluation a more sensitive diagnostic technique is needed which examines the whole body. Positron emission tomography (PET) using the radiolabeled glucose analog 18-fluoro-2-deoxy-glucose (FDG) offers a functional imaging approach for the entire body. Moreover, FDG-PET is shown to be able to detect various types of tumors among which is HNSCC.[4] Therefore, we have started a pilot study in which we evaluate the value of FDG-PET in screening for distant metastases and synchronous tumors below the clavicles in HNSCC patients. The FDG-PET results are compared to the results of CT scan of the thorax in HNSCC patients with aforementioned risk factors for distant metastases.

MATERIALS AND METHODS

Thirty-five consecutive HNSCC patients (13 women and 22 man) with high-risk factors for distant metastases underwent screening for distant metastases and synchronous second primary tumors between May 1998 and August 1999. The mean age was 59 years and ranged from 25 to 85 years. Primary tumor sites include oral cavity (n= 4: T1N2b, 2xT2N0, T2N3) oropharynx (n=8: T1N0, T2N2a, T2N2c, T2N2c, T3N0, T4N2c, T4N3, recurrence), hypopharynx (n=4: T4N2b, T4N3, 2x recurrence), larynx (n=7: T1N2c, T2N3, 2xT3N2c,

156

T3N3, T4N0, T4N1, 2xT4N2c), nasopharynx (n=3: T3N2c, T3N3, T4N3), cervical oesophagus (n=2: T3N0, T3N2c) and lymph node metastases of unknown primary tumor (n=6: N2c, 5xN3). Some patients were already known with secondary primary HNSCC at the time of screening. These patients had the following high risk factors for development of distant metastases: three or more lymph node metastases (n=10), bilateral lymph node metastases (n=13), lymph node metastases of 6 cm or larger (n=12), low jugular lymph node metastases (n=7), locoregional recurrence (n=3) and second primary tumor (n=7). Some patients had more than one risk factor.

In all 35 patients a spiral CT scan of the thorax was performed using a fourth-generation Siemens Somaton Plus (Siemens AG, Erlangen, Germany) after intravenous administration of contrast medium (Ultravist, Schering AG, Berlin, Germany). Contiguous axial scanning planes were used at 10 mm slice thickness without interslice gap. Radiological criteria for lung metastases were multiple, smooth and peripherially located lesions; for primary lung tumors, solitary speculated and mostly centrally located lesions. All patients underwent FDG-PET after a 6-hour fast. At 60 minutes after the intravenous administration of 10 mCi (370 MBq) of FDG imaging of the whole body was performed using a dedicated PET scanner (Siemens HR plus).

RESULTS

FDG-PET detected in one patient lung metastases (Figure) and primary lung cancer in two other patients. One primary lung cancer was histopathologically confirmed by thoracotomy and another primary lung cancer was confirmed by a follow-up CT scan. FDG-PET detected also a hepatocellular carcinoma, which was confirmed by ultrasound guided fine needle aspiration cytology and an intra-abdominal adenocarcinoma, which was confirmed histopathologically after laparotomy. Increased uptake sites in lung, liver and pelvis in 4 patients were not confirmed. Additional radiological examinations showed no abnormalities. During follow-up none of these patients developed metastases or second primary tumors at these sites. CT scan of the thorax was only positive in the patient with lung metastases and in one of the patients with a primary lung tumor.

The follow-up results of the 30 patients without confirmed distant metastases and second primary tumors below the clavicles were analyzed. Seventeen patients died of disease (median 9 months, rang 1 to 25 months) and 2 patients died due to other causes (median 6 months, range 2 to 9 months). The median follow up of the other 11 patients was 18 months (range 14 to 25 months). Five patients developed distant metastases. In 4 patients these distant metastases were found within 12 months. The sites of the distant metastases were lungs (n=2) and bone (n=3). One patients who developed distant metastases during follow-up had locoregional recurrence at the time of the detection of the distant metastases. Of the 4 patients without locoregional recurrence at the time of detection of distant metastases 3 were diagnosed within 12 months after screening. One patient developed pancreas cancer during follow-up.

DISCUSSION

In this study in HNSCC patients at risk for development of distant metastases the incidence of distant metastases found at presentation (3%) is lower than in our previous study (17%) [2], while the incidence of synchronous primary tumors (11%) is higher than reported in the literature (4%).[3]

Both FDG-PET and CT scan of the thorax detected lung metastases in one patient. However, both scans missed also lung and bone metastases in 4 patients as these appeared during follow-up in these patients. Both FDG-PET and CT scan of the thorax detected primary lung cancer in one patient. Only FDG-PET detected also primary lung cancer in another patient and intra-abdominal tumors in two other patients. Therefore, in 5 patients the selection of therapy was altered based on FDG-PET results, while this would be done only in 2 patients if this selection was based on the results of CT scan of the thorax.

Only a few studies have been reported on the detection of distant metastases or synchronous second primary tumors in head and neck cancer patients. Manolidis et al [5] reported on the FDG-PET results of 29 patients with various tumor types and stages. FDG-PET detected 9 of the 10 histopathologically confirmed distant metastases. There was one false-positive finding. During follow-up no distant metastases were found .in other patients. Hanasomo et al [6] reported on 8 patients who had FDG-PET for staging of distant metastatic disease. FDG-PET detected in 2 of the 4 patients distant metastases, while all 4 distant metastases were found by CT scan of the thorax. There was one false-positive FDG-PET finding. McGuirt et al [4] reported in a review article their results. Simultaneous pulmonary PET scanning with scanning of the head and neck region was done to look for second primary or metastatic cancer of the lung in 97 patients. In these patients 17 pulmonary lesions were detected, of which 6 proved to be malignant. They discontinued the extended scanning because of decreased quality of head and neck information resulting from the need to cover larger volumes, limiting scanning time for this area when the chest was also scanned. In another study [7] of the same group FDG-PET scans from midcranium to the diafragm were obtained on 56 patients with a variety of head and neck tumors on initial examination before definitive therapy. FDG-PET detected in 3 patients lung tumors, while CT scan of the thorax detected only 2 of these lung tumors. Six false-positive FDG-PET results were found. They concluded that no compelling reason was found for including the chest region as a routine practice. Nabi et al [8] reviewed the clinical course of 15 head and neck cancer patients with intrathoracic lesions detected by FDG-PET. In 9 of these patients malignant lesions were diagnosed histopathological or on repeated CT scans during follow-up. They recommend that the chest be routinely surveyed during FDG-PET evaluation of head and neck cancer patients. Stokkel et al [9] found in 12 of 68 head and neck cancer patients a synchronous primary tumor located in the head and neck or thorax. It is difficult to compare the results of aforementioned studies with the presented results in this study due to various tumor types and stages, lack of comparison with conventional diagnostic techniques (e.g. CT scan of the thorax) or low number of patients included.

In conclusion, FDG-PET can detect distant metastases and synchronous primary tumors in HNSCC patients and seems to be superior to CT scan of the thorax. Further investigations are needed to implement FDG-PET in the routine diagnostic work-up of HNSCC patients.

Figure. Whole body and axial view FDG-PET of a patient with a T2N3 supraglottic laryngeal carcinoma. Increased uptake is seen in the primary tumor, the lymph node metastases and the lung metastases (arrow).

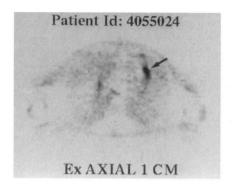

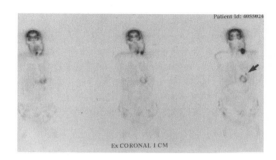

REFERENCES

1. Leon X, Quer M, Orus C, del Prado Venegas M, Lopez M. Distant metastases in head and neck cancer patients who achieved locoregional control. Head Neck 2000;22:680-686.
2. Bree R de Deurloo EE, Snow GB, Leemans CR. Screening for distant metastases in patients with head and neck cancer. Laryngoscope 2000;110:397-401.
3. Drooghe IJ, Vos M de, Cauwenberge PB van. Multiple primary tumours in head and neck cancer: results of a prospective study and future perspectives. Laryngoscope 1998;108:250-256.
4. McGuirt WF, Greven K, Williams D, Keyes JW, Watson N, Cappellari JO, Geisinger KR. PET scanning in head and neck oncology: a review. Head Neck 1998;20:208-215.
5. Manolidis S, Donald PJ, Volk P, Pounds TR. The use of positron emission tomography scanning in occult and recurrent head and neck cancer. Acta Otolaryngol 1998;suppl 534:5-11.
6. Hanasono MM, Kunda LD, Segall GM, Ku GH, Terris DJ. Uses and limitations of FDG positron emission tomography in patients with head and neck cancer. Laryngoscope 1999;109:880-885.
7. Keyes JW, Chen MYM, Watson NE, Greven KM, McGuirt WF, Williams DW. FDG PET evaluation of head and neck cancer: value of imaging the thorax. Head Neck 2000;22:105-110.
8. Nabi HA, Spaulding M, Farrell E, Lamonica D. Detection of synchronous lung lesions by FDG-PET imaging: infleunce on management of patients withe head and neck cancer. J Nucl Med 1998;39:248P.
9. Stokkel MPM, Moons KGM, Broek FW ten, Rijk PP van, Hordijk GJ. ^{18}F-Fluorodeoxyglucose dual-head positron emission tomography as a procedure for detecting simultaneous primary tumors in case of head and neck cancer. Cancer 1999;86:2370-2377.

FDG-PET FOR DETECTION OF UNKNOWN PRIMARY TUMORS

Lars Jenicke, Karl H. Bohuslavizki, Malte Clausen
Department of Nuclear Medicine, University Hospital Hamburg-Eppendorf, Martinistr. 52,
D-20246 Hamburg, Germany

Correspondence to: *Karl H. Bohuslavizki, MD, PhD, Department of Nuclear Medicine,*
University Hospital Hamburg-Eppendorf, Martinistr. 52, D-20246 Hamburg, Germany,
Phone: +49 40 42803–4047, Fax: +49 40 42803–6775 (e-mail: bohu@uke.uni-hamburg.de)

Cancer of unknown primary is a heterogeneous group of tumors with varying clinical features. The enlargement of cervical lymph nodes is often one of the first clinical manifestations of a tumor disease[1, 2]. Palpation and localization of these enlarged lymph nodes may be helpful in determining their dignity and the origin of the primary tumor site[3]. An additional ultrasound-guided fine-needle aspiration cytology may give evidence of tumor cells in cervical masses[2, 4]. Panendoscopy, computerized tomography (CT), and magnetic resonance imaging (MRI) complete the search for the unknown primary tumor site. However, despite of an accurate diagnostic work-up, the primary tumor site can not be detected in up to 12 % of all patients with cervical lymph node metastases[5-8]. Cytological examination of patients with cancer of unknown origin, i.e. so-called CUP-syndrome, often reveals squamous cell carcinoma or undifferentiated carcinoma[5]. This holds especially true for metastatic lymph nodes of the upper and middle cervical compartments. In contrast, lymph nodes of the inferior portion of the neck often contain adenocarcinoma.

Moreover, patients with CUP-syndrome comprise of a subgroup of patients presenting with metastases located extracervically, e.g. in the skeleton, the liver, in the brain or in the axillary region. Due to this heterogeneous entity of CUP-syndrome whole-body imaging by one single modality would be desirable in these patients.

The primary objective in patients with cervical lymph node metastases is the treatment of both cervical adenopathy and the primary tumor site. Therefore, treatment includes an irradiation of both sides of the neck as well as an irradiation of potential sites of the tumor bearing mucosa. Other authors advocate an ipsilateral neck treatment alone either by irradiation or by surgery[9]. The current variety of therapeutic approaches emphasizes the diagnostic and therapeutic difficulties in patients with CUP-syndrome confined to the neck. Nevertheless, an accurate diagnostic work-up is crucial[10] since both prognosis and survival rates mainly depend on the detection of the primary tumor site. In detail, five-year-survival-rates of patients with localized squamous cell carcinoma and bilateral cervical metastases are significantly higher as compared to patients with unknown primary tumor site and comparable lymph node status[1, 11-15]. Careful staging of CUP-syndrome is of utmost importance since the therapeutic approach mainly depends on the extent of the tumor. The five-year-survival-rate of patients with an occult primary and ipsilateral cervical lymph node metastases amounts to about 29-50%[16-20]. In case of bilateral cervical lymph node metastases ($T_XN_{2c}M_0$) five-year-survival-rate decreases to 17-28%[12-15]. An example of a patient is given in Fig. 1). However, when the primary tumor site can be localized in squamous cell carcinoma of the head and neck associated with bilateral lymph node metastases five-year-survival-rates again raise up to 55 %[11]. Consequently, the main goal and the justification of an extensive diagnostic work-up is to detect a potentially curable malignancy[10, 21] in order to substantially increase patients' survival rate[22].

Since the glucose analog ^{18}F-2-deoxy-D-glucose (FDG) is both accumulated and trapped within metabolically active cells, positron emission tomography (PET) using FDG can be used to identify increased glycolytic rates of several malignancies, e.g. colorectal cancer[23, 24], lung cancer[25-27], and primary breast cancer[28-31]. Moreover, CUP-syndrome is known to be a multi-system disease with potential metastatic spread in the whole body. Thus, whole-body imaging using FDG-PET offers the advantage to search both for metastases and for the primary tumor site. This is of utmost importance since in up to 40% of the patients with malignant cervical lymph nodes the primary is localized below the clavicles, with the most common site in the lungs[1, 10, 12]. An example of a patient is given in Fig. 2. In consequence, based on PET findings resources may be efficiently directed towards appropriate diagnostic and therapeutic procedures in order to substantially contribute to patients' quality of life and survival rate.

Initial studies demonstrated the value of FDG-PET for the detection of unknown primary of head and neck tumors[13, 32]. In 1997, Braams and coworkers[32] investigated 13 patients with cervical lymph node metastases of unknown origin. PET correctly identified the primary in four patients. Moreover, in one patient a plasmocytoma was identified as the primary tumor. Recently, Assar and coworkers[33] detected spots of increased uptake in 12 of 17 patients. They found a primary lung cancer in two of these 12 patients, which was localized in the upper lobe of the lung. In 10 of 12 patients biopsy directed by PET findings led to a confirmation of the primary carcinoma in 7 patients. In their study, FDG-PET detected the primary tumor in more than 50%. Accordingly, Schipper and coworkers[13] reported 25% true positive PET findings in 16 patients with cervical metastases of unknown origin[13, 34]. Recent studies showed, that a previously unknown primary tumor may be identified by FDG-PET in 8-53% of the patients[33, 35-41]. Values for sensitivity and specificity of FDG-PET ranged from 50-100% and 74-83% for the detection of unknown primary tumor site and from 86-100% and 73-90% for the diagnosis of lymph node metastases of unknown origin, respectively. Our data published recently[42, 43] are in good agreement with the literature.

In conclusion, FDG-PET is a valuable diagnostic tool in patients with CUP-syndrome since it may detect the unknown primary tumor in up to 50% of all patients investigated. Additionally, FDG-PET assists in both guiding biopsies for histological evaluation and selecting the appropriate treatment protocols in these patients.

162

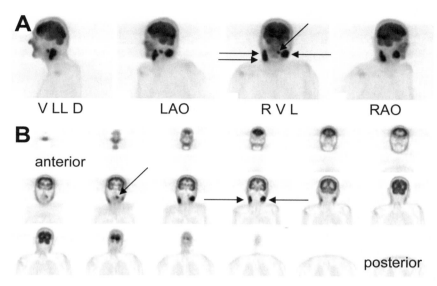

Figure 1. Maximum intensity projections (A) of the bust from left lateral (V LL D), left anterior olique (L A O), anterior (R V L), and right anterior oblique (R A O) views and coronal slices (B) from anterior to posterior. 51-year-old male patient presenting with bilateral cervical metastases of a squamous cell carcinoma unknown primary. Note massive focal increased FDG-uptake at the site of the known cervical metastases as well as an additional single focus in the left palatine tonsil (arrow). Histology confirmed squamous cell carcinoma of the palatine tonsil.

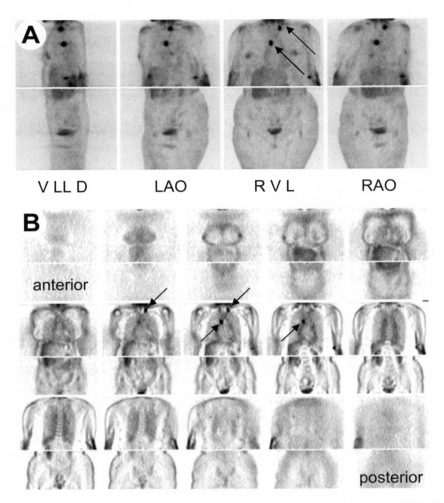

Figure 2. Maximum intensity projections (A) of the truncus from left lateral (V LL D), left anterior olique (L A O), anterior (R V L), and right anterior oblique (R A O) views and coronal slices (B) from anterior to posterior. 65-year-old male patient presenting with a left sided supraclavicular lymph node metastasis of a squamous cell carcinoma of unknown primary. Note an increased FDG uptake at the site of the known lymph node metastasis as well as in the right lung (arrows). Histology confirmed squamous cell carcinoma of the lung.

164

REFERENCES

1. Jones AS, Cook JA, Philips DE, Roland NR. Squamous carcinoma presenting as an enlarged cervical lymph node. Cancer 1993;72:1756-1761.

2. Liu YJ, Lee YT, Hsieh SW, Kuo SH. Presumption of primary sites of neck lymph node metastases on fine needle aspiration cytology. Acta Cytol 1997;41:1477-1482.

3. Haynes BF. Enlargement of lymph node and spleen. In: Isselbacher KJ, Braunwald E, Wilson JD, Martin JB, Fauci AS, Kasper DL, eds. *Harrison's principles of internal medicine.* 13 ed. New York: McGraw-Hill; 1994:323-329.

4. van den Brekel MWM, Castelijns JA, Stel HV, et al. Occult metastatic neck disease: detection with US and US-guided fine-needle aspiration cytology. Radiology 1991;180:457-461.

5. de Braud F, Heilbrun LK, Ahmed K, et al. Metastatic squamous cell carcinoma of an unknown primary localized to the neck. Advantages of an aggressive treatment. Cancer 1989;64:510-515.

6. Leipzig B, Winter ML, Hokanson JA. Cervical nodal metastases of unknown origin. Laryngoscope 1981;91:593-598.

7. Nordstrom DG, Tewfik HH, Latourette HB. Cervical lymph node metastases from an unknown primary. Radiat Oncol Biol Phys 1979;5:73-76.

8. Wang RC, Goepfert H, Barber AE, Wolf P. Unknown primary squamous cell carcinoma metastatic to the neck. Arch Otolaryngol Head Neck Surg 1990;116:1388-1393.

9. Reddy SP, Marks JE. Metastatic carcinoma in the cervical lymph nodes from an unknown primary site: results of bilateral neck plus mucosal irradiation vs. ipsilateral neck dissection. Int J Rad Oncol Biol Phys 1997;37:797-802.

10. Maiche AG. Cancer of unknown primary. A retrospective study based on 109 patients. Am J Clin Oncol 1993;16:26-29.

11. Clarke RW, Stell PM. Squamous carcinoma of head and neck in the young adult. Clin Otolaryngol 1992;17:18-23.

12. Jones AS, Phillips DE, Helliwell TR, Roland NJ. Occult metastases in head and neck squamous carcinoma. Eur Arch Otorhinolaryngol 1993;250:446-449.

13. Schipper JH, Schrader M, Arweiler D, Müller S, Sciuk J. Die Positronen-emissionstomographie zur Primärtumorsuche bei Halslymphknotenmetastasen mit unbekanntem Primärtumor. HNO 1996;44:254-257.

14. Snee PM, Vyramuthu N. Metastatic carcinoma from unknown primary site: the experience of a large oncology centre. Br J Radiol 1985;58:1091-1095.

15. Snow GB, Patel P, Leemans CR, Tiwari R. Management of cervical lymph nodes in patients with head and neck cancer. Arch Otorhinolaryngol 1992;249:187-194.

16. Barrie JR, Knapper WH, Strong EW. Cervical nodal metastases of unknown origin. Am J Surg 1970;120:466-470.

17. Davidson BJ, Spiro RH, Patel S, Patel K, Shah JP. Cervical metastases of occult origin: the impact of combined modality therapy. Am J Surg 1994;168:395-399.

18. Glynne-Jones RGT, Anand AK, Young TE, Berry RJ, Phil D. Metastatic carcinoma in the cervical lymph nodes from an occult primary: a conservative approach to the role of radiotherapy. J Rad Oncol Biol Phys 1990;18:289-294.

19. Spiro RH, de Rose G, Strong EW. Cervical node metastasis of occult origin. Am J Surg 1983;146:441-446.

20. Yang ZY, Hu JH, Yan JH, et al. Lymph node metastases in the neck from an unknown primary. Report on 113 patients. Acta Radiol Oncol 1983;22:17-22.

21. Schapira DV, Jarrett AR. The need to consider survival, outcome, and expense when evaluating and treating patients with unknown primary carcinoma. Arch Intern Med 1995;155:2050-2054.

22. Schlag PM, Hunerbein M. Cancer of unknown primary site. Ann Chir Gynaecol 1994;83:8-12.

23. Imdahl A, Reinhardt MJ, Nitzsche EU, et al. Impact of 18F-FDG-positron emission tomography for decision making in colorectal cancer recurrences. Langenbecks Arch Surg 2000;385:129-134.

24. Whiteford MH, Whiteford HM, Yee LF, et al. Usefulness of FDG-PET scan in the assessment of suspected metastatic or recurrent adenocarcinoma of the colon and rectum. Dis Colon Rectum 2000;43:759-770.

25. Dewan NA, Gupta NC, Redepenning LS, Phalen JJ, Frick MP. Diagnostic efficiacy of PET-FDG imaging in solitary pulmonary nodules. Chest 1993;104:997-1002.

26. Hübner KF, Buonocore E, Singh SK, Gould HR, Cotten DW. Characterization of chest masses by FDG positron emission tomography. Clin Nucl Med 1995;20:293-298.

27. Knight SB, Delbeke D, Stewart JR, Sandler MP. Evaluation of pulmonary lesions with FDG-PET. Chest 1996;109:982-988.

28. Scheidhauer K, Scharl A, Pietrzyk U, et al. Qualitative [^{18}F]-FDG positron emission tomography in primary breast cancer: clinical relevance and practicability. Eur J Nucl Med 1996;23:618-623.

29. Avril N, Dose J, Ziegler S, Janicke F, Schwaiger M. Diagnosis of breast carcinoma and locoregional lymph nodes with positron emission tomography. Radiologe 1997;37:741-748.

30. Crippa F, Agresti R, Seregni E, et al. Prospective evaluation of fluorine-18-FDG PET in presurgical staging of the axilla in breast cancer. J Nucl Med 1998;39:4-8.

31. Avril N, Rose CA, Schelling M, et al. Breast imaging with positron emission tomography and fluorine-18 fluorodeoxyglucose: use and limitations. J Clin Oncol 2000;18:3495-3502.

32. Braams JW, Pruim J, Kole AC, et al. Detection of unknown primary head and neck tumors by positron emission tomography. Int J Oral Maxillofac Surg 1997;26:112-115.

33. Assar AOS, Fischbein NJ, Caputo GR, et al. Metastatic head and neck cancer: role and usefulness of FDG PET in locating occult primary tumors. Radiology 1999;210:177-181.

34. Kole AC, Nieweg OE, Pruim J, et al. Detection of unknown occult primary tumors using positron emission tomography. Cancer 1998;82:1160-1166.

35. Greven KM, Keyes JW, Jr., Williams DW, 3rd, McGuirt WF, Joyce WT, 3rd. Occult primary tumors of the head and neck: lack of benefit from positron emission tomography imaging with 2-[F-18]fluoro-2-deoxy-D- glucose. Cancer 1999;86:114-118.

36. Hanasono MM, Kunda LD, Segall GM, Ku GH, Terris DJ. Uses and limitations of FDG positron emission tomography in patients with head and neck cancer. Laryngoscope 1999;109:880-885.

37. Jungehulsing M, Scheidhauer K, Damm M, et al. 2[F]-fluoro-2-deoxy-D-glucose positron emission tomography is a sensitive tool for the detection of occult primary cancer (carcinoma of unknown primary syndrome) with head and neck lymph node manifestation. Otolaryngol Head Neck Surg 2000;123:294-301.

38. Lassen U, Daugaard G, Eigtved A, Damgaard K, Friberg L. 18F-FDG whole body positron emission tomography (PET) in patients with unknown primary tumours (UPT). Eur J Cancer 1999;35:1076-1082.

39. Safa AA, Tran LM, Rege S, et al. The role of positron emission tomography in occult primary head and neck cancers [see comments]. Cancer J Sci Am 1999;5:214-218.

40. Shinohara M, Tomita M, Ohira S, Nishimura A. Evaluation of 18F-FDG positron emission tomography (PET) in the detection of unknown primary tumors. Hokkaido Igaku Zasshi 1999;74:249-256.

41. Stokkel MP, Terhaard CH, Hordijk GJ, van Rijk PP. The detection of unknown primary tumors in patients with cervical metastases by dual-head positron emission tomography. Oral Oncol 1999;35:390-394.

42. Bohuslavizki KH, Klutmann S, Kroger S, et al. FDG PET detection of unknown primary tumors. J Nucl Med 2000;41:816-822.

43. Bohuslavizki KH, Klutmann S, Sonnemann U, et al. F-18 FDG PET for detection of occult primary tumor in patients with lymphatic metastases of the neck region. Laryngorhinootologie 1999;78:445-449.

166

SENTINEL NODE BIOPSY TO UPSTAGE THE CLINICALLY NEGATIVE NECK FOR HEAD AND NECK SQUAMOUS CELL CARCINOMA

G. L. Ross, MRCSEd[1], T. Shoaib, FRCSEd[1], D. S. Soutar, ChM[1], I. G. Cammileri, FRCS (Plast)[1], H. W. Gray, FRCP[2], R. G. Bessent, MA, Dphil, FIPEM[3], D. G. MacDonald, FRCPath[4](Glasgow, United Kingdom)
[1]Plastic Surgery Unit, Canniesburn Hospital, Switchback Road, Bearsden, Glasgow, UK
[2]Department of Nuclear Medicine, Royal Infirmary, Glasgow, UK
[3]Departments of Clinical Physics and Nuclear Medicine, Royal Infirmary, Glasgow, UK
[4]Oral Pathology Unit, Glasgow Dental Hospital and School, Glasgow, UK

Source of financial support: This Research was funded by Canniesburn Research Trust and the White Lily Trust

Running title   Sentinel node biopsy in head and neck cancer

Key Words: Head and neck neoplasms, sentinel node biopsy, radical neck dissection, lymph node excision, Squamous cell carcinoma

Correspondence to: Gary Ross, Head and Neck Research Fellow, Plastic Surgery Unit, Canniesburn Hospital, Switchback Road, Bearsden,Glasgow, UK G61 1QL, Fax 00441412115652, Phone 00441413343283

ABSTRACT

Background. The role of sentinel node biopsy (SNB) in patients with oral and oropharyngeal squamous cell carcinoma patients to upstage the clinically N0 neck was investigated to determine whether the pathology of the sentinel node reflected that of the neck.

Methods. Patients with head and neck squamous cell carcinoma accessible to injection were enrolled into the study. SNB was performed after blue dye and radiocolloid injection. Preoperative lymphoscintigraphy and the peroperative use of a gamma probe identified radioactive sentinel nodes and visualization of blue stained lymphatics identified blue sentinel nodes. If the sentinel node was negative there was no further treatment to the neck. If the sentinel node was positive a therapeutic neck dissection was performed.

Results. SNB was performed on 39 clinically N0 necks. Sentinel nodes were harvested in 37/39. Five patients had positive sentinel nodes and twenty-six were staged sentinel node negative The sentinel node was the only node containing tumor in 3/5. There was a mean follow up of 7 months.

Conclusions. SNB can accurately upstage the clinically N0 patient with early nodal disease. Its use as a quality of care in head and neck squamous cell carcinoma requires the results of longer follow up observational trials.

INTRODUCTION

Head and neck squamous cell carcinoma spreads via lymphatics to the regional draining lymph nodes in the neck, and this spread is thought to be embolic in nature[1]. Since the presence of lymph node metastases is an important prognostic factor in head and neck cancer, decreasing survival by 50%[2], reliable staging of the neck in this disease is imperative to determine further management. In squamous cell carcinoma of the upper aerodigestive tract the investigation and treatment of the patient with a clinically N0 neck remains controversial[3]. Physical examination, magnetic resonance imaging, ultrasound scanning and computed tomography of the neck, have not proved reliable in assessing nodal involvement, with approximately 30% of patients with clinically clear necks (N0) containing occult metastases in neck dissection specimens[4]. Currently the only highly accurate means of identifying nodal disease is to perform a staging END[5] although other staging techniques such as ultrasound assisted fine needle aspiration cytology and Positron Emission Tomograpghy are currently being evaluated. For early disease, clinicians are reluctant to perform an END, since up to 80% of patients will not benefit, yet adopting a wait-and-see policy to all necks will result in a high proportion of patients subsequently developing late stage regional failure[6]. Since the treatment of early neck disease carries a better prognosis than late neck disease[6], the management of the clinically N0 neck remains one of the continuing debates in oral and oropharyngeal cancer[7].

The sentinel node concept states that a tumor spreads via lymphatics to the first echelon lymph node encountered in the lymph node basin and this spread is embolic in nature[8]. If the sentinel, or first echelon, node can be identified and examined for the presence of tumor metastases, the need to perform an elective staging lymph node dissection is negated[9]. The concept has been mainly applied to breast cancer[10] and malignant melanoma[11], and in these cancers, sentinel nodes free from tumor imply a regional lymph node basin free from tumor with a high degree of accuracy.

Initial results of the sentinel node procedure in head and neck cancer have reported mixed success. In a series of 16 cases, Pitman et al[12] were unable to find any blue nodes in patients injected with blue dye alone, and in a series of five cases using radiocolloid alone, Koch et al remained unconvinced of its role in the management of head and neck cancer patients[13]. The first case of a successful sentinel node biopsy in head and neck cancer using radiocolloid to trace the first echelon node was performed in 1996 by Alex and Krag on a patient with a supraglottic carcinoma[14] and in 1998, Bilchik et al reported the use of SNB in a variety of neoplasms, including head and neck cancer[15]. More recently, we described our method for successful SNB using blue dye and radiocolloid[16]. Werner et al have had success with the procedure in the clinically N0 neck[17] and Alex et al have published their experience using radiocolloid alone[18]

In malignant melanoma it was found that combining preoperative lymphoscintigraphy, vital dye and gamma probe facilitates sentinel node identification and possibly improves the accuracy of staging.[19-23]. The sentinel node can be identified in 90-100% of cases[19,24-28.] This triple diagnostic approach has become the standard of care in SNB. Initially we performed SNB on forty necks followed by END showing a sensitivity of 94%[29]. Having successfully implemented SNB as a diagnostic tool we obtained ethical approval to use SNB to stage the node negative neck.

MATERIALS AND METHODS

Thirty-six patients have entered the study to date. Patients undergoing sentinel node biopsy were admitted the day prior to surgery. The triple diagnostic procedure of preoperative lymphoscintigraphy and intraoperative blue dye and gamma probe has previously been described[27]. Sentinel nodes were identified in their lymph node level and were labeled according to color and presence of radioactivity. Radioactivity was confirmed within the sentinel node *ex-vivo* using the Neoprobe 1500 (Ethicon Endosurgery, UK). Once the sentinel nodes were excised the Neoprobe was used to search the resection bed to ensure that there were no residual areas of high radioactivity. A positive node containing metastases was temed a "positive sentinel node; a sentinel node containing measurable radioactivity was termed "hot", and one with blue stained afferent lymphatics termad "blue". Once the operator was satisfied of the complete removal of radioactive nodes, the wound was closed.

The sentinel nodes were fixed in 10% neutral buffered formalin and after fixation were bisected through their longest axis. If the thickness of the halves was more than approximately 2mm the slices were further trimmed to provide additional 2mm thick blocks. One Hematoxylin and Eosin (H&E) stained section was prepared from each histological block and examined for possible metastasis. Our full SNB protocol, which has not been completed in all patients as yet, involves step serial sectioning and immunohistochemistry for cytokeratins if the initial H&E examination is negative. Patients with negative SNB findings were followed up in outpatients every three months and no further treatment to the neck was carried out. If metastatic tumour was found, either on routine H&E, step sectioning or immunohistochemistry, a therapeutic neck dissection (TND) in the form of a modified radical neck dissections with preservation of the accessory nerve, sternocleidomastoid and the internal jugular vein was undertaken. In all cases where TND was undertaken, the pathological dissection followed fixation. All nodes over approximately 2.5mm in maximum diameter were identified in their anatomic groups. Each node was bisected through its longest axis and one half was processed for H&E examination

Patients have been followed for on average 7months (range 2-24 months) following SNB.

RESULTS

SNB was performed in thirty-six consecutive patients. The male: female ratio was 3:1 and the mean age was 55 years (range 33-88). Sentinel nodes were removed from thirty-four patients. Thirty-one N0 patients had SNB to stage the clinically negative neck and three N+ patients had SNB to stage the contralateral clinically negative neck and a TND for clinically suspected or confirmed nodal metastases on the ipsilateral neck, for tumours close to or invading the midline. Of the thirty-one patients, twenty-six had SNB performed unilaterally and five patients had SNB bilaterally.

The total number of sentinel nodes harvested was 73 (mean per patient 2.3) Figure 1 shows the number of positive nodes by T classification and figure 2 shows the neck levels from which sentinel nodes were harvested.

Forty-three nodes were hot and blue, 17 nodes were hot and 13 nodes were blue only. Figure 3 shows the number of positive sentinel nodes identified by each technique

Five patients were upstaged with sentinel node biopsy and these patients had a subsequent TND and post-operative radiotherapy. In three of TND's no further positive nodes were found

The median follow up of these patients is seven months (range 2-24 months) and so far there have been two patients who have developed neck recurrence having been staged sentinel node negative. The time interval to development of neck recurrence was five and seven months respectively.

DISCUSSION

When using a combination of blue dye and radiocolloid injection, our success rate in identifying sentinel nodes within the neck is 34/36 (94%). This compares favourably with the rate of sentinel node identification in patients undergoing sentinel node biopsy for cutaneous lesions of the head and neck.

The procedure in head and neck cancer may be more technically demanding than in head and neck melanoma. The close proximity of sentinel nodes to the primary site, especially when the primary site is the floor of mouth, renders gamma probe identification of radioactive nodes in the submandibular and submental triangles difficult. The two cases in which we were unable to identify the sentinel node were both floor of mouth tumours. In both cases no sentinel node was found on lymphoscintigraphy or intraoperatively with either the blue dye or the neoprobe. In an attempt to improve identification for floor of mouth tumours we use a series of malleable lead plates. These shield the injection site, reduce shine through and scatter from the primary site and aid radiolocalisation.

There were two patients who developed neck recurrence. These occurred five and seven months post SNB. The first was a recurrence in a neck of a patient who underwent bilateral SNB for a T4 tongue lesion extending from anterior to posterior third, the primary being treated by brachytherapy alone. The sentinel node was originally harvested from level 3 as a hot/blue node and the subsequent TND showed a single nodal recurrence in Level 2. The second patient had a unilateral SNB for a postero-inferior alveolar ridge T4 tumour. The sentinel nodes were both hot/blue and harvested from levels 1 and 2 respectively. The subsequent TND showed a single nodal recurrence in level 1.

The reasons for recurrence in these patients may be due to the size and depth of invasion of the tumour. In the first case the size of the tumor may have made surrounding it by injection impossible. The second patient had deep bony invasion and our injection technique would have been unable to surround the deep aspect of the tumour that most likely had the invasive front. Thus the involved lymphatic channel may have not been injected in either case. We postulate that for T4 tumours SNB may be of limited value.

It is likely that SNB will be most effective for T1/2 tumours of the oral cavity. We propose a multicentre study to investigate SNB in patients with T1 or T2 lesions of the oral cavity and oropharynx and clinically N0 necks. If the sentinel node is free of tumor, no elective treatment of the neck will be undertaken

The use of SNB in clinical practice is limited as a research tool at present until the results of observational multicentre trials are available. Details of our multicentre trial are available on the web-site www.canniesburn.org.

Figure 1. Sentinel node identification by neck level

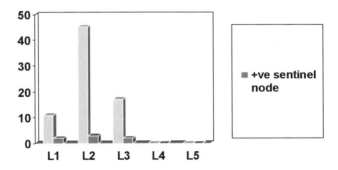

Figure 2. Sentinel nodes by T stage

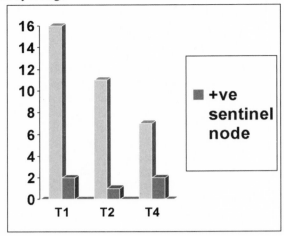

Figure 3. Sentinel node identification by each technique

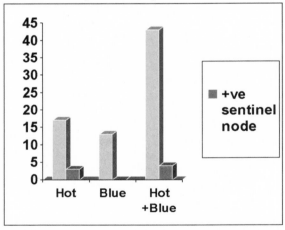

REFERENCES

1.   I.A. McGregor, F.M. McGregor in "Cancer of the Face and Mouth", 1st Edition. Churchill Livingstone, 1986.
2.   Alvi A. Johnson JT. Extracapsular spread in the clinically negative neck (N0): implications and outcome. Otolaryngology - Head & Neck Surgery. 1996; 114:65-70
3.   Pillsbury HC, III, Clark M. A rationale for therapy of the N0 neck. Laryngoscope 1997; 107:1294-315.
4.   Woolgar JA. Beirne JC. Vaughan ED. Lewis-Jones HG. Scott J. Brown JS. Correlation of histopathologic findings with clinical and radiologic assessments of cervical lymph-node metastases in oral cancer. International Journal of Oral & Maxillofacial Surgery. 1995; 24:30-7.
5.   Woolgar JA, Vaughan ED, Scott J, Brown JS. Pathological findings in clinically false negative and false positive neck dissections for oral carcinoma. Ann.R.Coll.Surg.Engl. 1994; 76:237-44.

6.   Haddadin KJ, Soutar DS, Oliver RJ, Webster MH, Robertson AG, MacDonald DG. Improved survival for patients with clinically T1/T2, N0 tongue tumors undergoing a prophylactic neck dissection. Head Neck 1999;21:517-25.

7.   Pillsbury HC 3rd. Clark M. A rationale for therapy of the N0 neck. Laryngoscope 1997; 107:1294-315

8.   Morton DL, Wen DR, Wong JH, Economou JS, Cagle LA, Storm FK et al. Technical details of intraoperative lymphatic mapping for early stage melanoma. Arch.Surg. 1992; 127:392-9.

9.   Reintgen D, Cruse CW, Wells K, Berman C, Fenske N, Glass F et al. The orderly progression of melanoma nodal metastases. Ann.Surg. 1994; 220:759-67.

10.   Krag DN, Weaver DL, Alex JC, Fairbank JT. Surgical resection and radiolocation of the sentinel lymph node in breast cancer using a gamma probe. Surg.Oncol. 1993; 2:335-9.

11.   Ross MI. Surgical management of stage I and II melanoma patients: approach to the regional lymph node basin. Semin.Surg.Oncol. 1996; 12:394-401.

12.   Pitman KT, Johnson JT, Edington H, et al. Lymphatic mapping with isosulfan blue dye in squamous cell carcinoma of the head and neck. Arch Otolaryngol Head Neck Surg 1998;124:790-3.

13.   Koch WM, Choti MA, Civelek AC, Eisele DW, Saunders JR. Gamma probe-directed biopsy of the sentinel node in oral squamous cell carcinoma. Arch.Otolaryngol.Head Neck Surg. 1998; 124:455-9.

14.   Alex JC, Krag DN. The gamma-probe-guided resection of radiolabeled primary lymph nodes. Surg.Oncol.Clin.N.Am. 1996; 5:33-41.

15.   Bilchik AJ, Giuliano A, Essner R, Bostick P, Kelemen P, Foshag LJ et al. Universal application of intraoperative lymphatic mapping and sentinel lymphadenectomy in solid neoplasms. Cancer J.Sci.Am. 1998; 4:351-8.

16.   Shoaib T, Soutar DS, Prosser JE, Dunaway DJ, Gray HW, McCurrach GM et al. A suggested method for sentinel node biopsy in squamous cell carcinoma of the head and neck. Head Neck 1999; 21:728-33.

17.   Werner JA, Dunne AA, Brandt D, Ramaswamy A, Kulkens C, Lippert BM et al. Studies on significance of sentinel lymphadenectomy in pharyngeal and laryngeal carcinoma. Laryngorhinootologie 1999; 78:663-70.

18.   Alex JC, Sasaki CT, Krag DN, Wenig B, Pyle PB. Sentinel lymph node radiolocation in head and neck squamous cell carcinoma. Laryngoscope 2000; 110:198-203.

19.   Gershenwald JE, Tseng CH, Thompson W, et al. Improved sentinel lymph node localization in patients with primary melanoma with the use of radiolabeled colloid. Surgery.1998; 124:203-210.

20.   Albertini JJ, Cruse CW, Rapaport D, et al. Intraoperative radiolymphoscintigraphy improves sentinel lymph node identification for patients with melanoma. Ann Surg. 1996; 223:217-224.

21.   Krag DN, Meijer SJ, Weaver DL, et al. Minimal-access surgery for staging of malignant melanoma. Arch Surg.1995; 130:654-658.

22.   Captain BA, Newell OE, Lime I, et al. Localising the sentinel node in Cutaneous melanoma: gamma probe detection versus blue dye. Ann Surg Oncol.1997; 4:156-160.

23.   Nieweg OE, Jansen L, Kroon BBR. Technique of lymphatic mapping and sentinel node biopsy for melanoma. Eur J Surg Oncol 1998; 24: 520-524.

24.   Haddad FF, Stall A, Messina J, et al. The progression of melanoma nodal metastasis is dependent on tumor thickness of the primary lesion. Ann Surg Oncol. 1999; 6:144-149.

25   Bostick P, Essner R, Glass E, Kelley MC, Sarantou T, Foshag LF et al. Comparison of blue dye and probe assisted intraoperative ltymphatic mapping in melanoma to identify sentinel nodes in 100 lymphatic basins. Arch Surg 1999; 134: 43-49.

26.   Leong SP, Steinmetz I, Habib FA, et al. Optimal selective sentinel lymph node dissection in primary malignant melanoma. Arch Surg.1997; 132:666-672.

27.   Lenisa L, Santinami M, Belli F, Clemente C, Mascheroni L, Patuzzo R et al. Sentinel node biopsy and selective lymph node dissection in cutaneous melanoma patients. J Exp Clin Cancer Res 1999; 18:69-74.

28.   Borgstein PJ, Meijer S, van Diest PJ. Are locoregional cutaneous metasteses in melanoma predictable? Ann Surg Oncol 1999; 6:315-321.

29.   The accuracy of sentinel node biopsy in the clinically N0 neck. Shoaib T, Soutar DS,Dunaway DJ, Camilleri IG,Gray HW, et al. The 5th International Conference on Head and Neck Cancer. San Francisco, July 29 - August 2, 2000.

SENTINEL NODE BIOPSY – A PREDICTIVE INTRAOPERATIVE STAGING PROCEDURE IN HNSCC

Anja-A. Dünne [1], D. Brandt [2], Ch. Külkens [1], A. Ramaswamy [3], B.J. Folz [1], B.M. Lippert [1], R. Moll [3], J.A. Werner [1]

[1]Department of Otolaryngology, Head and Neck Surgery, Philipps-University of Marburg, Germany
[2]Department of Clinical Nuclear Medicine Philipps-University of Marburg, Germany
[3]Department of Pathology Philipps-University of Marburg, Germany

Keywords: Sentinel Node, HNSCC; occult lymph node metastasis, N0-neck

ABSTRACT

Background. Few communications exist about the value of sentinel node (SN) biopsy for head and neck squamous cell carcinoma (HNSCC). We investigated the predictiveness of intraoperative SN biopsy in patients with clinically N0-neck suffering from HNSCC.

Patients and methods. A number of 37 previously untreated patients with clinically N0-neck suffering from HNSCC were staged by intraoperative SN biopsy. After intraoperative identification of the SN all patients were treated by neck dissection (ND) according to the primary side and the extent of suspected occult lymphogenic metastatic spread. Postoperatively histological results of the SN and the ND specimens were compared.

Results. In 31 patients the tumor-free SN reflected the regional lymph node status. In 6 patients an isolated metastasis could be proven in the intraoperatively identified SN.

Conclusions. Intraoperative SN biopsy is predictive for the detection of clinically occult lymph node metastases in HNSCC. Therefor SN biopsy might help to limit the extent of ipsilateral neck dissection, if used as an intraoperative staging procedure.

INTRODUCTION

Prognosis of patients suffering from squamous cell carcinoma of the upper aerodigestive tract (HNSCC) is defined to a lesser extent through the size of the primary tumor. It is rather the extent of metastatic disease, which in squamous cell carcinoma predominantly occurs in a lymphogenous pattern that predicts the course of the disease. The extraordinary relevance of lymphogenic metastatic spread with regard to prognosis becomes evident, if the partly drastic reduction of 5-year-survival-rates in cases of histologically confirmed neck node metastases is considered.

Based on the controverse discussion about optimized therapy for cases with no clinical evidence of lymphogenic metastazation, the question arrises whether the concept of the SN biopsy, as it is applied increasingly for melanoma and breast cancer, will also be of significance for HNSCC. The promising announcements concerning breast cancer, but also concerning other tumor entities like malignant melanoma, vulvar and penile carcinoma[1-3] are met by only scarce experiences with SN biopsy in head and neck squamous cell carcinoma (HNSCC)[4-11]. Based on their liminated number of patients, these investigations can not judge a final verdict about the status of SN biopsy in HNSCC.

The results of SN biopsy in 37 untreated patients with a clinically suspected N0-neck suffering from HNSCC shall help to answer questions, whether this method is applicable for the head and neck cancer and to its importance for tumors of this region.

PATIENTS AND METHODS

Two patients suffered from a squamous cell carcinoma of the lower lip, five patients from a carcinoma of the anterior oral cavity, thirteen patients from a oropharyngeal carcinoma and ten patients from a laryngeal carcinoma, while one pateint suffered from a hypopharyngeal carcinoma. Summerizing, there were six patients with T1, nineteen patients with T2 and six patients with T3-stage.

In all patients the application of 1.2mCi nanocolloid disolved in 0.2-0.3ml saline was performed by four pertumoral injections intraoperatively at the beginning of the operation which usually includes Neck dissection and the resection of the primary. During the Neck dissection, the sentinel node was identified using a 14-mm gamma-probe (Navigator Gamma Guidance System), marked or excised. One or two surrounding nodes with diminished activity were equally identified, marked or excised. These were defined as sentinel node two, sentinel node three or four with regard to their decrease of radiopharmaceutical uptake.

Postoperatively the histological results of the intraoperatively identified SN as well as of the nodes with diminished activity were compared with the histological results of ND specimens.

RESULTS

In all thirty-seven patients with pretherapeutic N0-neck, a sentinel node could be detected. In thirty-one cases, the histological investigation of the sentinel node showed no malignant cells. This fact was considered to be representative of the regional neck lymph node status.

For the remaining six patients an isolated tumor metastasis was detected in the intraoperatively identified sentinel node. In five of these six patients the first draining lymph node in the mean draining region showed the highest intranodal accumulation intraoperatively and was shown to contain an isolated tumor metastasis. But in one patient suffering from a carcinoma of the oropharynx, a lymph node in a neighbouring draining basin (SN$_2$) showing reduced uptake of the tracer substance, contained an isolated micrometastasis. This finding may suggest the existence of several first-draining lymph nodes due to a primary tumor draining into two neighbouring basins, due to its localization.

DISCUSSION

The SN concept is a diagnostic and therapeutic measure, which should be applied in cases, where lymphogenic metastasization is clinically not evident, but may become very likely. Because regional control and survival are poorer in patients who develop cervical metastases at a later point of time, it is important to identify those patients who are likely to harbor occult regional disease referring them to elective treatment. As a generale rule, elective treatment of the regional lymphatics is indicated, if the potential risk of occult disease exceeds twenty percent. Application of this principle, requires a reliable system for assessing the risk of cervical metastases, which should be based on characteristics of the primary tumor proven to be predictive[12].

If SN biopsy would be suitable for HNSCC not only a reduction of operation related morbidity but maybe also a reduction of treatment costs could be achieved. On the basis of the results of the presented 37 previously untreated patients with a clinically suspected N0-neck, it can be stated that SN biopsy in fact seems to be of relevance, if certain observations are taken into consideration.

The value of this is bound tightly on the undoubtable identification of the respective sentinel node. This demand poses a special challenge on the detection technique especially in the head and neck region with a total of about 300 neck lymph nodes. Differences in denseness of distribution patterns of initial lymphatics in the head and neck region, have a direct influence on the identification of the first draining lymph node. Based on the tight lymph node system in head and neck area it may be helpful to investigate several tracer accumulating lymph nodes in cases of clinically suspected N0-neck in order to prevent false negative results. These nodes should then be sent for separate histologic refurbishing, as long as this method is under clinical investigation. In the future the identified lymph nodes may as well be investigated intraoperatively by frozen sections.

Furthermore, the nature of the investigation, is bound tightly to the quality of the injection and thus to the experience of the investigator. An intraoperative injection technique may therefore lead to considerably superior results, due to a better exposure and less interference by the patient. This applies especially to oropharyngeal carcinomas at profound sites and, of course, to laryngeal and hypopharyngeal carcinomas.

Taking all these points into consideration, throughout intraoperative Sentinel node biopsy the first draining lymph node could be identified in all cases of N0- and N1-neck.

CONCLUSION

The results of our investigation encourage, that in the context of the controversal discussion of the optimal treatment concept in patients with N0-neck, in selected situations, this method may contribute in more security indication a selective type of neck dissection. Nevertheless, still no final judgement about the value of SN biopsy in HNSCC should be given. All published results have to be critically discussed and further investigations including a representative number of patients are required in order to clarify whether SN biopsy is of relevance in HNSCC patients. Until now, the common concepts of neck dissection should not be left behind.

REFERENCES

1. Jansen L Koops HS, Nieweg OE, Doting E, Kapteijn AE, Balm AJM. Sentinel node biopsy for melanoma in the head and neck region. Head Neck 2000;22:272-33.
2. Doting MHE, Jansen L, Nieweg OE, Piers DA, Tiebosch ATMG, Koops HS. Lymphatic mapping with intralesional tracer administration in breast carcinoma patients. Cancer 2000;88:2546-25.
3. De Cicco C, Sideri M, Bartolomei M, Grana C, Cremonesi M, Fiorenza M, Maggioni A, Bocciolone L, Mangioni C, Colombo N, Paganelli G. Sentinel node biopsy in early vulvar cancer. Br J Cancer 2000;82:295-299.
4. Alex JC, Krag ND. The gamma probe-guided resection of radiolabeled primary lymph nodes. Surg Oncol Clin N Am 1996;5:33-41.
5. Koch WN, Choti MA, Civelek C, Eisele DW, Saunders JR. Gamma probe directed biopsy of the Sentinel Node in oral squamous cell carcinoma. Arch Otolaryngol Head Neck Surg 1998;124:455-459.
6. Pitman KT, Johnson JT, Edington H, Barnes EL, Day R, Wagner RL. Lymphatic mapping with isosulfan blue dye in squamous cell carcinoma of the head and neck. Arch Otolaryngol Head Neck Surg 1998;124:790-793.
7. Shoaib T, Soutar DS, Prossar JE, Dunaway DJ, Gray HW, McCurrach GM. A suggested method for sentinel node Biopsy in squamous cell carcinoma of the head and neck. Head Neck 1999;21:728-733.
8. Werner JA, Dünne A-A, Brandt D, Ramaswamy A, Külkens C, Lippert BM, K. Joseph, R. Moll. Untersuchungen zum Stellenwert der Sentinel Node Biopsie bei Karzinomen des Pharynx und Larynx. Laryngorhinootol 1999;12:663-670.
9. Alex JC, Sysaki CT, Krag DN, Weinig B, Pyle PB. Sentinel Lymph Node radiolocalization in head and neck squamous cell carcinoma. Laryngoscope 2000;110:198-203.
10. Zitsch RP 3rd, Todd DW, Renner GJ, Singh A. Intraoperative radiolymphoscintigraphy for detection of occult nodal metastasis in patients with head and neck squamous cell carcinoma. Otolaryngol Head Neck Surg 2000;122:662-666.
11. Chiesa F, Mauri S, Grana C, Tradati N, Calabrese L, Ansarin M, Mazzarol G, Paganelli G. Is there a role for sentinel node biopsy in early N0 tongue tumors? Surgery 2000;128:16-21.
12. Eicher SA, Weber RS. Surgical management of cervical lymph node metastases. Curr Opin Oncol 1996;8:215-220

SENTINEL LYMPH NODE DETECTION
IN HEAD AND NECK CANCER

Steffen Höft[1],MD, Claus Muhle[2], MD, Winfried Brenner[2], MD, Heinrich Rudert[1], MD, Steffen Maune[1], MD

[1]Dept. of Otorhinolaryngology, Head and Neck Surgery
[2]Clinic of Nuclear Medicine, University Clinics Kiel, Germany

Correspondence to: Steffen Höft, MD, Dept. of Otorhinolaryngology, Head and Neck Surgery, Arnold-Heller-Str. 14, 24105 Kiel, Phone.: ++ 49 / 4 31 / 5 97 22 40, Fax: ++ 49 / 4 31 / 5 97 22 72 (e-mail: hoft@hno.uni-kiel.de)

INTRODUCTION

In the management of malignant tumors of the head and neck detection of lymphatic metastases is pivotal for the planning of a treatment strategy. Evidence of metastatic disease results in a therapy of the neck. However, lack of evidence of metastatic disease does not rule out occult metastatic disease. Therefore elective neck dissection is performed if the risk of occult metastatic disease exeeds 15-20%.[1] Patients with occult metastases benefit from this strategy as it results in further therapy of the neck. Yet, the majority of patients will suffer from the morbidity of a neck dissection without gaining advantages as the preoperative diagnosis of a N0-neck will be confirmed. Nonetheless these patients will suffer from the morbidity of a neck dissection. Therefore an improved staging of the neck is necessary to select patients without metastatic disease in whom an elective neck should be avoided.

In the treatment of malignant melanomas and breast cancer gamma-probe guided detection of the sentinel lymph node (SLN) has been shown to be of prognostic value for staging of the lymphatic metastases.[2, 3] The aim of this study was to investigate the feasbilty of the sentinel lymph node concept in head and neck cancer.

MATERIAL AND METHODS

10 patients with squamous cell carcinomas of the head and neck were included in the study. There were 1 female and 9 male patients. The average age was 59.2 years. Primary tumors

were located in the larynx (n = 5), mobile tongue (n = 3), tonsil (n = 2). All patients had been staged N0 by ultrasound using a SONOLINE Versa Pro (Siemens, Erlangen, Germany) with a 7.5 MHz linear array transducer. In two patients an ultrasound-guided fine needle aspiration cytology was performed to confirm the preoperative N0-status.

For lymphoscintigraphy up to 50 MBq Tc-99-colloid (Solco®Nanocoll, Solco, Basel, Switzerland) dissolved in 0.1 – 0.2 ml were injected peritumorally. Particle size was less than 80 nm in diameter. Patients with easily accessible tumors were injected preoperatively, whereas patients with laryngeal tumors were injected intraoperatively.

Sentinel lymph node biopsy, elective neck dissection and tumorexcision were performed in one setting. Elective neck dissection was bilateral in 6 patients and ipsilateral in 4 patients. For elective neck dissection cutaneous flaps were raised. SLNs were localized using a gamma-probe (Navigator GPS, RMD, Watertown, MA, USA). SLNs were then biopsied and sent for pathohistologic examination. Neck dissection specimens were harvested after biopsy of the sentinel lymph nodes and checked again for SLNs after having been removed from situs. Thereafter they were also sent for pathohistologic examination. SLNs and neck dissection specimens were compared regarding occult metastatic disease.

RESULTS

In 10 patients between 1 and 11 SLNs were detected intraoperatively (table 1). In two patients one SLN each was detected in the neck dissection specimen when it was examined again with the gamma-probe after having been harvested. In one patient the lymph node was located in level I in the other patient it was located in level II.

patient	sentinel lymph nodes ipsilateral	contralateral	all	metastases in SLN	level
1	9	1	0	0	
2	1	0	0	0	
3	3	0	0	0	
4	5	0	0	0	
5	4	-	1	1	III
6	11	0	1	1	I
7	1	-	0	0	
8	7	-	0	0	
9	4	0	0	0	
10	5	-	0	0	

Table 1: Depicting number of sentinel lymph nodes (SLN) detected in the ipsi- and contralateral side of the neck, number of occult metastases found in the neck dissection specimen and in the SLN and the correlating level of the neck.

Time interval between peritumoral injection and application of the gamma-probe varied between 90 and 415 minutes. The longer the time-interval between Nanocoll®-injection and SLN-biopsy the more lymph nodes accumulated tracer (diagram 1).

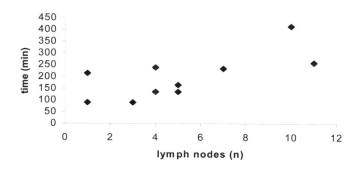

Diagram 1: Correlating time-intervall between peritumoral injec-tion and lymph node biopsy to the number of lymph nodes accumulating tracer intraoperatively.

In 8 patients pathohistologic diagnosis was N0. 2 patients had to be upstaged to N1. The metastasis in each case was located in a SLN detected with the gamma-probe intraoperatively. In one case the primary tumor was located in the mobile tongue and the metastasis was found in level III of the neck. In the other case a metastasis of a carcinoma of the tonsil was detected in level I of the neck. There was no instance that a SLN was negative for metastatic disease whereas another lymph node contained metastatic disease.

DISCUSSION

In the staging of squamous cell carcinoma of the head and neck considerable attention is focused on the neck. Standard staging procedures include ultrasound, computed tomography, and magnetic resonance imaging. Detection of metastases by these morphologic methods is depending on an increased size or structural changes of a lymph node as a symptom of metastatic disease.[4] In positron emission tomography as a functional diagnostic tool metastases of less than 5 mm cannot be detected.[5] Therefore small metastases may not be visualized by any of these means. Lymphoscintigraphy with subsequent biopsy of the SLN offers a different approach for the detection of occult metastases. For squamous cell carcinomas of the head and neck lymphoscintigraphy has been shown to have potential for the detection of occult metastatic disease in patients staged N0.[6] There have been first reports of SLN biopsy in carcinomas of the head and neck. [7-12]

In two patients a SLN each that had not been detected in vivo was detected after neck dissection specimens had been removed from situs. This may be contributed to the lapse of time between first application of the gamma-probe and the removal of the neck dissection specimen allowing the tracer to advance from first echelon nodes representing true sentinel nodes to subsequent lymph nodes. This is supported by the fact that the longer the time interval between injection and biopsy of SLNs was, the more lymph nodes accumulating tracer were detected. Additionally, there is the possibility that a SLN was not detected because of the background-activity of the primary tumor covering up the SLN.

Examination with a gamma-camera could differentiate SLNs accumulating tracer at an early point of time after injection from lymph nodes accumulating tracer at a later point of time suggesting that they may be second echelon lymph nodes. However, in the present study 50% of the patients suffered from laryngeal carcinoma. In these patients general anesthesia is needed to perform a peritumoral injection. To avoid a second general anesthesia peritumoral injection, elective neck dissection and tumor resection are performed in one setting. Therefore a lymphadenography applying a gamma-camera is not possible. Consequently, neither a mapping of subsequent lymph nodes nor an aberrant lymphatic drainage can be ruled out and all lymph nodes accumulating tracer have to biopsied.

Background-activity from tumor site poses a problem especially in levels I and II of the neck. This is due to the fact that the mandibula is limiting the range of motion of the gamma-probe making it more difficult to point the gamma-probe away from the primary site. Additionally most tumor sites are located in close proximity to these levels of the neck.

In this study all occult metastases were detected by sentinel lymph node biopsy during neck dissection. There were no metastases missed. Therefore further studies to validate the prognostic value of the sentinel lymph node concept in predicting metastatic disease in head and neck cancer seem to be promising.

CONCLUSION

The diagnostic value of the SLN-concept seems to be valid in head and neck cancer taking into account the small number of patients. A long time interval between injection and gamma-probe application results in numerous lymph nodes accumulation activity that may not necessarily be SLNs.

REFERENCES

1.   Weiss MH, Harrison LB, Isaacs RS. Use of decision analysis in planning a management strategy for the stage N0 neck. Arch Otolaryngol Head Neck Surg 1994;120:699-702.
2.   Morton DL, Wen D-R, Wong JH, et al. Technical details of intraoperative lymphatic mapping for early stage melanoma. Arch Surg 1992;127:392-399.
3.   Nwariaku FE, Euhus DM, Beitsch PD, et al. Sentinel lymph node biopsy, an alternative to elective axillary dissection for breast cancer. Am J Surg 1998;176:529-531.
4.   Van den Brekel MWM, Stel HV, Casteljins JA, et al. Cervical lymph node metastasis: assessment of radiologic criteria. Radiology 1990;177:379-384.
5.   Kau RJ, Alexiou C, Laubenbacher C, Werner M, Schwaiger M, Arnold W. Lymph node detection of head and neck squamous cell carcinomas by positron emission tomography with fluorodeoxyglucose F 18 in a routine clinical setting. Arch Otolaryngol Head Neck Surg 1999;125:1322-1328.
6.   Höft S, Maune S, Klutmann S, Bohuslavizki KH, Brenner W, Werner JA. Lymphoscintigraphy for detection of metastases in head and neck squamous cell carcinoma. Eur J Lymph Rel Prob 1999;7:93-96.
7.   Pitman KT, Johnson JT, Edington H, et al. Lymphatic mapping with isosulfan blue dye in squamous cell carcinoma of the head and neck. Arch Otolaryngol Head Neck Surg 1998;124:790-793.
8.   Koch WM, Choti MA, Civelek AC, Eisele DW, Saunders JR. Gamma probe-directed biopsy of the sentinel node in oral squamous cell carcinoma. Arch Otolaryngol Head Neck Surg 1998;124:455-459.
9.   Shoaib T, Soutar DS, Prosser JE, et al. A suggested method for sentinel node biopsy in squamous cell carcinoma of the head and neck. Head Neck 1999;21:728-733.

10. Werner JA, Dünne A-A, Brandt D, et al. Untersuchungen zum Stellenwert der Sentinel Lymphonodektomie bei Karzinomen des Pharynx und Larynx. Laryngo-Rhino-Otol 1999;78:663-670.
11. Alex JC, Sasaki CT, Krag DN, Wenig B, Pyle PB. Sentinel lymph node radiolocalization in head and neck squamous cell carcinoma. Laryngoscope. 2000;110:198-203.
12. Chiesa F, Mauri S, Grana C, et al. Is there a role for sentinel node biopsy in early N0 tongue tumors? Surgery 2000;128:16-21.

ASSESSMENT OF THE N0 NECK USING ULTRASOUND GUIDED CYTOLOGY OF SENTINEL LYMPH NODES IN HEAD AND NECK CANCER PATIENTS

Eline J.C. Nieuwenhuis[1], Michiel W.M. van den Brekel[1], Ruud H. Brakenhoff[1], Rik Pijpers[2], Charles R. Leemans[1], Gordon B. Snow[1], Jonas A. Castelijns[3]
[1]Department of Otolaryngology/Head and Neck Surgery
[2]Department of Nuclear Medicine
[3]Department of Radiology

Correspondence to: *E. J. C. Nieuwenhuis, Vrije Universiteit Medical Center, P.O. Box 7057, 1007 MB Amsterdam, The Netherlands, Phone: +31 20 44 43690, Fax: +31 20 44 43688 (e-mail: ejc.nieuwenhuis@azvu.nl)*

INTRODUCTION

In head and neck squamous cell carcinoma (HNSCC) the lymph node status of the neck is the most important prognosticator. A clinically negative neck (N0) at palpation is at risk of harboring occult metastases. Because of the low morbidity of elective neck dissection, this policy is widely accepted if the risk of occult metastases is estimated to be higher than 20%.[1] Although both computed tomography (CT) and magnetic resonance imaging (MRI) of the neck have been found to be superior to palpation in detecting cervical metastases, these modalities still have a relatively low accuracy for the N0 neck.[2-3] Furthermore, CT and MRI have the disadvantages of being expensive and not readily accessible for repeated use for follow-up of patients. In contrast, ultrasound guided fine needle aspiration cytology (USgFNAC) has a high sensitivity and specificity in experienced hands. Moreover, it is a quick, safe and cheaper technique compared to CT and MRI.[4-6] USgFNAC can help to reduce the risk of occult metastases, which justifies local excision of the tumor and a wait-and-see policy for the neck. In a retrospective study USgFNAC for initial staging as well as follow-up of the neck was evaluated. Almost 20% of oral cancer patients treated by transoral excision only on the basis of negative USgFNAC findings developed a neck node metastasis during follow-up, of whom 71% still could be salvaged by therapeutic neck dissection.[7]

Obviously, selection of the correct node for aspiration is very important and currently based on known patterns of lymphatic spread as well as on size and site of lymph nodes. However, these criteria are prone to errors, causing false-negative cases at USgFNAC. The sensitivity of USgFNAC could be improvement with better selection of lymph nodes at risk, i.e. selective aspiration of the sentinel node (SN).

The aim of this study is to investigate whether the combined use of an SN procedure and USgFNAC of the lymph nodes at risk can decrease the false-negative rate in patients treated with transoral excision and a wait-and-see policy for the neck.

PATIENTS AND METHODS

Fourty-four patients with a T1 (n=27) or T2 (n=17) N0 HNSCC of the oral cavity or oropharynx were included in the study, 21 men and 23 women. All patients were treated between May 1998 and August 2000. Primary tumors were localized in the floor of mouth (n=13), mobile tongue (n=27), buccal mucosa (n=2), and inferior alveolar process (n=2).

All patients received 15-20 MBq ^{99m}Tc-labeled colloidal albumin (CA) suspended in 0.4 ml saline (Nanocoll®, Sorin Biomedica, Sallugia, Italy, particle size 3-80 nm), by 3 to 4 submucosal peritumoral injections. Directly after injection of ^{99m}Tc-labeled colloidal albumin dynamic planar imaging (20 frames of 60 s) of the neck was performed using a large field of view gamma camera (Dual Head Genesys Imaging System, ADAC Laboratories, Milpitas, CA). Subsequently, static scintigraphy was performed during 120 sec in anterior projection to reduce overprojection and radio-active scatter from the injection site over the sentinel nodes in the neck. A handheld gamma probe (Navigator, Gamma Guidance System, RMD, Watertown, MA) was then used to detect the localization of the SN, after which its location was marked on the overlying skin. Within 1 hour after scintigraphy the SN was identified by ultrasound using a 7-MHz linear array transducer (Acuson Company, Mountain View, CA, USA, and ATL, HDI 3000, Bothell, WA, USA). In 10 patients additional static images were acquired 2-4 hours post-injection Subsequently, USgFNAC was performed of the visualized SNs as well as other enlarged lymph nodes. After preparation of the cytological smears, the needle and syringe were washed in phosphate buffered saline to obtain residues that were used for radioactivity counting in a gamma counter (Wallac, Turku, Finland) in order to confirm that the aspirated lymph node was an SN, i.e. contained radiolabeled CA. All 44 patients were planned for transoral excision of the primary tumor and a wait-and-see policy for the neck, including USgFNAC every 3 months. The initial cytological findings were correlated to the outcome of the neck, which ranged from 6 to 32 months (median 18 months).

RESULTS

In 40 out of 44 patients at least one SN was visualized by lymphoscintigraphy after peritumoral injection of ^{99m}Tc-CA. One SN was visible in 24 patients, 2 SNs in 15 patients, and 3 SNs in 1 patient. Bilateral drainage was seen in 2 patients, whereas the remaining SNs were located ipsilateral. In 4 out of 44 patients dynamic scintigraphy did not enable identification of the SN, probably due to radioactive scatter from the injection site. These 4 patients all presented with primary tumors in the anterior oral cavity. However, in 3 out of these 4 patients a SN was identified afterwards by measurement of radioactivity in at least one of the aspirated residues of enlarged lymph nodes. Hence, in only 1 out of 44 patients we did not succeed in identifying a single SN. In 10 patients static imaging was acquired 2-4 hours post injection, which showed complementary hot spots in 4 patients.

In 10 out of 44 patients 12 SNs would not have been aspirated on the basis of the size criteria. From 4 of these 12 SNs insufficient material was aspirated for a cytological diagnosis, whereas diagnostic smears were obtained from the other 8 SNs; these were all tumor-negative at cytology. Cytology of the SN was tumor-positive in 3 cases. Two of these 3 patients received additional neck surgery and one patient was treated with radiotherapy. Of the remaining 41 patients cytology was reported to be tumor-negative, and these patients therefore received the planned transoral excision of the primary tumor and wait-and-see policy for the neck. By USgFNAC during follow-up, it was shown that 10 of these 41 patients (24%) developed a lymph node metastasis in the neck within 1.5 to 7 months after treatment of the primary tumor. All 10 patients underwent therapeutic neck dissection, and 9 patients also received postoperative radiotherapy. In total, 9 of the 10 patients (90%) were salvaged; one patient died of distant metastases. No regional recurrences in the treated necks were observed. The other 31 patients did not develop a lymph node metastasis during follow-up. Follow-up of these 31 patients ranged from 6 to 32 months (median 18 months).

DISCUSSION

The SN concept is based on the principle that the site of a primary tumor has a specific lymph drainage pattern, orderly organized in subsequent nodes. The first echelon lymph node or SN can be visualized using peritumoral injection of radiolabeled particles and subsequent lymphoscintigraphy. The histopathological examination of the SN should be predictive for the N-stage of the neck, i.e. if the SN is tumor-negative, then all other nodes should be negative, whereas when other nodes are tumor-positive, the SN should be involved as well. In patients with breast cancer and melanoma the concept and predictive value of the SN has been confirmed in large studies.[8-10] Based on these studies, it has convincingly been demonstrated that the SN can predict the regional lymph node status and furthermore, that biopsy of the SN can prevent unnecessary elective regional lymph node dissections.

Sentinel node biopsy in head and neck cancer has been investigated previously.[11-13] All studies encountered several difficulties particular for the head and neck region. The main difficulty arises from the proximity of lymph nodes to the site of injection. In our study, this was clearly illustrated in the 4 patients with tumors localized in the anterior oral cavity. On the other hand, non visualization of an SN implies that extra attention should be focused to level I at ultrasonography. Another problem is that the tracer travels quickly; in 22 of the 40 (55%) patients lymphoscintigraphy identified the SN(s) within the first minute of imaging. Therefore, it is very important to perform dynamic lymphoscintigraphy in order to discriminate between a true SN and spill to second echelon nodes.

In this study the combination of USgFNAC with an SN procedure did not reveal any clinical improvement. Although in 10 patients additional nodes were aspirated as a result of the SN procedure, this had no consequence for the therapeutical management of these patients, since all cytological findings were negative. Cytology of the aspirated SNs did change the surgical treatment of 3 patients, but these SNs would all have been selected for aspiration on the basis of size criteria at US. Despite the disappointing additional value of SN aspiration, we reached a negative predictive value of 76% (31/41), which implies that 24% (10/41) of the patients developed a neck node metastases. These data are is in agreement with our earlier results.[7]

The salvage rate of patients who develop a lymph node metastasis during follow-up is of crucial importance for the clinical impact of a wait-and-see policy. Surgery and postoperative radiotherapy could salvage 9 of the 10 patients who developed neck failures during follow-up. These false negative SN-USgFNAC can be due either to aspiration from a wrong part of the sentinel node (sampling error) or a false negative cytology. Molecular detection of small tumor deposits might improve the sensitivity of USgFNAC. We are currently investigating whether real-time RT-PCR of the lymph node aspirate residues can improve sensitivity of USgFNAC.

In conclusion, a combined approach of lymphoscintigraphy and USgFNAC of SN(s) in patients with an N0 HNSCC is a technically demanding procedure. Although the SN procedure does improve lymph node selection, the sampling error in these small nodes, smaller than the regular size criteria, does not improve the clinical results. We were therefore not able to decrease the false-negative rate of USgFNAC with the addition of SN aspiration, compared to our former policy where only enlarged (more than 4mm) lymph nodes were examined. However, the moderate rate of occult metastases and high salvage rate after therapeutic neck treatment justifies further use of a wait-and-see policy with USgFNAC only for the N0 neck in HNSCC patients.

| Case (sex) | Localization | USgFNAC | | Histopathology | | |
		Interval (months)	Level (size in mm)	No of meta (ENS)	Involved levels	Follow-up (months)
1 (m)	Floor of mouth	6,5	1 (10)	7 (6)	1-4	75, DOC
2 (v)	Mobile tongue	1	3 (15)	5 (5)	1-4	65, NED
3 (m)	Floor of mouth	4	3 (5)	5 (4)	1-4	34, DOC
4 (m)	Mobile tongue	3	2 (6)	2 (1)	2-3	20, DOD
5 (m)	Soft palate	3,5	2 (25 and 8)	2 (1)	2	56, NED
6 (m)*	Floor of mouth	5	2 (8)	2 (0)	1-2	52, NED
7 (m)*	Floor of mouth	2	1 (5) and 4 (16)	6 (5)	1,3-5	14, DOC
8 (v)*	Mobile tongue	8	2 (9)	3 (1)	2	11, NED
9 (m)*	Mobile tongue	1,5	3 (10)	2 (2)	1-2	16, NED
10 (v)*	Mobile tongue	1,5	2 (10)	2 (1)	2	14, NED
11 (m)	Buccal mucosa	2	1 (9)	1 (0)	1	6, NED

Table 1. Characteristics of the 11 patients who developed neck metastases.

The interval between transoral resection and the positive USgFNAC findings are indicated in column 3, level and size of lymph node metastases in column 4. ENS, extranodal spread. Follow-up after therapeutic treatment of the neck. DOC, dead of other cause; NED, no evidence of disease; DOD, dead of disease.
*lymph node metastases detected by USgFNAC

REFERENCES

1. Weiss MH, Harrison LB, Isaacs RS. Use of decision analysis in planning a management strategy for the stage N0 neck. Arch Otolaryngol Head Neck Surg 1994;120:699-702.
2. Atula TS, Varpula MJ, Kurki TJ, Klemi PJ, Grenman R. Assessment of cervical lymph node status in head and neck cancer patients: palpation, computed tomography and low field magnetic resonance imaging compared with ultrasound-guided fine-needle aspiration cytology. Eur J Radiol 1997;25:152-161.

3. Stern WBR, Silver CE, Zeifer BA, Persky MS, Heller KS. Computed tomography of the clinically negative neck. Head Neck 1990;12:109-113.

4. Van den Brekel MW, Castelijns JA, Stel HV et al. Occult metastatic neck disease: detection with US and US-guided fine- needle aspiration cytology. Radiology 1991;180:457-661.

5. Righi PD, Kopecky KK, Caldemeyer KS, Ball VA, Weisberger EC, Radpour S. Comparison of ultrasound-fine needle aspiration computed tomography in patients undergoing neck dissection. Head Neck 1997;19:604-610.

6. Takes RP, Righi P, Meeuwis CA et al. The value of ultrasound with ultrasound-guided fine-needle aspiration biopsy compared to computed tomography in the detection of regional metastases in the clinically negative neck. Int J Radiation Oncology Biol Phys 1998;40:1027-1032.

7. Van den Brekel MW, Castelijns JA, Reitsma LC, Leemans CR, van der Waal I, Snow GB. Outcome of observing the N0 neck using ultrasonographic-guided cytology for follow-up. Arch Otolaryngol Head Neck Surg 1999;125:153-6.

8. Borgstein PJ, Pijpers R, Comans EF, van Diest PJ, Boom RP, Meijer S. Sentinel lymph node biopsy in breast cancer: guidelines and pitfalls of lymphoscintigraphy and gamma probe detection. J Am Coll Surg 1998;186:275-283.

9. Morton DL, Thompson JF, Essner R et al. Validation of the accuracy of intraoperative lymphatic mapping and sentinel lymphadenectomy for early-stage melanoma: a multicenter trial. Multicenter Selective Lymphadenectomy Trial Group. Ann Surg 1999;230:453-463.

10. Muller MG, Borgstein PJ, Pijpers R et al. Reliability of the sentinel node procedure in melanoma patients: analysis of failures after long-term follow-up. Ann Surg Oncol 2000;7:461-468.

11. Shoaib T, Soutar DS, Prosser JE et al. A suggested method for sentinel node biopsy in squamous cell carcinoma of the head and neck. Head Neck 1999;21:728-733.

12. Jansen L, Koops HS, Nieweg OE et al. Sentinel node biopsy for melanoma in the head and neck region. Head Neck 2000;22:27-33.

13. Koch WM, Choti MA, Civelek AC, Eisele DW, Saunders JR. Gamma probe-directed biopsy of the sentinel node in oral squamous cell carcinoma. Arch Otolaryngol Head Neck Surg 1998;124:455-459.

SENTINEL NODE BIOPSY IN PATIENTS UNDERGOING NECK DISSECTIONS

T. Shoaib, G.L. Ross, D.S. Soutar, I. Camilleri, H.W. Gray, R.G. Bessent, D.G. MacDonald
Plastic Surgery Unit, Canniesburn Hospital, Switchback Road, Bearsden, Glasgow. G61 1QL. United Kingdom.

INTRODUCTION

Sentinel node biopsy (SNB) is a new technique in the management of cancers. The technique, which has been studied most in melanoma and breast cancer, involves the identification of the first lymph node draining a tumour and the examination of that node for the presence of nodal metastases. If the sentinel lymph node (SLN) does not contain tumour, the implication is that the whole regional lymph node basin is free from tumour and a formal lymph node dissection can be avoided.

Few studies on sentinel node biopsy have been performed in head and neck cancer. This study was performed to determine whether the SLN could be identified in patients with head and neck cancer, undergoing neck dissections, and to determine if the SLN was an accurate reflector of the pathological status of the neck. If these aims were met, the technique could be applied as a staging procedure, and avoid an elective neck dissection in a subsequent study.

METHODS

Patients with biopsy proven, single focus, mucosal malignancies of the upper aerodigestive tract were included in the study.

SLN's were firstly identified by injection of Patent Blue V dye only. Subsequently patients were injected with radiocolloid and blue dye. The radiocolloid initially used was Albures (a large diameter colloid) for all primary tumour sites. Subsequently, Albures was reserved for tumours of the tongue and floor of mouth while Nanocoll (a small diameter colloid) was used for tumours at other sites. The presence of SLN's in the neck was recorded, as was the levels within the neck, the presence of blue dye and amount of radioactivity within the SLN's. The pathological stage of the remaining neck dissection specimen was also noted.

RESULTS

SNB using blue dye alone was performed in 16 cases. SLN's were found in only seven cases of 16 and no SLN's contained tumour by routine pathology. In these seven cases, tumour was present in the remaining neck specimen in three cases, and in these three the SLN's did not contain tumour. Parts of these results were previously published in *Head and Neck*.

SNB using a combination of blue dye and radiocolloid was performed in 40 clinically N0/x necks (from 37 patients). Twenty necks were staged pathologically N0 (pN0) and 20 were pathologically involved with metastases (pN+). In the pN+ cases, SLN's were found in 36 cases and the SLN's was found to contain tumour, using routine pathology, in 16 cases of 17 where a sentinel node was found. These results are in press for publication in *Cancer*.

SNB was performed in 27 clinically N+ necks (from 25 patients) in patients where neck dissections were also performed, using blue dye and radiocolloid. In 18 cases Albures was the radiocolloid used and in 9 cases Nanocoll was used. In the group injected with Albures, SLN's were identified in 15, tumour was found in the neck dissection in 12 cases, and the SLN's contained tumour in two of these 12. In the group injected with Nanocoll, SLN's were found in eight of nine, the neck contained tumour in eight and the SLN's also contain tumour in seven of eight. These results are being prepared for formal publication.

CONCLUSIONS

In head and neck cancer, SNB to stage the neck is best performed in the clinically N0 neck using a combination of radiocolloid and blue dye injection. The use of the SNB procedure in the clinically involved neck is not accurate but the sensitivity of the procedure increases when a small diameter colloid is used. The presence of radioactivity in the neck is a reflection of lymphatic transport from the injection site to the SLN's and the choice of radiocolloid should be dependent on the anatomical site of the primary malignancy. It is possible to locate SLN's in the neck, when no other elective neck surgery is performed, using a smaller incision than that for a neck dissection. The true sensitivity of SNB in this context is unknown but will become apparent with time. In patients with head and neck cancer, with tumours accessible to injection without the need for general anaesthesia, the SLN accurately stages the neck and we believe the procedure should be investigated in larger multicentre trials. These conclusions are in press for publication in *Current Opinion in Otolaryngology – Head and Neck Cancer*.

PATTERNS OF METASTASES IN CUTANEOUS, OCULAR AND MUCOSAL MELANOMA

B. J. Folz, MD[1]; M: Koellisch, MD[2]; Burkard M. Lippert, MD[1]; Christoph Kuelkens, MD[1]; Jochen A. Werner, MD[1]

[1]Department of Otolaryngology, Head and Neck Surgery, Philipps-University Marburg, Germany, (Chairman: Prof. Dr. J. A. Werner)
[2]Otolaryngology Office, Loewenwall 13, Braunschweig, Germany

Correspondence to: Benedikt J. Folz, Department of Otolaryngology, Head and Neck Surgery, Philipps-University Marburg, Deutschhausstr. 3, D-35037 Marburg, Germany, Tel.: ++49-6421-2862850, Fax: ++49-6421-2866367 (e-mail: folz@mailer.uni-marburg.de)

INTRODUCTION

Melanoma in humans occur as cutaneous, mucosal and ocular melanoma as well as melanoma of unknown primary. The distribution of the different melanoma types are shown in a synopsis (Table 1), which has been delineated from a publication by Chang[1], in which he evaluated data based on almost 85.000 melanoma cases. According to this publication malignant mucosal melanoma is the rarest type of melanoma with the worst prognosis. One reason for the poor prognosis might be a different biological behaviour of mucosal melanoma in comparison to other types of melanoma. The presented study was initiated to evaluate, whether differences in biologic behaviour of cutaneous, ocular and mucosal melanoma with regard to metastases could be delineated.

PATIENTS AND METHODS

A total number of 40 patients suffering from mucosal melanoma of the head and neck from two different tertiary referral centers could be evaluated for the study. Clinical data were obtained from the patients´ charts and were evaluated with the statistical software packages SPSS PC 3.0 and CSS:Statistica. The data were then compared to data of cutaneous and ocular melanoma, which were obtained from publications with similar intention.

RESULTS

Initial lymph node metastases of mucosal melanoma were found in 12 of 40 patients, and distant metastases were found in 5 patients at initial presentation. 23 of 40 patients experienced local recurrence, which was accompanied by lymph node metastases in 6 patients. The overall survival-rate was 16 months after diagnosis of the local recurrence. Delayed nodal metastases were found in 11 of 40 patients, the time intervall after diagnosis of the initial tumor varying from 5 months to 6 years. Delayed distant metastases were found in 9 of 40 patients and once distant metastases were diagnosed the patients survived for a median time interval of 13 weeks. There was no uniform pattern in the localization of distant metastases, which could be found in the axillary nodes, the inguinal nodes, the skin, the bones, the viscera, the mediastinum, the lungs, the oro- and nasopharynx, the brain and the liver. On initial presentation a single metastatic site could be found in 11 of 40 patients with mucosal melanoma. Overall the metastases were found most often in the lymph nodes with a total of 26 of 40 patients affected. Second most common site, but with significantly fewer numbers were the lungs with 3 of 40 patients and the bones with 2 of 40 patients. Liver metastases were found in only one patient.

In cutaneous melanoma more than 3 sites of metastases were found in 55% of the patients in a study published by Albert from 1996[2]. The ranking of the metastatic site was lung metastases on first rank with 51% of the patients affected. On rank 2 lymph node metastases could be found in 45% of the patients and skin metastases in 36% of the cases. The liver was affected in 24% of the cases.

In ocular melanoma one metatstatic site could be found in 55% of the patients[2]. Most commonly the metastases of ocular melanoma could be found in the liver with 90% of the patients affected. The lungs were affected in 20% of the cases and the bones were affected in 16% of the cases. Lymph node metastases were rather uncommon in ocular melanoma with only 6% of the patients affected.

See Figure 1.

DISCUSSION

Survival and the occurence of metastases in some types of melanoma seem to be strongly dependent on local recurrence. Kingdom[3] found in his survey of 17 patients with mucosal melanoma of the nose and the paranasal sinuses a local recurrence rate of up to 80%. Recurrence occured after a disease-free interval of 3-40 months and 80-85 % of the recurrences were manifest within 10-16 months[3, 4]. These observations are similar to our own observations, which have been published in a previous communication[5]. In the current study local recurrence was found in 23 of 40 patients. An explanation to the high rate of recurrence was offered by Freedman[6], who postulated the occurence of multi-centric disease as a reason for the high recurrence rate. In cutaneous melanoma the local recurrence rate seems to be dependent on the histologic type of melanoma. Cohn-Cedermark[7] observed, that patients suffering from nodular melanoma experience local recurrence sooner than those suffering from superficial spreading melanoma, however survival after recurrence was not related to histogenic type. Milton[8] observed that in cutaneous melanoma patients with thick lesions

194

gave rise to a higher proportion of recurrences in the vicinity of the scar, whereas patients with thin lesions gave rise to regional or distant metastases. Local and locoregional recurrence in contrast does not seem to be a problem in ocular melanoma, where systemic metastases occur more frequently[9].

Elective lymph node dissection is not recommended by some authors for mucosal melanoma[10, 11]. In contrast elective neck dissection has been recommended for cutaneous melanoma recently[12]. However it seems to be undisputable to perform neck dissection in mucosal melanoma in cases of proven lymph node metastases[13, 14]. In ocular melanoma neck dissection should be reserved for patients with clinically demonstrable lymphadenopathy after the exclusion of distant disease, which may only be few, due to the fact that cervical lymph node metastases are often associated with distant metastases in this type of tumor[15]. According to Lee[16] lymph node or distant metastases are rare exceptions to the rule in early stages of mucosal melanoma. In our survey 12 of 40 patients presented with initial lymph node metastases, which seems to contradict this observation. Distant metastases were found in 5 of 40 patients initially. We attribute the relatively high number of diagnosed lymph node and distant metastases in our study to refined methods in staging with CT-scans, ultrasound imaging, fine-needle aspiration cytology and MRI-scanning.

The comparison of the above mentioned data suggest that cutaneous, ocular and mucosal melanoma in fact show distinct patterns of metastases. As most common site for cutaneous melanoma metastases the lungs could be identified[2], whereas ocular melanoma metastases rather favour the liver[17]. In mucosal melanoma of the head and neck metastases are most commonly found in the draining lymph nodes of the neck and the axilla. Nodal recurrence of mucosal melanoma is associated with local recurrence in 25% of the patients, and local recurrence seems to be the most predictive factor for the poor overall-survival-rates in mucosal melanoma with a median survival time of 16 months after local recurrence and a local recurrence rate of more than 50%. However, once distant metastases have occured the survival-rates in all three types of melanomas mentioned here are quite similar with 24 weeks for cutaneous melanoma, 18 weeks for uveal melanoma and 13 weeks for mucosal melanoma.

Table 1. Synopsis of Melanoma Distribution in Humans; delineated from Chang, 1998

Melanoma Type	Percentage of Melanoma	5-year-survival
Cutaneous Melanoma	91.2%	80.8%
Ocular Melanoma	5.2%	74.6%
Melanoma of Unknown Primary	2.2%	29.1%
Mucosal Melanoma	1.3%	25.0%

REFERENCES

1. Chang AE, Karnell LH, Menck HR. The National Cancer Data Base report on cutaneous and noncutaneous melanoma: a summary of 84,836 cases from the past decade. The American College of Surgeons Commission on Cancer and the American Cancer Society. Cancer. 1998; 83:1664-78.
2. Albert DM, Ryan LM, Borden EC. Metastatic ocular and cutaneous melanoma: a comparison of patient characteristics and prognosis. Arch Ophthalmol. 1996, 114:107-8.

3.   Kingdom TT, Kaplan MJ. Mucosal melanoma of the nasal cavity and paranasal sinuses. Head Neck 1995, 17:184-189

4.   Hoyt DJ, Jordan T, Fisher SR. Mucosal melanoma of the head and neck . Arch Otolaryngol Head Neck Surg 1989, 115:1096-1099

5.   Folz BJ, Niemann AM, Lippert BM, Hauschild A, Werner JA. Mucous membrane melanomas of the upper aerodigestive tract. An analysis of 34 cases. Laryngorhinootologie. 1997, 76:289-94.

6.   Freedman HM, De Santo LW, Devine KD, Weiland LH. Malignant melanoma of the nasal cavity and paranasal sinuses. Arch Otolaryngol 1973, 97:322-325

7.   Cohn-Cedermark G, Mansson-Brahme E, Rutqvist LE, Larsson O, Singnomklao T, Ringborg U. Metastatic patterns, clinical outcome, and malignant phenotype in malignant cutaneous melanoma. Acta Oncol. 1999, 38:549-57.

8.   Milton GW, Shaw HM, Farago GA, McCarthy WH. Tumor thickness and the site and time of first recurrence in cutaneous malignant melanoma (stage 1). Br J Surg 1980, 67:543-6

9.   Sutherland CM, Chmiel JS, Haik BG, Henson DE, Winchester DP. Patient characteristics, methods of evaluation and treatment of ocular melanoma in the United States for the years 1981 and 1987. Surg Gynecol Obstet 1993, 177:497-503

10.   Panje WR, Moran WJ. Melanoma of the upper aerodigestive tract: a review of 21 cases. Head Neck Surg 1986, 8:309-312

11.   Snow GB, van der Esch EP, van Slooten EA. Mucosal melanoma of the head and neck. Head Neck Surg 1978, 1:24-30

12.   Karakousis CP. Therapeutic node dissections in malignant melanoma. Semin Surg Oncol 1998, 14:291-301

13.   Eneroth CM, Lundberg C. Mucosal malignant melanoma of the head and neck. Acta Otolaryngol 1975, 80:452-458

14.   Shah JP, Juvos AG, Strong EW: Mucosal melanomas of the head and neck. Am J Surg 1977, 134:531-535

15.   Tojo D, Weing BL, Resnick KI. Incidence of cervical metastasis from uveal melanoma: implications for treatment. Head Neck 1995, 17:137-139

16.   Lee SP, Shimizu KT, Tran LM, Juillard G, Calcaterra TC. Mucosal melanoma of the head and neck: the impact of local control on survival. Laryngoscope 1994, 104:121-126

17.   Patel JK, Didolkar MS, Pickren JW, Moore RH. Metastatic pattern of malignant melanoma. A study of 216 autopsy cases. Am J Surg. 1978, 135:807-10.

196

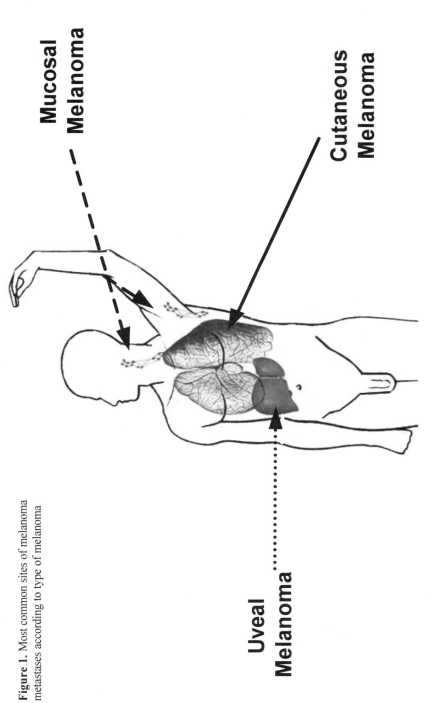

Figure 1. Most common sites of melanoma metastases according to type of melanoma

Mucosal Melanoma

Cutaneous Melanoma

Uveal Melanoma

SENTINEL NODE BIOPSY FOR MELANOMA IN THE HEAD AND NECK REGION

Liesbeth Jansen, MD[1], Heimen Schraffordt Koops, MD PhD[2], Omgo E. Nieweg, MD PhD[1], M.H. Edwina Doting, MD[3], B. Acca E. Kapteijn, MD PhD[1], Alfons J.M. Balm, MD PhD FACS[1], Albert Vermey, MD PhD FACS[4], John Th. Plukker, MD PhD[2,4], Cornelis A. Hoefnagel, MD PhD[5], D. Albertus Piers, MD PhD[6], Bin B.R. Kroon, MD PhD[1]

[1]Department of Surgery and [5]Department of Nuclear Medicine, The Netherlands Cancer Institute/ Antoni van Leeuwenhoek Hospital, Plesmanlaan 121, 1066 CX Amsterdam, the Netherlands
[2]Department of Surgical Oncology and [4]Head and Neck Surgery, [3]Department of Surgery and [6]Department of Nuclear Medicine, Groningen University Hospital, P.O. Box 30.001, 9700 RB Groningen, the Netherlands

Running title: Sentinel Node Biopsy Head and Neck Melanoma.

Key words: melanoma; sentinel node biopsy; head and neck; lymph node metastases

Correspondence to: Liesbeth Jansen, MD, Department of Surgery, The Netherlands Cancer Institute / Antoni van Leeuwenhoek Hospital, Plesmanlaan 121, 1066 CX Amsterdam, the Netherlands, Phone: 31-20-5122552; Fax: 31-20-5122554 (e-mail: LbJansen@nki.nl)

INTRODUCTION

Sentinel node biopsy has had a major impact on the practice of treating patients with cutaneous melanoma. The sentinel node is the first lymph node that receives lymphatic drainage from a malignant tumour and is therefore the first node to contain metastases if lymphatic dissemination occurs. Sentinel node biopsy is used to select patients for regional lymph node dissection. In our experience, the sentinel node can be identified in virtually all patients with melanoma on the trunk or limbs[1]. Sensitivity was estimated to be 89%[1]. Sentinel node status is a strong predictor of recurrence and survival[1]. About 6% of melanomas in our population is located in head or neck. The use of sentinel node biopsy in this subgroup has not been widely accepted. Lymphatic mapping may be more difficult to perform in this area because of the complex and unpredictable lymphatic drainage routes. In 34% to 84% of the patients, drainage is discordant with clinical prediction[2-4] and bilateral drainage is seen in approximately 10% of the patients[5]. The following study was designed to determine the clinical value of sentinel node biopsy for melanoma in the head and neck region[6].

MATERIALS AND METHODS

Thirty consecutive patients with clinically localised cutaneous melanoma in the head and neck region were included in this prospective study, performed in two tertiary care institutions from 1994 through 1997. The mean age of patients was 51 years (range 23-79 years). The primary melanoma was located on the face in six cases, on the scalp in eight, on the ear in four and in 12 cases in the neck. Median Breslow thickness was 3.0 mm (mean 3.8 mm, range 1.2 - 12.0 mm). The level of invasion was Clark IV or V in 23 cases. Sixteen patients had a nodular melanoma. Ulceration was present in nine lesions (30%). Thus, a large proportion of patients had unfavourable prognostic factors.

Lymphoscintigraphy was performed one day before surgery. Dynamic and static images were made up to two hours after injection of 50 MBq ^{99m}Tc-labelled human albumen colloid in 0.1 - 0.4 ml intracutaneously completely surrounding the tumour site. Images were always made in two directions, using a gamma camera with low energy, high resolution collimators.

Sentinel node biopsy was performed by a general surgeon, experienced in lymphatic mapping, together with a head and neck surgeon, with a technique described in detail elsewhere[1]. Intraoperatively, 0.5 - 1.0 ml patent blue dye and a gamma probe (Neoprobe® 1000/1500) was used. If a sentinel node was found to be located in the parotid gland, it was removed only if it was likely that this could be done without damaging facial nerve branches.

Sentinel nodes were examined at at least six levels with hematoxylin and eosin staining and immunohistochemistry stains for S-100 and HMB-45.

Formal lymph node dissection was performed according to the standards of neck dissection classification[7] if (micro)metastases were found in a sentinel node. Median follow-up was 26 months (range 1 - 48). No patient was lost to follow-up.

RESULTS

An average 2.3 sentinel nodes were visualised per patient (range 1-4) with lymphoscintigraphy in 27 of 30 patients. Approximately 60% of all sentinel nodes became visible within ten minutes after injection and 86% within thirty minutes. Scintigraphy did not visualise a sentinel node in three cases where the melanoma was located in the neck. Twenty-five patients showed drainage to lymph nodes on the ipsilateral side of the neck and two patients showed bilateral drainage. In 10 cases, unexpected drainage was visualized to sentinel nodes in levels that were not adjacent to the skin area where the primary melanoma was located. For example, drainage was seen from a melanoma caudally in the lateral neck to a node in level II/III and from the face to a level III node.

An average of 2.6 sentinel nodes was excised per patient(range 1-5) in 27 patients. No sentinel node was identified in three cases. About half of the sentinel nodes excised (37/70= 53%) were both blue and radioactive. Thirty sentinel nodes (43%) were radioactive but not blue and three (4%) were only blue.

In 18 patients (60%), there was a discrepancy between the number of sentinel nodes seen on scintigraphy and the true number as identified during the operation. Four times a sentinel node was located in the body of the parotid gland and was left untouched. In two cases no radioactive or blue node was identified at the site of exploration. In two cases radioactive tissue was excised in which no lymph node was found histologically. Eighteen sentinel nodes were recovered during the operation that had not been depicted on lymphoscintigraphy because they were located too close to another sentinel node or to the injection site to be seen separately on the scan.

The sentinel node was tumour-positive in eight patients. Six of these patients underwent formal lymph node dissection. Two patients in whom a parotid sentinel node contained metastasis and a subdigastric sentinel node was negative underwent subtotal parotidectomy with subdigastric biopsy. In none of these eight patients additional tumour-positive nodes were found.

Four of the 19 patients with negative sentinel nodes had a recurrence. Two may have had a false-negative biopsy because they returned with lymph node metastases in the same basin as where the tumour-negative sentinel node had been removed 11 and 17 months earlier. One patient had a local recurrence and one had distant metastases. Of the eight patients with a tumour-positive sentinel node, one had a distant recurrence and two had a regional recurrence. The three patients in whom no sentinel node was identified did not have a recurrence thus far (follow-up 28-37 months).

DISCUSSION

This study confirms the findings by Morton[5], O'Brien[3] and Carlson[8] that early metastatic disease of melanoma in the head and neck can be identified with lymphatic mapping and sentinel node biopsy, but not without a considerable number of technical difficulties.

Lymphoscintigraphy did not reveal sentinel nodes in three of 30 cases. In each of these cases, the melanoma was located in the neck and the "hot spot" at the injection site may have obscured an underlying sentinel node. As much as 16 sentinel nodes were found that were too close to another hot node to be seen on the scan. This problem occurred more often than in axilla or groin because in the head and neck many more lymph nodes are close together[9]. On the other hand, there is the problem that in the neck area often a large number of non-sentinel nodes is visualised soon after injection. This problem may be solved by using a smaller volume of tracer, a smaller amount of radioactivity or a tracer with a greater particle size

The surgeons also had more difficulties identifying the sentinel node in the neck than in axilla or groin. In half of our cases the sentinel node was either blue or radioactive. The surgeon therefore needs to be experienced in both the blue dye technique and the gamma probe detection[10]. In other parts of the body, sentinel nodes are more often both blue and radioactive[1]. Morton suggested to inject the blue dye repeatedly[5] to increase the percentage of blue nodes. In four patients a sentinel node in the parotid gland was left untouched because it was unlikely that this could be done without damaging facial nerve branches. Further studies are needed to evaluate the benefit of sentinel node biopsy to justify risking damage to the facial nerve branches. Carlson et al.[8] used loupe magnification for nodes in the parotid area to avoid this problem.

There were two false-negative sentinel node biopsies among 10 patients with lymph node metastases. This compares unfavourably to similar studies[5,8,11-13] reporting no false-negative results in series with up to 14 patients with metastases. One must bear in mind that the numbers of patients with metastases are small and that mean follow up is less than three years in each of these studies. It may be too early to draw final conclusions on sentinel node biopsy for head and neck melanoma, but our results suggest that it is not as successful as it is in other locations. Besides that, it is still unclear whether sentinel node biopsy improves survival and regional tumour control. Morton et al. have initiated a multicentre trial to investigate this.

In conclusion, sentinel node biopsy for melanoma in head and neck is a technically demanding procedure. Although sentinel node biopsy may help determine whether a neck dissection is necessary in certain patients, further investigation is required before this technique can be recommended for the standard management of cutaneous head and neck melanoma.

REFERENCES

1.   Jansen L, Nieweg OE, Peterse JL, Hoefnagel CA, Valdés Olmos RA, Kroon BBR. Reliability of sentinel lymph node biopsy for staging melanoma. Br J Surg. 2000;87:484-489.
2.   Wells KE, Cruse CW, Daniels S, Berman CG, Norman J, Reintgen DS. The use of lymphoscintigraphy in melanoma of the head and neck. Plast Reconstr Surg. 1994;93:757-761.
3.   O'Brien CJ, Uren RF, Thompson JF et al. Prediction of potential metastatic sites in cutaneous head and neck melanoma using lymphoscintigraphy. Am J Surg. 1995;170:461-466.
4.   Shah JP, Kraus DH, Dubner S, Sarkar S. Patterns of regional lymph node metastases from cutaneous melanomas of the head and neck. Am J Surg. 1991;162:320-323.
5.   Morton DL, Wen DR, Foshag LJ, Essner R, Cochran AJ. Intraoperative lymphatic mapping and selective cervical lymphadenectomy for early-stage melanomas of the head and neck. J Clin Oncol. 1993;11:1751-1756.
6.   Jansen L, Schraffordt Koops H, Nieweg OE et al. Sentinel node biopsy for melanoma in the head and neck region. Head Neck. 2000;22:27-33.
7.   Robbins KT. Pocket guide to neck dissection classification and TNM staging of head and neck cancer. Alexandria, VA: American Academy of Otolaryngology - Head and Neck Surgery Foundation, Inc. 1991.
8.   Carlson GW, Murray DR, Greenlee R et al. Management of malignant melanoma of the head and neck using dynamic lymphoscintigraphy and gamma probe-guided sentinel lymph node biopsy. Arch Otolaryngol Head Neck Surg. 2000;126:433-437.
9.   Jansen L, Nieweg OE, Kapteijn BAE et al. Reliability of lymphoscintigraphy in indicating the number of sentinel nodes in melanoma patients. Ann Surg Oncol. 2000;7:624-630.
10.   Kapteijn BAE, Nieweg OE, Liem IH et al.Localizing the sentinel node in cutaneous melanoma: gamma probe detection versus blue dye. Ann Surg Oncol. 1997;4:156-160.
11.   Wells KE, Rapaport DP, Cruse CW et al. Sentinel lymph node biopsy in melanoma of the head and neck. Plast Reconstr Surg. 1997;100:591-594.
12.   Bostick P, Essner R, Sarantou T et al. Intraoperative lymphatic mapping for early-stage melanoma of the head and neck. Am J Surg. 1997;174:536-539.
13.   Alex JC, Krag DN, Harlow SP et al. Localization of regional lymph nodes in melanomas of the head and neck. Arch Otolaryngol Head Neck Surg. 1998;124:135-140.

IMMUNE RESTORATION IN CANCER PATIENTS VIA CYCLOOXYGENASE INHIBITION: REDUCED EXPRESSION OF THE CHEMOKINE RECEPTOR CCR2

S. Lang, MD[1], Barbara Wollenberg, MD[1], C. Clausen[1], I. Löhr[1], R. Zeidler, PhD[1], D. Hölzel, PhD[2]

[1] Department of Otorhinolaryngology, Head and Neck Surgery; Grosshadern Medical Center, Ludwig-Maximilians-University Munich, Germany
[2] Institute for Medical Informatics, Biometry, and Epidemiology

Running title: Reduced CCR2 Expression in Cancer Patients

Key Words: Cyclooxygenase Inhibition; SCCHN; Head and Neck Cancer; Chemokine Receptor; CCR2

Acknowledgement. This work was supported by the Deutsche Forschungsgemeinschaft, the Rudolf Bartling-Stiftung, and the Dr. Sepp und Hanne Sturm-Gedächtnisstiftung donated to S. Lang and R. Zeidler.

Correspondence to: Dr. Stephan Lang, MD, Ludwig-Maximilians-University of Munich, Grosshadern Medical Center, Department of Otorhinolaryngology, Head and Neck Surgery, Marchioninistr. 15, 81377 Munich, Germany, Phone.:+49-89-7095-3896, Fax:+49-89-7095-6896

ABSTRACT

Background. Prostaglandin E2 (PGE$_2$) is produced by various types of malignomas and elevated PGE$_2$ serum levels, known to act immunosuppressively, can regularly be found in cancer patients. The mechanism of PGE$_2$-mediated immunosuppression however is not fully elucidated yet.

Methods. We investigated CCR2 expression on monocytes from 21 SCCHN patients and 18 healthy control donors by FACS analysis.

Results. Monocytes from SCCHN patients with large tumor burden showed a reduced CCR2 expression in comparison to monocytes from healthy donors. This downregulation was most probably due to soluble factors present in the patient's sera, since expression of CCR2 on monocytes from healthy donors was similarly reduced after incubation in sera from SCCHN patients.

Conclusion. In conjunction with our previously published data showing that cyclooxygenase inhibition restores chemokine receptor expression on monocytes *in vitro,* our results provide the rationale for the use of NSAIDs in chemoprevention or immunoadjuvant therapy of head and neck cancer.

INTRODUCTION

Accumulation of leukocytes is the hallmark of pathological conditions, including inflammatory reactions and tumors. In particular, T lymphocytes as well as cells of the monocyte/macrophage lineage have the potential to elicit antitumor reactions. In order to exert their immunological function, leukocytes emigrate from the blood across the wall of microvessels and accumulate in inflammatory tissues as well as in the vicinity of tumors. This process, called diapedesis, is mandatory for leukocytes to kill e.g. bacteria. Emigrated immune effector cells also recognize and eliminate malignantly transformed cells and control tumor growth. Although leukocytes were known to accumulate at the site of immune reactions, attractants that control this accumulation have been identified only recently.

Today, chemokines are recognized as stimuli that largely control leukocyte migration. Chemokines are small proteins that, under pathological conditions, are mostly produced by tissue cells and infiltrating leukocytes. The chemokine family is remarkably homogeneous with four cysteins forming two essential disulfide bonds. CXC and CC chemokines are distinguished according to the position of the first two cysteins. CCR2 is a seven-transmembrane domain chemokine receptor expressed on monocytes and lymphocyte subsets that recognizes monocyte chemotactic proteins-1 (MCP-1, -2 and –3). This interaction has been shown to be important for monocyte recruitment at the side of inflammation.[1]

Patients with SCCHN have a tumor-suppressed immune system partially due to the immunosuppressive effects of prostaglandins, especially prostaglandin E2 (PGE2), which are known to be elevated in SCCHN.[2] PGE2 is a metabolite of arachidonic acid and is synthesized by either of the two cyclooxygenase isoformes, Cox-1 and Cox-2.[3] Cox-1 is constitutively expressed in most tissues and is thought to carry out „housekeeping" functions such as cytoprotection of the gastric mucosa.[3] In contrast, Cox-2 is normally undetectable in normal tissues but upregulated in transformed cells. For example, Fosslien et al. found Cox-2 to be absent from normal mucosa, expressed moderately in dysplastic lesions, and being highly upregulated in malignant tissue.[3] Consequently, Cox-2 has been ascribed a neoangiogenetic and tumor-promoting effect.[4]

We have described recently that the chemokine receptor CCR5 and the ß2-Integrin Mac-1 were downregulated on primary monocytes after incubation in conditioned supernatants from human carcinoma cell lines derived from squamous cell carcinomas of the head and neck (SCCHN). We provided evidence that this downregulation was attributable – at least in part – to PGE2 produced by these cell lines and showed that this reduced expression accounted for impaired function of these monocytes, i.e. reduced migration and adhesion capacity.[5] We show here that the expression of another chemokine receptor, CCR2, is suppressed on monocytes from tumor patients in vivo.

MATERIAL AND METHODS

Monocyte isolation. Peripheral blood mononuclear cells (PBMC) from tumor patients and healthy volunteers were separated by Ficoll-Hypaque (Seromed; Berlin, Germany) gradient centrifugation. Monocytes were enriched by plastic adhesion for two hours at 37°C in RPMI and non-adherent cells were removed by washing with PBS. Adherent cells yielded approximately 60% CD14+ monocytes as confirmed by flow cytometry.

Co-culture of monocytes with allogeneic serum. Expression of the surface molecules on monocytes from tumor patients and healthy donors was investigated after cross-incubation with autologous or allogeneic sera from patients and healthy donors. By doing so we checked for an immunoinhibitory effect of tumor-serum on the monocytes and a possible restoration of receptor expression in case of serum derived from healthy donors. Thus, 5×10^5 monocytes were cultivated in the presence of tumor- or control-derived serum for two days under standard culture conditions. Finally, the adherent monocytes were harvested using a cell scratcher and subjected to FACS analysis.

FACS analysis. Staining of cells was performed as previously described[5]. Briefly, cells were incubated with an anti-CCR2 antibody (Pharmingen, Hamburg, Germany) for 30 min in PBS/2% FCS on ice. After washing in PBS, cells were incubated with a secondary FITC-labeled antibody. After a final washing cells were analyzed with a FACSCalibur (Becton Dickinson, Heidelberg, Germany).

Statistical analysis. Significance of differences was calculated using the Wilcoxon-test. P values <0.05 were considered to be significant.

RESULTS

CCR2 is downregulated on monocytes from SCCHN patients
We investigated CCR2 expression on monocytes from SCCHN patients (n=21) and healthy control donors (n=18) by FACS analysis. Monocytes from SCCHN patients with large tumor burden, i.e. stage pT3,4 with loco-regional lymphnode metastases (n=7), showed a significantly reduced CCR2 expression (p=0.0469) in comparison to monocytes from healthy donors as demonstrated in a representative experiment in Figure 1. This downregulation was most probably due to soluble factors present in the patient's sera, since expression of CCR2 on monocytes from healthy donors was similarly significantly reduced (p=0.0061) after incubation in sera from stage pT3,4 pN+ patients (n=7).

DISCUSSION

The results presented here demonstrate that monocytes from patients with SCCHN display a defective CCR2 expression. Reduced CCR2 expression was specific, since other surface molecules like MHC class I or the co-stimulatory molecule, CD80, were not affected (data not shown). The selective reduction of CCR2 expression resembles the suppression of CCR5 on monocytes by prostaglandin E2, as we have shown previously.[5]

Reduced CCR2 expression on peripheral monocytes and tumor associated macrophages is also found in patients with ovarian carcinoma.[6] These monocytes only poorly migrated in response to the chemokine MCP-1 thus implicating functional defects. The observed more prominent decrease of CCR2 expression from SCCHN patients with T3 or T4 tumors implies the possibility that factors released from the tumor itself may leak into the circulation to control or even inhibit excessive transmigration of monocytes. Down-regulation of CCR2 may be of particular interest taking in account that MCP-1 is a main determinant of macrophage infiltration into tumors.[1] Since diapedesis is pivotal for efficient tumor cell elimination, downregulation of CCR2, and consequently, reduced function of monocytes/macrophages may represent a new strategy of tumor escape from immune responses.

In summary, our data demonstrate that soluble factors present in the sera of SCCHN patients suppress CCR2 expression on monocytes. As we have shown recently that cyclooxygenase inhibition restores CCR5 expression *in vitro*,[5] these new findings provide additional arguments for an *in vivo* application of NSAIDs for immune restoration.

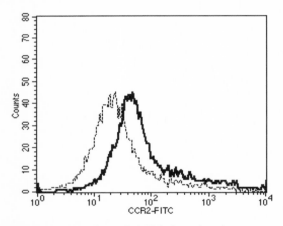

Figure 1. Expression of CCR2 is reduced on monocytes from tumor patients. PBMC-derived monocytes were enriched by plastic adhesion in cell culture medium an analyzed for surface CCR2 expression by FACS. Expression of CCR2 was found to be reduced on monocytes from tumor patients (dotted line) in comparison to monocytes from healthy donors (black line). Mean fluorescence values for patient's monocytes and monocytes from healthy donors were 117 and 325, respectivly.

REFERENCES

1.   Luster AD. Chemokines – Chemotactic cytokines that mediate inflammation. New Engl J Med 1998; 338(7):436-445.
2.   Culo F, Kaplan I, Katic V, Kolak T, Bakula B. Production of prostaglandin E by squamous cell carcinoma of the head and neck and adenocarcinoma of gastrointestinal tissue. Med Oncol Tumor Pharmacother 1992;9:35-39.

3.	Fosslien E. Molecular Pathology of Cyclooxygenase-2 in neoplasia. Ann of Clin Lab Science 2000;30:3-20.
4.	Tsujii M, Kawano S, Tsuji S, Sawaoka H, Hori M, Dubois RN. Cyclooxygenase regulates angiogenesis induced by colon cancer cells. Cell 1998;93:705-716.
5.	Zeidler R, Csanady M, Gires O, Lang S, Schmitt B, Wollenberg B. Tumor cell-derived prostaglandin E2 inhibits monocyte function by interfering CCR5 and Mac-1. FASEB J 2000;14:661-668.
6.	Sica A, Saccani A, Bottazzi B, Bernasconi S, Allavena P, Gaetano B, Fei F, LaRosa G, Scotton C, Balkwill F, Mantovani A. Defective Expression of the monocyte chemotactic protein-1 receptor CCR2 in macrophages associated with human ovarian carcinoma. J Immunol 2000;164:733-738.

T CELLS SPECIFIC FOR THE WILD-TYPE P53$_{264-272}$ PEPTIDE IN PATIENTS WITH HEAD AND NECK CANCER - IMPLICATIONS FOR IMMUNOSELECTION OF EPITOPE-LOSS TUMOR VARIANTS.

Thomas K. Hoffmann[1,2], Henning Bier[1], Ulrich Hauser[1], Albert D. Donnenberg[2,3,4], Sydney D. Finkelstein[3,5], Albert B. DeLeo[2,5], Theresa L. Whiteside[2,5,6].

[1]Department of Otorhinolaryngology, Head & Neck Surgery, Heinrich-Heine-University, D-40225 Düsseldorf, Germany.
[2]University of Pittsburgh Cancer Institute,
[3]Department of Medicine,
[4]Department of Immunology and Infectious Disease, Graduate School of Public Health,
[5]Department of Pathology, and
[6]Department of Otolaryngology at the University of Pittsburgh, Pittsburgh, Pennsylvania 15213, U.S.A.

Running title: p53 as an immune-target in head & neck cancer

Key words: p53; head and neck cancer; tetramer, immunotherapy

Acknowledgement: Supported in part by grant D/99/08916 of the Dr. Mildred Scheel Stiftung für Krebsforschung [T.K.H.] and by the National Institutes of Health Grant PO-1 DE-12321 [T.L.W., A.D.L.].

Corresponence to: Thomas K. Hoffmann, M.D., Department of Otorhinolaryngology, Head & Neck Surgery, Heinrich-Heine-University, Moorenstr. 5, D-40225 Düsseldorf, Germany, Phone.: ++49-211-811 7570, Fax: ++49-211-811 8880 (e-mail: t-k-h@web.de)

ABSTRACT

Background. Mutations in the p53 gene and accumulation of mutated p53 protein are frequently found in squamous cell carcinomas of the head and neck (SCCHN). Since accumulation of p53 is associated with enhanced presentation of wild-type sequence (wt) p53 peptides to immune cells, the development of "pan"-vaccines against SCCHN has focused on wt p53 epitopes.

209

Methods. We used the HLA-A2.1-restricted wt p53$_{264-272}$ epitope pulsed on autologous dendritic cells to generate cytotoxic T lymphocytes (CTL) *ex vivo* from circulating precursor T cells of HLA-A2.1$^+$ patients with SCCHN. **Results.** CTL specific for the wt p53$_{264-272}$ peptide were generated from PBMC obtained from 3/7 patients. Paradoxically, none of the respective three tumors could adequately present the epitope. In contrast, patients who did not generate peptide specific CTL had tumors which accumulated altered p53 and potentially could present the p53$_{264-272}$ epitope. These findings suggest that *in vivo* CTL specific for the wt p53$_{264-272}$ peptide may play a role in the elimination of epitope expressing tumor cells. This immunoselection hypothesis was confirmed when p53$_{264-272}$ specific T cells were enumerated in the peripheral circulation of SCCHN patients using tetrameric p53$_{264-272}$ / HLA-A2.1 complexes in multicolor flow cytometry. **Conclusions.** Immunoselection of tumors which become resistant to anti-p53 immune responses has important implications for future p53-based vaccination strategies.

INTRODUCTION

Current standard treatment of squamous cell carcinomas of the head and neck (SCCHN) consists of surgery and/or radiotherapy and/or chemotherapy[1]. However, prognosis of patients with SCCHN remains to be poor[2]. Novel treatment strategies are needed to improve patient survival, and tumor vaccine development is considered a promising therapeutic strategy. Since mutations of p53 frequently occur in SCCHN[3,4,5], the altered and accumulated tumor suppressor gene product could be an attractive candidate for tumor vaccination strategies[6,7]. Initially, the effort to develop p53-based vaccines focused on missense mutations, which are tumor specific in nature. However, they have limited clinical usefulness, because of the requirement that they need to occur within epitopes which are presented by human leucocyte antigen (HLA) molecules expressed by the individual patient. On the other hand, the majority of p53 mutations involves the alteration of a single amino acid. Therefore, in p53 accumulating tumors, the majority of p53 epitopes processed and presented to immune cells can be expected to be wild-type and potential candidates for the development of broadly-applicable cancer vaccines[8-17].

We used the HLA-A2.1-restricted, human wild type sequence (wt) epitope p53$_{264-272}$ in order to induce an anti-p53 response *ex vivo* with peripheral blood mononuclear cells (PBMC) obtained from patients with SCCHN. For this *in vitro* sensitization (IVS), dendritic cells (DC) were used as potent antigen presenting cells after being pulsed with the p53$_{264-272}$ peptide. T cells which were obtained after IVS were evaluated with regard to the presence of p53 mutations and protein expression in the patients′ tumors. These *in vitro* experiments were completed by investigations in which p53$_{264-272}$ specific T cells were determined in the peripheral circulation of SCCHN patients using novel tetrameric p53$_{264-272}$ peptide / HLA-A2.1 complexes in a multicolor flow cytometry assay.

METHODS

Generation of anti-p53 CTL using peptide pulsed autologous DC
PBMC were isolated from HLA-A2.1$^+$ SCCHN patients and healthy controls. DC were generated from monocytes in the presence of GM-CSF and IL-4, pulsed with the p53$_{264-272}$

peptide (LLGRNSFEV), and co-cultured with autologous PBMC in the presence of low dose IL-7 and IL-2. After weekly restimulations, reactivity of generated T cells was tested in γ-IFN ELISPOT as well as cytotoxicity assays against various targets: peptide pulsed T2 cells and cell lines of SCCHN, naturally presenting the p53$_{264-272}$ epitope. Specificity was confirmed in antibody (Ab) blocking experiments and by tetramer staining.

Tetrameric peptide / HLA-A2.1 complexes ("tetramers")
The streptavidin-phycoerythrin (PE)-labeled tetramers were applied in four-color flow cytometry assays as previously described by us in detail[18].

p53 analysis in SCCHN
Exons 5 through 8 of the p53 gene were analyzed using a PCR based technique[19]. For p53 protein, immunohistochemistry with D0-7 was performed.

RESULTS

In vitro generation of anti-p53 CTL
Generated T cells were HLA class I-restricted and reacted against T2 cells pulsed with p53$_{264-272}$ peptide and, to a lesser extent, against HLA-A2.1 matched SCCHN cell lines which naturally present the epitope[20]. In contrast, SCCHN cell lines which do not express the epitope were only minimally lysed and their killing was not blocked by anti-HLA-A2 Ab. Tetrameric p53$_{264-272}$/HLA-A2.1 complexes were used to confirm the anti-p53$_{264-272}$ specificity of CTL present in bulk IVS cultures. In one SCCHN patient up to 35 % out of all CD8$^+$ lymphocytes were found to be CD8$^+$/tetramer$^+$ after 4 IVS.

Table 1 summarizes the results obtained with PBMC of SCCHN patients after IVS with the p53$_{264-272}$ peptide. T cells of 3/7 patients were found to be reactive against peptide-loaded T2 cells as well as against tumor cells naturally presenting the wt p53$_{264-272}$ epitope. This reactivity was HLA class I-restricted, as it was blocked by anti-HLA class I or -HLA-A2 Ab.

p53 analysis in patients´ tumor and association to anti-p53 response
Immunohistochemistry for p53 as well as sequencing of the p53 gene in the patients' tumors were performed in order to investigate a possible association between p53$_{264-272}$ specific CTL response and p53 status of the tumor. Although it is generally considered that HLA-A2$^+$ tumor target cells sensitive to lysis by CTL recognizing the wt p53$_{264-272}$ epitope do accumulate mutant p53, this phenotype is not an absolute prerequisite for CTL recognition. In particular, mutation at codon 273 is known to prevent the processing and presentation of p53$_{264-272}$ epitope, due to interference with the proteasome pathway[21] (Table 1). In the four patients who did not show CTL responses to wt p53$_{264-272}$ epitope (#1, #2, #3 and #4), mutated p53 was detected in all tumors. The tumors of patients #1, #2 and #3 accumulated p53 and could present the epitope, whereas the tumor of patient #4 had a mutation in codon 213, resulting in a stop codon prior to the epitope. In the three patients who showed CTL responses (#5, #6 and #7), the tumors had wt p53 and no protein accumulation (#5, #6), while the tumor of patient #7 accumulated p53 with a missense mutation at codon 273, known to prevent the processing and presentation of p53$_{264-272}$ epitope[21]. All three tumors were, therefore, unlikely to present the wt p53$_{264-272}$ epitope. Thus, it would appear that the presence of a CTL response

to the epitope under study is more prevalent in patients bearing a tumor unable to present this particular epitope.

In vivo frequency of p53$_{264-272}$ specific T cells in SCCHN patients
We next extended the study to 30 SCCHN patients and 30 healthy individuals (all HLA-A2.1$^+$) and determined the frequency of p53$_{264-272}$ specific T cells by multicolor flow cytometry, using tetramer technology. First, patients who responded to IVS with the p53 peptide had higher frequencies of p53$_{264-272}$ specific precursor T cells than „non-responders". Furthermore, SCCHN patients had significantly higher proportions of p53$_{264-272}$ specific CD8$^+$ T cells in the circulation as compared to normal donors. Patients with particularly high frequencies of wt p53$_{264-272}$ specific T cells had p53 negative tumors. In contrast, tumors of patients with very low frequencies of wt p53$_{264-272}$ specific T cells showed p53 overexpression in most cases.

CONCLUSIONS

We are currently involved in the exploration of immunological approaches for the adjuvant treatment of SCCHN. Either by using unknown tumor antigens[22] or a known tumor associated antigen[20], we were able to induce anti-tumor responses *in vitro*. However, it was not always possible to induce an anti-tumor response with PBMC obtained from SCCHN patients. In case of p53 we expected that PBMC of SCCHN patients whose tumors accumulate p53 would yield anti-p53 responses and not of those whose tumor can not present the p53$_{264-272}$ epitope. Surprisingly, anti-p53 CTL were generated from PBMC of patients with tumors unlikely to present the wt p53$_{264-272}$ epitope (wild type p53 expression or p53 mutation which prevents presentation of the epitope), but not from PBMC of patients whose tumors most likely could present the epitope (accumulation of mutant p53). These findings suggest that *in vivo*, CTL specific for the wt p53$_{264-272}$ peptide may play a role in the elimination of tumor cells expressing this epitope and in immunoselection as well as outgrowth of "epitope-loss" tumor cells (Figure 1).

Figure 1. Model for immuno-selection of epitope loss tumor variants. The initial tumor consists of a p53 heterogeneity with some parts accumulating p53 (p53$^+$) whereas others do not accumulate p53 (p53$^-$). The p53 accumulating cells are subsequently subjected to significant selection pressure by certain expandable wt p53 specific CTL. This, subsequently, could lead to the outgrowth of p53 protein „negative" tumors.

Immunoselection of epitope loss tumor variants

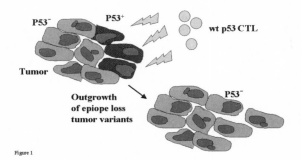

Figure 1

212

This immunoselection hypothesis was further supported by the reciprocal relationship between frequency of p53$_{264-272}$ specific T cells and p53 tumor status, suggesting that in the presence of wt p53$_{264-272}$ specific T cells epitope-loss tumor variants are selected *in vivo*[23]. Such an immunoselection might contribute to tumor escape from the immune system and has important implications for future p53-based immunization strategies, since potential „responders" appear to lack suitable targets. However, PBMC of patients whose tumors had a high potential to express the target-antigen were low in number and were not expandable by IVS. These cells can be considered to have been tolerized[24,25,26], and it seems to be necessary to break PBMC tolerance in these individuals in order to introduce a p53 based immunotherapy. We subsequently sought to increase the immunogenicity of the wt p53$_{264-272}$ peptide by introducing single amino acid exchanges and indeed were able to increase response frequencies *in vitro*[27]. Most importantly, these variant peptides or altered peptide ligands were found capable to induce specific T cells in a proportion of PBMC obtained from SCCHN patients who did not respond to the parental peptide. Importantly, this was the case in a patient whose autologous tumor was able to present the p53 epitope.

The possibility that immunoselection of epitope-loss tumor cells might occur during p53-based immunotherapy merits consideration in designing future clinical trials. It implies that the use of vaccines capable of targeting multiple tumor-associated antigens may be necessary to prevent tumor escape from the immune system[28].

Table 1. PBMC obtained from SCCHN patients were stimulated with peptide-pulsed DC. Effector cell reactivity was tested in ELISPOT or cytotoxicity assays, and T-cell specificity for the p53$_{264-272}$ epitope was confirmed using tetramer technology. The results after the 3rd IVS are shown in the second column. p53 mutations were determined by sequence analysis and p53 protein expression by immunohisto-chemistry. The R 273 H mutation has been shown to prevent presentation of p53$_{264-272}$ epitope[21].

Table 1 Summary of responses to wt p53$_{264-272}$ in patients with SCCHN and the p53 status of patients with SCCHN.

SCCHN	response to IVS	p53 mutation	p53 accumulation
1	-	R-248-W	+
2	-	V-157-F	+
3	-	E-286-K	+
4	-	213 stop	-
5	+	wt	-
6	+	wt	-
7	+	R-273-H	(+)

The R-273-H

L 264	→	Presentation of p53$_{264-272}$
L 265		
G 266		
R 267		
N 268	mutation →	L 264
S 269		L 265
F 270		G 266
E 271		R 267
V 272		N 268
R 273		S 269 → Presentation of p53$_{264-272}$ ✗
		F 270
		E 271
		V 272
		H 273

213

REFERENCES

1. Vokes E E. Combined-modality therapy of head and neck cancer. Oncology 1997;11:27-30.
2. Parker SL, Tong T, Bolden S, Wingo PA. Cancer Statistics. CA Cancer J Clin 1996;46:5-12.
3. Hollstein M, Sidransky D, Vogelstein B, Harris CC. p53 mutations in human cancers. Science 1991;253:49-53.
4. Hollstein M, Shomer B, Greenblatt M, Soussi T, Hovig E, Montesano R, Harris CC. Somatic point mutations in the p53 gene of human tumors and cell lines: updated compilation. Nucleic Acids Res 1996;24:141-146.
5. Raybaud Diogene H, Tetu B, Morency R. p53 overexpression in head and neck squamous cell carcinoma: review of the literature. Eur J Cancer B Oral Oncol. 1996;32b: 143-149.
6. Harris C C. Structure and function of the p53 tumor suppressor gene: clues and rational cancer therapeutic strategies. J Natl Cancer Inst 1996;88:1442-55.
7. DeLeo A B. p53-based immunotherapy of cancer. Critical Rev Immunol 1998;18:29-35.
8. Houbiers J G A, Nijman HW, Drijfhout JW, Kenemans P, van der Velde CJH, Brand A, Momburg F, Kast WM, Melief CJM. In vitro induction of human cytotoxic T lymphocyte responses against peptides of mutant and wild-type p53. Eur J Immunol 1993;23:2072-2077.
9. Nijman HM, van der Burg SH, Vierboom MP, Houbiers JG, Kast WM, Melief CJ. p53, a potential target for tumor-directed T cells. Immunol Lett 1994;40:171-178.
10. Zeh HJ, LederGH, Lotze MT, Salter RD, Tector M, Stuber G, Modrow S, Storkus WJ. Flow-cytometric determination of peptide-class-I complex formation. Identification of p53 peptides that bind to HLA-A2. Human Immunol 1994;39:79-85.
11. Theobald M, Biggs J, Dittmer D, Levine AJ, Sherman LA. Targeting p53 as a general tumor antigen. Proc Natl Acad Sci 1995;92:11993-11997.
12. Mayordomo JI, Loftus DJ, Sakamoto H, DeCesare CM, Appasamy PM, Lotze MT, Storkus WJ, Appella EA, DeLeo AB. Therapy of murine tumors with p53 wild-type and mutant sequence peptid-based vaccines. J Exp Med 1996;183:1357-1365.
13. Ropke M, Hald J, Guldberg P, Zeuthen J, Norgaard L, Fugger L, Svejgaard A, van der Burg S, Nijman HW, Melief CJ, Claesson MH. Spontaneous human squamous cell carcinomas are killed by a human cytotoxic T lymphocyte clone recognizing a wild-type p53-derived peptide. Proc Natl Acad Sci 1996;93:14704-14707.
14. Vierboom M P, Nijman HW, Offringa R, van der Voort EI, van Hall T, van den Broek L, Jan Fleuren G, Kenemans P, Kast WM, Melief CJ. Tumor eradication by wild type p53 specific cytotoxic T lymphocytes. J Exp Med 1997;186:695-703.
15. Gnjatic S, Cai Z, Viguier M, Chouaib S, Guillet JG, Choppin J. Accumulation of the p53 protein allows recognition by human CTL of a wild-type p53 epitope presented by breast carcinomas and melanomas. J Immunol 1998;160:328-333.
16. McCarty TM, Liu X, Sun JY, Peralta EA, Diamond DJ, Ellenborn JDI. Targeting p53 for adoptive T-cell immunotherapy. Cancer Res 1998;58:2601-2605.
17. Chikamatsu K, Nakano K, Storkus WJ, Appella E, Lotze MT, Whiteside TL, DeLeo AB. Generation of anti-p53 cytotoxic T lymphocytes from human peripheral blood using autologous dendritic cells. Clin Cancer Res 1999;5:1281-1288.
18. Hoffmann TK, Donnenberg V, Friebe U, Meyer M, Rinaldo CR, DeLeo AB, Whiteside TL, Donnenberg AD. Competition of peptide-MHC class I tetrameric complexes with anti-CD3 provides evidence for specificity of peptide binding to the TCR complex. Cytometry 2000;41:321-328.
19. Finkelstein SD, Przygodzki R, Pricolo V, Sakallah SA, Swalsky PA, Bakker A, Lanning R, Bland KI, Cooper DL. Prediction of biologic aggressiveness in colorectal cancer by p53/K-ras-2 topographic genotyping. Mol. Diagnosis 1996;1:5-12.
20. Hoffmann TK, Nakano K, Elder E, Dworacki G, Finkelstein SD, Apella E, Whiteside TL, DeLeo AB. Generation of T cells specific for the wild-type sequence $p53_{264-272}$ peptide in cancer patients – implications for immunoselection of epitope-loss variants. J Immunol 2000;165:5938-5944.
21. Theobald M, Ruppert T, Kuckelkorn U, Hernandez J, Häussler A, Antunes Ferreira E, Liewer U, Biggs J, Levine AJ, Huber C, Koszinowski UH, Kloetzel PM, Sherman LA. The sequence alteration associated with a mutational hotspot in p53 protects cells from lysis by cytotoxic T lymphocytes specific for a flanking peptide epitope. J Exp Med 1998; 188:1017-1028.
22. Hoffmann TK, Meidenbauer N, Dworacki G, Kanaya H, Whiteside TL. Generation of tumor-specific T lymphocytes by cross-priming with human dendritic cells ingesting apoptotic tumor cells. Cancer Res 2000;60:3542-3549.

23. Hoffmann TK, Donnenberg A, Finkelstein S, Chikamatsu K, Donnenberg V, Friebe-Hoffmann U, Appella E, Whiteside TL, DeLeo AB. Immunosection of epitope loss tumor variants by wild type sequence p53$_{264-272}$ specific T cells in the peripheral circulation of patients with squamous cell carcinoma of the head and neck. Submitted for publication.

24. Matzinger P. Tolerance, danger, and the extended family. Annu Rev Immunol 1994 12:991.

25. Theobald M, Biggs J, Hernández J, Lustgarten J, Labadie C, Sherman LA. Tolerance to p53 by A2.1-restricted cytotoxic T lymphocytes. J Exp Med 1997;185:833-839.

26. Hernández J, Lee PL, Davis MM, Sherman LA. The use of HLA-A2.1/p53 peptide tetramers to visualize the impact of self tolerance on the TCR repertoire. J Immunol 2000;164:596-602.

27. Hoffmann TK, Nakano K, Maeurer M, Chikamatzu K, Loftus DJ, Appella E, Whiteside TL, DeLeo AB. Variant peptides of the wild-type sequence p53$_{264-272}$ epitope overcome the unresponsiveness of T cells in cancer patients – implications for immunotherapy. Submitted for publication.

28. Marincola FM, Jaffee EM, Hicklin DJ, Ferrone S. Escape of human solid tumors from T-cell recognition: molecular mechanisms and functional significance. Adv Immunol 2000;74:181-273.

CHEMOTHERAPY-INDUCED APOPTOSIS IS NOT DEPENDENT ON FAS/FAS LIGAND INTERACTIONS IN SQUAMOUS CELL CARCINOMA OF THE HEAD AND NECK (SCCHN)

Hilmar Balló[1], Cristoph Sproll[1], Ursula Koldovsky[2], Vera Balz[1], Henning Bier[1]
[1]Dept. of ORL/Head & Neck Surgery, Heinrich-Heine-University, Düsseldorf, Germany
[2]Dept. Of Gynecology, Heinrich-Heine-University, Düsseldorf, Germany

Correspondence to: Dr. med. Hilmar Balló, Dept. of ORL/Head & Neck Surgery, Heinrich-Heine-University, Moorenstr. 5, 40225 Düsseldorf, Phone: 0049-211 8117577, Fax: 0049-211 8118880 (Ballo@uni-duesseldorf.de)

ABSTRACT

It is well established that antineoplastic drugs display their cytotoxic action via apoptosis and that p53 wild type expression may be an important factor for the sensitivity to anticancer agents. Moreover, the finding of a p53 responsive element within the Fas gene, a central mediator of apoptosis, has led to a mechanistic explanation of how p53 may contribute to tumour progression and drug resistance. To further investigate the role of the Fas system in chemotherapy, we determined a) Fas and FasL expression (FACS-analysis), b) cytotoxicity (colorimetric MTT-assay), c) apoptosis (FACS-analysis with annexin), and d) effects of apoptosis inhibitors in established cell lines of SCCHN upon treatment with the anticancer drugs Cisplatin and Bleomycin. In addition, p53 sequence analysis of the whole coding region was performed. Irrespective of their p53 status, upregulation of Fas and FasL was demonstrated in SCCHN lines after treatment with anticancer drugs. The addition of caspase-inhibitors, but not antagonistic anti-Fas antibodies, interfered with the induction of apoptosis, thus suggesting alternative signaling pathways. Our data provide evidence that the Fas system is not inevitably engaged in the cytotoxic action of antineoplastic agents in SCCHN.

INTRODUCTION

The mechanisms of drug induced apoptosis are poorly understood. Recent studies suggest that p53 may be required in cells treated with chemotherapeutic agents. The precise mechanism of p53 mediated apoptosis is still unclear. Nuclear accumulation of p53 results in transcription of several genes that are involved in apoptosis, like bcl2/bax, mdm2, TGF-α_and Fas (CD95).

217

The Fas system, comprising the Fas receptor (APO-1/CD95), and its ligand FasL (CD95L) is a central mediator of programmed cell death in both physiological and pathological processes. Fas is expressed on a great variety of cell-types throughout the body while the expression of FasL was initially believed to be restricted to activated immunocompetent cells. Later FasL expression has also been described in other tissues for example stromal cells in the eye or testis and recent findings provide evidence for a role of the Fas system in the regulation of tumor progression[1-5].

The Fas system is also considered to be involved in the cytotoxic action induced by DNA damaging anticancer drugs. Upregulation of Fas upon treatment with anticancer drugs has been related to p53 wild type expression for several tumor cell lines[6]. Nevertheless, the significance of this Fas upregulation on the induction of apoptosis in solid tumors remains unclear. Identification of a p53 responsive element within the Fas gene led to a mechanistic explanation of how p53 can contribute to tumor progression or drug resistance[7]. In this context p53 acts as a transcriptional factor for Fas expression. In order to investigate the role of the Fas system in head and neck cancer, we assessed the expression of Fas and FasL in a panel of established cell lines. Furthermore, we performed functional experiments to test whether drug-induced apoptosis involves the Fas system and if so, whether this is dependent on p53 wild type expression.

MATERIAL AND METHODS

Cell lines and cell culture
The human head and neck squamous cell carcinoma cell lines (HNSCC) UD-SCC-1-6 were established and characterized in our laboratory[8]. Furthermore, tumor cell lines HLac79[9] and UM-SCC-11B, -14C -17A and -22B[10] were investigated. 8029Na and 8029DDP are recloned sublines of HLac79, established in our laboratory. All cell lines were kept under standard conditions in a fully humidified atmosphere at 37°C and 5% CO_2.

RT-PCR
RT-PCR was performed on total cellular RNA extracted from the cell lines. After subjecting mRNA to first strand cDNA synthesis, PCR for Fas and FasL was performed with specific primers, described by Gastman et al.[11] leading to a 683 bp sequence for Fas and for FasL described by O'Connell et al.[12] leading to a 344 bp sequence. Primers for p53 were described by Murakami et al.[13]. The RT-PCR-products were submitted to electrophoresis on a 1% agarose gel and visualized by ethidium bromide staining.

Sequence analysis of amplified p53 cDNA
RT-PCR-products were purified with the QIAquick PCR Purification Kit (QIAGEN GmbH/Hilden/Germany) according to the manufacturers protocol. 4 _l of purified RT-PCR-product were mixed with 8 _l PRISM AmpliTaq FS Ready Reaction Dye Terminator sequencing kit (Applied Biosystems, Weiterstadt, Germany) and 6 nmol of specific oligo-nucleotide primer. After ethanol-precipitation, the sequencing products were analyzed on an Applied Biosystems model 373 automated sequencer. Identified mutations were confirmed by repeated RT-PCR-analysis.

Immunohistochemistry

Immunohistochemistry was performed on tumor cell monolayers. Fas was detected with mouse monoclonal antibody APO-1 (DAKO/Carpinteria/USA) and FasL with rabbit polyclonal antibody N-20 (Santa Cruz Biotechnology/Santa Cruz/USA). The Vectastain ABC Kit (Vector Laboratories/Burlinggame/USA) was used according to the manufacturers instructions. Monolayers were fixed with methanol and acetone, incubated with primary antibodies for 1 hour, followed by exposure to biotinylated secondary antibody for 30 minutes and ABC complex. Reaction products were visualized by immersing the slides in diaminobenzidine-tetrachloride or 3-amino-9-ethylcarbazol and finally counterstaining the cells with Mayer´s hemalaune.

MTT-Assay

Tumor cells were seeded in a density of 6000 cells/well in 96-well plates and kept under standard conditions in a moist atmosphere. On day 3, IC-50 of cisplatin or bleomycin +/- caspase-inihbitors (Calbiochem/Darmstadt/Germany) in a concentration of 10 mmol or antagonistic anti-Fas blocking antibody ZB4 (Beckham-Coulter/Fullerton/USA) was added to the tumor cells 24h prior to the addition of CH-11 (1000 ng/ml). Isotype-matched antibody was used as a negative control. For the 13 cell lines tested, IC-50 ranged between 1,0_g/ml and 7,5_g/ml for cisplatin (medac/Hamburg/Germany) and 3,4_g/ml and 288_g/ml for bleomycin (Heinrich Mack/Illertissen/Germany). The effect on tumor cells of antibody CH-11 was also tested alone. After antibody incubation for 36 or 48h growth inhibition was measured in a colorimetric MTT-assay.

Flow cytometric analysis

Surface expression of Fas and FasL was measured after detachment of the cells with trypsin/EDTA. The cells were treated with anti-Fas-IgG-FITC (Beckham-Coulter/Fullerton/USA) or anti-FasL NOK-1 (Pharmingen/Franklin Lakes/USA), followed by secondary FITC-labeled antibody. Normal mouse anti-human-IgG served as negative control. Apoptosis was measured using the Annexin-Kit (Beckham-Coulter/Fullerton/USA) according ot the manufacturers instructions.

RESULTS

Fas and FasL were detectable by immunohistochemistry in all cell lines. Fas expression was membranously pronounced while FasL was detected intracytoplasmatic. Moreover, we successfully identified mRNA for both Fas and FasL by RT-PCR in all cell lines. To further investigate the funtional capacity of the Fas system in our experimental system, we incubated the cell lines with the agonistic antibody CH-11, in order to induce apoptosis in Fas expressing cells.

It turned out that the majority of the tumor cell lines were resistant to CH-11 mediated apoptosis. Treatment with CH-11 alone led to growth inhibition of 40-60% in UD-SCC-6, UM-SCC-17A and HLac79 and by lower percentage in UM-SCC14-C. For all other cell lines only a minor or no cytotoxic effect was observed.

P53 sequence analysis showed that only two cell lines (UD-SCC-2, UM-SCC-17A) expressed wild type p53. In the remaining 11 cell lines the p53 gene harbors deletions or missense mutations.

To further investigate whether the Fas system was involved in drug induced apoptosis in HNSCC and its dependancy to p53, we measured Fas and FasL surface expression after pretreatment with cisplatin or bleomycin by FACS-analysis. FACS-analysis revealed an upregulation of Fas and to a lower extent of FasL after anticancer drug treatment. This effect was not dependant on the p53 status of the tumor cell line. Furthermore, we tried to confirm the results obtained by FACS-analysis by additional functional experiments using the MTT-assay. Herewith, we were able to reproduce the resistance to CH-11 mediated apoptosis. After pretreatment with either cisplatin or bleomycin some tumor cell lines became more sensitive for CH-11 mediated apoptosis, like 8029NA or UD-SCC-1 (both with mutated p53), resulting in an additive effect. The addition of caspase-inhibitors partly reversed the anticancer drug effects, indicating at least that cisplatin and bleomycin exert their effects via apoptosis. In contrast, the addition of antagonistic Fas antibody ZB4 did not inhibit cell death after drug treatment.

In order to confirm that cell death after drug treatment is due to apoptosis, we reexamined the MTT-results by FACS-analysis using the Annexin-Apoptosis-Kit. Early apoptotic events were detectable when cells were treated with either cisplatin or bleomycin or with combinations of the anticancer drug plus CH-11, irrespective of the p53 status of the cell line. Again, apoptosis induced by these agents was blockable by caspase-inhibitors, but not by the antagonistic Fas antibody.

DISCUSSION

We have detected Fas and FasL in HNSCC by immunohistochemistry, RT-PCR and FACS-analysis. Despite Fas expression, the majority of the cell lines tested turned out to be resistant to CH-11 induced apoptosis. Only the cell lines UD-SCC-6, UM-SCC-17A and Hlac79 showed growth reduction of 40-60% after treament with CH-11 alone. Fas resistance in HNSCC could be due to yet not determined loss of proapoptotic or gain of antiapoptotic factors. Another possibility is the expression of decoy receptor 3 or FLICE-inhibitory-protein. Both components were shown to be highly expressed in lung cancer[14,15]. A role for the Fas system has been suggested in drug induced apoptosis in several cell types[16-19]. Nevertheless this remains a matter of debat, because there are numerous reports that do not support the link between the Fas system and the cytotoxic action of anticancer drugs[20-23]. An involvement of the Fas signalling pathway in drug induced apoptosis requires an upregulation of Fas and FasL, leading to fratricide or autocrine mechanisms of cell death. Indeed, we demonstrated increased Fas and FasL expression on all HNSCC after pretreatment with anticancer drugs. In some cases, this led to an enhanced cytotoxicity of CH-11 as in UD-SCC-1, UD-SCC-6 and 8029NA. Antagonistic Fas antibody ZB4 was not able to block drug induced apoptosis, as caspase-inihbitors did. Interestingly, this effect seems to be independant on the p53 status of the cell line. This is in contrast to reports suggesting that the Fas gene is under transcription control of functional p53[6,7,24]. UD-SCC-2 and UM-SCC17-A, however, the only wildtype p53 expressing cell lines in our panel, showed no increase in CH-11 mediated apoptosis, as the mutated cell lines UD-SCC-1, UD-SCC-6 and 8029NA. These findings suggest that the Fas-system is only partly related to drug induced apoptosis in HNSCC. Furthermore, its dependance on p53 wildtype expression remains questionable. Currently we are investigating the functional capacity of p53 in our HNSCC in order to obtain a more detailed insight in drug induced apoptosis and its relation to the Fas system.

REFERENCES

1. Bennett MW, O'Connell J, O'Sullivan G C, Roche D, Brady C, Kelly J, et al. Expression of Fas ligand by human gastric adenocarcinomas: a potential mechanism of immune escape in stomach cancer [see comments]. Gut 1999;44(2):156-62.

2. O'Connell J, Bennett MW, O'Sullivan GC, Collins JK, Shanahan F. Resistance to Fas (APO-1/CD95)-mediated apoptosis and expression of Fas ligand in esophageal cancer: the Fas counterattack. Dis Esophagus 1999;12(2):83-9.

3. Medema JP, de Jong J, van Hall T, Melief CJ, Offringa R. Immune escape of tumors in vivo by expression of cellular FLICE- inhibitory protein [see comments]. J Exp Med 1999;190(7):1033-8.

4. Bodey B, Bodey B, Jr., Siegel SE, Kaiser HE. Fas (Apo-1, CD95) receptor expression in childhood astrocytomas. Is it a marker of the major apoptotic pathway or a signaling receptor for immune escape of neoplastic cells? In Vivo 1999;13(4):357-73.

5. Hahne M, Rimoldi D, Schroter M, Romero P, Schreier M, French LE, et al. Melanoma cell expression of Fas(Apo-1/CD95) ligand: implications for tumor immune escape. Science 1996;274(5291):1363-6.

6. Owen-Schaub LB, Zhang W, Cusack JC, Angelo LS, Santee SM, Fujiwara T, et al. Wild-type human p53 and a temperature-sensitive mutant induce Fas/APO-1 expression. Mol Cell Biol 1995;15(6):3032-40.

7. Muller M, Strand S, Hug H, Heinemann EM, Walczak H, Hofmann WJ, et al. Drug-induced apoptosis in hepatoma cells is mediated by the CD95 (APO- 1/Fas) receptor/ligand system and involves activation of wild-type p53. J Clin Invest 1997;99(3):403-13.

8. Ballo H, Koldovsky P, Hoffmann T, Balz V, Hildebrandt B, Gerharz CD, et al. Establishment and characterization of four cell lines derived from human head and neck squamous cell carcinomas for an autologous tumor- fibroblast in vitro model. Anticancer Res 1999;19(5B):3827-36.

9. Zenner HP, Lehner W, Herrmann IF. Establishment of carcinoma cell lines from larynx and submandibular gland. Arch Otorhinolaryngol 1979;225(4):269-77.

10. Carey TE, Van Dyke DL, Worsham MJ, Bradford CR, Babu VR, Schwartz DR, et al. Characterization of human laryngeal primary and metastatic squamous cell carcinoma cell lines UM-SCC-17A and UM-SCC-17B. Cancer Res 1989;49(21):6098-107.

11. Gastman BR, Johnson DE, Whiteside TL, Rabinowich H. Caspase-mediated degradation of T-cell receptor zeta-chain. Cancer Res 1999;59(7):1422-7.

12. O'Connell J, O'Sullivan GC, Collins JK, Shanahan F. The Fas counterattack: Fas-mediated T cell killing by colon cancer cells expressing Fas ligand. J Exp Med 1996;184(3):1075-82.

13. Murakami Y, Hayashi K, Sekiya T. Detection of aberrations of the p53 alleles and the gene transcript in human tumor cell lines by single-strand conformation polymorphism analysis. Cancer Res 1991;51(13):3356-61.

14. Pitti RM, Marsters SA, Lawrence DA, Roy M, Kischkel FC, Dowd P, et al. Genomic amplification of a decoy receptor for Fas ligand in lung and colon cancer. Nature 1998;396(6712):699-703.

15. Irmler M, Thome M, Hahne M, Schneider P, Hofmann K, Steiner V, et al. Inhibition of death receptor signals by cellular FLIP. Nature 1997;388(6638):190-5.

16. Tillman DM, Petak I, Houghton JA. A Fas-dependent component in 5-fluorouracil/leucovorin-induced cytotoxicity in colon carcinoma cells. Clin Cancer Res 1999;5(2):425-30.

17. Fulda S, Sieverts H, Friesen C, Herr I, Debatin KM. The CD95 (APO-1/Fas) system mediates drug-induced apoptosis in neuroblastoma cells. Cancer Res 1997;57(17):3823-9.

18. Friesen C, Fulda S, Debatin KM. Deficient activation of the CD95 (APO-1/Fas) system in drug-resistant cells. Leukemia 1997;11(11):1833-41.

19. Friesen C, Fulda S, Debatin KM. Cytotoxic drugs and the CD95 pathway. Leukemia 1999;13(11):1854-8.

20. McGahon AJ, Costa Pereira AP, Daly L, Cotter TG. Chemotherapeutic drug-induced apoptosis in human leukaemic cells is independent of the Fas (APO-1/CD95) receptor/ligand system. Br J Haematol 1998;101(3):539-47.

21. Ferreira CG, Tolis C, Span SW, Peters GJ, van Lopik T, Kummer AJ, et al. Drug-induced apoptosis in lung cnacer cells is not mediated by the Fas/FasL (CD95/APO1) signaling pathway. Clin Cancer Res 2000;6(1):203-12.
22. Gamen S, Anel A, Lasierra P, Alava MA, Martinez-Lorenzo MJ, Pineiro A, et al. Doxorubicin-induced apoptosis in human T-cell leukemia is mediated by caspase-3 activation in a Fas-independent way. FEBS Lett 1997;417(3):360-4.
23. Villunger A, Egle A, Kos M, Hartmann BL, Geley S, Kofler R, et al. Drug-induced apoptosis is associated with enhanced Fas (Apo-1/CD95) ligand expression but occurs independently of Fas (Apo-1/CD95) signaling in human T-acute lymphatic leukemia cells. Cancer Res 1997;57(16):3331-4.
24. Muller M, Wilder S, Bannasch D, Israeli D, Lehlbach K, Li-Weber M, et al. p53 activates the CD95 (APO-1/Fas) gene in response to DNA damage by anticancer drugs. J Exp Med 1998;188(11):2033-45.

DEREGULATION OF CYCLIN D1 AND P16 AND THEIR RELATION TO CISPLATIN SENSITIVITY IN SQUAMOUS CELL CARCINOMA CELL LINES OF THE HEAD AND NECK

Jan Åkervall[1], David Kurnit[2], Meredith Adams[1], Jeremy Prager[1], Bob Zhu[1], Susan Fisher[3], Carol Bradford[1], and Thomas Carey[1].
[1]Department of Otolaryngology, Head and Neck Surgery
[2]Departement of Human Genetics, University of Michigan, Cardinal Bernardin Cancer Center, Loyola University, Chicago, Illinois.

Acknowledgements: This study was supported by NIH (grant nos. 1 R01 DE13346 and 1 R01 CA83087) and the Swedish Cancer Foundation.

ABSTRACT

We investigated amplifications and overexpression of cyclin D1, and homozygous deletions of p16 in relation to sensitivity to Cisplatin in 23 established squamous cell carcinoma of the head and neck (SCCHN). The purpose of the study was to identify biological markers that can predict response to therapy. Cyclin D1 is a proto-oncogene and the protein has a distinct role in the G1 to S transion of the cell cycle. The tumour suppressor gene protein p16 acts as a negative inhibitor of cyclin D1, but is frequently inactivated in SCCHN. Chemosensitivity was assessed by MTT assay in 23 established UMSCC cell lines. The cyclin D1 amplification status was evaluated by real-time PCR (data verified by differential- and conventional PCR) using a chromsome 18q microsatellite marker probe as a internal normal copy gene control. Cyclin D1 expression on the protein level was tested by western blotting.

Cyclin D1 amplification was seen in 7 of 23 (30%) and cyclin D1 overexpression in 12 of 19 (63%) of the cell lines. As expected, all cell lines showing amplifications also revealed overexpression (p=0.004, Fisher's exact test). Homozygous deletions were determined in 12 of the 23 (53%) cell lines. Mean sensitivity to Cisplatin was 9.2 ID50 (range 2.7 to 36.7). Five of 8 cell lines, showing cyclin D1 amplifications, were highly sensitive to Cisplatin (3 to 4.8 ID50), the remaining 3 revealed intermediate sensitivity. There was a statistical trend (P=0.10, Fisher's exact test) that cell lines overexpressing cyclin D1 protein responded better to Cisplatin. There was no correlation between either cyclin D1 DNA amplification or homozygous p16 deletions and sensitivity to Cisplatin. The findings in the present study indicate that cyclin D1 might be a marker for prediction of chemotherapy in HNSCC.

223

INTRODUCTION

No survival benefit has been associated with induction chemotherapy[1], partly due to the time delay to efficient treatment observed among non-responders[2]. These data indicate the need for biological markers that can predict response to chemotherapy, in order to minimize morbidity and in the long run enhance survival rates.

Cyclin D1 (CCND1/PRAD-1) is a cell cycle regulating gene, located at chromosome 11, band q13, involved in the G1 to S transition of the cell cycle. The cyclin D1 protein and cdk4/6 phosphorylates pRb, and releases transcription factor complex DP1/E2F that starts tracsription of early response genes, *e.g.*, p16. p16 acts as a negative inhibitor on the cyclin D1-cdk4/6 complex.

The cyclin D1 gene is frequently amplified and overexpressed in a variety of human carcinomas, *e.g.*, SCCHN[3], therefore postulated to be an oncogene. Tumours or cell lines overexpressing cyclin D1 have a higher percentage of cells in S-phase, which hypothetically make them more vulnerable to chemotherapeutic agents acting on S-phase cells.

We investigated a possible relation between cyclin D1 amplification and overexpression, and homozygous deletions of p16, in relation to sensitivity to Cisplatin, in order to identify a marker for prediction of response to therapy.

MATERIAL AND METHODS

Twenty-three established UMSCC cell lines were analysed for chemosensitivity by MTT assay, amplification of cyclin D1 and homozygous deletion of p16 by real time PCR[4,5], and cyclin D1 protein expression by Western blotting. All techniques were performed using standard protocols. Control experiments in another 40 UMSCC cell lines and in 19 fibroblast cell lines were performed to verify the real time PCR data.

RESULTS

ID50 values showed an average of 9.8 (2.7-36.7). Amplification of cyclin D1 was observed in 7 of 23 (30%) cell lines, with an average amplification level of 7.0 (2.1 –24.0).). Real time PCR analysis of p16 revealed homozygous deletions in 15 of 23 (65%) cell lines. No p16 copy number exceeded 1.1.

Western blotting revealed cyclin D1 expression (+, ++ or +++) in 12 of 19 (63%) UMSCC. Five cell lines were strongly overexpressed (+++) and all of these also showed cyclin D1 DNA amplification. All cases showing cyclin D1 DNA amplification were overexpressed, and DNA amplification explained 7 of 12 (75%) of the cases overexpressing cyclin D1. There was a statistic correlation between cyclin D1 DNA amplification and cyclin D1 overexpression on the protein level (p=0.003, Fisher's exact test).

There was a statistical trend for a correlation between cyclin D1 overexpression (+, ++, or +++) and good response to Cisplatin (lowest 25th percentile, ID50<4.4)(p=0.10, Fisher's exact test). However, no correlation was observed between chemosensitivity and any of the following parameters: cyclin D1 amplification, homozygous deletions of p16 or a combination of these two.

Twelve of 40 (30%) control UMSCC showed cyclin D1 amplification, and homozygous deletion of p16 was observed in 25 of the 40 (62.5%) UMSCC. No one of the 19 tested fibroblast cell lines did show either cyclin D1 amplifications or homozygous deletions of p16.

DISCUSSION

In the present study, we investigated a possible association between deregulation of the cell cycle regulating genes cyclin D1 and p16 in relation to sensitivity to Cisplatin in 23 UMSCC cell lines. The frequencies of cyclin D1 amplification and homozygous deletion of p16 (30% and 65%, respectively) were in accordance with the 40 control UMSCC cell lines (30% and 62.5%, respectively). The findings are also in accordance with earlier studies, in which most authors have reported cyclin D1 amplification rates at 18-40%[3], and rates for homozygous deletions of p16 in 25-66% of SCCHN[6]. Corresponding data for cyclin D1 overexpression, 63% in the present study, is also in accordance with the literature[3].

As been shown earlier, cyclin D1 amplification leads to overexpression of the protein[3]. In the present study, the two parameters were strongly associated with each other (p=0.003, Fisher's exact test), and all cases showing high amplification levels also revealed high levels of protein expression.

There was a statistical trend towards an association between cyclin D1 overexpression and good response to Cisplatin (p=0.10, Fisher's exact test).

Despite great technical improvements in surgery and radiation therapy, the prognosis for patients with HNSCC has not changed significantly over the last decades, indicating that no further improvement is to be expected from standardized treatment protocols based on TNM-classification and clinical parameters solely. Individualization from a biological standpoint will hopefully bring morbidity and mortality down, as over- as well as undertreatment can be avoided. One way to define such individualized treatment regimens is to correlate different biological phenotypes and genotypes to response to certain therapeutic agents. The present study indicates that cyclin D1 overexpression might be such a predictive marker. However, further investigations are needed to analyze a possible association between cyclin D1 overexpression and response to 5-fluorouracil as well as to a combination of this drug and Cisplatin.

REFERENCES

1. Pignon, JP et al., 2000. Chemotherapy added to locoregional treatment for head and neck squamous-cell carcinoma: three meta-analyses of updated individual data. MACH-NC Collaborative Group. Meta-Analysis of Chemotherapy on Head and Neck Cancer. Lancet. 355: 949-55.
2. Akervall, J. et al., (in press). Overexpression of cyclin D1 correlates with neoadjuvant treatment with Cisplatin 5-fluorouracil in squamous cell carcinoma of the head and neck. Acta Oncologica.
3. Akervall, J. 1998. Prognostic factors in squamous cell carcinoma of thee head and neck, with emphasis on 11q13 rearrangements and cyclin D1 overexpression. (Thesis)

4. Higuchi, R et al., 1993. Kinetic PCR: Real time monitoring of DNA amplification reactions. Biotech 11:1026-30
5. Lee, LG et al., 1993. Allelic discrimination by nick translation PCR with fluorogenic probes. Nucl Acids Res 21:3761-66
6. Liggett, WH et al., 1998. Role of the p16 tumour suppressor gene in Cancer. J Clin Oncol 16:1197-1206.

FLAVOPIRIDOL, MECHANISM OF ACTION IS INDEPENDENT OF BCL-2

Emily P. Slater[1], Tatjana V. Achenbach[1], Stephanie E. Lehmann[2], Jochen A. Werner[2], Rolf Müller[1]
[1]Institute of Molecular Biology and Tumor Research, Marburg, Germany
[2]Department of Otolaryngology, Head and Neck Surgery, Marburg, Germany

Acknowledgments: This work was supported in part by a grant from the Dr. Mildred Scheel Stiftung (to R.M. and E.P.S.) The authors wish to thank Elvira Nalbatow and Roswitha Peldszus for excellent technical assistance.

Correspondence to: Emily Slater, Institue of Molecular Biology and Tumor Research, Philipps-University, D-35033 Marburg (e-mail: slater@imt.uni-marburg.de)

ABSTRACT

Squamous cell carcinomas of the head and neck region (HNSCC) are notorious for their poor response to chemotherapeutic intervention. A characterization of eight different cell lines isolated from primary tumors as well as metastases revealed the over-expression of Bcl-X_L, an anti-apoptotic member of the Bcl-2 family, in all cell lines. Nevertheless, treatment with the relatively new chemotherapeutic, Flavopiridol led to cell killing in all cell lines, with IC50 values ranging from 60 to 300 nM. To better understand the mechanism of cell killing we compared cell lines with varying levels of Bcl-2. Cell lines with high levels of the anti-apoptotic protein, endogenous or achieved through over-expression, still responded to the drug. In addition down-regulation of the protein by anti-sense oligonucleotide treatment had no effect on Flavopiridol-induced cell killing. Treatment with Flavopiridol led to activation of caspases in the absence of cytochrome *c* release. Thus, Flavopiridol can be considered a suitable candidate drug for testing in the treatment of refractory carcinomas of the head and neck.

TEXT

Most drugs currently used in anti-cancer therapy are thought to kill target cells by triggering apoptosis, thus, defects in the apoptotic machinery can be a major obstacle. Apoptosis or programmed cell death has been studied extensively over the past decade. Whereas the molecular mechanisms underlying drug-induced apoptosis are still ill defined, p53 mediated mitochondrial damage seems to play a major role in this process. Caspases, a growing family of cysteine proteases that cleave specific substrates at aspartic acid residues have also been identified as major components of this pathway. All caspases are synthesized as inactive proenzymes that must be activated by proteolytic cleavage at specific aspartate residues. A well-characterized pathway of caspase activation involves release of cytochrome c from the mitochondria that together with APAF-1 and ATP leads to the proteolytic cleavage and activation of procaspase 9. The downstream effector proteases include caspase 3, whose activation leads to the typical hallmarks of apoptosis, such as chromatin condensation and membrane blebbing. Pro-apoptotic as well as anti-apoptotic Bcl-2 family members modulate the cytochrome c-triggered pathway by acting at the mitochondria where they are believed to regulate the release of cytochrome c.

Cell surface death receptors such as CD95 (APO-1/Fas) are also involved in drug-induced apoptosis. Thus, DNA-damaging agents can induce expression of the CD95/Fas ligand system or effect clustering of CD95 in the plasma membrane through other mechanisms. This triggers the recruitment of caspase 8 to the receptor complex leading to its autocatalytic cleavage. Active caspase 8 in turn effects the activation of the executioner caspases, such as caspase 3, followed by the proteolysis of a plethora of target proteins and ultimately cell death.

The synthetic flavone, Flavopiridol inhibits the activation of multiple cyclin-dependent kinases, and this inhibition leads to an arrest of the cell cycle [1]. In addition, flavopiridol has been shown to be an efficient inducer of apoptosis in a variety of tumor cells [1,2], although the precise molecular mechanisms remain obscure. A major problem with conventional therapy is the fact that tumor cells usually evolve potent anti-apoptotic mechanisms that counteract the induction of death in response to treatment, such as the loss of p53 or the over-expression of multi-drug resistance genes, such as *mrp-1* [3]. This can be due to the selective pressure imposed by pro-apoptotic oncogenic alterations that accumulate during tumor development or, as in relapsed cancers, result from the selection of treatment-resistant variants. Intriguingly, Flavopiridol-induced apoptosis is refractory to these genetic alterations [4,5].

In an attempt to explain the mechanism of resistance of squamous cell carcinomas of the head and neck region to chemotherapeutic intervention, eight different cell lines isolated from primary tumors as well as metastases were analyzed for the expression of known apoptotic and drug resistance genes. Western blot analysis indicated that all cell lines expressed high levels of the anti-apoptotic Bcl-2 family member, Bcl-X$_L$ (data not shown). Despite the high expression of this anti-apoptotic protein, Flavopiridol was able to kill these cell lines with IC50 values ranging from 60 to 300 nM (data not shown). For this reason we decided to investigate the role of anti-apoptotic Bcl-2 family members in Flavopiridol-induced cell killing using Bcl-2 as a model.

To assess the role of endogenous Bcl-2 expression for Flavopiridol-induced apoptosis, three cell lines expressing varying levels of the Bcl-2 protein were tested (Figure 1A). HeLa cells, a

228

cervical carcinoma cell line, express hardly detectable levels of the Bcl-2 protein. HL-60 cells, a promyelocytic leukemia cell line, express low, but detectable levels. The small cell lung cancer cell line, SW2, expresses very high levels of the anti-apoptotic protein. All cell lines contain low levels of the pro-apoptotic protein, Bax. After treatment with 500 nM Flavopiridol for 18 h, cell killing was analyzed. Whereas the HeLa and HL-60 cell line were killed either by Camptothecin or Flavopiridol, the SW2 cell line showed only significant killing following treatment with Flavopiridol.

To obtain direct evidence that the Bcl-2 expression does not prevent cell killing by Flavopiridol, HeLa cells were transiently transfected with an expression vector resulting in over-expression of Bcl-2 and then treated with the chemotherapeutics as described in Fig. 1A. Transfected cells were identified by co-transfection with cDNA encoding a green fluorescent protein (GFP). Upon comparison of the total cell population to those cells transfected with GFP and Bcl-2, there was no apparent difference in the level of cell killing after treatment with Flavopiridol. In contrast, the effect obtained with Camptothecin-treatment was significantly decreased in the presence of Bcl-2 over-expression (Figure 1B).

To confirm and extend these observations, SW2 cells were treated with an anti-sense oligonucleotide directed against Bcl-2 to down-regulate the level of the protein (Figure 1C, Western blot). Whereas the percent killing with Camptothecin (Cam) or cis-Platin increased in the presence of the anti-sense oligonucleotide, there was no change in the percent killing induced by Flavopiridol (Figure 1C).

To elucidate the pathways involved in Flavopiridol-induced cell killing, Flavopiridol- or Camptothecin-treated HeLa and SW2 cells were analyzed for the activation of caspases critical for apoptosis. HeLa cells which express low levels of the Bcl-2 protein (Figure 1A) demonstrate activation of caspases 9, 8 and 3 in response to both Flavopiridol and Camptothecin, however the kinetics of activation are different. In the case of Flavopiridol, activation of caspase 8 occurs early followed by activation of 3 and then 9. With Camptothecin caspase 9 activation occurs early followed by 3 and then 8. PARP (poly-ADP ribose polymerase) cleavage occurs in both cases, but cytochrome c release occurs early for Camptothecin and late for Flavopiridol. This would suggest that the mitochondrial pathway including release of cytochrome c followed by caspase 9 activation and ultimately 3 would be the mechanism for Camptothecin. In contrast, Flavopiridol appears to activate caspase 8 first, which could in turn activate 3, with caspase 9 playing only a minor role (Figure 2A). SW2 cells that are known to express high levels of Bcl-2 (Figure 1A) show no release of cytochrome c with either drug treatment. Clearly, cytochrome c release is not required for killing by Flavopiridol. Interestingly, these cells express no caspase 8. Surprisingly, caspase 3 is activated in the absence of caspase 8 and without prior activation of caspase 9 (Figure 2B). Caspase 3 is either activated by an as yet unidentified caspase or possibly by Flavopiridol itself. These results taken together indicate that caspases are instrumental in Flavopiridol-induced apoptosis and that this drug uses multiple pathways to achieve cell killing. Flavopiridol not only uses "classical" pathways of drug-induced apoptosis, but also seems to trigger hitherto unidentified mechanisms.

Implications of Flavopiridol for cancer therapy

We have shown that Flavopiridol-induced apoptosis is not blocked by Bcl-2 over-expression, one of the most common problems encountered with cancer cells (Figures 1 and 2)[6]. In addition, Flavopiridol could trigger apoptosis even in the absence of Caspase 3[6] or Caspase 8, since it can utilize alternate pathways for the induction of cell death. Caspases 3 and 8 are also lacking in certain human tumors, which could render them resistant to conventional chemotherapy. In aggressive neuroblastoma, where n-Myc is amplified, the expression of the apoptotic effector Caspase 8 is suppressed [7]. The examination of eighteen neuroblastoma cell lines revealed 13 that lacked expression of Caspase 8 mRNA and protein. However, only one cell line had a deletion of the gene for Caspase 8. The resistance to apoptosis observed following drug-treatment (Doxorubicin) or the addition of Fas and TNF ligands could be reversed by the re-introduction of Caspase 8 into deficient neuroblastoma cells and embryonic fibroblasts lacking Caspase 8. So clearly, Flavopiridol would be an advantage in chemotherapy. Taken together with the p53-independence and refractoriness to multi-drug resistance, Flavopiridol could make an invaluable contribution to clinical oncology. In this context, the strong synergism of Flavopiridol with other drugs, such as Taxol [8], might be of particular importance.

CONCLUSION

The efficacy of Flavopiridol was found to be due to its refractoriness to several mechanisms of drug resistance. It is independent of the multi-drug resistance gene, p53 and, as described here, largely independent of the anti-apoptotic family member Bcl-2. Neither the over-expression of the protein nor the anti-sense mediated down-regulation of Bcl-2 had any effect on the induction of apoptosis. Furthermore, Flavopiridol was found to induce apoptosis via different pathways of caspase activation. Caspase 3 was found to be an important executioner in Bcl-2 independent apoptosis and membrane depolarization occurred in the absence of cytochrome c release[6]. It would appear that Flavopiridol acts directly on, as of yet, unidentified components of the mitochondria and, therefore, can circumvent the resistance induced by Bcl-2 expression.

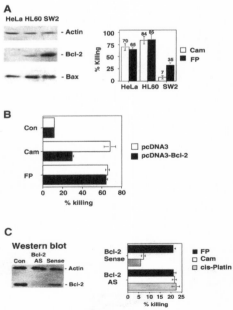

Figure 1: Modulation of the expression levels of Bcl-2 protein does not affect the response to Flavopiridol. **A**. Three cancer cell lines expressing Bax and varying levels of Bcl-2 and their responsiveness to the chemotherapeutic agents Camptothecin (Cam) and Flavopiridol (FP). **B**. Over-expression of Bcl-2 in HeLa cells results in decreased killing by Camptothecin (Cam), but no change with Flavopiridol (FP). **C**. Down-regulation of the level of Bcl-2 protein using anti-sense (AS) oligonucleotides directed against Bcl-2 resulted in increased killing of SW2 cells by Camptothecin (Cam) and cis-Platin, but no change with Flavopiridol.

230

Figure 2: Cleavage of procaspases and PARP and release of cytochrome *c* in HeLa cells (**A**) and in SW2 cells (**B**) treated with Camptothecin (Cam) or Flavopiridol (FP) for the times indicated.

A

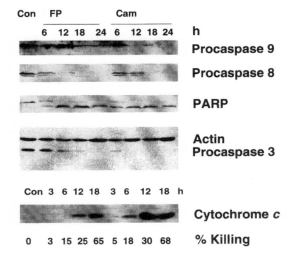

Con	FP	Cam	
	6 12 18 24	6 12 18 24	h

Procaspase 9

Procaspase 8

PARP

Actin
Procaspase 3

Con 3 6 12 18 3 6 12 18 h

Cytochrome *c*

0   3 15 25 65 5 18 30 68   % Killing

B

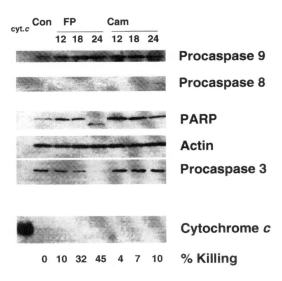

cyt.c Con FP   Cam
            12 18 24 12 18 24

Procaspase 9

Procaspase 8

PARP

Actin

Procaspase 3

Cytochrome *c*

0 10 32 45 4 7 10   % Killing

REFERENCES

1. Schrump DS, Matthews W, Chen GA, et al. Flavopiridol Mediates Cell CycleArrest and Apoptosis in Esophageal Cancer Cells. Clin Canc Res 1998; 4: 2885-2890.
2. Patel V, Senderowicz AM, Pinto DJ, et al. Flavopiridol, a novel cyclin-dependent kinase inhibitor, suppresses the growth of head adn neck squamous cell carcinomas by inducing apoptosis. J Clin Invest 1998; 102: 1674-1681.
3. Reed JC. Dysregulation of Apoptosis in Cancer. J Clin Oncol 1999; 17: 2941-2953.
4. Shapiro GI, Koestner DA, Matranga CB, et al. Flavopiridol induces cell cycle arrest and p53-independent apoptosis in non-small cell lung cancer cell lines. Clin Cancer Res 1999; 5: 2925-2938.
5. Hooijberg JH, Broxterman HJ, Scheffer GL, et al. Potent interaction of Flavopiridol with MRP1. Br. J. Cancer 1999; 81: 269-276.
6. Achenbach TV, Muller R, Slater EP. Bcl-2 independence of Flavopiridol-induced apoptosis. Mitochondrial depolarization in the absence of cytochrome c release. J Biol Chem 2000; 275:32089-97.
7. Teitz T, Wei T, Valentine MB, et al. Caspase 8 is deleted or silenced preferentially in childhood neuroblastomas with amplification of MYCN. Nature Medicine 2000; 6: 529-535.
8. Motwani M, Delohery TM, Schwartz GK. Sequential dependent enhancement of caspase activation and apoptosis by Flavopiridol on paclitaxel-treated human gastric and breast cancer cells [In Process Citation]. Clin Cancer Res 1999; 5: 1876-83.

232

BIOKINETIC STUDY AND THERAPEUTIC EFFICACY
OF FERROFLUID BOUND ANTICANCER AGENT

Ch. Alexiou[1], W. Arnold[1], P. Hulin[1], R. Klein[1], A. Schmidt[1], Ch. Bergemann[2], F.G. Parak[3],
[1]Department of Otolaryngology, Head and Neck Surgery, Klinikum rechts der Isar, Technical University of Munich, 81675 Munich
[2]Chemicell, 10777 Berlin
[3]Physics-Department E 17, Technical University of Munich, 81675 Munich, Germany

Supported by the Margarete Ammon Foundation, Munich, and grants from the Technical University of Munich, Germany.

Correspondence to: *Department of Otolaryngology, Head and Neck Surgery, Klinikum rechts der Isar, Technical University of Munich, Ismaningerstrasse 22, 81675 Munich, Germany, Phone: 49-89-4140-2370; Fax: 49-89-4140-4853 (e-mail: C.Alexiou@lrz.tu-muenchen.de)*

ABSTRACT

Ferrofluids coated with starch polymers can be used as biocompatible carriers in a new field of locoregional tumor therapy called "magnetic drug targeting". Bound to medical drugs, such magnetic nanoparticles can be enriched in a desired body compartment using an external magnetic field. In the present study, we confirm the concentration of ferrofluids in VX2 squamous cell carcinoma tissue of the rabbit using histological investigations and MR imaging. The biodistribution of these magnetic nanoparticles was studied by the use of Jod[123] and Fe[59] labeled particles. The therapeutic efficacy of "magnetic drug targeting" was studied using the rabbit VX2 squamous cell carcinoma model. Mitoxantrone coupled ferrofluids were injected intraarterially into the artery supplying the tumor (femoral artery). The magnetic field (1,7 Tesla) was focused to the tumor placed at the medial portion of the hind limb of New Zealand White rabbits. Complete tumor remissions could be seen without any negative side effects by using only 20% of the normal systemic dosage of the chemotherapeutic agent mitoxantrone.

INTRODUCTION

Biocompatible ferrofluids are superparamagnetic nanoparticles, that may be used as a delivery system for anticancer agents in locoregional tumor therapy, called „magnetic drug targeting". Through this form of target directed drug application, one attempts to concentrate a pharmacological agent at its site of action in order to minimize unwanted effects in the organism and to increase its locoregional effectiveness.

Ferrofluids are used in medicine since the 1960es for e.g. the magnetically controlled metallic thrombosis of intracranial aneurysms and magnetically guided selective embolization of the renal artery in case of a renal tumor [1,2].

Ferrofluids are also used as a contrast agent for MRI. Superparamagnetic iron oxide particles (SPIO) are a new class of MR contrast agents that have been shown to significantly increase the detectibility of hepatic and splenic tumors. No acute or subacute toxic effects were detected by histologic or serologic studies in rats and beagle dogs who received a total of 3000 µmol Fe/kg, 150 times the dose proposed for MR imaging of the liver. These results indicate that ferrofluids are fully biocompatible potential contrast agent for MRI[3]. These particles are selectively taken up by cells of the mononuclear phagocytosing system (e.g. Kupffer's cells in the liver and macrophages in the spleen, lymph nodes, or bone marrow), depending on the particle design (e.g. coating or size). The value of these particles in the diagnostic evaluation of liver and spleen tumors has already been shown in animal experiments and clinical studies [4, 5].

Ultrasound, CT, and MR imaging do not allow reliable differentiation between hyperplastic and tumorous lymph nodes or detection of small metastases in normal-sized lymph nodes. SPIO are also used for MR lymphography for the detection of lymph node metastases. In tumor-bearing rabbits, different degrees of metastatic displacement of lymph nodes were discernible, and even small metastases (3 mm in diameter) could be visualized[6].

Ferrofluids are also used for a specific cell seperation method called "immunomagnetic cell seperation"[7] and Ferrofluids are also an important subject in the development of an implantable artificial heart[8].

MATERIALS AND METHODS

Ferrofluids
The ferrofluids used in the experiments were obtained from Chemicell (Berlin, Germany; German patent application no. 19624426.9) and consisted of a biocompatible colloidal dispersion formed by wet chemical methods from iron oxides and hydroxides to produce special multidomaine particles [9]. These ferrofluids are covered with hydrophilic starch polymers coupled with endstanding functional groups (e.g. phosphate) allowing ionic binding to many therapeutic drugs. Figure 2 shows a schematic drawing of a magnetic nanoparticle covered by starch polymer. The hydrodynamic diameter of the whole particle is about 100 nm. Organic as well as inorganic agents (R) can ionically bound to the functional group, in this case phosphat. The chemotherapeutic agent mitoxantrone (Novantron®, Lederle, Wolfratshausen, Germany) is ionically bound to the endstanding groups of the starch coating.

234

The drug has to be released from the carrier system before it can take effect. The release of the drug starts within 20 minutes and reaches the maximum after approximately 1 hour.

Chemotherapeutic agent

The chemotherapeutic agent used in the experiments, mitoxantrone ((Novantron®, Lederle, Wolfratshausen, Germany) is a synthetic anthracendion that inhibits DNA and RNA synthesis by intercalating in DNA molecules, which causes strand breaks. The body surface area and the dose of mitoxantrone (10 mg/m^2 of body surface area) used for the experiments were calculated according the instructions of Kirk and Bistner's handbook of veterinarian procedures and emergency treatment[10].

Magnetic field

An electromagnet with a magnetic flux density of a maximum of 1,7 Tesla was used to produce an inhomogenous magnetic field. The magnetic flux density was focused onto the region of the tumor with a specially adapted pole shoe that was placed in contact with the surface of the tumor. On the tip of the pole shoe, the gradient has its maximum[11]. The magnetic field was focused on the tumor during the ferrofluid injection and for 60 min in total.

VX2 squamous cell carcinoma

The VX2 squamous cell carcinoma was obtained from Deutsches Krebsforschungszentrum (Heidelberg, Germany). The animals soon (within 2-3 weeks) develop central tumor necroses, locoregional lymph node metastases, and hematogenous metastases.

Animals

The experimental animals were female New Zealand White rabbits (2000-2500 g body weight, 12-15 weeks old; Charles River, Sulzfeld, Germany).

Surgical intervention

Fragments of viable VX-2 tissue 1 mm in size were taken from the tumor periphery in donor animals. These fragments were placed in a special medium (RPMI 1640, 2,0 g/l Na HCO3, L-Glutamin, Seromed™, Biochrom, Berlin, Germany) and were immediately implanted under sterile conditions into the hind limb of anesthetized recipient rabbits in the supply area of the femoral artery. The chemotherapy experiments were performed when the tumors had reached a volume of approximately 3500 mm^3.

For application of the chemotherapy, the animals were anesthetized with an intramuscular injection of ketamine 35 mg/kg body weight (Narketan 10™, Chassot, Bern, Switzerland) and xylazine 5 mg/kg body weight (Xylapan™, Chassot, Bern, Switzerland), the femoral artery was cannulized and an indwelling catheter (Venflon, 0.8 mm, Ohmeda Co., Helsingburg, Sweden) was placed after separation of the femoral vein and the saphenous nerve approximately 2 cm distal to the inguinal furrow. The mitoxantrone bound ferrofluid was administered by perfusor over a period of 10 min. To prevent thrombosis, prophylaxis consisting of heparin sodium (Heparin-Natrium-25.000 Ratiopharm™, Ratiopharm, Ulm, Germany) was given preoperatively, once postoperatively and twice daily for 5 days postoperatively (200 IU kg/ body weight, s.c.).

RESULTS

1. Localization of ferrofluids in the tumor tissue after "magnetic drug targeting"
The enrichment of ferrofluids in tumor tissue focused by the external magnetic field was documented in vivo by histological analysis and MRI.

Tumor tissue was investigated with Prussian blue, which is a specific stain used to identify iron. A dark-blue crystalline salt $Fe_4(Fe(CN)_6)_3$ obtained by precipitation from ferric salt treated with a solution of ferrocyanic acid or a ferrocyanide. Histological findings of VX2-squamous cell carcinoma tissue after "magnetic drug targeting" showed ferrofluid particles distributed throughout the entire tumor. The histological examinations of tumor sections confirmed an intravascular as well as an intratumoral enrichment of the ferrofluids. After a 3-month observation period, no ferrofluids were histologically evident.

The distribution and the enrichment of the intraarterially injected ferrofluids were investigated in vivo by MRI after "magnetic drug targeting". In MRI the magnetic particles strongly reduce the transverse relaxation time (T2) and lower significantly the longitudinal relaxation time (T1). The MRI was made 6 h after treatment with "magnetic drug targeting" and the concentration of ferrofluids was seen by extinction of signal in the area of the tumor.

Biodistribution was studied by the use of Iod^{123} and Fe^{59} labeled nanoparticles. The scintigraphically detected Iod^{123}- signal after intraarterial (artery leading the tumor, femoral artery) application has been shown to be significantly higher in the magnetically focused region compared to the application without external magnetic field (figure 1).

Quantitative analysis by Fe^{59}-labeled ferrofluids showed more than 90% ferrofluid enrichment in the tumor focused by the magnetic field compared to other tissues (e.g. spleen, lung, liver, heart, ren, gallbladder) after one and six hours by magnetic field.

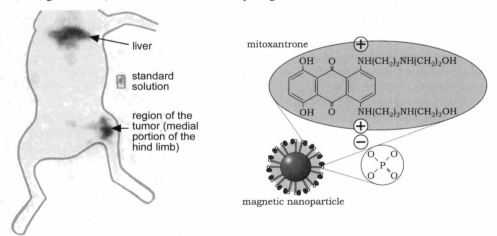

Figure 1.Enrichment of Jod^{123} labeled nanoparticles in the area of interest (VX2-tumor) after "magnetic drug targeting". The images were taken 30 min later still showing stable concentration of ferrofluids within the tumor tissue.

Figure 2. Structural formula of mitoxantrone bound to magnetic nanoparticle

236

2. Animal experiments with "magnetic drug targeting"

Tumor bearing rabbits (VX-2 squamous cell carcinoma) in the area of the hind limb, were treated by a single intraarterial injection (A. femoralis) of mitoxantrone coupled ferrofluids (figure 2), while focusing an external magnetic field (1,7 Tesla) onto the tumor for 60 minutes. With a reduction of the dose of mitoxantrone to 20% of the regular systemic dose complete tumor remission could be achieved in these animals without any negative side effects, like e.g. leucocytopenia, alopecia or gastrointestinal disorders. After "magnetic drug targeting" the tumor size decreased and showed a complete remission within 15 days (median value; range from 12 to 57 days). There were no clinical or histopathological signs of recurrent cancer during an observation period of 3 month.

Control groups that have had a comparable dose of intraarterial mitoxantrone without "magnetic drug targeting" showed an increase of the tumor growth and developed metastases after 30 days. Intraarterial doses of mitoxantrone (75% and 100% of the systemic dose) result in tumor remission but also the development of severe negative side effects (leucocytopenia, unilateral alopecia, ulcers).

DISCUSSION

The difference between success or failure of chemotherapy depends not only on the drug itself but also on how it is delivered to its target. Because of the relatively non-specific action of chemotherapeutic agents, there is almost always some toxicity to normal tissue. Therefore, it is of great importance to be able to selectively target the antineoplastic agent to its tumor target as precisely as possible, to reduce the resulting systemic toxic side effects from generalized systemic distribution and to be able to use a much smaller dose, which would further lead to a reduction of toxicity.

The goal of the present study was to concentrate ferrofluids coupled with cytostatic agents in a desired target area using a magnetic field. The principle of "magnetic drug targeting" consists of two steps: The first step is the delivery of the mitoxantrone bound magnetic nanoparticles to the desired body compartment (tumor), the second is the release of the drug from its carrier. An additional helpful factor is that microvascular permeability in neoplastic tissues is increased (8-fold compared with normal tissue) as is diffusion (33-fold)[12], which allows chemotherapeutic agents much easier to penetrate into tumor tissue. The metabolism of ferrofluid particles takes place in the liver and spleen in analogy to iron metabolism.

At present, i.a. delivery of chemotherapeutic agents is approved and well accepted for treatment of liver metastases[13] and has occasionally been used for other tumor types also (e.g., inoperable head and neck tumors); but it has often necessitated complicated, time-consuming operative procedures, including general anaesthesia[14].

These data demonstrate the accumulation of ferrofluids in tumor tissue by focusing an external magnetic field. The strong and specific therapeutic efficacy in tumor treatment with mitoxantrone bound ferrofluids may indicate that this system could be used as a delivery system for anticancer agents, like radionuclids, cancer-specific antibodies, anti-angionetic-factors, genes etc.

REFERENCES

1. Alksne JF, Fingerhut A, Rand R. Magnetically controlled metallic thrombosis of intracranial aneurysms. Surgery 1966; 60: 212-218.
2. Hilal SK, Michelsen WJ, Driller J, Leonard E. Magnetically guided devices for vascular exploration and treatment. Radiology 1974;113: 529-534.
3. Weissleder R, Hahn PF, Stark DD et al. MR imaging of splenic metastases: ferrite-enhanced detection in rats. AJR 1987; 149: 723-726.
4. Weissleder R, Stark DD, Engelstad BL et al. Superparamagnetic iron oxide: pharmacokinetics and toxicity. AJR 1989;152: 167-173.
5. Weissleder R, Elizondo G, Wittenberg J, Lee AS, Josephson L, Brady TJ. Ultrasmall superparamagnetic iron oxide. An intravenous contrast agent for assessing lymph nodes with MR imaging. Radiology 1990;175: 494.
6. Taupitz M, Wagner S, Hamm B, Dienemann D, Lawaczeck R, Wolf KJ. MR lymphography using iron oxide particles. Detection of lymph node metastases in the VX2 rabbit tumor model. Acta Radiol. 1993; 34: 10-15.
7. Hardingham JE, Kotasek D, Sage RE, Eaton MC, Pascoe VH. Detection of circulating tumor cells in colorectal cancer by immunobead-PCR is a sensitive prognostic marker for relapse of disease. Molec. Med. 195;1: 789-794.
8. Mitamura Y, Wada T, Keisuke S. A ferrofluidic actuator for an implantable artificial heart. Artif. Organs 1992; 16 (5): 490-495.
9. Lübbe AS, Bergemann C, Huhnt W et al. Preclinical experiences with magnetic drug targeting: tolerance and efficacy. Cancer Res 1996; 56: 4694-4701.
10. Bistner SI, Ford RB, Raffe MR (eds.). Kirk and Bistner's Handbook of Veterinarian Procedures and Emergency Treatment, Ed 6, p. 907. Philadelphia: W.B. Saunders Co., 1995.
11. Alexiou C, Arnold W, Klein RJ et al. Locoregional cancer treatment with Magnetic Drug Targeting. Cancer res. 2000; 60: 6641-6648.
12. Gerlowski LE, Jain RK. Microvascular permeability of normal and neoplastic tissues. Microvasc. Res. 1986; 31: 288-305.
13. Link KH, Kornmann M, Formenti A et al. Regional chemotherapy of non-resectable liver metastases from colorectal cancer-literature and institutional review. Langenbecks Arch, Surg. 1999; 384: 344-353.
14. Scheel J. Die intraarterielle Chemotherapie. In: H.H. Naumann, J. Helms, C. Herberhold, E. Kastenbauer (eds.), Oto-Laryngologie in Klinik und Praxis, pp. 457-460. Stuttgart: Thieme, 1998.

238

METASTASES OF SQUAMOUS CELL CARCINOMA OF THE ORAL TONGUE

Correspondence to: *Jeffrey N. Myers M.D., Ph.D., Department of Head and Neck Surgery, University of Texas M.D. Anderson Cancer Center, 1515 Holcombe Boulevard, Houston, TX 77030, Phone: (713) 792-6920, FAX: (713) 794-4662 (e-mail: jmyers@notes.mdacc.tmc.edu)*

ABSTRACT

Squamous cell carcinoma of the oral tongue (SCCOT) is amongst the most common tumors arising in the upper aerodigestive tract (UADT) and it is responsible for a significant number of cancer deaths worldwide every year. Improvements in surgical technique and enhanced technology for the delivery of radiation therapy have not made a significant impact on the mortality rate for this disease entity. Regional nodal disease is the primary mode of treatment failure, but patients with SCCOT are also at risk for distant metastases. The presence of nodal metastases and extracapsular extension of tumor outside the lymph node (ECS) are the most reliable predictors of dying from disease. Furthermore, patients with these adverse pathologic criteria have higher rates of regional and distant relapse. These findings indicate that more intensified treatment approaches including systemically active agents are warranted in SCCOT patients with ECS. These data also suggest that surgical specimens from this patient population should serve as important reagents for discerning the biologic bases of SCCOT tumor progression. Enhanced knowledge of the mechanisms of SCCOT tumor progression should in turn enhance our ability to prognosticate and treat this disease.

SQUAMOUS CELL CARCINOMA OF THE ORAL TONGUE (SCCOT): THE CLINICAL PROBLEM

SCCOT: Incidence and Prognosis

SCCOT is among the most common tumors of the upper aerodigestive tract (UADT) accounting for 6000 new cases and 1750 cancer deaths in the United States each year. The standard treatment for SCCOT in the U.S. is surgery. Post-operative, adjuvant radiation therapy is recommended for patients determined to be at high-risk for treatment failure based on clinicopathologic criteria. Despite improvements in surgical and radiation therapy techniques, high-risk patients fail treatment, locally, local-regionally, or regionally. The 5-year overall survival for stage III and IV patients has not improved significantly and remains at 54% and 34%, respectively. Most often, patients develop treatment failure with regional recurrence, but distant metastases can also occur in patients with SCCOT.

Significance of Regional Metastasis and ECS on Survival of Patients with SCCOT

To determine the impact of cervical metastasis with and without ECS, we retrospectively reviewed the records of more than 338 patients with SCCOT treated with surgery at The University of Texas M.D. Anderson Cancer Center from 1982-1998.

The overall and disease-specific survival were significantly reduced by the presence of nodal metastases on pathologic review of the surgical specimen (pN+) ($p < 0.00001$). The median overall survival for pN0 patients was 120 months versus 42 months for pN+ patients, with 5-year overall survivals of 72% and 42% respectively. The 5-year disease-specific survival was 88% for pN0 patients and 59% for those pN+. The survival data of those patients who were pathologically node positive were further analyzed by dividing this group into those with and without ECS. The 5-year overall survival was found to be 51% for pN+ECS- and 30% for pN+ECS+($p = 0.014$). The 5-year disease-specific survivals were 65%(pN+ECS-) and 48%(pN+ECS+) ($p = 0.02$) (Figure 1).

Significance of Regional Metastasis and ECS on Regional and Distant Relapse

When local, regional, and distant recurrence were taken together, those patients who were pN+ECS- had higher recurrence rates (34.2%) than those who were pN0 (19.8%), and those with pN+ECS+ (51.1%) had the highest total recurrence rate ($p < 0.01$). When analyzed by type of recurrence, local recurrence was found to occur at a similar rate across these groups pN0 (12.4%) pN+ECS-(19.2%) and pN+ECS+ (13.3%)($p = 0.46$, OR=1.34). Regional recurrence was significantly more frequent in the pN+ECS-group (14/73= 19.2%) than the pN0 group (14/121=11.6%) and occurred more often still in the pN+ECS+ group (13/45=28.9%) ($p = 0.04$, OR=1.95). Similarly, distant metastasis (DM) occurred most often in the pN+ECS+ group (11/45=24.4%) [$p = 0.015$, OR=3.61(1.2-10.61)]. To determine the association of DM with regional recurrence, all patients with DM (26/337=7.7%) were analyzed for the presence or absence of local and/or regional recurrence. More patients had DM in the absence (18/337=5.3%) rather than the presence of local/regional failure (8/337=2.4%).

SCCOT: Novel Approaches to Therapy of Patients with ECS

The higher rates of distant and regional failure seen in patients with nodal disease and ECS has led investigators to develop clinical trials of post-operative adjuvant chemoradiation which have yielded intriguing results. In a non-randomized prospective trial carried out from June 1982 until December 1992, 371 patients were treated surgically for SCCHN, and all had free margins, but the presence of ECS. Of these patients 53 (14%) had surgery only, 187 (50%) had surgery + radiation (50-60Gy), and 131 (35%) had surgery+radiation followed by chemotherapy with 5-fluorouracil(5-FU) and methotrexate[1]. All patients were followed for at least 30 months and the disease free survival rates were found to be 17% (surgery only), 40% (surg+XRT) and 58% (surg+XRT+CTX) ($p < 0.001$). In a prospective Phase II study, RTOG 88-24, 52 patients with surgically treated stage IV SCCHN or + margins were treated with 60 Gy in 30 fractions over 6 weeks with cisplatin 100mg/m^2 being administered on days 1, 23, and 43[2]. Actuarial analysis at 3 years revealed a 48% overall survival and 81% local-regional control rate. However, severe and life-threatening toxicities were seen in 20% and 12% of patients, respectively. Based on these results which were better than historical controls, the

240

RTOG has carried out a prospective randomized trial comparing RT alone to RT+cisplatin. Results of this study are pending at this time.

In a phase III trial from Toulouse in France, 83 patients operated on for Stage III or IV SCCHN or who had ECS were randomized to receive RT alone consisting of 65-70Gy to the primary sites and 65-74Gy to involved nodal basins or to receive RT+chemotherapy[3]. Chemotherapy consisted of cisplatin 50mg IV weekly for 7-9 cycles and the group of patients who received it along with radiation had statistically significant enhancements in overall survival, and disease free survival than the RT only group. The promising results of these studies indicate that systemic therapy although associated with greater toxicity than radiation only can improve regional control and survival.

We have developed a novel adjuvant therapy trial for oral cavity cancer patients with ECS. The protocol uses post-operative radiotherapy given in combination with cisplatin and C225, a humanized monoclonal antibody that targets the epidermal growth factor receptor (EGF-R). Patients with SCC of the oral cavity who have been primarily treated with surgery and are found to be high risk on the basis of pathologic criteria including: 1) Pathologic nodal status of N2b or greater 2)Extranodal extension of tumor or 3) Positive Margins will be treated 2 weeks prior to the initiation of radiation therapy with a course of cisplatin 100mg/m^2 and C225 at MTD. They will be then be treated with external beam radiation therapy to a dose of 60Gy given in 30 fractions to the primary site and neck(s). Cisplatin is concurrently administered at 100 mg/m^2 on days 1 and 22. C225 at MTD is delivered on day 1 and weekly up to 8 total doses. The patients will be observed for acute, sub-acute, and late toxic effects as well as for local, regional, and distant recurrence for a minimum of 3 years.

SCCOT: BIOLOGIC APPROACHES TO STUDYING SCC METASTASES

Six Acquired Capabilities of Metastatic Cancer Cells
Over the past several decades, remarkable advances in multiple fields of cancer research have allowed for better understanding of the molecular and cellular pathogenesis and progression of oral cavity cancer. Recently, Hanahan and Weinberg have constructed a conceptual framework within which one can organize studies of tumor development and progression[4]. In this model, these authors describe six essential hallmarks that cells need to acquire in order to become successful tumor cells. These hallmarks are: 1) acquisition of autonomous proliferative signaling, 2) inhibition of growth inhibitory signals, 3) evasion of programmed cell death 4) immortalization, 5) acquisition of a nutrient blood supply (angiogenesis), and 6) acquisition of the ability to invade tissue. Since all of these steps are thought to be essential for tumor progression, one must consider these in parallel when analyzing a particular tumor type of markers tumor progression.

The goals of our research program in SCCOT Metastases are to identify the cellular and molecular mechanisms of regional and systemic metastases. There are several main approaches to this including the study of archival and human tumor specimens from SCCOT patients who are pathologically N0, N+ECS-, or N+ECS+. These specimens are compared for cellular endpoints associated with the necessary acquired capablities of cancers including immunohistochemical staining for PCNA as a marker for proliferation, TUNEL as a marker for apoptosis, and CD31 as a marker of angiogenesis. In addition, analysis of expression of key mediators of angiogenesis, invasion, immortalization, proliferation, and apoptosis are ongoing and utilize in situ hybridization and RNAse protection assays amongst other methods to assess relative gene expression.

Animal Models of SCCOT Tumor Invasion and Metastasis

Another major focus of our work has been to develop an orthotopic murine tumor model of SCCOT metastasis. The major goals of this work is to provide a model for evaluating mechanisms which are potentially important for the development of regional and distant metastases. Another major objective of this project is to a develop a preclinical model in which novel therapeutics can be evaluated.

To establish the feasibility of tumor establishment and identification of cervical metastases in mice we used the B16/C57bl 6 syngeneic metastatic tumor model and showed that it is possible to generate primary tumor implants in the tongue and to identify cervical metastases of the submucosaly implanted tumors. Having confirmed the feasibility of submucosal lingual injection, we selected 3 oral cavity squamous cell carcinoma cell lines, which had previously been established MDA 1986, Tu 159, and Tu 167 in the Head and Neck Laboratory at the UTM.D. Anderson Cancer Center, for growth in the tongues of nude mice. All three of these cell lines formed histologicaly verified tumors in 5/5 animals when $5X10^6$ cells were inoculated submucosaly in the tongue. The orthotopically-grown SCCOC tumors resulting from submucosal injection of Tu167have a histologic appearance very similar to that of primary human SCCOT specimens.

We next evaluated the orthotopic concept that human tumors grow better in nude mice when grown at a site most closely resembling their primary site of origin. To do this, SCCOC tumor cells were injected sumucosally in the tongues of nude mice and were also injected subcutaneously with a corresponding number of each cell type and tumorigenecity was determined. For Tu 159 5/5 animals developed tumor at the following dose of tumor cells inoculated in the tongue: $5X10^4$; $1X10^5$; $5X10^5$; $1X10^6$ and $5 X10^6$. Subcutaneous tumors developed in none of the animals inoculated subcutaneously with $5X10^4$ cells, and in only 1/5 animals and 3/5 animals inoculated with $1X10^5$ or $5X10^5$ cells, respectively. All animals injected with the two highest doses of Tu159 formed subcutaneous tumors. This experiment shows Tu 159 to have high tumorigenicity and reveals at least an order of magnitude difference in the minimal tumorigenic dose of this oral cavity tumor when implanted in oral tongue versus subcutaneous implantation.

Analysis of the Tu167 has demonstrated a similar trend in which tumors have been found in all animals injected submucosally with $1X10^5$; $5X10^5$; $1X10^6$ or $5 X10^6$ cells. Only 1/5 animals developed subcutaneous tumors when injected with $1X10^5$; $5X10^5$; or $1X10^6$ cells, indicating at least a fifty-fold difference in minimal tumorigenic dose between submucosa and subcutis with this cell line.

The results of the tumorigenicity study of the Tu 1986 cell line show that the MDA 1986 cell line is very potent in tumor formation, particularly at the orthotopic site, with as few as 5000 cells leading to tumor formation in all animals. At least $1X10^5$ cells were needed to form subcutaneous tumors in 100% of animals with the MDA 1986 cell line, which again supports the orthotopic concept.

After gross and microscipic examination of primary tumor cervical lymph node specimens from 45 animals, 2 animals have been observed to have tumor metastatic to the cervical lymph nodes detectable by microscopic determination only for a metastatic rate of 4.4% (Figure 2a). The presence of lymph node metastasis highlights the utility of this model system for characterizing the biologic processes and specific molecules critical for the development of cervical metastases. The low rate of metastases seen indicates that it will be possible to generate cell lines of varying metastatic potential using both *in vitro* and *in vivo* selection methods. Furthermore, lingually injecting Tu167AK6 a cell line selected in vitro from the Tu167 floor of mouth cell line for resistance to anchorage independent cell death, resulted in pulmonary metastases (Figure 2b). Thus, this orthotopic model recapitulates the most common metastatic pathways of SCCOT seen in patients, and therefore serves as a useful preclinical model for identifying mechanisms of metastasis and for evaluating novel forms of therapy.

SCCOT and Anoikis: An Analysis of Acquired Capabilities in SCCOT Tumor Progression

The acquisition of resistance to cell death has been postulated to be critical for tumor development and progression by Weinberg and Hanahan[4] The role of evasion of cell death has been studied in a number of tumor systems and there are abundant data to support that the acquisition of apoptosis resistance enhances tumor progression[4-8].

One form of apoptosis evasion which is believed to be associated with tumorigenecity, invasion, and metastasis is evasion of attachment regulated programmed cell death, ARPCD, or anoikis[9]. Normal epithelia are supported by basement membranes which provide survival and proliferative signals. Terminal differentiation for these cells includes detachment from the basement membrane, changes in cell morphology, keratin accumulation (in the case of oral and cutaneous epithelia), and, ultimately, cell death[10]. The successful growth of oral epithelia and tumors derived from them in tissue culture requires adherent growth conditions on tissue culture dishes which support extra-cellular matrix deposition from cells and exogenously added serum components[11-14]. The de-attachment of epithelia from the extra-cellular matrix and placement in suspension culture leads to massive cell death in epithelia of different types[14-18]. The rates of anoikis of several epithelial cell lines have been evaluated and many have acquired resistance to anoikis.

In order to evaluate the role of acquisition of anoikis-resistance in the progression of squamous cell carcinoma of the oral cavity (SCCOC), we have selected the anoikis-sensitive Tu167, a cell line derived a human floor of mouth SCCOC, for growth in suspension culture. We compared the resultant anoikis-resistant cell line, JMAR, for *in vitro* growth and survival parameters and tumorigenicity in an orthotopic nude mouse model of SCCOC. These studies have shown more rapid tumor growth and an increased rate of distant metastases in those implanted with the anoikis-resistant cell line.

CONCLUSIONS

Nodal metastases and ECS are important predictors of treatment failure in patients with SCCOT. Novel treatment strategies are needed to prevent regional and distant relapse and to improve survival of this patient population. Therefore, patients with SCCOT with these adverse pathologic criteria should be considered for treatment protocols, which intensify local, regional, and systemic treatment. Furthermore, tumor biopsies and surgical specimens from these patients should be intensively scrutinized at the cellular and molecular level in order to identify the mechanisms of tumor progression. Such studies should yield additional prognostic markers and potentially identify novel targets for therapy. Furthermore, the development of appropriate tumor models should facilitate further verification of the molecular mechanisms of SCCOT metastasis and enable the pre-clinical assessment of novel treatment strategies to proceed.

Figure 1.

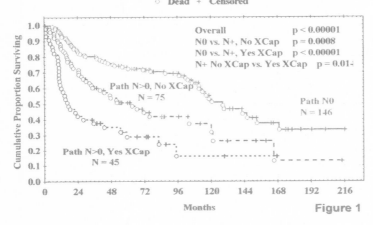

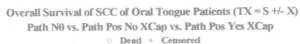

Figure 2.

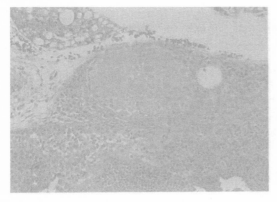
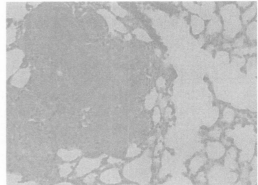

244

REFERENCES

1. Johnson JT, Wagner RL, Myers EN. A long-term assessment of adjuvant chemotherapy on outcome of patients with extracapsular spread of cervical metastases from squamous carcinoma of the head and neck. *Cancer* 1996; 77:181-185.
2. Al-Sarraf M, Pajak TF, Byhardt RW, Beitler JJ, Salter MM, Cooper JS. Postoperative Radiotherapy With Concurrent Cisplatin Appears to Improve Locoregional Control Of Advanced, Resectable Head And Neck Cancers: RTOG 88-24. *Int J Radiation Oncology Biol. Phys.* 1997; 37(4); 777-782.
3. Bachaud JM, Cohen-Jonathan E, Alzieu C, David JM, Serrano E, Daly-Schveitzer N. Combined Postoperative Radiotherapy and Weekly Cisplatin Infusion for Locally Advanced Head and Neck Carcinoma: Final Report of A Randomized Trial. *Int J Radiation Oncology Biol Phys* 1996; 36(5): 999-1004.
4. Hanahan D WRA. The hallmarks of cancer. *Cell.* 2000; 100(1):57-70. Review. No abstract available.
5. Reed J. Dysregulation of Apoptosis in Cancer. *J Clin Oncology* 1999; 17(9):2941-2953.
6. Glinsky G, Glinsky V. Apoptosis and metastasis: a superior resistance of metastatic cancer cells to programmed cell death. *Cancer Letters* 1996; 101:43-51.
7. Takaoka A, Adachi M, Okuda H, et al. Anti-cell death activity promotes pulmonary metastasis of melanoma. *Oncogene* 1997; 14:2971-2977.
8. Oka K, Qi B, Yutsudo M. Tumorigenic Conversion Resulting from Inhibition of Apoptosis in a Nontumorigenic HeLa-derived Hybrid Cell Line. *Cancer Research* 1999; 59(April 15, 1999):1816-1819.
9. Yawata A, Adachi M, Okuda H, et al. Prolonged cell survical enhances peritoneal dissemination of gastric cancer cells. *Oncogene* 1998; 16:2681-2686.
10. Rak J, Mitsuhashi Y, Sheehan C, et al. Collateral Expression of Proangiogenic and Tumorigenic Properties in Intestinal Epithelial Cell Variants Selected for Resistance to Anokisis. *Neoplasia* 1999; 1(1):23-30.
11. Haake A, Polakowska R. Cell Death by Apoptosis in Epidermal Biology. *J Invest Dermatol* 1993; 101(2):107-112.
12. Xu L, Schantz SP, Edelstein D, Sacks PG. A simplified method for the routine culture of normal oral epithelial (NOE) cells from upper aerodigestive tract mucosa. *Methods Cell Science* 1996; 18:31-39.
13. Hoffman H, Merkle S, Carey T. Head and Neck Squamous Carcinoma Cell Lines Capable of Serum-Free Growth In Vitro Head and Neck Cancer, Volume II, vol. II: B. C. Decker, Inc., 1990; 94-97.
14. Sacks PG. Cell, tissue, and organ culture as *in vitro* models to study the biology of squamous cell carcinomas of the head and neck. *Cancer and Metastasis Reviews* 1996; 15:27-51.
15. Kantak S, Kramer R. E-cadherin regulates anchorage-independent growth and survival in oral squamous cell carcinoma cells. *J Biol Chem* 1998; 273(27):16953-61.
16. Thomas F, Contreras J, Bilbao G, Ricordi C, Curiel D, Thomas J. Anoikis, extracellular matrix, and apoptosis factors in isolated cell transplantation. *Surgery* 1999; 126(2):299-304.
17. Gniadecki R, Hansen M, Wulf H. Two Pathways for Induction of Apoptosis by Ultraviolet Radiation in Cultured Human Keratinocytes. *J Invest Dermatol* 1997; 109(2):163-169.
18. Grossmann J, Maxson J, Whitacre C, et al. New Isolation Technique to Study Apoptosis in Human Intestinal Epithelial Cells. *Am J Pathol* 1998; 153(1):53-62.
19. Von Herbay A, Rudi J. Role of Apoptosis in Gastric Epithelial Turnover. *Microscopy Research and Technique* 2000; 48:303-311.

LYMPH NODE METASTASES OF ORAL AND OROPHARYNGEAL SQUAMOUS CELL CARCINOMA

Frank Waldfahrer, Heinrich Iro
Department of Otorhinolaryngology, Head and Neck Surgery

Correspondence to: *University Erlangen-Nuremburg, Waldstrasse 1, D-91054 Erlangen, Germany (mail to: heinrich.iro@hno.imed.uni-erlangen.de)*

Lymph node metastases are a common phenomenon in oral and oropharyngeal cancer so that the neck must always be included in every therapeutic consideration – without any exception. In the Erlangen series of more than 4000 patients treated between 1970 und 1990 62% of the patients with oral cancer and 71% of the patients with oropharyngeal cancer showed enlarged neck nodes at first presentation. It is quite clear that especially small nodes lead to difficulties seperating reactive inflammation from malignant disease.

Many prognostic factors have been identified in the context of lymph node metastases in head and neck cancer. There is no doubt that T category and tumor localisation influences regional metastasis. Number and volume of neck metastases are important prognostic factors, too. But beneath these well-known TNM relevant factors we were able to identify some additional prognostic factors, proven by multivariate analysis using a cox model. These factors are extracapsular spread of lymph node metastases ($p<0,0001$) as a histopathologic criterion and fixation of lymph nodes ($p<0,0001$) as an easy-to-handle clinical factor.

The clinically positive neck
In cases of clinical suspicious nodes most head and neck oncologists will agree that surgical treatment – neck dissection – is the treatment of the first choice, especially if the primary tumor will be removed surgically too. Of course, radiation therapy and /or antineoplastic chemotherapy are important alternatives.

In non-midline cancer usually at least the homolateral neck is scheduled to undergo neck dissection. By the way, in cases of midline cancer it is generally accepted to perform bilateral neck dissection.

Elective neck dissection on the opposite site in nod-midline cancer?
But in the context of non-midline cancer some questions are still unsolved. These questions deal with the treatment of the opposite site in case of absence of clinically positive nodes.

Dealing with this question we performed an analysis of our tumor registry selecting only patients with non-midline cancer. We found 433 patients treated between 1970 and 1990 who underwent surgical treatment of at least the homolateral neck side. Clinically, 62% showed suspicious nodes only on the tumor side, while bilateral disease was present in 8%. Only contralateral involvement occured in less than 1%.

The most important result of this analysis is the share of contralateral metastases in correlation to the homolateral neck status. In patients without homolateral metastases we found contralateral metastases in 2,3% compared with 2,6% in patients with homolateral metastases. These contralateral metastases were occult in most cases (Figure 1).

So it is to conclude, that contralateral metastases in non-midline cancer are certainly not common, but also occur in patients with homolateral negative necks. Therefore it is not suitable to decide on performing opposite neck dissection in dependance from the homolateral pathohistological results. Summarizing, performing contralateral neck dissection is a general (conceptional), not a particular decision.

Comparison between clinical and pathohistological staging
When comparing the clinical findings with the postoperative – pathohistological – findings concerning lymph node metastases an important problem can be recognized: enlarged nodes resemble not always lymph node metastases but sometimes only reactive changes.

Beneath false-positive preoperative findings false-negative findings play a much more important role as undertreatment might have fatal consequences on survival of the patient. In this context we should discuss the question of elective neck treatment in oral and oropharyngeal cancer. The decision for or against elective neck treatment depends on the suspected rate of occult lymph node metastases. This topic has been discussed extensively in the literature. It is still in discussion which rate of occult metastases might be accepted when preferring a policy of watchful waiting.

To determine the rates of occult metastases in oral and oropharyngeal cancer we analyzed our tumor registry again. We found 208 out of 614 patients with oral and 207 out 774 patients with oropharyngeal cancer to have a N0 neck.

More than half of the patients with oral cancer recieved elective neck dissection, while only 35% of the patients with oropharyngeal cancer did.

In oral cancer we found occult lymph node metastases in 27% and in oropharyngeal cancer in 36%. In addition, extracapsular spread was determined in 9% in oral cancer and in 15% in oropharyngeal cancer

In a further step we analyzed the relevance of the T category on occult neck nodes.

Even in small – that meens in T1 cancer – we found occult metastases in about 20% of the cases. The probability of occult metastases increases with higher T category as it was suspected.

These high rates of occult neck nodes should induce the consequence to perform elective neck treatment in all cases of oral and oropharyngeal cancer – even when the primary tumor is small.

However, when discussing our data it must be consideresd that ultrasonographic examinations were not performed as routine procedures through the whole period. It is few doubt that modern imaging procedures and in particular diagnostic fine needle aspiration biopsy would help to achieve lower rates for occult neck metastases.

CONCLUSION

It should not be any further doubt that an elective treatment of the neck should be considered regularly in any cases of oral and oropharyngeal cancer. Another point is in what way this elective treatment should be performed. One important argument for a neck dissection in contrast to elective irradiation is the possibility of pathohistological assessment and the option for a subsequent radiotherapy in cases of positive nodes. Especially in cases in which a transcervical approach is performed to resect the primary tumor no serious arguments are obvious against surgical treatment of the neck.

In cases of non-midline cancer we should consider that the absence of homolateral metastases is no suitable proof for the absence of contralateral node involvement.

Further readings can be provided by the authors.

Figure 1. Contralateral lymph node metastases in non-midline cancer

433 Patients with Non-Midline Cancer

- **433 Pat.**   **homolateral neck dissection**
- **81 Pat.**   **additional contralateral neck dissection**

Homolateral Neck:
- **61% positive (265/433), 39% negative (168/433)**

- **Patients <u>with</u> homolateral metastases (n=265)**
    - 18% (47/265) occult
    - 2,6% (7/265)   contralateral metastases (4/7 occult)
- **Patients <u>without</u> homolateral metastases (n=168)**
    - 55% (92/168) with cN+ -> false positive clinical staging
    - 2,3% (4/168)   contralateral metastases (3/4 occult)

Department of Otorhinolaryngology, Head and Neck Surgery, Erlangen 1970-1990

CERVICAL METASTASES IN PHARYNGEAL CARCINOMAS:
TREATMENT AND PROGNOSTIC FACTORS

K. Kunev, T. Hadjieva, I. Chalakov, Yu. Rangachev, L. Popov,
Department of Otorhinolaryngology, Medical University, Sofia, Bulgaria
Department of Roentgenology, Medical University, Sofia, Bulgaria

ABSTRACT

For a period of 12 years the authors have studied 501 patients with pharyngeal carcinoma, of which 60.73% with carcinoma of nasopharynx, 23.76% with carcinoma of mesopharynx and 15.51% with hypopharyngeal carcinoma. The localisation of metastases and therapeutical approach are reviewed in detail. The results are dependent on the localisation and the spread of the primary tumor. The existence of cervical metastases is a poor prognostic sign for achieving tumor control. The assessed prognostic factors are volume, localisation and morphologic characteristics of the metastases, engagement of the node's capsule and of the surrounding tissues. The authors discuss the therapeutical approach in different localisations and the possibilities for achieving better and longer lasting tumor control.

INTRODUCTION

The malignant tumors of the pharynx are of special interest with their clinical development, diagnostic problems, immunological properties, and their interaction with the pharyngeal space, larynx, skull cavity, and the therapeutic problems which they set on.

It is characteristic that the patients with malignant tumors of the pharynx which were observed were hospitalized in comparative late stage of the disease, with wide spread of the process and availability of near of distant metastases. Very frequent the initial discret symptomatic is interpreted like a symptom of other illness, and this is not in assistance of the early diagnosis. At the moment of manifestation of the disease the stage is too advanced and the therapeutic possibilities are too small. Some of the malignant tumors of the pharynx are characterized by their local aggressive growth which can lead to intracranial spread.

The clinic of the disease depends on anatomical disposition of the pharynx and the biological pecularity of the malignant tumors. The morphological pecularities of the malignant tumors of

251

the pharynx are characterized by their great variety and the dominating of one of other form in the different localisations of sublocalisation.

Yet in the previous century was evaluated that the surmont of the barrier of primary localisation and the spreading of the carcinoma of the pharynx in the regional lymph nodes of the neck is a very unfavourable moment in a fight to achieve a tumor control. During the 50[s] of the 19th century Chelins[1] said the "tumor once disseminated and left his primary localisation, who engaged the submandibular glands is impossible to be cured." This point of view was attacked already in the 19th century from the innovation methods for the treatment of regional metastases of malignant tumors of the head.

In 1906 George Crile took notice that the metastases in the lymph nodes of the neck remaining enough time localised, giving a possibility to be treated.

The aim of this study was to analyze the metastases in carcinoma of the pharynx their treatment and their prognostic moments to achieve a tumor control.

MATERIAL AND METHODS

Over a period of 15 years were treated 501 patients of pharyngeal carcinoma. In the first group with nasopharyngeal malignant tumors were 60.73% from all patients. In the second group with mesopharyngeal malignant tumors were included 23.76% and the last 15.51% from the patients were with malignant hypopharyngeal tumors.

Of 279 patients with nasopharyngeal carcinoma men were more often concerned than women and the correlation between them was 3:1. Men were 66.54% and women were 33.46%. The majority of the patients were between 51 and 60 years old. The youngest patient with carcinoma of the nasopharynx was 14 years old, and the oldest was 85 years old. There were generally 279 patients with malignant tumors of the nasopharynx. Of these, 175 patients were with metastases in locoregional lymph nodes.

131 patients were with mesophanryngeal carcinoma. 71% from these patients were men, 29% were women. The majority of the patients also were between 51 and 60 years old. 56 from them were with cervical metastases.

91 patients were with hypopharyngeal carcinoma. There also prevailed men. Men were 78.02% and women were 21.98%. The most common age of the patients with hypopharyngeal carcinoma was also between 51 and 60 years. Cervical metastases were found in 46 patients and in 45 not.

The cervical metastases are divided into 6 zones according to their localisation. Zone 1 encompasses the submental and submandibular lymph nodes. Zone 2, 3, 4 desribe the deep jugular nodes – upper, middle, lower. The margin between zones 2 and 3 is the hyoid bone, and the margin between zones 3 and 4 is where the omohyoid muscle crosses the carotid sheath. Zone 5 is the posterior triangle and zone 6 is paratracheal lymph nodes.

OUTCOMES

Nasopharynx: Of 279 patients with malignant tumors of the nasopharynx which we followed 62.93% were with cervical metastases. 62.35% from women with malignant tumors of the nasopharynx were with cercival metastases. Of these 62.35%, 22.5% were with N1 stage, 21.5% with stage N2 and 19.35% with stage N3. 63.24% from men with malignant tumors of the nasopharynx were with cervical metastases. With N2 stage were 23.24%. More rare were men with N3 stage – 22.16% and the most rare were men with N1 stage – 17.76% (fig. 1). The most common localisation of the cervical metastases in the malignant tumors of the nasopharynx which we observed were at the level of the common carotid artery, and the most engaged lymph nodes were in the zones two and three. We observed rare engagement of the lymph nodes in zone one. We established metastases in this zone in 14 patients. 32 patienst were with bilateral cervical metastases, and 17 of them were with cervical metastases which engaged zone two, three and four. In the other 14 patients the cervical metastases were engaged all groups. Separate affect of the supraclavicular lymph nodes we did not observe.

Of the 175 patients with malignant tumors of the nasopharynx and cervical metastases 73.14% were with histopathologically proven poorly differentiated nonkeratizing squamous cell carcinoma and lymphoepithelioma Regaud-Schmincke. Non differentiated nasopharyngeal carcinoma gave much more often cervical metastases than the well-differentiated keratizing squamous cell carcinoma. We used for the radiation therapy installation "Rokus". In the initial stage we used conventional fractionated RT. Later we used hyperfractionated radiotherapy. The median focal dose of the primary focus was up to 64 Gy. We followed up the state of regional lymph nodes. We ascertained that regression of the malignant tumors of the nasopharynx and cervical metastases came most frequently after the first 10-12Gy. The regression was dependant on biology oft the tumor and from the immunological status of the patient. Patients with unsatisfactory immunological status had a worse prognosis.

We observed persistence of the locoregional metastases after complete finished course of radiotherapy in 19.86% from the patients. Of these patients 30 were with stage IV according to the American Joint Committee on Cancer (AJCC) staging system – 1997 year, and 17 were with stage III. 35.1% of these patients were with well-differentiated squamous cell carcinoma, 24.3% were moderate-differentiated squamous cell carcinoma, there was one case with cylindroma, and the others were with undifferentiated carcinomas. Metastases which persist were with size great than 6cm. We observed 16 patients with recurrent nasopharyngeal carcinoma. Of these 16 patients 5.71% were with stage II, 6.45% with stage III and 6.62% with stage IV. The patients with recurrent nasopharyngeal carcinoma were with very poor prognosis independently from our re-treatment, the survival time was between 6 and 12 months. Four of these patients were with lung metastases. Our preference method for re-treatment was surgery – radical neck dissection. 17 patients with persistent disease after radiotherapy were treated by surgery. Other 20 patients were inoperable and were re-treated with palliative and symptomatic therapy. Both radiotherapy and chemotherapy were used for young patients with III and IV staged disease. The one year survival rate was 87%. After five years the rate falls to 50% and after 10 years were almost the same.

Mesopharynx: Of 75 patients with malignant tumors of the mesopharynx the local alterations in the primary focus were very advanced. 52.75% of them were with cervical metastases classified as follows: stage N1 – 18.32%, N2 – 14.5% and stage N3 – 9.93% (fig. 2).

Hypopharynx: Of all patients with malignant tumors of the hypopharynx 49.45% were not with cervical metastases. 50.55% were with cervical metastases which we classified as follows: N1-metastase in a single ipsilateral lymph node, 3cm or less in a greatest dimension – 20.88%. N2 stage – metastases in ipsilateral, contralateral or bilateral lymph nodes more than 6cm in greatest dimension – 10.99%, and N3 stage metastases in a lymph node more than 6cm in a greatest dimension – 18.68% (fig. 3).

The treatment of the cervical metastases were surgery or radiotherapy, depending on the condition of the primary tumor and the engaging of the surrounding tissue from the metastases.

CONSIDERATION

The progress in the knowledge of the biology of the tumor of the head and neck, the new tendencies that these are diseases with chronic progress with determinate prognostic moments in their development. These findings binding us to considering in dynamic of the natural development and the prognostic factors to control the progress and to achieve tumor control. In initial stage of the development of the tumor in his intraepithelial form, the leading role for the carcinoma belongs to the environment. The necessary prerequisite for the arising of the nasopharyngeal carcinoma is EBV-infection, systematic use of tobacco and alcohol and in recent years the carcinoma of the oral cavity and the chewing of tobacco.

The factors on the part of the patient are cumulate hereditary, insufficiency, anomalies in DNA, disturbance in glutadion metabolism and impossibility for immune answer.

The impossibility to achieve adequate tumor control in patients with weak of missing immunity is a very poor prognostic factor. In the patients with compromise immunity the monocite cells producing a great number of prostaglandins which influence upon the immune processes[2]. At the appearance of metastases the immune processes are changing[3].

The presence of metastases is poor prognostic factor[4]. He draw the conclusion that the possibility to achieve a tumor control decrease with about 50% when tumor engaged the regional lymph nodes. The prognosis of course is unfavourable in patients with conglomerates of lymph nodes or with multiply lymph nodes, the destruction of the capsule of the lymph node and the attitude of the metastases to surrounding tissues[4, 5]. The fast and aggressive development of the cervical metastases is unfavourable prognostic moment. Indisputably, the condition of the regional lymph nodes is a considerable moment in a possibility to achieve a tumor control. And the exact estimate of the condition of the neck is from exclusively importance for the presence of micrometastases.

The choice of method of treatment of course is also from exclusive importance for the prognostis of the disease. The conduct is dependent on the biology of the tumor, its spread, its morphological characteristic and the immune condition of the patient.

254

Nasopharynx

	Contralateral Metastases	Homolateral Metastases
N1	53 patients with metastases in zones II and III **N3**	21 patients with bilateral metastases
N2	11 patients with bilateral metastases in zones II and III	14 patients with metastases in zones I, II, III, IV
	6 patients with contralateral metastases in zones II and III	17 patients with homolateral metastases in zones II, III, IV
	46 patients with homolateral metastases in zones II and III	7 patients with metastases in zones II, III, IV and V
	Distant metastases PUL – 6 patients and OS – 2 patients	

Figure 1. Cervical metastases in malignant tumors of the nasopharynx

Mesopharynx

	Contralateral metastases	Homolateral Metastases
N1	24 patients with metastases in zones II and III **N3**	4 patients with bilateral metastases
N2	6 patients with bilateral metastases in zones II and III	2 patients with metastases in zones II, III, IV and V
	3 patients with contralateral metastases in zones II and III	7 patients with homolateral metastases in zones III, IV and V
	10 patients with homolateral metastases in zones II and III	7 patients with metastases in zones II, III, IV and V

Figure 2. Localisation of the cervical metastases in malignant tumors of the mesopharynx

Hypopharynx

	Contralateral metastases	Homolateral Metastases
N1	19 patients with metastases in zones II and III **N3**	3 patients with bilateral metastases inzones II and III
N2	5 patients with bilateral metastases in zones II and III	10 patients with homolateral metastases in zones II, II and IV
	4 patients with homolateral metastases in zones II, III and IV	4 patients with homolateral metastases in zones II, III, IV and V
	1 patient with contralateral metastases in zones II and III	
	Distant metastases PUL – 5 patients	

Figure 3. Localisation of the cervical metastases in malignant tumors of the hypopharynx

REFERENCES

1. Shah, J. P., 1994, Cervical lymph node, Metastases-Diagnostic, Therapeutic, Prognostic, Implications of the head and neck, 1994, NY
2. Berlinger, N. T., Deficient immunit in head and neck cancer due to excessive monocite production of prostaglandins, Laryngoscope, 1984, 94, 11, 1407-1410
3. Schuller, D. E., R. P. Rock, J. Rinehart, A. R. Rodemans-Benen, T-Lymphostasis as a prognostic indicator in head and neck cancer, Arch, Laryngol., 1986, 112, 9, 938-941
4. Shah, J. P., R. A. Cendin, H. W. Farr., Carcinoma of the oral cavity – factors affecting treatment; Failure the primary site and neck, Am. J. Surg., 1976, 132, 504-507
5. Richard, J. M., H. Sancho-Garnier, C. Micheau, Prognostic factors in cervical lymph node, Metastases in upper respiratory and digestive tract carcinomas, Laryngoscope, 1987, 97, 97-101
6. Shah, J. P. Cancer of the upper aerodigestive tract, NY, Appieton-Century-Crofts, 1982
7. Spiro, R. H., The management of neck nodes in head and neck cancer: A surgeon's view, Bull. of NY Acad. of medicine, 1985, 61,7

OBSERVING THE N0 NECK IN T2 ORAL AND OROPHARYNGEAL CARCINOMA USING ULTRASOUND GUIDED CYTOLOGY

Eline J.C. Nieuwenhuis[1], Jonas A. Castelijns[2], Michiel W.M. van den Brekel[1], Gordon B. Snow[1], Charles R. Leemans[1]
[1]Department of Otolaryngology/Head and Neck Surgery
[2]Department of Radiology

Correspondence to: C.R. Leemans, Vrije Universiteit Medical Center, P.O. Box 7057, 1007 MB Amsterdam, The Netherlands, Phone: +31 20 44 43690, Fax: +31 20 44 43688 (e-mail: chr.leemans@azvu.nl)

INTRODUCTION

Head and neck squamous cell carcinoma (HNSCC) metastasizes primarily to the cervical lymphatic system. The most important prognosticators of lymph node metastases for patients with HNSCC are the number of metastases, size and presence of extranodal spread. For example, the failure rate at distant sites, with controlled locoregional disease, varies from 6.9% in pN0 cases to 46.8% for patients with more than 3 lymph node metastases in their neck dissection specimen.[1] In many institutions throughout the world the neck is mainly staged by palpation. As a consequence of the low sensitivity of palpation, a neck without palpable lymph nodes (N0) is at high risk of harboring occult metastases. The management of the N0 neck is a source of continuous controversy among clinicians. Many head and neck surgeons favor the opinion that the N0 neck should be treated electively when the risk of occult metastases is estimated to be higher than 20%.[2] For the majority of patients, this policy results in overtreatment of the neck, while no benefit in survival has been demonstrated in 3 prospective studies compared to delayed neck dissection for lymph node metastases.[3-5]

Although current diagnostic imaging techniques such as computed tomography (CT), magnetic resonance imaging (MRI) and ultrasonography (US) in general have increased diagnostic accuracy, these modalities still have a relatively low accuracy for the N0 neck.[6] In contrast, ultrasound guided fine needle aspiration cytology (USgFNAC) has a higher sensitivity and specificity and is more cost-effective than CT and MRI. We found that in experienced hands the sensitivity for the N0 neck can reach 73% with a specificity of 100%.[7] Others reported sensitivities in the range of 42% to 50%.[8,9] Since 1992, we gradually changed our policy towards the neck for patients with T1-T2 oral carcinomas, who could be treated by transoral tumor excision. In case of negative USgFNAC at initial staging, these patients are treated by local excision of the primary tumor and are spared an elective lymph node dissection. Instead, these patients are followed by palpation and USgFNAC at regular intervals (wait-and-see policy). In a retrospective study USgFNAC for initial staging as well as follow-up of the neck was evaluated. Approximately 20% of patients with small oral and oropharyngeal carcinomas treated by transoral excision only on the basis of negative USgFNAC findings developed a neck node metastasis during follow-up.[10] Taken into account that such groups of patients are usually reported to have a 40% incidence rate of lymph node metastases, these data indicate that USgFNAC in this study detected approximately 50% of occult metastases. Possible causes of false negative results are aspiration of the wrong node, aspiration of the wrong part of a node containing a small metastasis (sampling error) and false interpretation of the cytopathologist. Furthermore, USgFNAC is not an easy technique and may have a long learning curve with a high interobserver variance.

Whereas many clinicians support an observation policy for the neck in T1 HNSCC, the management of the neck in T2 HNSCC is more controversial. Regular follow-up with USgFNAC after transoral excision might enable early detection and possibly high salvage rate of neck failures, which justifies a wait-and-see policy. Therefore, we assessed the clinical outcome of all patients treated between 1993 and 2000 by transoral excision only for a T2 oral or oropharyngeal tumor with negative USgFNAC findings at initial staging.

PATIENTS AND METHODS

A study was performed in 56 patients treated by transoral excision between 1993 and June 2000 for a T2 N0 histologically proven squamous cell carcinoma of the oral cavity or oropharynx. All patients had negative USgFNAC findings at initial staging. Population consisted of 30 men and 26 women, with an median age of 64 years. Primary tumor localizations were floor of mouth (FOM) (n=22), mobile tongue (n=23), buccal mucosa (n=7), and inferior alveolar process (n=1), soft palate (n=3). None of the patients were previously treated.

Ultrasonographic examinations of levels 1 through 5 of both sides of the neck were performed, using a 7.5 MHz linear array transducer (Acuson Company, Mountain View, CA, USA, and ATL, HDI 3000, Bothell, WA, USA). Lymph nodes with a minimal diameter of 3 mm or larger in level I, and 4 mm or larger in the other levels were aspirated. USgFNAC of the enlarged lymph nodes was performed, using a syringe holder (Cameco, Taeby, Sweden) and a 0.6 x 25mm needle. After each aspiration, smears were prepared and sent for cytological examination. In 13 of the 56 patients initial ultrasonography did not show enlarged lymph nodes, and thus no aspirates were obtained. In 26 patients only ipsilateral lymph nodes were aspirated, whereas from the remaining 17 patients enlarged lymph nodes were detected and aspirated bilaterally. Follow-up visits were performed every 6 weeks, including USgFNAC every 12 weeks for the first year. Follow-up ranged from 9 months to 8 years (median 52 months).

RESULTS

Out of 56 patients, 11 (19,6%) developed lymph node metastases in the neck during follow-up. Five regional failures were detected with USgFNAC, whereas in 6 patients USgFNAC confirmed clinical suspicion of the neck metastases. The size of the tumor positive lymph nodes at USgFNAC was ≤ 1cm in 8 of 11 patients (72,7%). These neck failures were located ipsilaterally in 10 cases and bilaterally in one case. This patient presented with a FOM carcinoma extending to the midline. In 9 out of 11 patients the lymph node metastases were detected within 6 months after treatment of the primary tumor and in 2 out of 11 patients between 6 and 12 months. All 11 patients were treated by neck dissection, of whom 9 also received postoperative radiotherapy based on the histopathological examinations of the neck dissection specimen, i.e. ≥ 2 tumor-positive lymph nodes or the presence of extranodal spread. In one patient there was no indication for postoperative radiotherapy and one patient refused radiotherapy. Histopathological examination of the 11 neck dissection specimens revealed 37 tumor positive lymph nodes in total (median 2), of which 26 (70,3%) lymph nodes in 9 (81,8%) neck dissection specimens showed extranodal spread.

Ten of the 11 patients (90,9%) who developed lymph node metastases in the neck were salvaged. No regional recurrences in the treated necks were observed. One patient developed metastases in the untreated contralateral neck side and died of his disease. Three other patients died of other causes, without evidence of recurrence of their index tumor, 14-75 months after treatment of the neck metastases. The other 7 patients with neck failures are still alive without evidence of disease, with a follow-up ranging from 6 to 65 months after therapeutic neck dissection. In the 11 patients with neck metastases of their tumor, no local recurrences were seen, whereas 2 patients developed a 2nd primary tumor.

Of the 45 patients who did not develop metastases in the neck, 4 patients (8,9%) developed local recurrences and 6 patients (13,3%) developed a 2nd primary tumor.

DISCUSSION

In a previous study, we found USgFNAC to be more accurate than palpation, CT or MRI for the assessment of the N0 neck.[11] As a consequence, it can be helpful in selecting patients for either a therapeutical neck dissection or a wait-and-see policy for the neck. Comparison between these two policies has been the topic in three prospective studies, but none of these studies showed a significant difference in survival.[3-5] The failure rate in the neck in this study is 19,6%, which compares favorably to the failure rates ranging from 24% to 57% quoted in the literature for patients treated with transoral excision only and a wait-and-see strategy for the neck.[3-5,12] These differences could be attributed to the fact that in none of these other studies imaging was used initially.

The salvage rate in case of neck metastases after a wait-and-see policy for the neck is of crucial importance. We found that USgFNAC often enables detection of small lymph node metastases. Five of the 11 neck failures were detected before being palpable, and most of these nodal metastases were smaller than 1 cm. Furthermore, all neck failures were detected within 12 months after transoral excision of the primary tumor, which stresses the importance of regular follow-up including USgFNAC every 3 months for at least the first year. Surgery and postoperative radiotherapy could salvage 90,9% (10/11) of the patients who developed neck failures during limited follow-up. However, in the literature others reported salvage rates varying from 27% to 82% after development of cervical metastases.[3-5,12] Again, in these studies only palpation was used at initial staging of the neck and during follow-up.

In conclusion, USgFNAC at initial staging reduces the risk of occult neck metastases for small oral cavity or oropharynx tumors, which justifies a wait-and-see strategy for the N0 neck. Regular follow-up with USgFNAC contributed to the timely detection of lymph node metastases in the neck and a high salvage rate.

Table 2. Characteristics of the 11 patients who developed neck metastases

Case (sex)	Localization	USgFNAC Interval (months)	Level (size in mm)	Histopathology No of meta (ENS)	Involved levels	Follow-up (months)
1 (m)	Floor of mouth	6,5	1 (10)	7 (6)	1-4	75, DOC
2 (v)	Mobile tongue	1	3 (15)	5 (5)	1-4	65, NED
3 (m)	Floor of mouth	4	3 (5)	5 (4)	1-4	34, DOC
4 (m)	Mobile tongue	3	2 (6)	2 (1)	2-3	20, DOD
5 (m)	Soft palate	3,5	2 (25 and 8)	2 (1)	2	56, NED
6 (m) *	Floor of mouth	5	2 (8)	2 (0)	1-2	52, NED
7 (m) *	Floor of mouth	2	1 (5) and 4 (16)	6 (5)	1, 3-5	14, DOC
8 (v) *	Mobile tongue	8	2 (9)	3 (1)	2	11, NED
9 (m) *	Mobile tongue	1,5	3 (10)	2 (2)	1-2	16, NED
10 (v) *	Mobile tongue	1,5	2 (10)	2 (1)	2	14, NED
11 (m)	Buccal mucosa	2	1 (9)	1 (0)	1	6, NED

The interval between transoral resection and the positive USgFNAC findings are indicated in column 3, level and size of lymph node metastases in column 4. ENS, extranodal spread. Follow-up after therapeutic treatment of the neck. DOC, dead of other cause; NED, no evidence of disease; DOD, dead of disease.
* lymph node metastases detected by USgFNAC

REFERENCES

1.   Leemans CR, Tiwari R, Nauta JJ, van der Waal I, Snow GB. Regional lymph node involvement and its significance in the development of distant metastases in head and neck carcinoma. Cancer 1993;71:452-456.

2.   Weiss MH, Harrison LB, Isaacs RS. Use of decision analysis in planning a management strategy for the stage N0 neck. Arch Otolaryngol Head Neck Surg 1994;120:699-702.

3.   Vandenbrouck C, Snacho-Garnier H, Chassagne D, Saravane D, Cachin Y, Micheau C. Elective versus therapeutic radical neck dissection in epidermoid carcinoma of the oral cavity-results of a randomized clinical trial. Cancer 1980;46:386-90.

4.   Fakih AR, Rao RS, Patel AR. Prophylactic neck dissection in squamous cell carcinoma of oral tongue: a prospective randomized study. Semin Surg Oncol 1989;5:327-30.

5.   Kligerman J, Lima RA, Soares JR et al. Supraomohyoid neck dissection in the treatment of T1/T2 squamous cell carcinoma of oral cavity. Am J Surg 1994;168:391-4.

6.   Atula TS, Varpula MJ, Kurki TJ, Klemi PJ, Grenman R. Assessment of cervical lymph node status in head and neck cancer patients: palpation, computed tomography and low field magnetic resonance imaging compared with ultrasound-guided fine-needle aspiration cytology. Eur J Radiol 1997;25:152-161.

7.   Van den Brekel MW, Castelijns JA, Stel HV et al. Occult metastatic neck disease: detection with US and US-guided fine- needle aspiration cytology. Radiology 1991;180:457-461.

8.   Righi PD, Kopecky KK, Caldemeyer KS, Ball VA, Weisberger EC, Radpour S. Comparison of ultrasound-fine needle aspiration computed tomography in patients undergoing neck dissection. Head Neck 1997;19:604-610.

9.   Takes RP, Righi P, Meeuwis CA et al. The value of ultrasound with ultrasound-guided fine-needle aspiration biopsy compared to computed tomography in the detection of regional metastases in the clinically negative neck. Int J Radiation Oncology Biol Phys 1998;40:1027-1032.

10.   Van den Brekel MW, Castelijns JA, Reitsma LC, Leemans CR, van der Waal I, Snow GB. Outcome of observing the N0 neck using ultrasonographic-guided cytology for follow-up. Arch Otolaryngol Head Neck Surg 1999;125:153-156.

11.   Van den Brekel MWM, Castelijns JA, Stel HV, Golding RP, Meyer CJ, Snow GB. Modern imaging techniques and ultrasound-guided aspiration cytology for the assessment of neck node metastases: a prospective comparative study. Eur Arch Otorhinolaryngol 1993;250:11-17.

12.   Khafif RA, Gelbfish, GA, Tepper P, Attie, JN. Elective radical neck dissection in epidermoid cancer of the head and neck. A retrospective analysis of 853 cases of mouth, pharynx, and larynx cancer. Cancer 1991; 67:67-71.

WAIT – AND – SEE POLICY – CHANCE OR RISK IN THE N0 NECK ?

Christian Popella, Hiltrud Glanz, Christoph Arens
Dept. of ENT, Head and Neck Surgery, University-Clinics Giessen, Germany, (Director: Prof. Dr. H. Glanz)

Keywords: N0 neck, neck dissection, wait-and-see policy

Correspondence to: Ch. Popella, MD, Department ENT, Head and Neck Surgery, University-Clinics Giessen, Feulgenstrasse 10, 35385 Giessen, Germany, Phone: ++49-641-99-43707, Fax. ++49-641-99-43709 (e-mail: christian.popella@hno.med.uni-giessen.de)

ABSTRACT

Background. Presupposing that the neck remains negative after preoperative imaging techniques like ultrasound, CT or MRI, the decision to perform a neck dissection is always an individual one, influenced by the primary tumor and patient-related factors. Criteria relating to the tumor are site, size, depth on infiltration and grading of the primary tumor.

Methods. We investigated 261 patients, who had a primary tumor in the oral cavity, oropharynx, hypopharynx, larynx, lip, skin of face and auricle, after a period of 10 years retrospectively. The tumor stages ranged from T1 to T3. In all patients, a wait-and-see strategy was pursued. Not only tumor-related factors but also sonographical findings were analyzed in the cases of recurrences.

Results. 16 patients (2%) demonstrated late neck metastases, 5 patients died tumor-related. Most late metastases occured after tumor stage pT1 but with low grade differentiation.

Conclusion. Some sites like tongue, pharynx and lip and certain histological and sonographical findings indicate therapeutical guidelines. A regular tumor follow-up allows the detection of metastases in an early stage with good prognosis in a selected indication of a wait-and-see policy.

INTRODUTION

Wait an see policy – is it a chance or a risk for patients with an N0 neck? The decision whether to include the neck lymph nodes in the concept of a tumor therapy in cases of smaller squamous cell carcinoma is always an individual one and depends on different primary tumor- related and patient-related factors. Criteria relating to the tumor are site, size, and grading. The patients themselves must be reliable concerning the follow up, if a wait and see policy should be pursued. This strategy allows avoidance of side effects and complications of treatment on one hand. On the other hand it always involves the risk of undertreatment with fatal consequences.

MATERIALS AND METHODS

Presupposing that the neck lymph nodes remain unsuspicious of metastases in the preoperative assessment like palpation, sonography, CT or MRI, we did not perform a neck dissection in 261 previously untreated cancer patients within the period from 1990 to 2000. The primary tumor was located in the mucosa of the oral cavity, oropharynx, hypopharynx, larynx, lips and in the skin of face and auricle. The tumor stages ranged from pT1 to pT2 and in some selected cases to pT3. All tumors were treated by primary surgery without postoperative irradiation.

RESULTS

None of the 167 patients with glottic cancer suffered from late regional metastases, even in 39 pT2 and 6 pT3 stages. A second group without any late neck metastases were 19 patients with squamous cell carcinomas of the skin of the auricle. 3 patients showed an advanced stage, too (pT3).

Due to the highly selected indication of a wait and see policy we had only 16 patients with late neck metastases, that not allows a statistical but a descriptive and critical analysis of these cases. Half of the patients remarked the enlarged lymph nodes themselves, the other half was diagnosed in the follow up. First patients with cancer of the mucosa: 4 out of a total of 19 patients with tongue cancer developed late neck metastases within 5 to 41 months and 3 out of 22 patients with lip cancer within 3-10 months. In the oropharynx (7 cases) late metastases occurred two times within 12-15 months. 1 patient with cancer of the floor of mouth (10 cases) had a late neck failure after 3 months and 1 patient out of 2 patients with hypopharyngeal cancer after 12 months. In 1 patient with a supraglottic cancer (9 cases) the late metastases occurred after 46 months without any evidence of a second primary tumor. Pathohistology showed a very highly differentiated tumor with a very low mitotic rate.

Concerning the patients with skin cancer, late metastases occurred in 2 out of 2 patients with a cheek cancer after 6 respectively 5 months and in 2 out of 4 patients with cancer of the forehead within 3 and 5 months, respectively.

In general the interval between treatment of the primary tumor and the metastases occurrence ranged from 1 to 24 months in patients with a primary stage pT1 and a histological middle or low grade differentiation. As already mentioned, only the 2 patients with very late metastases after more than 40 months showed a high grade differentiation.

Preoperative imaging techniques: Most of the patients were investigated by sonography preoperatively. In 7 cases a lymph node could be detected but was classified as a reactive unspecifically enlarged node. The largest diameter ranged from 10 to 20 mm. In 3 cases the shape was round and in 4 cases the hilus structure was not demonstrable. Retrospectively, these lymph nodes should have been considered suspicious of metastatic growth. 7 further patients, however, had no demonstrable lymph nodes, that means occult metastases and in 2 patients with skin cancer no sonography was performed.

Treatment and outcome: In most of the patients delayed metastases were treated by a selective or modified radical neck dissection , sometimes combined with a parotidectomy preserving the facial nerve and postoperative irradiation. Nevertheless, 5 out of these 16 patients (31%) died tumor-related. Regarding all 261 cancer patients with an N0 neck, however, we observed a tumor-related death in 2 % only.

DISCUSSION

In principle, the treatment of the N0 neck is based on a neck dissection, a radiation therapy or a wait-and-see policy. The factors that contribute to a therapy decision are probability of occult metastases, efficacy of therapy in primary and salvage surgery, quality-of-life-measures and patients preferences[1]. The precise role of an elective neck dissection is less clear. Some authors investigated oral and laryngeal cancer patients and found a frequency rate of occult metastases in neck dissection specimen of 20-41 % and recurrences in wait-and-see policy in up to 36 %. They recommend an elective neck treatment because of an improved survival outcome[2-6]. Other authors indicate a neck dissection if the probability of micrometastases exceeds 10 %[7, 8] or 20 %[1, 9]. Several authors have advocated the use of various histologic parameters to predict metastatic potential like T category, tumor differentiation, perineural and lymphatic vessel invasion, molecular markers and others[7, 8, 10, 11].

In our study, we can presume the following risk factors:
1. Site of primary tumor: If the primary tumor is located in an area with a lower lymphatic drainage like vocal fold or external ear, the risk of occult metastases is rather low. Other regions richly supplied with lymphatics, like skin of face and forehead or oral cavity, lips and pharynx, are involved with a higher danger of late metastases.

2. Grading: Middle- and low-grade differentiated tumors have a higher risk of occult metastases in the first 2 years, but in high grade tumors we must suspect late metastases even after 2 years.

3. Sonography: Preoperative detectable lymph nodes with typical sonographical criteria, like round shape, loss of hilus structure and enlargement in longest diameter, should be examined with special care and in shorter intervals. A cytological or histological clarification should be performed early.

4. Patient: A wait-and-see policy should be performed only in patients who are reliable in regular follow-up examinations because occult metastases can become a risk if they are diagnosed in a delayed stage.

REFERENCES

1. Weiss MH, Harrison LB, Isaacs RS. Use of decision analysis in planning a management strategy for the stage N0 neck. Arch Otolaryngol Head Neck Surg 1994; 120:699-702
2. McGuirt WF Jr, Johnson JT, Myers EN, Rothfield R, Wagner R. Floor of mouth carcinoma. The management of the clinically negative neck. Arch Otolaryngol Head Neck Surg 1995; 121:278-282
3. Hicks WL JR, Kollmorgen DR, Kuriakose MA et al. Patterns of nodal metastasis and surgical managementof the neck in supraglottic laryngeal carcinoma. Otolaryngol Head Neck Surg 1999; 121:57-61
4. Lydiatt DD, Robbins KT, Byers RM, Wolf PF. Treatment of stage I and II oral tongue cancer. Head Neck 1993; 15:308-312
5. Yii NW, Patel SG, Rhys-Evans PH, Breach NM. Management of the N= neck in early cancer of the oral tongue. Clin Otolaryngol 1999; 24:75-79
6. Haddadin KJ, Soutar DS, Oliver RJ, Webster MH, Robertson AG, MacDonald DG. Improved survival for patients with clinically T1/T2, N0 tongue tumors undergoing a prophylactic neck dissection. Head Neck 1999; 21:517-525
7. Schipper J, Gellrich NC, Marangos N, Maier W. The importance of the B-mode ultrasound studies in patients with cancer of the upper aerodigestive tract and in N0 lymph node stage. Laryngo Rhino Otol 1999; 78:561-565
8. Steiner W, Hommerich CP. Diagnosis and treatment of the N0 neck of carcinomas of the upper aerodigestive tract. Report of an international symposium, Gottingen, Germany, 1992. Eur Arch Otorhinolaryngol 1993; 250:450-456
9. Van den Brekel MW, Castelijns JA, Reitsma LC, Leemans CR, van der Waal I, Snow GB. Outcome of observing the N0 neck using ultrasonographic-guided cytology for follow up. Arch Otolaryngol Head Neck Surg 1999; 125:153-156
10. Pillsbury HC 3rd, Clark M. A rationale for therapy of the N0 neck. Laryngoscope 1997; 107:1294-1315
11. Ozdek A, Sarac S, Akyol MU, Unal OF, Sungur A. Histopathological predictors of occult lymph node metastases in supraglottic squamous cell carcinomas. Eur Arch Otorhinolaryngol 2000; 257:389-392

SELECTIVE NECK DISSECTION IN THE MANAGEMENT OF THE NECK IN SQUAMOUS CELL CARCINOMA OF THE UPPER AERODIGESTIVE TRACT

Petra Ambrosch, MD
Department of Otorhinolaryngology, Head and Neck Surgery, University of Goettingen, Goettingen, Germany

Correspondence to: Priv.-Doz. Dr. Petra Ambrosch, Dept. of Otorhinolaryngology-Head and Neck Surgery of the University of Goettingen, Robert-Koch-Str. 40, D-37075 Goettingen, Germany. Phone: +49/551/39-2807, Fax: +49/551/39-2809, (*e-mail: ambrosch@med.uni-goettingen.de*)

ABSTRACT

Objective: The purpose of this study was to evaluate the efficacy of selective neck dissection (SND) in elective and therapeutic treatment of the neck.

Methods: A retrospective review of 503 previously untreated patients undergoing 711 SNDs as a part of initial therapy for squamous cell carcinoma of the larynx, oral cavity, oro- and hypopharynx from 8/1986 to 6/1997 at a single institution was undertaken. Lymph nodes were pathologically negative in 249 and positive in 254 patients. Postoperative radiotherapy was given to 14.5% of the node-negative and 62.2% of the node-positive patients. The median follow-up interval was 41 months.

Results: The 3 year regional recurrence rates estimated according to Kaplan-Meier were as follows: pN0 4.7%, pN1 4.9%, pN2 12.1%. A comparison of recurrence rates with respect to extent of neck disease and postoperative radiotherapy demonstrated a tendency to an improved regional control in irradiated patients with one metastasis and a distinctly improved regional control in patients with multiple metastases or metastases with extracapsular spread.

Conclusion: The results achieved with SND compare favorably with the results reported for modified radical neck dissection. The application of SND might be extended to more-advanced neck disease.

INTRODUCTION

It is well recognized that the status of the cervical lymph nodes is the most important prognostic factor in squamous cell carcinoma of the upper aerodigestive tract. The presence, number, size, level and extranodal spread of cervical lymph node metastases considerably reduces locoregional control and survival rates of the patients. The generally accepted indications for performing SND are the clinically negative neck in patients with a high risk of occult neck metastases and the therapeutic management of N1 disease. In the literature there is disagreement about the applicability of the method in patients with more extensive neck disease. The purpose of this study was to evaluate the therapeutic value of SND performed electively and therapeutically.

PATIENTS AND METHODS

The medical records of all patients undergoing neck dissection at the Dept. of Otorhinolaryngology-Head and Neck Surgery of Goettingen University, Goettingen, Germany, between 8/1986 and 6/1997, were reviewed. Five-hundred and fifty six patients with previously untreated squamous cell carcinoma of the oral cavity, the oropharynx, the hypopharynx or the larynx and N0-N2 neck disease were identified. Thirty-three of the 556 patients underwent either MRND or RND and were excluded, so that a total of 523 patients had SND. Further excluded were 20 (3.8%) patients who experienced locoregional recurrences during follow-up, as the failure in the neck may be assumed to be a result of failure to control the primary tumor with subsequent reseeding in the neck. The remaining 503 patients ranged in age from 16 to 92 years (median age, 56 years); 430 were male, and 73 were female. Staging was done according to the 1992 UICC/AJCC criteria.

All patients were treated curatively by end- or transoral laser microsurgical resection of the primary tumor and a delayed, discontinuous uni- or bilateral neck dissection. Primary site characteristics and numbers of SNDs carried out are listed in Table 1. Early and advanced pT categories were equally distributed with 52.7% for pT1 and pT2 versus 47.3% for pT3 and pT4, respectively.

A total of 711 dissections were performed. Various types of SND were performed according to the primary site and the extent of neck disease (Fig. 1). In oral primaries, the lymph nodes of the levels I, II and III were usually removed. In the majority of laryngeal, oropharyngeal and hypopharyngeal primaries the lymph nodes of the levels II and III were dissected. Prompted by our clinical impression that there is a low incidence of metastases in level IV, the lymph nodes of this level were not removed routinely, but only, when during surgery metastases were clinically suspected or proven by frozen section.

Although the modalities of radiotherapy changed over the years, postoperative radiotherapy was always delivered to the primary site, the dissected and the contralateral neck. One hundred and ninety-four patients were subjected to postoperative radiotherapy. In general, indications included advanced pT stage of the primary tumor with microscopically positive margins despite re-resection, one or more lymph node metastases and lymph node metastases with extracapsular spread (ECS). Another indication was the treatment of occult retropharyngeal lymph node metastases in primaries, which are likely to metastasize to those nodes (e. g., carcinoma of the oro- or hypopharynx with midline origin). Since many patients declined adjuvant radiotherapy, fewer patients were irradiated than met the above criteria.

The median follow up interval was 41 months (range, 2 to 149 months). Control of neck disease after SND was the main endpoint assessed. Regional recurrence rates were calculated by the Kaplan-Meier method.[1]

RESULTS

Accuracy of Preoperative Staging of the Neck
Among the 220 patients who had elective SND, the surgical specimens contained metastases in 49 (22.3%) patients. On the other hand, enlarged lymph nodes suspected to be metastases proved to be pathologically negative in 78 (27.6%) of 283 patients.

Histopathologic Findings
The surgical specimens of 432 neck sides were pathologically node-negative. One or more lymph node metastases were found in 279 neck dissection specimens. With the method of histopathological work up used, one or more metastases with ECS were detected in 68 (24.4%) node-positive neck dissections. The distribution of the pN categories was as follows: pN0 49.5%, pN1 17.5%, pN2a 2.2%, pN2b 25.8%, pN2c 5.0%.

Postoperative Radiotherapy
Among the 249 patients with histopathologically uninvolved lymph nodes, 36 (14.5%) patients received postoperative radiotherapy. The indications were advanced pT stage with positive resection margins despite re-resection and the prophylactic treatment of retropharyngeal lymph nodes. To 158 out of 254 (62.2%) patients with histologically proven lymph node metastases postoperative radiotherapy was given. The percentages of patients irradiated in the different pN categories were as follows: pN1 45.5%, pN2a 72.7%, pN2b 67.7%, pN2c 88.0%.

Neck Recurrences
In the group of patients with pathologically tumor-free neck dissection specimens (n=249), 12 patients developed late neck metastases in the dissected neck and 2 patients in the contralateral undissected neck. The contralateral metastases were regarded as censored observations. The 3 year neck recurrence rate estimated according to Kaplan-Meier was 4.7% [2.0%; 7.5%].

Eleven patients with neck recurrence in the dissected neck developed the recurrence within the dissected area and one patient with an oral cavity carcinoma developed metastases in the submandibular nodes, which were initially not removed. Salvage therapy was successful in 10 patients. Two patients died due to uncontrolled disease in the neck. One patient with a contralateral neck recurrence died due to neck metastasis and one is alive with no evidence of disease.

In the group of patients with pathologically tumor-positive neck dissection specimens (n=254), 21 patients developed recurrent neck metastases in the dissected neck. Two patients developed late neck metastases in the opposite undissected side of the neck; these metastases were regarded as censored observations. In patients staged pN1 (n=88), the Kaplan-Meier 3 year neck recurrence rate was 4.9% [0.2%; 9.7%]. In patients staged pN2 (n=166), the Kaplan-Meier 3 year neck recurrence rate was 12.1% [6.6%; 17.7%].

Seventeen patients with recurrent neck metastases developed the recurrence in the ipsilateral dissected field; two of them had bilateral recurrences after initial unilateral neck dissection. Four recurrences were found in the dissected neck outside the dissected area: two in the submandibular nodes of patients with oral or oropharyngeal carcinomas, one in the posterior triangle nodes of a patient with supraglottic carcinoma, and one in the retropharyngeal lymph nodes in a patient with carcinoma of the uvula.

Only in 5 of 21 (24%) patients with recurrent metastases in the dissected neck subsequent treatment was successful. Fourteen patients died from neck recurrence and 2 are alive with tumor. The two patients with contralateral neck recurrences are alive with no evidence of disease.

The Kaplan-Meier 3 year neck recurrence rate for patients initially treated with surgery alone (n=309) was 8.5% [5.3%; 11.8%]. The Kaplan-Meier 3 year neck recurrence rate for patients who received combined therapy (n=194) was 4.7% [1.3%; 8.1%]. In patients with pN1 disease the 3 year neck recurrence rates were comparable after surgical and combined therapy, in patients with pN2 disease, however, the 3 year recurrence rate after surgery only, was three-fold increased compared with the rate after combined therapy (Table 2).

DISCUSSION

Since the early metastasizing of head and neck carcinomas follows predictable routes, SND in the clinically N0 neck has become an accepted treatment method. In the most recent literature an expanded role in the treatment of selected patients with more advanced neck disease is credited to SND[2-5], but generally MRND or even RND are preferred.

In the present study, SND was indicated as an elective or therapeutic procedure. Out of 220 patients thought to be clinically negative, occult metastases were confirmed pathologically in 22.3%. The relatively high rate of undetected metastases compares with the experience of others[6-9] and is a strong argument in favor of elective neck surgery.

Undeniably, the most important outcome measure for the efficacy of SND is the control of disease in the neck. For the histopathologic tumor-negative neck a Kaplan-Meier 3 year recurrence rate of 4.7% was found in our study. If one does not consider failures outside the dissected area, due to poor selection of the type of dissection, the regional failure rate is even lower. This result is in accordance with other reports. Several studies about SND have documented the incidence of neck recurrences to be 3% to 7% in the pN0 neck.[4, 6, 8, 10-13] There seem to be no great differences in the results reported for SND and MRND in pathologically tumor-negative necks.[8, 9, 14]

As the majority of head and neck surgeons perform MRND or RND in cases of proven metastases, there is only limited information available on the efficacy of SND as a therapeutic procedure, and its value is discussed controversially. The published series that used SND include 20%-30% node-positive patients, who were treated electively and turned out node-positive postoperatively. Many head and neck surgeons use SND as a "staging procedure" and in the case of metastases, either proven by frozen section biopsy[15] or clinically suspected, surgery is continued as modified radical or radical neck dissection. Others apply postoperative radiotherapy in node-positive patients who underwent SND.[6, 12]

In the pN+ neck treated with SND the regional recurrence rates reported were about 15% to 20%. Byers et al.[14] found an incidence of 20% recurrences in the dissected neck after surgery and 15% after surgery and radiotherapy. Spiro et al.[6] observed a failure rate in the neck of 7% in occult metastases. When neck nodes were involved both clinically and pathologically, neck recurrence was documented in 6%. Comparable results have been published by others.[3, 4, 11, 12]

The series using therapeutic MRND usually include patients with more advanced neck disease. To attempt a comparison, we report here the recurrences in relation to the histopathologic status of the neck. In our study, a Kaplan-Meier 3 year neck recurrence rate of 4.9% for the pN1 neck and of 12.1% for the pN2 neck was found. These results compare with the results reported by Leemans et al.[16] for the node-positive neck after MRND: the overall failure rate was 9.7%; the recurrence rate in necks with 1 or 2 metastases was 9.1%, and 11.3% in necks with ≥3 metastases.

Recurrences outside the dissected area are only rarely observed.[4, 7, 8, 12] However, in the majority of the reports, no data are available as to whether metastases recurred within or outside the previously dissected fields. In our study, 5 of 33 (15.2%) regional failures were located outside the dissected levels. Three recurrences in level I are regarded as the result of a surgeon's error in choosing the proper extent of SND. The retropharyngeal nodes, which are not included in neck dissection, were the site of recurrence in another case. Only one recurrence in level V would have fallen within a comprehensive neck dissection. In our opinion, the very low incidence of recurrences in levels IV and V observed by us does not justify a concept of treating all patients with MRND.

Histologic factors increasing the likelihood of neck recurrence are the presence of extracapsular spread and the involvement of multiple nodes at multiple levels. Postoperative radiotherapy was recommended if the surgical specimen contained a single metastasis[16]; others favor the use of postoperative radiotherapy, if the dissection specimen contains three or more positive nodes without ECS.[11] The addition of postoperative radiotherapy is considered to improve disease control at the primary site and in the neck.

In our study, the 3 year neck recurrence rate in the necks of patients initially treated with surgery alone was 8.5%. The 3 year neck recurrence rate after combined therapy was 4.7%. In the pN1 neck the 3 year recurrence rates were 3.0% with the addition of postoperative radiotherapy and 6.3% without postoperative radiotherapy. Given these data, a prospective randomized trial to assess the efficacy of postoperative radiotherapy in the pN1 neck seems desirable, since there was only a tendency to an improved regional control after combined therapy. However, in the pN2 neck the 3 year neck recurrence rates were 7.0% in patients who had postoperative radiotherapy and jumped up to 24.0% in patients without radiotherapy. This observation prompted us to strongly recommend postoperative radiotherapy in patients with at least two positive nodes. Patients with N2 neck disease should be counselled to agree with postoperative radiotherapy and to complete this treatment prior to undergoing neck dissection.

CONCLUSION

In our study we could demonstrate that the surgically demanding SND, if performed with the greatest possible care, is efficient in the elective and therapeutic treatment of the cervical lymph nodes. The main advantage is that selective approaches further reduce postoperative disfigurement and dysfunction, which can still be significant after MRND. With respect to regional control our results achieved with SND with or without postoperative radiotherapy were comparable to the results reported after MRND and RND with or without postoperative radiotherapy.

Table 1. Distribution of Primary Site Locations, pT Categories and SND (n=503 Patients)

	Primary Site Oral Cavity	Oropharynx	Hypopharynx	Larynx	Total
	n	n	n	n	n
pT Category					
pT1	22	20	21	8	71
pT2	45	53	39	57	194
pT3	25	42	11	67	145
pT4	7	26	17	43	93
Total	99	141	88	175	503
Neck dissection					
Ipsilateral	53	91	66	85	295
Bilateral	46	50	22	90	208

Table 2. Neck Recurrences by Pathologic Node Status and Postoperative Radiotherapy

pN	Combined Therapy n	3 y neck recurrence rate	95% CI	Surgery only n	3 y neck recurrence rate	95% CI
pN0	36	0.0%	-	213	5.5%	[2.3%; 8.6%]
pN1	40	3.0%	[0.0%; 8.9%]	48	6.3%	[0.0%; 13.1%]
pN2	118	7.0%	[1.5%; 12.5%]	48	24.0%	[11.6%; 36.4%]

Figure 1. Distribution of the Types of SND performed in pN0 Patients (n=249) and in pN+ Patients (n=254)

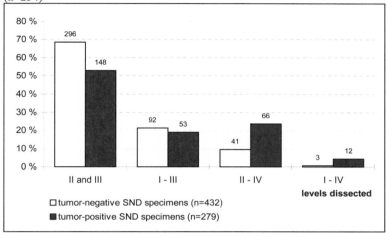

REFERENCES

1.   Kaplan EL, Meier P: Nonparametric estimation from incomplete observations. J Am Stat Assoc 1958;58:457-481.
2.   Ambrosch P, Freudenberg L, Kron M, et al.: Selective neck dissection in the management of squamous cell carcinoma of the upper digestive tract. Eur Arch Otorhinolaryngol 1996;253:329-335.
3.   Traynor SJ, Cohen JI, Gray J, et al.: Selective neck dissection and the management of the node-positive neck. Am J Surg 1996;172:654-657.
4.   Pellitteri PK, Robbins KT, Nauman T: Expanded application of selective neck dissection with regard to nodal status. Head Neck 1997;19:260-265.
5.   Kerrebijn JGF, Freeman JL, Irish JC, et al.: Supraomohyoid neck dissection. Is it diagnostic or therapeutic. Head Neck 1999;21:39-42.
6.   Spiro RH, Morgan GJ, Strong EW, et al.: Supraomohyoid neck dissection. Am J Surg 1996;172:650-653.
7.   Davidson J, Khan Y, Gilbert R, et al.: Is selective neck dissection sufficient treatment for the N0/Np+ neck? J Otolaryngol 1997;26:229-231.
8.   Pitman KT, Johnson JT, Myers EN: Effectiveness of selective neck dissection for management of the clinically negative neck. Arch Otolaryngol Head Neck Surg 1997;123:917-922.
9.   Brazilian Head and Neck Cancer Study Group: Results of a prospective trial on elective modified radical classical versus supraomohyoid neck dissection in the management of oral squamous carcinoma. Am J Surg 1998;176:422-427.
10.   Byers RM, Wolf PF, Ballantyne AJ: Rationale for elective modified neck dissection. Head Neck Surg 1988;10:160-167.
11.   Medina JE, Byers RM: Supraomohyoid neck dissection: rationale, indications, and surgical technique. Head Neck 1989;11:111-122.
12.   Spiro RH, Gallo O, Shah JP: Selective jugular node dissection in patients with squamous carcinoma of the larynx or pharynx. Am J Surg 1993;166:399-402.
13.   Henick DH, Silver CE, Heller KS, et al.: Supraomohyoid neck dissection as a staging procedure for squamous cell carcinomas of the oral cavity and oropharynx. Head Neck 1995;17:119-123.
14.   Byers RM: Modified neck dissection: a study of 967 cases from 1970-1980. Am J Surg 1985;150:414-421.
15.   Manni, JJ, vdHoogen FJA: Supraomohyoid neck dissection with frozen section biopsy as a staging procedure in the clinically node-negative neck in carcinoma of the oral cavity. Am J Surg 1991;162:373-376.

16.   Leemans CR, Tiwari R, van der Waal I, et al.: The efficacy of comprehensive neck dissection with or without postoperative radiotherapy in nodal metastases of squamous cell carcinoma of the upper respiratory and digestive tracts. Laryngoscope 1990;100:1194-1198.

THE EVIDENCE BASE FOR TREATMENT OF THE NECK

Johan Wennerberg, M.D., Ph.D.

Acknowlegement: This study was supported by Swedish Cancer Society (4013-B99-03PCC and 1304-B99-13XBC), The King Gustaf V Jubilee Fund (grant no: 00:530) and Government grant to clinical research.

Correspondence to: Dept of Otorhinolaryngology, Head and neck surgery, University Hospital of Lund, S-221 85 Lund, Sweden, Fax: ++46 46 2110968 (e-mail: johan.wennerberg@onh.lu.se

INTRODUCTION

Our way of acting as doctors has for centuries relied on the belief in authorities, experts and textbooks as the sound base. In the beginning of the seventies a Canadian working party first began to emphasise the importance of systematic examination of the scientific foundation for our decision-making[1] Later on this have been followed by The US Task Force for Preventive Services[2]. In Great Britain the same line was pursued by the Cochrane Centre in Oxford and the Cochrane Collaboration[3]. The levels of evidence is usually graded in three or four levels (table 1)[4].

The radical neck dissection (RND) was described by Crile in 1906[5]. It was strongly advocated by Hayes Martin in the 1950s[6]. Ten years later Suarez described the functional neck dissection[7] and in the late 1960s and 1970s Bocca popularised it and expanded the use to patients with non-fixed lymph node metastases[8].

But neck treatment is not only surgery. In Sweden SBU - The Swedish Council on Technology Assessment in Health Care in the mid 1990s evaluated the use of Radiotherapy for Cancer[9, 10]. Parallel to the surgical treatment of the neck prophylactic and curative radiotherapy to the neck improved. A dose of 50 Gy/5w was shown to eliminate 90 % of subclinical disease, with a failure frequency of less than 5%[11, 12]. For clinical lymph node metastases (N1-3), radiotherapy alone can provide tumour control in 70% of tumours ≤ 1 cm and in 30% of tumours ≤ 4 cm[13].

In the section on "Head and neck cancer: Regional lymph nodes" SBU concluded that the literature review shows: "-that radiotherapy plays a decisive role in preventing subclinical metastases in the regional lymph nodes from progressing to clinical." And "- that radiotherapy, usually in combination with surgery, has a major impact on clinical lymph node metastases."

The sound base for decisions on treatment of the neck in patients with malignant tumours of the head and neck ought to be well designed and conducted studies. But, what evidence do we actually rely on when we decide the treatment of a node-negative or node-positive neck?

MATERIAL AND METHODS

Procedures for evaluating the scientific literature:

The procedure applied was the same as used *by SBU - The Swedish Council on Technology Assessment in Health Care* in their evaluation of Radiotherapy for Cancer[9, 10] and revised in an ongoing update of the present knowledge.

For the present survey studies published 1966 to 2000 were searched through MEDLINE and other appropriate databases (table 1). All abstracts were read and relevant articles identified and further studied. Some literature reviews were also studied. References cited in the reviewed literature were used to identify and review older, yet important reports. Each publication was classified according to weight of scientific evidence (table 2)[4].

RESULTS

Seven reports with potentially high scientific value addressing some aspect of neck dissection (1980-1999) were identified[14-20]. All were randomised controlled trials (RCTs). Three studies comprised more than 100 patients[17, 19, 20]. Two papers reported the calculated power of the studies[14, 18]. Only one fulfilled a majority of predefined criteria, and this study was closed prematurely[18].

Nine reports with potentially high scientific value addressing some aspect of radiotherapy (RT) to the neck (1978-1995) were identified[21-29]. Eight were randomised controlled trials, three comprising more than 100 patients[24, 25, 28]. One was published in Chinese with only an abstract in English not giving enough details to evaluate the results[29]. One was a retrospective "all or none" report[21]. None of seven evaluable RCT studies presented the calculated power of the study.

Neither for neck dissection nor for radiotherapy to the neck are there any confirmatory RCTs

From the studies above we have data that support the believe that:
- In oral cavity T1-3 N0 (with RT to primary) immediate RND is not superior to follop-up (FU) + salvage RND[14].
- In oral cavity T1-2 N0 resection + supraomohyoidal neck dissection (SOND) (with RT if ECS+) is superior to resection + salvage surgery/RT[16]

276

- In oral tongue T1-2 N0 prophylactic RND improves DFS[15].
- In resectable oral cavity and oropharynx squamous cell carcinoma (SCC) resection + post op RT is superior to RT alone[18].
- In resectable oral SCC T2-4, N0 there is no difference neither in local or neck recurrences nor survival between patients treated with prophylactic SOND or modified RND[19].
- In resectable supraglottic or transglottic SCC T2-4, N0 there is no difference neither in local or neck recurrences nor survival between patients treated with prophylactic type III RND or lateral neck dissection (levels II-IV)[20].
- Elective irradiation to clinical N0 neck reduces subsequent development of metastases (and increases DFS in supragl lx ca)[21, 25].
- Preoperative radiation with 15-20 Gy do not decrease locoregional failure or increase DFS in oral and pharyngeal HNSCC stage II-IV[22, 24].
- Postoperative radio-chemotherapy to stage III-IV H&N ca with pN+ ECS (extra capsular spread) reduces loco-regional failure better than RT alone[27].
- Preoperative radio-chemotherapy reduces locoregional failure and increases survival in oral and oropharyngeal SCC (compared to no adjuvant Rx)[28].

DISCUSSION

Elective (prophylactic) as well as curative treatments of the neck are carried out weekly and daily in hospitals treating cancers of the head and neck all over the world. Tumours in this region are common, Carcinomas of the oral cavity and pharynx is the 6th most common tumour in a worldwide perspective. The annual incidence is estimated to approximate 380.000 new cases a year. It is reasonable to believe that several ten thousands of neck treatments are performed every year.

In contrast to this the number of studies with potentially high scientific evidence dealing with treatment of the neck is remarkably small. The majority of the RCTs comprise less than 100 patients and taking into account that the 95% confidence interval for 25 out of 50 is 35,5 - 64,5 %, one can not expect to detect moderate, but clinically relevant differences in such a small sample.

We e.g. still don't know:
- If prophylactic RT (+/- CHX), prophylactic neck dissection or "wait and see" with salvage surgery is to prefer in the N0 neck.
- RND is superior to modified RND in the N+ neck.
- The value of post operative RT to the pN+ neck, with and without ECS +.

In conclusion, the answer to the question: "What is the evidence-base for neck treatments?", is: "Weak and frail". The solution to overcome this shortcoming is multicentre collaboration in prospective randomised trials.

Table 1. Search strategy (1966-2000):

Citations found	Query as sent	
181 161	Head and neck neoplasms (MeSH Terms)	OR
	Head and neck neoplasms (Text Word)	OR
	Carcinoma, squamous cell (MeSH Terms)	OR
	Carcinoma, squamous cell (text Word)	OR
40 760	Lymphatic metastasis (MeSH Terms)	OR
	Lymphatic metastasis (Text Word)	OR
	Lymph node excision (MeSH Terms)	OR
	Lymph node excision (Text Word)	
11 613	Combination of the above	
110	AND Randomized controlled trial	

(A corresponding search 1960-65 gave no matches)

Table 2.

High scientific evidence:
Adequate size and study type, well conducted and analysed. E.g. a randomised controlled study (RCT) or "all or none"
(Met when <u>all</u> patients died before the Rx became available, but some now survive on it; or when some patients died before the Rx became available, but <u>none</u> now died on it.)
Fulfils beforehand-defined criteria.

Moderate scientific evidence:
Large studies with controls from matched groups. Fulfils partly beforehand-defined criteria.

Low scientific evidence:
Studies with selected controls, *e.g.* retrospective comparisons between patient groups, which has and has not respectively a defined treatment. Fulfils poorly beforehand-defined criteria.

REFRENCES

1. Canadian Task Force on the periodic health examination. The periodic health examination. Can Med Assoc J 1979;121:1193-1254.
2. US Preventive Services Task Force. Guide to clinical preventive services. Baltimore: Williams & Wilkins; 1989.
3. The Cochrane Collaboration. In.: http://www.cochrane.de/.
4. National Health Service (NHS). Levels of Evidence and Grades of Recommendations. In.: Http://cebm.jr2.ox.ac.uk/docs/levels.html.
5. Crile G. Excision of cancer of the head and neck. With special reference to the plan of dissection based on 132 patients. JAMA 1906;47(1780-6).
6. Martin H, Valle BD, Ehrlich H, Cahan WG. Neck dissection. Cancer 1941;4(441-99).
7. Suarez O. Le probleme chirurgical du cacner du larynx. Ann Otol Rhinol Laryngol 1962;79:22-34.
8. Bocca E, Pignataro O. A conservative technique in radical neck dissection. Ann Otol Rhinol Laryngol 1967;81:975-87.
9. SBU. Radiotherapy for cancer. Volume 1. Acta Oncologica 1996;35(Suppl. 6):1-100.
10. SBU. Radiotherapy for cancer. Volume 2: A critical review of the litterature. Acta Oncologica 1996;35(Suppl. 7):1-152.
11. Fletcher GH. Elective irradiation of subclinical disease in cancers of the head and neck. Cancer 1972;29:1450-4.
12. Bataini J, Bernier J, Jaulerry C, Brunin F, Pontvert D. Impact of cervical disease and its definitive radiotherapeutic management on survival: experience of 2013 patients with squamous cell carcinomas of the oropharynx and pharyngolarynx. Laryngoscope 1990;100:716-23.

13. Varghese C, Sankaranarayanan R, Nair B, Nair M. Predictors of neck node control in radically irradiated squamous cell carcinoma of the oropharynx and laryngopharynx. Head Neck 1993;15:105-8.

14. Vandenbrouck C, Sancho-Garnier M, Chassagne D, Saravane D, Cachin Y, Micheau C. Elective versus therapeutic radical neck dissection in epidermoid carcinoma of the oral cavity. Cancer 1980;46:386-90.

15. Fakih AR, Rao RS, Patel AR. Prphylactic neck dissection in squamous cell carcinoma of oral tongue: A prospective randomized study. Semin Surg Oncol 1989;5:327-30.

16. Kligerman J, Lima RA, Soares JE, Prado L, Dias FL, Freitas EQ. Supraomohyoid neck dissection in the treatment of T1/T2 squamous cell carcinoma of oral cavity. Am J Surgery 1994;168:391-4.

17. Bier J. Radical neck dissection versus conservative neck dissektion for squamous cell carcinoma of the oral cavity. Recent Results Cancer Res 1994;134:57-62.

18. Robertson AG, Soutar DS, Paul J, Webster M, Leonard AG, Moore KP, et al. Early closure of a randomized trial: Surgery and postoperative radiotherapy versus radiotherapy in the management of intra-oral tumours. Clin Oncol 1998;10:155-60.

19. Brazilian Head and Neck Cancer Study Group. Results of a prospective trial on elective modified radical classical versus supraomohyoid neck dissection in the management of oral squamous carcinoma. Am J Surgery 1998;176:422-7.

20. Brazilian Head and Neck Cancer Study Group. End results of a prospective trial on elective lateral neck dissection vs type III modified radical neck dissection in the management of supraglottic and transglottic carcinomas. Head & Neck 1999;8:694-702.

21. Lindberg RD, Fletcher GH. The role of irratiation in the management of head and neck cancer: analysis of results and causes of failure. Tumori 1978;64:313-25.

22. Strong MS, Vaughan CW, Kayne HL, Aral IM, Ucmakli A, Feldman M, et al. A randomized trial of preoperative radiotherapy in cancer of the oropharynx and hypopharynx. Am J Surgery 1978;136(4):494-500.

23. Hintz B, Charyulu K, Chandler JR, Sudarsanam A, Garciga C. Randomized study of control of the primary tumor and survival using preoperative radiation, radiation alone, or surgery alone in head and neck carcinomas. J Surgical Oncology 1979;12:75-85.

24. Tertz JJ, King ER, Lawrence W. Preoperative irradiation for head and neck cancer: Results of a prospective study. Surgery 1981;89(4):449-53.

25. Skolyszewski J. An evaluation of elective irradiation of neck nodes in patients with cancer of the supraflottic larynx. Tumori 1981;67:129-33.

26. Kokal WA, Neifeld JP, Eisert D, Lipsett Ja, Lawrence W, Beatty JD, et al. Postoperative radiation as adjuvant treatment for carcinoma of the oral cavity, larynx,, and pahrynx: Preliminary report of a prospective randomized trial. J Surgical Oncology 1988;38:71-6.

27. Bachaud J-M, David J-M, Boussin G, Daly N. Combined postoperative radiotherapy and weekly cisplatin infusion for locally advanced squamous cell carcinoma of the head and neck: preliminary report of a randimized trial. Int J Radiation Oncology Biol Phys 1991;22:243-6.

28. Mohr C, Bohndorf W, Carstens J, Härle F, Hausamen JE, Hirche H, et al. Preoperative radiochemotherapy and radical surgery in comparison with radical surgery alone. Int J Oral Maxillofac Surg 1994;23:140-8.

29. Tang P, Zhang B, Xu G. [Pre-operative radiotherapy for N0 supraglottic carcinoma: a randomized study]. Chung Hua Erh Pi Yen Hou Ko Tsa Chih 1995;30(4):203-5.

279

CLASSIFICATION OF NECK DISSECTION:
ARE WE MAKING ANY PROGRESS?

Javier Gavilán, MD, Professor and Chairman, Department of Otolaryngology, La Paz University Hospital, Madrid, Spain.

Correspondence to: *Prof. Javier GavilánIlíada, 17, 28220-Majadahonda, Madrid, Spain, Fax: 34 91 727 7050 (e-mail: jgavilan@mx4.redestb.es)*

The main purpose of this presentation is to address the issue of neck dissection classification from a conceptual, non-conventional perspective. The following paragraphs reflect the personal view of the author and should not be considered a consensus of opinion. However it is true that for many surgeons outside the United States, the classifications currently used to describe the different types of neck dissection look too complex to be useful from a practical standpoint. Trying to provide a conceptual approach to the problem is the main goal of this paper.

HISTORY OF NECK DISSECTION

Although in 1888 the Polish surgeon F. Jawdinsky described en-block neck dissection, it is George Washington Crile (1864-1943) of Cleveland, Ohio, who is considered the "grandfather" of modern surgery for neck metastasis. In 1906, he published the results of treatment of 132 head and neck cancers of which 60 patients enjoyed a three-year survival – four times better than a comparable group with cervical metastases who did not have a neck dissection[1]. This landmark paper established the basis for effective treatment of such lesions by describing a block resection of the cervical lymph node bearing tissue, either in continuity with the primary tumor or as a secondary operation for subsequent metastasis.

The "radical neck dissection" described by Crile was strongly influenced by the oncologic premises of the time proposed by Halsted. The concept of the "bloc" that was in vogue for the treatment of breast cancer required removal of the primary site with draining lymphatics and nodes in continuity. In breast surgery the pectoralis muscle was part of the "bloc". In the radical neck dissection the sternocleidomastoid muscle was removed to provide better access to the underlying lymphatics. No oncologic benefits beyond access were claimed. In the radical breast operation the axillary vein was removed to give better clearance to lymph nodes. In the radical neck dissection the entire venous system of the lateral neck was included for the same reason.

The analogous thinking behind head and neck and breast cancer procedures persisted for nearly a century. Following reconsideration of the basis for breast cancer surgery there was reconsideration of head and neck cancer surgery. The concept "bigger is better" began to be reexamined. Two issues contributed to the reorientation of surgery for neck metastasis: 1) It became evident that radical neck dissection was too aggressive for the N0 neck, and 2) the need to perform bilateral operations according to the location of the primary tumor gained acceptance among head and neck surgeons.

At this point, less than radical operations could evolve from two different approaches: modifications of the standard procedure or new operations not based on the surgical principles of radical neck dissection. The difference between these concepts is crucial and has not been understood in the literature.

MODIFIED NECK DISSECTIONS

Modified operations use the same basic principles, rationale, and surgical technique of the original procedure from which they derive. In this case, modified neck dissections are technical variations of the radical operation described by Crile in which preservation of one or more important anatomic structures is attempted. The sternocleidomastoid muscle, the internal jugular vein and the spinal accessory nerve are among the basic structures preserved in these procedures.

NEW CONCEPTS

Functional neck dissection, described in the 1960' by the Argentinean Osvaldo Suárez[2], provided a new approach to neck dissection. This procedure is based on the anatomic compartmentalization of the neck. The lymphatic system of the neck is contained within a fascial envelope which, under normal conditions, may be removed without resecting other neck structures such as the internal jugular vein, sternocleidomastoid muscle, or spinal accessory nerve.

FUNCTIONAL NECK DISSECTION AS A CONCEPT

Although the two approaches herein specified —modifications and new procedures— may look similar to many, there is a great conceptual difference between them. In the first case the surgical technique is modified to preserve some neck structures, whereas in the second, a different approach is used to treat the neck with disease confined to the lymphatic system[3].

To help clarifying the situation it must be understood that the neck can be approached in two different ways, i.e. functional and radical. The functional approach consists of a fascial dissection which follows the anatomic planes defined by the fascial system of the neck. Thus, it requires that the tumor cells are contained within the lymphatic system of the neck. On the other hand, the radical approach is a block dissection that is indicated when the anatomic planes have been violated by the tumor.

This difference may appear terminological and irrelevant when it comes to compare "functional" versus "modified radical". It may be said that although the rationale is different, the end result is the same: the lymphatic system is removed from the neck preserving the remaining neck structures. However, the situation becomes more complex when the extent of the resection appears in the surgical scenario.

EXTENSION OF NECK DISSECTION

Until now, no mention has been made to the extent of the resection because only conceptual facts have been addressed. Several factors influence the limits of the dissection in every single case. The accurate knowledge of the lymph flow and the pattern of nodal metastasis from different primary tumors are among the most important. Other factors that may influence the extent of the resection refer to questions such as morbidity, time, and cost. While the concerns about morbidity and time should only have minor influence since we are only dealing with removal of lymphatic structures, cost -and other economic implications- have had a major impact on the current system of classification, especially in the United States. The need to have a detailed description of every surgical procedure for reimbursement purposes in the United States influences the exhaustive classifications currently proposed.

Fragmentation of the two basic concepts into multiple surgical techniques on the basis of the extension of the resection constitute the basis for the development of selective neck dissections.

SELECTIVE NECK DISSECTIONS

Selective neck dissections are the logical outgrowth of the functional concept and represent a movement away from the "more is better" philosophy of the beginning of the twentieth century. However, their main disadvantage is that they focus more on nodal groups than on the system as a whole. It should be remembered here that division of the neck into nodal groups is only an artificial attempt to simplify the complexity of the lymphatic system of the neck. Nodal regions give a useful schematic view of the neck that may be used to unify criteria among different surgeons and institutions, but they are no more than a human approach to a natural problem with the intention to make nature more understandable. In other words, although the nodal group system may be considered a "true" in the field of neck dissection, they are not "the only truth". The lymphatic tissue of the neck is distributed in several chains that follow the sinuous path of vessels and nerves. Encasing the complexity of this system into separate boxes may not reflect the full nature of the issue.

An additional concern of the nodal group system is the increasing number of regions that we are recently suffering. The 5 original regions described by surgeons at Memorial hospital have been increased to a total of 9 by subdivision of some areas. With 9 nodal regions, 7 primary locations, 4 T stages, 4 N stages, and 2 sides of the neck we "only" have 2016 different situations. Although not all mathematical possibilities are clinical realities, what becomes obvious is that the current number of different procedures very much exceeds the capability of many head and neck surgeons and most training doctors. I must recognize that I am among the large number of surgeons who do not feel comfortable with the current classifications.

CLASSIFYING NECK DISSECTION: A CONCEPTUAL APPROACH

Over the last 35 years we have been involved in head and neck surgery and during this time we have used a conceptual approach to neck dissection classification. We teach two ways of treating the neck -functional and radical- and, after the operation, carefully report the structures that have been preserved or removed, as well as the approximate extent of the dissection. This system is frequently criticized for being too simplistic and its detractors argue that it does not allow comparisons among different institutions. However, before the reader makes up his/her mind and positions for or against this proposal I would like to raise three questions that must be personally answered by every surgeon involved in neck dissection.

THE QUESTIONS

1. Is it possible to compare among different surgeons/institutions with the current classifications?
2. Are we all able to identify the limits of every nodal region at surgery?
3. Are we improving our practice –either from the teaching or clinical standpoint- with a vast number of different situations and surgical procedures?

MY ANSWERS

Before you answer these questions let me express my opinion.

1. I do not think we can compare surgical procedures from different surgeons/institutions with the current classification. Of course, we can use the same name for a given operation. But I do not think this operation is the same when performed by different surgeons. The name will be the same but the procedure is surely different because…

2. … I do not think that we use the same real limits for the nodal regions at surgery. It is very easy to draw lines on a paper and describe theoretic limits on a book, but at surgery, with retractors all over, pulling hands from assistants, and surgical maneuvers to facilitate the operation, all these limits become distorted. Again, we can use the same name for the operation, but very probably the surgical specimen will look different.

3. I do not think we are making any progress by including so many different operations neither from the clinical nor –even less- from the teaching standpoint.

284

CONCLUSIONS

To sum up this approach to the issue of neck dissection classification, I think that, at least for teaching purposes, we should use concepts and describe the structures that have been removed or preserved. We recommend using nodal regions as an "orientation" for comparisons but emphasize the need to avoid "region fundamentalism" and "level hypertrophy" which in our opinion does not lead to improved practice.

Neck dissection classification is a controversial field and opinions from different approaches should be integrated in order to create a widely accepted system of neck surgery grouping.

REFERENCES

1. Crile G. Excision of cancer of the head and neck. With special reference to the plan of dissection based on 132 patients. JAMA 1906; 47: 1780-1786.
2. Suárez O. El problema de las metastasis linfáticas y alejadas del cáncer de laringe e hipofaringe. Rev Otorrinolaringol 1963; 23: 83-99.
3. Gavilán J, Herranz J, DeSanto LW, Gavilán C. Functional and Selective Neck Dissection. New York: Thieme, in press.

OPERATIONS FOR PRESERVATION AND CORRECTION
OF THE FUNCTION BY THE MANAGEMENT
OF LARYNX-HYPOPHARYNX CANCERS
AND THEIR METASTASES

György Lichtenberger, M.D., Ph.D.
Professor and Chairman
Department of Otorhinolaryngology, Head and Neck Surgery, Szent Rókus Hospital and
Institutions, Budapest, Hungary*

Running title: G. Lichtenberger: Operations for preservation and

Key words: preservation, restoration, correction, carcinoma, Bioplastique

Correspondence to: *Prof. György Lichtenberger, MD, PhD, Department of Otorhinolaryngology, Head and Neck Surgery, Szent Rókus Hospital and Institutions, Gyulai Pál u. 2., H-1085 Budapest, Hungary, Phone: (36-1) 266-1466, Fax: (36-1) 266-2768*

ABSTRACT

The primary tumor of the larynx and their metastases are in a tight connection because the larynx-hypopharynx cancer is a disease of two poles, which gives in certain percent of the cases regional metastases except the vocal cord cancers. The aim of the treatment of the primary tumor and its metastases became in the last decades the preservation of the function as much as possible in all the cases where it still allows an ablastic operation. The further purpose was to introduce methods for restoration or correction of the eventually occurred functional deficiencies after tumor operations. Author performed operations with outer exposure of the larynx and endoscopic minimally invasive techniques without tracheostomy with which the functional problems, the voice, breathing and swallowing disturbances could be solved or, at least, corrected.

Analyzing the results of the 113 cases after performing above operations, author concluded, that these interventions ensure for the patients improved quality of life after tumor surgery, the permanent suffering from complaints had ceased, and also the more radical surgery sacrifing hole organs became superfluous.

INTRODUCTION

The primary tumor of the larynx and their metastases are in a tight connection because the larynx-hypopharynx cancer is a disease of two poles, which gives in certain percent of the cases regional metastases except the vocal cord cancers.

The aim of the treatment of the primary tumor and its metastases became in the last decades the preservation of the function as much as possible in all the cases where it still allows an ablastic operation. Some decades ago our first aim was to apply treatment modalities for maintaining or preserving the function instead of laryngectomy and the radical neck dissection. The further purpose was to introduce methods for restoration or correction of the eventually occurred functional deficiencies after tumor operations.

Besides the introduction of the classical vertical and horizontal partial laryngectomy and their combinations, the operating repertoire has been enlarged in the last decades with different variants of laser cordectomy. For the treatment of supraglottic cancer in the past we performed open supraglottic laryngectomy. In the case of enlarged supraglottic cancer involving also the base of the tongue with regional neck metastasis we nowadays perform open supraglottic laryngectomy with resection of the base of tongue, as well. If there are definitive multiplex metastases, then we perform the MRND so that we remove all the structures on the neck, but preserve the accessory spinal nerve. In No neck case, in the past we followed mostly the "wait and see" policy checking the neck regularly. Recently we perform much more the MRND preserving the sternocleidomastoid muscle, the jugular vein and the accessory spinal nerve.

Steiner[1] and Rudert[2] worked out the indications and operating methods for modern laser endoscopic supraglottic laryngectomy without tracheostomy. They remove the supraglottic part of the larynx step by step in different pieces in the cases of bigger tumors, as well. Some years ago we started to replace also the classical supraglottic horizontal laryngectomy with endoscopic supraglottic laser laryngectomy without tracheostomy. Studying these endoscopic methods the books of Steiner[1] and Rudert and Werner[2] were beside their publications very useful as guidelines. We are aware that enlarged supraglottic tumors can endoscopically only be resected in different pieces. Otherwise it is very difficult to have an appropriate overview during and at the end of the operation.

The supracricoid laryngectomy with cricohyoidopexy is an operating method, which - I think - is the last option to preserve the laryngeal function before laryngectomy. In most of the cases it is possible to reconstruct the laryngeal structures in such a way that the lumen of the larynx is sufficiently wide by inspiration and the closing function is also perfect by deglutition (Fig. 1A-B-C-D). However by performing supracricoid laryngectomy it is an advantage also in connection of the deglutition to have the chance to perform MRND with preservation of the sternocleidoid muscle, the jugular vein, spinal accessory nerve, and to be able to preserve the stylohyoid and the digastric muscles, as well.

288

MATERIAL AND METHODS

Methods for restoration or correction of the function after larynx carcinoma operations. Despite the fact that the aim of the organ sparing techniques was the preservation of the function as much as possible after the operations of the primary cancer and their metastases, there may occur functional disturbances, or deficiencies.

We performed operations with outer exposure of the larynx and endoscopic minimally invasive techniques without tracheostomy with which the functional problems, the voice, breathing and swallowing disturbances could be solved or, at least, corrected (Table I).

To cease swallowing difficulties after supraglottic laryngectomy or supracricoid laryngectomy, the ary-region may be augmented submucousally, preventing aspiration (Fig. 2 A-B). In the case of the very rare swallowing disability after supraglottic laryngectomy cricopharyngeal myotomy may bring the solution.

In the case of enlarged larynx-hypopharynx tumors and their metastases the patients have the chance to survive only after radical operation, such as laryngectomy or laryngo-pharyngectomy with RND or MRND.

For voice rehabilitation we introduce a simple primary and secondary puncture technique, instead of the Singer-Blom[3] method. Using this ET (esophago-tracheal)-puncture technique[4] the risk of injuring the back wall of the pharynx or esophagus is eliminated.

This technique reduces many problems that occurred previously by the Singer-Blom[3] puncture, however there are other problems independent of the implantation, as well. The most serious of these are - we think - the spasm of the cricopharyngeus muscle and the leakage around the prosthesis. To solve these problems we performed the well known myotomy, which is a very effective intervention, and to stop leakage around the prosthesis we were the first who introduced Bioplastique augmentation with very good results.

RESULTS

To solve or, at least, reduce the functional disturbances occurring after the operation of larynx-hypopharynx cancers and their metastases we performed individual interventions corresponding with the complaints. To give information about the rate of the failures after the primary tumor operations wouldn't have been possible, because most of these patients have been admitted to our department after primary surgery. The operations for restoration or correction of the function and the results are to be seen in the Table I.

DISCUSSION

In the last decades there was a development in the organ and function sparing and reconstructing methods. Beside the conventional techniques the number of minimally invasive endoscopic procedures increased, as well. There were however functional deficiencies occurred after tumor surgery. To restore or, at least, correct the function it is necessary to know a wide range of classical and endoscopic procedures and to introduce methods for until not used purpose. The final result is in some cases only improvement of the situation, but for the patient it is already a big step forward. In some cases the problem is multifactorial. Therefore in such cases combined methods and two stage operations are necessary.

CONCLUSION

The importance of the methods introduced for the solution or correction of the functional deficiencies occurred after tumor surgery is that these interventions improve the quality of life of the patients. A significant part of these patients could avoid more radical operations sacrifying hole organs, and became free from the symptoms and complaint.

Table I. Operations for restoration or correction of the function after surgery of the larynx-hypopharynx cancers and their metastases I. (Cases and results)

1. Management of voice production disturbances

Thyroplasty with Titan implantation by Friedrich[5] for the management of the insufficient glottic closure 2 cordectomy
Improved the voice in both cases but the results are not to compare with the results that could be achieved w same technique by the management of the paralyzed vocal cords.
Solution of the anterior commissura web introducing special endoscopic operation by Lichtenberger[6]   7
Surgically successful 6 out of 7 cases, but functionally improved only 5 out of 7 cases.
Solution of the posterior commissura scarred adhesion by special endoscopic operation   1
Successful solution and nearly normal lumen, decannulation.
ET (esophago-tracheal) puncture[4] for voice prosthesis implantation   71
All the punctures were performed without problems and complications fixing the prosthesis in the appro place.
Myotomy to solve the spasm of the cricopharyngeal muscle resulting in speaking inability   7
Fluent speech after myotomy in 5 cases
Botulinum injection to solve the spasm of the cricopharyngeal muscle resulting in speaking inability   2
Fluent speech after Botox injection in 2 cases

2. Solution of breathing disturbances

Management of the laryngeal stenosis developed after hemilaryngectomy, with transposition of the hyoid 4 bone
Successful management of all 4 cases
Management of orifiziel tracheal stenosis developing after tracheotomy which was performed to partial 2 laryngectomy
The stenoses have been solved successfully in both cases using auricular cartilage transplant
Laminotomy by Réthi[7] to build up the scarred stenosed lumen of the larynx after supracricoid laryngectomy 2 and MRND due to severe postoperative infection
Sufficient wide lumen allowing the decannulation in 1 case.
The lumen became wider but still further operation is necessary due to granulation tissue in the cricoid level in 1 case.

3. Management of swallowing disorders

Collagen injection submucousally in the ary-region to prevent aspiration after supraglottic laryngectomy	3

The problem has been solved in 2 case. The swallowing ability improved in 1 case after the injection

Autolog fat injection submucousally in the ary-region to prevent aspiration after supracricoid laryngectomy	2

The swallowing ability thoroughly improved and the problem have been solved in 1 case. The swallowing ability only slightly improved. A second augmentation is necessary in 1 case.

Teflon-injection in the residual vocal cord to prevent aspiration after ¾ subtotal laryngectomy	1

The swallowing ability improved and the patient became able to eat after the removal of the nasogastric tube without difficulties

Myotomy of the cricopharyngeal muscles for management of swallowing disability after supraglottic laryngectomy combined with resection of the base of tongue and RND and MRND	2

The problems have been solved and complaints disappeared in both cases

Collagen injection around the voice prosthesis to cease the leakage around the prosthesis	2

Temporary good results in both cases

Bioplastique injection around the voice prosthesis to cease leakage around the prosthesis	5

Definitive good results in 4 cases and the leakage has been reduced in 1 case

Figure 1 A-B-C-D
The lumen of the larynx after supracricoid laryngectomy in deep inspiration, normal inspiration at the beginning of phonation and by phonation.

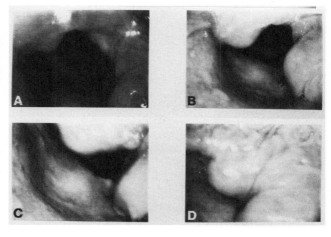

Figure 2A. Supracricoid larynx. Left arytenoid region partly removed.

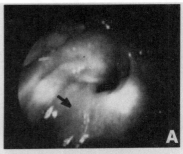

Figure 2B. Supracricoid larynx. Left arytenoid region after filling the submucosa with autolog fat.

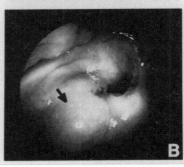

REFERENCES

1. Steiner W. Endoskopische Laserchirurgie der oberen Luft- und Speisewege. 1st Ed. Stuttgart-New York: G. Thieme Publisher; 1997. p. 74-83.
2. Rudert H, Werner JA. (Hrsg.) Lasers in otorhinolaryngology, and in head and neck surgery. Karger, Basel; 1995.
3. Singer MI, Blom ED. An endoscopic technique for restoration of voice after laryngectomy. Ann Otol Rhinol Laryngol 1980;89:529-533.
4. Lichtenberger G. New and Simple Endo-extra Oesophagotracheal Method of Developing the Fistula for the Implantation of a Voice Prosthesis. Diagnostic and Therapeutic Endoscopy 1997;3:189-191.
5. Friedrich G. Titanium Vocal Fold Medializing Implant: Introducing a Novel. Implant System for External Vocal Fold Medialization. Ann Otol Rhinol Laryngol 1999;108:79-86.
6. Lichtenberger G. Laryngomikrochirurgische Behandlung der in Glottishöhe liegenden Synechien. HNO (Berlin) 1985;33:213-215.
7. Réthi A. Chirurgie der Verengungen der oberen Luftwege. Stuttgart: G. Thieme; 1959.

EVALUATION OF THE PATIENTS WITH DISTANT NODAL METASTASES AFTER LARYNGECTOMY

Magdalena Józefowicz-Korczyńska PhD MD, Maciej Gryczyński PhD MD, Marek Łukomski PhD MD, Anna Murlewska PhD MD, Wioletta Pietruszewska MD
Department of Otolaryngology, Medical University of Lodz, Poland

Key words: laryngeal cancer, distant nodal metastases

Correspondence to: *Magdalena Józefowicz-Korczyńska, Department of Otolaryngology, Medical University of Lodz, 90-153 Lodz, 22 Kopcińskiego Str., Lodz, Poland, Phone: +48 42 678 57 85, Fax: +48 42 678 11 76*

ABSTRACT

Background. One of the most common reason of failure in laryngeal cancer treatment is metastases in regional neck lymph nodes. The purpose of our investigation was the evaluation of the patients with distant nodal metastases after laryngectomy

Methods. 930 patients with laryngeal cancer were surgically treated from 1985 to1994. In 782 cases total laryngectomy and in 148 partial laryngectomy were performed. A 5-year survival was 58%. We observed distant nodal metastases in 140 (15,1%) patients, who were analysed in this study.

Results. The most common localisation of primary larynx tumour was the supraglottic region in 90 (64,3%) patients. Laryngeal tumour extended beyond its limits to the surrounding tissue in 16 (11,4%). The most frequent T - status was T4, which was observed in 65 (46,4%) patients, and N0 status in 46 (53,5%) patients. After clinical confirmation of distant nodal metastases, 18 (11,4%) were not qualified for secondary neck surgical treatment and were palliativly radiated. In 122 (87,1%) patients secondary neck dissection were performed. The most common was radical or modified neck dissection. In patients with distant nodal metastases local recurrences (11,4% vs. 9%) and distant metastases to lung (6,4% vs. 2%) were more common observed than in the whole group of 930 surgically treated patients (p.<0,05). It could indicate on more aggressive phenotype of cancer cells in these patients. Survival rate in re-operated patients was 16,7%. The best solution of distant nodal metastases problem is the possibility of wide diagnosis of neck lymph nodes in patients with laryngeal cancer using either direct (TK, US) or indirect procedure as molecular biology that need further investigation.

INTRODUCTION

In the cervical and head lymphatic system there are about 300 nodes which constitute 30% of all human lymph nodes. Such their number, variety of structures in neck as well as reach feat tissue, strong muscles and sometimes short neck are often the reason for difficulties in clinical evaluation of lymph nodes lesion in this area. Classical treatment for regional node metastases is radical neck dissection by Jawdyński-Crile technique. This surgical procedure and its numerous modification with most often used by Bocca[1] is performed both for clinical resection of primarily confirmed neck tumour as well as prophylactic procedure in aggressive or highly advanced head and neck tumour. Several changes have been suggested for standard radical neck dissection and these surgical procedures have been defined by the American Academy of Otolaryngology- Head and Neck Surgery[2]. The risk for metastases after surgical treatment is high in subjects after incomplete resection, both microscopic and macroscopic primary or metastatic tumour. It refers to high and low histologically - advanced tumour, especially in subjects with supraglottic location of cancer. Management of the neck lymph nodes in patients with laryngeal cancer is more serious problem than primary tumour treatment. One of the most important factors in prognosis of the patients with laryngeal cancer is as well the evidence of neck lymph nodes metastases, which are observed during first assessment of primary tumour as distant nodal metastases.

The purpose of our investigation was the evaluation of our patients with distant nodal metastases after laryngectomy

MATERIAL AND METHODS

We analysed 930 patients with laryngeal cancer who underwent surgical treatment in Department of Otolaryngology, Medical University of Lodz from 1985 to 1994. In 782 cases total laryngectomy and in 148 partial laryngectomy were performed. During primary operation in 481 (51,7%) patients there were no operations of neck lymph nodes. Radical neck dissection in 195 (21,1%), modified neck dissection in 96 (10,3%) and selective neck dissection in 158 (17%) patients were performed. A 5-year survival in the whole group of 930 patients was 58%. We observed distant nodal metastases in 140 (15,1%) patients.

In group of patients with distant nodal metastases there were 136 (97,1%) male and 4 (2,9%) female. The age ranged from 38 to 78 years (mean 58,6) (Tab. I).

Table I. All patients were smokers and 122 (87,1%) person smoked more than 20 cigarettes a day for longer than 20 years. The patients were retrospectively assessed according to clinical staging system of the American Joint Committee on Cancer (AJCC, 1992). We evaluated nodal metastases in relation to primary T and N status, treatment management and 5 years follow-up. All the surgical specimens were subjected to histopathological examination.

Characteristic of the whole group of the patients with laryngeal cancer (N=930) and the subgroup with distant nodal metastases after laryngectomy (N=140).

Feature	Patients with laryngeal cancer (N=930)	Patients with distant nodal metastases (N=140)
Age: <65 year	753 (81,0%)	59 (42,1%)
>65 year	177 (19%)	81 (57,9%)
Sex: Female	65 (7,0%)	4 (2,9%)
Male	865 (93,0%)	136 (97,1%)
Localisation : supraglottic	511 (55%)	90 (64,3%)
glottic	419 (45%)	30 (35,7%)
Tumor size: T1-T2	214(23,0%)	25 (17,9%)
T3	409 (44,0%)	50 (35,7%)
T4	307 (33,9%)	65 (46,4%)
N status: N 0	642 (69,0%)	75 (53,6%)
N 1-3	288 (31,0%)	65 (46,4%)
Distant metastases: M0	911 (98,0%)	131 (93,6%)
M1	19 (2,0%)	9 (6,4%)
Local recurrences	84 (9,0%)	16 (11,4%)
Histologic grading: G1	279 (30,0%)	35 (25,0%)
G2	577 (62,0%)	90 (64,3%)
G3	74 (8,0%)	15 (10,7%)

RESULTS

We evaluated 140 (100%) patients with distant nodal metastases after laryngectomy. Clinical recurrences in cervical lymph nodes occurred from one to 72 months (mean 11 months) after first surgical procedure. The most common localisation of primary larynx tumour was the supraglottic region in 90 (64,3%) patients. Laryngeal tumour extended beyond its limits to the surrounding tissue in 16 (11,4%). The most frequent T - status was T4, which was observed in 65 (46,4%) patients, and N0 status in 46 (53,5%) patients. In group of patients with distant nodal metastases extracapsular extension in 41 (29,3%) patients and perivascular invasion in 15 (10,7%) patients were noted. During the primary tumour operation we did not perform any neck surgical procedure in N0 status (74 patients – 52,9%). In 25 (17,9%) patients with clinically palpable, small and mobile lymph nodes selective unilateral or bilateral neck dissections were performed. Evidence of neck lymph node metastases after these operations were confirmed in 20 (80,0%) cases. Radical or modified neck dissections were performed in 41 (29,3%) patients. After clinical confirmation of distant nodal metastases, 18 (11,4%) were not qualified for secondary neck surgical treatment and were palliativly radiated. There was no any successful therapy in these cases and patients die in a short period of time. In 122 (87,1%) patients secondary neck dissection were performed. The most common was radical neck dissection (Table II). In our group (140 patients) distant metastases to lung were observed in 9 (6,4%) patients. Five year follow-up was only 16,7%, which is a very poor results but it is comparable to other authors' findings[5].

Table II. Comparison the type of primary laryngectomy and surgical neck dissection procedure with secondary distant nodal metastases operation.

Primary Tumour Operation +Neck Dissection	Secondary neck dissection				
	RND or MND unilateral	RND or MND bilateral	RND or MDS + contrlat. SND	Radiotherapy	Total
Primary ND (N0)	61 (43,6%)	2 (1,4%)	8 (5,7%)	3 (2,1%)	74 (52,9%)
SND unilateral	4 (2,9%)	0 (0%)	0 (0%)	3 (2,1%)	7 (5,0%)
SND bilateral	10 (7,1%)	8 (5,7%)	0 (0%)	0 (0%)	18 (12,9%)
RND unilateral Or MNS	23 (16,4%) (contrlat.)	0 (0%)	0 (0%)	8 (5,7%)	31 (22,1%)
RND or MND +contrlat. SND	6 (4,3%) (contrlat.)	0 (0%)	0 (0%)	4 (2,9%)	10 (7,1%)
Total	104 (74,3%)	10 (7,1%)	8 (5,7%)	18 (11,4%)	140 (100%)

Legend: ND - neck dissection; RND - radical neck dissection; SND - selective neck dissection; MND - modified neck dissection

DISCUSSION

The prognosis of laryngeal cancer worsens dramatically with the discovery of primary or secondary lymph node metastases or the presence of local recurrences. In our group of patients with distant nodal metastases the most common localisation of primary larynx tumour was supraglottic region (64,3%) and N0 nodal status in over 50% of the patients. It is well known that there are a lot of pathways of lymphatic drainage in this area and it is necessary to think about selective neck dissection in such cases. The management of clinically negative neck in patients with squamous cell carcinoma of the larynx is still controversial. We did not performed selective neck dissection in N0 patients during primary larynx operation. Treatment strategies in such cases ranged from watchful waiting to elective neck dissection or even elective neck irradiation and have supporters[3-5] and opponents[6, 7] who prefer more passive management. According to the supporters, selective procedure protects the patients from regional subclinical recurrences of neoplasm and would improve survival. They also confirm that the results of surgical treatment of local or nodal recurrences after first larynx procedures are poor and a 5-year survival is not more than 30%. The opponents' reports that selective neck dissection does not increase the number of patients with longer survival period after these operations. Varela at all[7] in their results found histological confirmation of metastases presence in neck lymph nodes in 27% patients, which shows that in 75% patients neck dissection was unnecessary. They also underline the fact that selective neck dissection does not protect the operated patients from further development of disease and only to a small degree can stop neoplasmatic evolution. The same results were gained by Ramadan and Allen[5]. The decision about prophylactic neck dissection should be carefully considered in each case especially in patients with supraglottic localisation of larynx cancer[8]. We accepted this method performing surgical neck dissection in case of clinically palpability before and intra-operatively finding nodes. Moreover, after analysis of these 10 –years follow-up results we had new strategy and in supraglottic or hypopharynx carcinoma T3-T4 and N0, neck node dissection in level I to IV are performed. The clinically palpable lymph nodes does not always mean the presence of metastases but only active immunologic reaction to pathological changes and accompanying inflammatory process in larynx. In our[9] and other authors'[3] researches we found that clinical evidence neck nodes metastases were histopathologically confirmed in about 80% cases. Some authors reports that in the clinically palpable neck nodes, metastases exists twice more frequently, than in unpalpable ones[4]. In patients with distant nodes metastases local recurrences (11,4% vs.9%) and distant metastases (6,4% vs. 2%) were more common observed than in the whole group of 930 surgically treated patients (p.<0,05). It could indicate on more aggressive phenotype of cancer cells in these patients. The best solution of distant nodal metastases problem is the possibility of wide diagnosis of neck lymph nodes in patients with laryngeal cancer using either direct (TK, US) or indirect procedure as molecular biology, which could give the answer about the aggressiveness of primary tumour. This management might prevent local and nodal recurrences and would help the surgeon to plan surgical procedure and conduct long term observation.

REFERENCES

1.   Bocca E, Pignataro O: A conservation technique in radical neck dissection. Ann Otol Rhinol Laryngol 1967, 76:975-987.
2.   Robbins KT, Medina JE, Wolfe GT, Levine PA, Sessions RB, Pruet CW: Standardizing neck dissection terminology. Arch Otolaryngol Head Neck Surg 1991,117:601-605.
3.   Buckley JG, MacLennan K: Cervical node metastases in laryngeal and hypopharyngeal cancer: a prospective analysis of prevalence and distribution. Head –Neck. 2000,22,380-385.
4.   Ericher SA, Weber RS: Surgical management of cervical node metastases. Current Opinion in Oncology. Head –Neck, 1996,8,215-220.
5.   Ramadan HH, Allen G C: The influence of elective neck dissection on neck relapse in No supraglottic carcinoma. Am J Otolaryngol 1993,14,278—281.
6.   Khafif R A, Gelbfish G, A Tepper P., Attie J N: Elective radical neck dissection in epidermoid cancer of the head and neck. A retrospective analysis of 853 cases of mouth pharynx and larynx cancer. Cancer, 1991,1,67-71.
7.   Varela AS, Gonzales CF, Valerias RM, Regueiro VM,Caballero LT: Efficiency of funcional elective neck dissection for treatment of cancer of larynx. Rev Laryngol Otol Rhinol, 1996, 117,1,41-45.
8.   Ferlito A, Rinalto A. Selective neck dissection for laryngeal cancer in the clinically negative neck: is it justified?. J Laryngol Otol.1997,11,454-458.
9.   Józefowicz-Korczyńska M., Łukomski. M.: Bilateral neck nodes adenopathy in patients with laryngeal carcinoma - clinical evaluation. Otolaryng. Pol. 1997,51,25,27-30.

SURGICAL THERAPY IN ADVANCED LYMPH NODE METASTASES OF THE NECK

F. Bootz (Leipzig, Germany)

Correspondence to: *Prof. Dr. Friedrich Bootz, Department of Otorhinolaryngology, University of Leipzig, Liebigstr. 18a, 04103 Leipzig (email: bootz@medizin.uni-leipzig.de)*

Advanced lymph node metastases of head and neck cancer are a sign of advanced disease and thus associated in general with a poor prognosis. This fact in addition to the size of metastasis and possible infiltration of adjacent tissue are important features in decision-making of the appropriate therapy.

Before planning surgery of advanced lymph node metastases in the neck a few questions has to be answered beforehand:

- Is the primary tumour resectable?
- Is the metastasis resectable?
- Are there further metastases?
- Is there any influence on the prognosis applying surgery?
- How will quality of life be in relation to prognosis?

If the primary tumour is not resectable in general, radiotherapy will be performed. In these cases there is no need for surgical treatment of even advanced lymph node metastases. If there is complete tumour control after radiotherapy and there is still a remnant of the lymph node metastases, this can be removed surgically if it is resectable. If primary tumour treatment is done by surgery, lymph node metastases are also included, provided they are resectable. There is a discussion about resectability of neck metastases, concerning infiltration of carotid artery, of the base of skull, of the thoracic inlet, of deep neck muscles and of lower cranial nerves and brachial plexus. If further metastases are detected either as local metastases in the neck or distant metastases, the prognosis is getting rather poor and the indication for surgery has to be restricted. If there are bilateral large neck metastases surgery normally is limited, because there is no influence on the prognosis, the same is true for non resectable distant metastases. In these cases, a patient does not profit from surgery.

There are different opinions about resection of carotid artery. If metastases infiltrate the carotid artery, it sometimes can be pealed of the artery, but in general leaves malignant tumour-cells behind. This again can be the cause of local recurrence. If there is deep infiltration of the artery and there is a need of resection, it has to be checked beforehand, whether the blood supply of the brain by the contra lateral vessels is sufficient. This is done by the balloon occlusion test and in addition by brain-szintigraphy. There is no conformance about the need of reconstruction after resection of the carotid artery. Some authors suggest, that in any case there should be a reconstruction performed with a vein-graft, but on the other side it is obvious, that there might be a serious risk of spontaneous rupture or blow out.

The N-stage and the number of neck metastases do have an influence on the prognosis. The more advanced the metastases the poorer the prognosis. Also histology has an influence on the prognosis, especially perineural invasion, extracapsular spread and vascular invasion, which are characteristics of advanced lymph node metastases, do have a poor prognosis. Recurrences after prior treatment also do have a poor prognosis. In these cases there will be a negative selection, especially of aggressive tumour cells which after therapy might grow very rapidly.

We also have to consider quality of life in relation to prognosis. Especially, if we sacrifice nerves as for example the accessory nerve or we perform an extended radical neck dissection with cosmetic impairment, especially if this is performed bilaterally. And in addition to radiotherapy carotid artery blow out can occur. If prognosis is not very much influenced by these procedures the aspect of quality of life should be considered and if necessary surgery should be avoided. The extension of neck dissection depends on the infiltration and the size of the neck metastases. If the internal jugular vein is involved as well as the sternomastoid muscles, these structures have to be resected as well as the spinal accessory nerve. If these structures even in large neck metastases can be preserved this should be done. In radical neck dissection, where the carotid artery is completely exposed, because of resection of the sternomastoid muscles, some authors suggest to cover the artery with a muscle flap, which is harvested from the levator scapulae muscle and swung in a door like fashion over the artery.

If there is recurrent metastasis after surgery another surgical procedure can be performed to remove the recurrence if there is control of primary tumour or if primary tumour recurrence can be treated surgically as well. It is a challenging situation if both internal jugular veins are affected by metastases. A classic radical neck dissection cannot be performed on the other side synchroniously, since there is a high risk of severe oedema and brain swelling which can lead to new neurological deficits. In these cases the comitant vein on one side should be left behind even if radical resection is not possible. In these cases however, you should consider whether surgery does have any benefit for the patient. Skin infiltration of large metastases is not a contraindication for surgery per se. In many cases, however if there is skin infiltration, the tumour also shows deep infiltration which then again might limit surgery. If metastases can be removed, the affected skin also must be resected and needs further plastic reconstructive procedures. Only in a few cases skin can be closed primarily. But this again, especially if postoperative radiotherapy has to be applied, might lead to wound brake down with exposure of the carotid artery. In these cases flap reconstruction is needed. There are local and regional flaps as, for example, the pectoralis major flap, the deltopectoral flap, or, what we do prefer, microvascular free flaps, as the radial forearm flap and the latissimus dorsal flap. The radial forearm flap proved to be a very reliable skin transfer, which is also resistant to wound infection. If there are deep defects the more bulky scapular-flap or even the musculo-cutaneus Latissimus dorsi flap can be used. The Latissimus dorsi flap however has the disadvantage of mismatching of colour and texture of the flap skin to the surrounding skin. But the muscles can be used for coverage of the carotid artery. In cases where microvascular free flaps cannot be applied because of missing blood vessels or because of severe damage by radiotherapy, pedicled flaps can be recommended preferably the pectoralis major flap.

If surgery cannot be applied in the treatment of advanced lymph node metastases and especially recurrent lymph node metastases in the neck, brachy-therapy can be another option. The tubes for brachytherapy are introduced under MRI control to guarantee a parallel position and thus a perfect isodose during radiotherapy.

If decision is made for surgery in advanced lymph node metastases, one always should bear in mind, whether there is an increase of prognosis and whether mutilation and diminished quality of life correlates to the benefit in prognosis.

DANGEROUS AND LETHAL COMPLICATIONS
OF NECK DISSECTION

Harald Eufinger, MD, DD, PhD, Jutta Lehmbrock, MD
Department of Oral and Plastic Maxillofacial Surgery, Ruhr-University Bochum

Keywords: chylothorax; chyle fistula; complications; neck dissection; pneumothorax

Correspondence to: Harald Eufinger, MD, Department of Oral and Plastic Maxillofacial Surgery, Ruhr-University Bochum, In der Schornau 23-25, D-44892 Bochum, Germany. (e-mail: harald.eufinger@ruhr-uni-bochum.de)

ABSTRACT

Background. Due to the high number of important anatomical structures a neck dissection may lead to various complications both during surgery and postoperatively.

Methods. Life-threatening complications should be analyzed within a large patient series with standardized neck dissection. Between 1990 and 1999 395 neck dissections were performed in 357 patients: 195 left-sided - 105 of these radical, 200 right sided - 107 of these radical.

Results. In 4 cases life-threatening complications occurred: A severe hemorrhage at the jugular foramen during radical neck dissection and a tension pneumothorax leading to cardiovascular failure were managed intraoperatively. Postoperative deaths resulted from chyle fistulas with a chylothorax in one case and an extreme chyle flow of up to 7 l per day related to a cirrhosis of the liver in another.

Conclusions. Dramatic courses of chyle fistulas and rare complications should be considered in neck dissection both forensically for informed consent and clinically.

Neck dissection, either radical or conservative or functional, is a routine procedure in head and neck surgery and serves both therapeutic and diagnostic purposes. Due to the large wound surface and the high number of important anatomical structures a neck dissection may lead to

303

various complications both during surgery and postoperatively. It was the aim of our study to analyze life-threatening complications within a large series of standardized neck dissection.

METHODS

Between 1990 and 1999 395 neck dissections were performed in 357 patients. All dangerous or lethal complications caused by the neck dissection itself were included except for infections, late hemorrhages caused by infection, and general pulmonary or cardiovascular problems. Early postoperative bleedings, which always occurred under intensive care conditions and which could always be controlled without vital danger, were also excluded.

RESULTS

195 of the 395 neck dissections were left-sided, 105 of these radical, and 200 right-sided, 107 of these radical. The incision according to McFee was a standard with very few exceptions as well as the resection of the sternocleidomastoid muscle so that even in conservative neck dissections only the accessory nerve and the internal jugular vein were spared. No patient died during surgery, but 2 situations were vitally dangerous. In the postoperative period 2 patients died from complications, which were related to the intraoperative lesion of the thoracic duct in both cases. This basically unavoidable complication of a chyle fistula was observed in 19 patients after left-sided neck dissection and 3 times on the right side.

Patient 1. In a 75-year-old woman with left-sided radical neck dissection a chyle fistula occurred when a metastasis was resected in the lower neck. It was ligated and covered with fibrin glue. Because of severe chye flow the suction drainage was removed on the third postoperative day, and compressive dressings were applied. A few hours later dyspnoe occurred, which was clinically and radiologically due to a chylothorax requiring chest tube drainage. Due to persistent chyle flow in this thoracic drainage of up to 1 l per day under both enteral and parenteral nutrition a thoracotomy with ligation of the thoracic duct was performed 10 days later. Shortly afterwards the chyle flow recurred with increasing rates of more than 2 l per day so that another thoracotomy was indicated 14 days later. But even then the chyle flow persisted with ongoing chest tube drainage, and the patient died 2 days later on the 30th postoperative day.

Patient 2. In a 63-year-old man with radical neck dissection the ligation of the cranial internal jugular vein got loose and the vessel end could not be caught anymore. Finally the bleeding could only be controlled by compression after 3 hours and a blood loss of about 6 l with substitution of 8 units of blood. A postoperative CT scan could exclude any intracranial spread of the bleeding.

Patient 3. In a 66-year-old man with a conservative neck dissection a chyle fistula occurred. It was ligated intraoperatively, the area was furthermore covered with a muscular flap and fibrin glue, and the success of this treatment was even controlled under tilted OR-table position. However, the postoperative flow of chyle was extreme and reached a maximum of 7.2 l per day in spite of parenteral nutrition. A surgical revision on the 7th day including the use of the microscope failed already intraoperatively since the flow was just too extreme. So the persisting chyle flow of up to 6.5 l per day required thoracotomy and intrathoracic duct ligation on the 25th day. Afterwards the chyle flow persisted unchanged in the chest tube drainage. Before, acute abdominal problems had indicated a laparotomy on the 21st day, which had demonstrated ascites and a histologically confirmed cirrhosis of the liver. This cirrhosis had not been detected preoperatively and was regarded to be the reason for the extreme chyle production. The patient died from a septic shock on the 35th postoperative day after a precisely documented loss of a total of 144 liters of chyle in 34 days of intensive care. Such a high loss of chyle has a strong impact on the balance of proteins even under parenteral nutrition: Approximately 2.5 g proteins per 100 ml of chyle could be demonstrated under parenteral nutrition by repeated electrophoresis of the liquids in the drainage including elements of blood coagulation and immunoglobulines.

Patient 4. A 66-year-old man showed a very rare complication: During preparation in the lower neck a minimal lesion of the pleura occurred with small bubbles of air synchronous to ventilation, which subsided spontaneously after about 1 min. Auscultation did not reveal anything abnormal and the further course of the anesthesia was uneventful first. About 45 min later cardiovascular and pulmonary function deteriorated because of a tension pneumothorax with mediastinal shift, which required immediate chest tube placement. Afterwards conditions normalized immediately.

DISCUSSION

Generally left-sided, right sided and bilateral chylothorax represent well-described complications after left-sided neck dissection,[1-3] which occur typically without intraoperative pneumothorax. In contrast, the complications "pneumothorax"[4] and "jugular foramen hemorrhage"[5] have been described very rarely, a "tension pneumothorax" in neck dissection has not been described yet.

The frequency of chyle fistulas in left-sided neck dissection is reported at approximately 1-30 %[6-8] and is much less frequent in right sided neck dissection, where the ductus lymphaticus dexter drains much less chyle compared to the thoracic duct.[8] Even the successful intraoperative management of chyle fistulas leads to a considerable frequency of recurrences.[6,8,9] Then they may persist over several weeks and are treated individually by drainage, compressive dressings, low-fat diets or parenteral nutrition, protein substitution and surgical revision including intrathoracic duct ligation.[1,3,6-10] Physiologically chyle flow may reach 2 l per day, but for patients with cirrhosis of the liver much higher rates have been described.[11]

Hemorrhages during or after neck dissection are frequent and can be controlled fast and easily in the majority of cases. In close proximity to the skull base, however, the surgical access during neck dissection is limited and therefore the bleeding might become very dangerous.[5] The same refers to the pneumothorax: This rare complication can be controlled easily during surgery of the intubated patient, but may lead to life-threatening cardiovascular failure if a tension pneumothorax results, which requires immediate diagnosis and chest tube placement.[12]

In none of these 4 unusual case reports, which add up to a frequency 1 % of all evaluated interventions, the reported complications had been specifically mentioned in the respective informed consent. In conclusion a chyle fistula in left-sided neck dissection and a severe bleeding during and after surgery should always be included in informed consent of the patient. This must not be a rule for chylothorax, pneumothorax and tension pneumothorax, and for the distinct nomination of the jugular foramen as the location of a bleeding. However, the rare complications reported here need to be considered clinically so that the surgeon and the anesthetist can deal with them effectively.

REFERENCES

1. Cavallo CA, Hirata RM, Jaques DA. Chylothorax complicating radical neck dissection. Am Surg 1975;41:266-268.
2. La Hei ER, Menzie SJ, Thompson JF. Right chylothorax following left radical neck dissection. Aust N Z J Surg 1993;63:77-79.
3. Saraceno CA, Farrior RT. Bilateral chylothorax. Rare complication of neck dissection. Arch Otolaryngol 1981;107:497-499.
4. Madan SC, Rosenthal SP, Bochetto JF. Pneumomediastinum and pneumothorax following lower neck surgery. Arch Surg 1969;98:153-159.
5. Shugar MA, Gavron JP, Campbell JM. Management of jugular foramen hemorrhage during radical neck dissection. Laryngoscope 1982;92:106-107.
6. Rollon A, Salazar C, Mayorga F, Marin R, Infante P. Severe cervical chyle fistula after radical neck dissection. Int J Oral Maxillofac Surg 1996;25:363-365.
7. Spiessl B. Plattenepithelkarzinom der Mundhöhle. Thieme: Stuttgart; 1966. p 167.
8. Vajda L, Akuamoa-Boateng E, Cesteleyn L. Behandlung der iatrogenen Ductus-thoracicus-Läsion. In: Pfeifer G, Schwenzer N, editors. Fortschritte der Kiefer- und Gesichts-Chirurgie XXX. Thieme: Stuttgart New York; 1985. p 182-183.
9. Gregor RT. Management of chyle fistulization in association with neck dissection. Otolaryngol Head Neck Surg 2000;122:434-439.
10. Ramos W, Faintuch J. Nutritional management of thoracic duct fistulas. A comparative study of parenteral versus enteral nutrition. J Parenter Enteral Nutr 1986;10:519-521.
11. Rosser BG, Poterucha JJ, McKusick MA, Kamath PS. Thoracic duct-cutaneous fistula in a patient with cirrhosis of the liver: successful treatment with a transjugular intrahepatic portosytemic shunt. Mayo Clin Proc 1996;71:793-796.
12. Barton ED. Tension pneumothorax. Curr Opin Pulm Med 1999;5:269-274.

INTRAOPERATIVE MONITORING OF SPINAL ACCESSORY NERVE IN NECK-SURGERY

Fuchs M, Mehnert S, Stumpf R, Keiner S, Bootz F

INTRODUCTION

Iatrogenic injuries of the spinal accessory nerve may occur during surgery of the neck and result in functional impairment particularly of trapezoid muscle. They are the most common causes of trapezius palsy[1-3]. A damage can cause a reduction in mobility of the shoulder and abduction of the arm above the horizontal line, causing a permanent disability in some cases. Moreover, by the time these impairments cause pain and muscle tension in the shoulder and arm. Patients who underwent neck dissection are frequently concerned, particularly after radical neck dissection[4-6].

In its anatomical course the accessory nerve divides into an internal and external ramus immediately after leaving the jugulare foramen. Since the external ramus enters immediately the sternomastoid muscle and after this runs through the posterior neck triangle to the anterior edge of the trapezoid muscle this part is particularly endangered. It is known that the three portions of trapezoid muscle are additionally innervated by branches of the cervical plexus in various dimensions[7]. Soo et al.[8] described the exact motor innervation by comparison of motor action potentials and latencies after stimulation of accessory nerve and of the roots of the cervical plexus. Krause introduced a method anastomosing a subfascial branch of the deep cervical plexus to the distal stump of the accessory nerve during radical neck dissection. The results showed a good recovery of all three portions of trapezius muscle[9]. Weisberger et al. used a cable graft from the greater auricular nerve for reconstruction after sacrifice of the spinal accessory nerve during radical neck dissection resulting in an improved shoulder function[10].

The attempt in selective neck dissection is to avoid nerve injury. Beside the knowledge of surgical anatomy of the neck for a careful preparation electro-physiological methods for monitoring of cranial nerves during surgery were established during the last years. Various studies have examined and confirmed their efficiency to reduce the frequency as well as the extend of postoperative paralysis[11].

Online-EMGs of the muscle groups innervated by spinal nerves during operation accomplish three tasks:

- visual and acoustic warning of the surgeon at preparation close to the nerve
- identification of a suspected structure as cranial nerve by stimulation
- prognostic value of stimulated muscle potentials concerning the degree of post-operative paralysis

This intraoperative monitoring is available and frequently used in the facial nerve during surgery of the parotid gland[12,13] and the recurrent nerve during thyroid gland surgery[14,15].

Since there is little experience in the literature this study examines the applicability of a continuous intraoperative electromyography monitoring of the spinal accessory nerve. Expecting a comparable reduction of postoperative accessory nerve paralyses, our aims of a first analysis were:

- to find an optimal adaptation of intraoperative nerve monitoring to the conditions of the spinal accessory nerve,
- to describe the electro-physiological conditions to get reliable information of online-EMGs
- to examine the value of online-EMGs to predict frequency and extend of postoperative paralyses.

METHODS

Altogether we examined 33 patients (31 male, 2 female) who underwent a selective neck dissection in the context of surgery of malignant tumours of the head and neck. In 21 patients both sides were operated, so the total number of investigated neck-sides is 54.

In all cases a clinical examination and neuromyography of spinal accessory nerve and EMGs of sternocleidomastoid and trapezoid muscle were carried out before operation and 7 – 14 days as well as 3 – 4 months after surgery. (fig. 1)

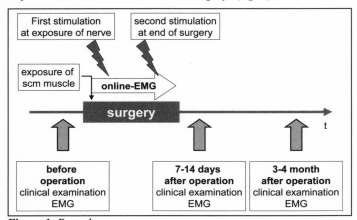

Figure 1: Procedure

Monitoring of spinal accessory nerve during surgery is performed by online-EMGs of the sternocleidomastoid and trapezoid muscle. Before desinfection of the operation area we inserted two unipolar needle electrodes in an angle of 30 degrees and in a distance of 1 cm in both trapezoid muscles and fixed them with tape. After exposure of the sternomastoid muscle two other needle electrodes were inserted in the middle of the muscle in the same distance and fixed with sutures.

Online-EMGs can be observed on a monitor during the whole operation. Simultaneously the surgeon gets acoustic information if EMG-potentials are derived. We used a two channel EMG "Neurosign 100" by Inomed and monitored spontaneous activity during dissection. In addition we captured the EMG-answers after stimulation of the nerve as soon as it was discovered during dissection and at the end of surgery in 42 neck-sides. In cases (12 neck-sides) with lymph node conditions not requiring a dissection near the spinal accessory nerve, the nerve was exposed only at the end of operation and stimulated at this time. In every case of stimulation we started with the minimal threshold amperage of 0,01 mA and increased the intensity step by step until an EMG-potential was registered. To avoid nerve damage the maximum amperage was 0,5 mA even if there was response. We located the thresholds with reliable responses and captured the potentials themselfs to carry out subtle differentiated analyses of their form in later examinations.

RESULTS

Measuring before surgery did not reveal clinical signs of a paralysis in any case. With the EMG we discovered restricted interference pattern with a particularly high frequency at the N2-necks in 14 of 54 measurements (i.e. neck sides) and no reduction of the amplitude in any case.

Postoperative clinical examination revealed a reduction of arm movement in 7 cases and reduction of muscle power in 6 cases. We detected restricted interference pattern in 23 neck-sides and a reduction of amplitudes in 6 neck-sides particularly again in the N2-necks with the EMG.

During intraoperative monitoring amperages between 0,05 mA and 0,5 mA were needed to trigger reliable answering potentials. The sternocleidomastoid muscle supplies more reliable answers than the trapezoid muscle even at lower amperages. Only in approximately one half of the cases it was possible to detect a potential of the trapezoid muscle, compared to almost all cases in sternocleidomastoid muscle (fig. 2).

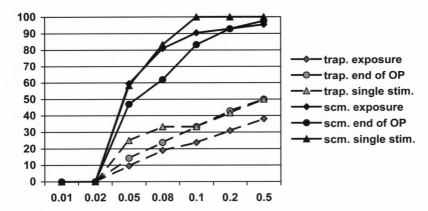

Figure 2: Threshold value of stimulation amperage [mA] to trigger reliable answering potentials in sternocleidomastoid and trapezoid muscle [cases in %]

Finally we determined the differences between both threshold amperages during operation (discovery of nerve – end of operation) in 42 neck-sides and compared it with postoperative clinical and EMG-results. In cases with no difference we found deficits in EMG in 35% and clinical deficits in 13%. If a higher amperage was necessary to generate a reliable answering potential at the end of operation deficits in EMG occur in 60% and in movement and muscle power in 20%.

SUMMARY

A continuous intraoperative electromyography monitoring is also applicable to the spinal accessory nerve. We obtained first results of the clinical application and derived information to optimize its application. So the capturing of stimulation answering potentials was more reliable from the sternomastoid than from the trapezoid muscle.

Comparing pre- and postoperative results we found reductions of the movement or muscle power most frequently in patients with a N2 classification.

An increase of threshold concerning stimulation amperage at the end of surgery could be a predictive of postoperative function. To support this assumption detailed analyses of the shape of the potentials are necessary.

REFERENCES

1. Donner TR, Kline DG. Extracranial spinal accessory nerve injury. Neurosurgery 1993;32:907-910
2. Harpf C, Rhomberg M, Rumer A, Rainer C, Hussl H. Iatrogene Läsion des Nervus accessorius bei der cervicalen Lymphknotenbiopsie. Chirurg 1999;70: 690-693
3. Wiater JM, Bigliani LU. Spinal accessory nerve injury. Clin Orthop 1999;368:5-16
4. Cheng PT, Hao SP, Lin YH, Yeh AR. Objective comparison of shoulder dysfunction after three neck dissection techniques. Ann Otol Rhinol Laryngol 2000;109:761-766
5. Terrell JE et al. Pain, quality of life and spinal accessory nerve status after neck dissection. Laryngoscope 2000;110:620-626

6. Koybasioglu A, Tokcaer AB, Uslu S, Ileri F, Beder L, Ozbilen S. Accessory nerve function after modified radical and lateral neck dissection. Laryngoscope 2000; 110:73-77

7. Kierner AC, Zelenka I, Heller S, Burian M. Surgical anatomy of the spinal accessory nerve and the trapezius branches of the cervical plexus. Arch Surg 2000;153:1428-1431

8. Soo KC, Strong EW, Spiro RH, Shah JP, Nori S, Green RF. Innervation of the trapezius muscle by the intra-operative measurement of motor action potentials. Head Neck 1993;15:216-221

9. Krause HR. Reinnervation of the trapezius muscle after radical neck dissection. J Craniomaxillofac Surg 1994;22:323-329

10. Weisberger EC, Lingeman RE. Cable grafting of the spinal accessory nerve for rehabilitation of shoulder function after radical neck dissection. Laryngoscope 1987;97:915-918

11. Romstock J, Strauss C, Fahlbusch R. Continuous electromyography monitoring of motor cranial nerves during cerebellopontine angle surgery. J Neurosurg 2000;93:586-593

12. Terrell JE et al. Clinical outcome of continuous facial nerve monitoring during primary parotidectomy. Arch Otolaryngol Head Neck Surg 1997;123:1081-1087

13. Wolf SR, Schneider W, Suchy B, Eichhorn B. Intraoperatives Fazialismonitoring in der Parotischirurgie. HNO 1995;43:294-298

14. Djohan RS, Rodriguez HE, Connolly MM, Childers SJ, Braverman B, Podbielski FJ. Intraoperative monitoring of recurrent laryngeal nerve function. Am Surg 2000;66:595-597

15. Timon CI, Rafferty M. Nerve monitoring in thyroid surgery: is it worthwhile? Clin Otolaryngol 1999;24:487-490

311

THE INNERVATION OF THE TRAPEZIUS MUSCLE –
NEW FINDINGS AND THEIR CLINICAL IMPLICATIONS

A. C. Kierner[1], I. Zelenka[2], M. Burian[3]
[1]ENT-Department, University Hospital Frankfurt a.M, Germany
[2]Department of Anatomy 2, University Vienna, Austria
[3]ENT-Department, University Hospital Vienna, Austria

Correspondence to: *Antonius C. Kierner, ENT-Department University Hospital Frankfurt a. M., Theodor Stern-Kai 7, D-60 590 Frankfurt a. M., Phone: ++49-69-6301-5163, Fax: 0049-69-6301-5435 (email: Kierner@em.uni-frankfurt.de)*

INTRODUCTION

Since the radical neck dissection has been first described by Crile in 1906[1] there has been a lot of controversy between surgeons and anatomists about the trapezius muscle innervation. Clinical studies have shown that even if the spinal accessory nerve (SAN) is identified and saved during surgery, up to 71% of the patients suffer from a trapezius muscle paresis postoperatively[2-4]. Since it is generally agreed by now that the so called shoulder syndrome due to trapezius muscle paresis is a severe and disabling complication for patients after neck dissection this question still gains actuality[5, 6]. Surprisingly, there is still considerable controversy on how to identify the SAN intraoperatively and data dealing with the nerves' topograhical anatomy are sparse, confusing or even contradictory[7-11]. Additionally it remains unclear how the SAN and the cervical plexus branches contribute in the innervation of the different parts of the trapezius muscle.

The aim of this study was to give an exact and detailed description of the anatomy of all nerves involved in the trapezius muscle innervation and to determine how much these nerves contribute in the innervation of the three different parts of the abovementioned muscle. Special emphasis was laid on the nerve supply of the clinically most important descending part of the muscle.

METHODS

92 posterior triangles of the neck (PTN) of 46 perfusion fixed individuals who had donated their bodies to the Institute of Anatomy where dissected with special emphasis laid on
1. the topographical anatomy of the SAN as related to the surgery of the neck and
2. the number and topograhy of the trapezius branches of the cervical plexus.

Additionally 20 trapezius muscles were stained with Sihler´s technique[12], which makes muscle tissue translucent by staining the nerves within it.

The fine branch of the SAN passing to the descending part of the trapezius muscle as found by gross dissection was identified during 20 modified radical neck dissections as well, up to now.

Furthermore intraoperative electromyography of the three parts of the trapezius muscle was performed in patients undergoing neck dissection.

RESULTS

In 43 PTN the SAN was found to cross the internal jugular vein in the anterior triangle of the neck ventrally in 56% and dorsally in 44%. Furthermore, the distance between the clavicle and the point where the SAN enters the PTN was measured in 90 PTN. The mean distance measured was 8.2cm (±1.01). In 29%, i.e. almost one third of the cases the SAN did not pass through the sternocleidomastoid (SCM) muscle at all.

In 44 PTN between 1 and 3 Rr. trapezii of the cervical plexus could be found. Only one R. trapezius was present in 9%, two could be found in 61% and three in 30%. So, with 61% two Rr. trapezii represent the most frequent case, in 90% showing a special topographical relationship to the transverse cervical artery: A thinner branch is crossing the artery superficially and a thicker one is crossing it profundly and more caudal.

The macroscopic findings presented herein have recently been published[13].

In all 20 muscles stained with Sihlers´ technique the Rr. trapezii were found to merge with the SAN passing together to the transverse and ascending part of the trapezius muscle. Additionally, one single branch arising from the SAN was the only nerve passing towards the descending part in all 20 muscles investigated.

When this fine cranial branch of the SAN was stimulated intraoperatively, EMG potentials could be seen in the descending part of the trapezius muscle whereas stimulation of the main nerve distal to the ramification lead to contractions in the ascending and transverse parts of the muscle solely.

DISCUSSION

The fine cranial branch of the SAN passing to the descending part of the trapezius muscle has been described for the first time as far as we know. The intraoperatively performed EMGs stimulating this branch, in our opinion clearly proved its putative function and importance for the integrity of the shoulder girdle. Furthermore, no conclusive data on the number, topographical anatomy and variance of the trapezius branches of the cervical plexus could be found up to now. In this respect the typical anatomical relationship found between the trapezius branches of the cervical plexus and the transverse cervical artery has to be emphasised. This is one of the reasons why in our opinion it is neither possible nor oncologically justified to identify and safe the cervical plexus branches intraoperatively[14].

Our data clearly show that the clinically important descending part of the trapezius muscle is innervated by a branch of the SAN solely, whereas the ascending and transverse parts gain nerve supply from both, the SAN and the cervical plexus. Additionally by staining the muscles according to Sihler´s technique it became obvious that the so called segmental branches are identical with the dorsal cutaneous nerves arising from the spinal nerves and do not ramify in the trapezius muscle. Therefore, an additional innervation by these branches as suggested by some authors seems rather unusual[8].

Considering the often cited "subfascial branches" we have to say, that any other branches than subfascial ones are anatomically impossible in the PTN[9,15]. Similarly, any other crossing between the IJV and the SAN as a ventral or dorsal one is impossible, too, the terms medial or lateral often used in this respect are therefore not only confusing but simply wrong.

Baring in mind all this, we hope that the data presented herein will help to minimize the rate of unexpected trapezius muscle paresis after surgery in the posterior triangle of the neck.

REFERENCES

1. Crile G.W. Excision of cancer of the head and neck. JAMA 1906;47:1780-1786
2. Carenfelt C., Eliasson K. Occurence, duration and prognosis of unexpected accessory nerve paresis in radical neck dissection. Acta Otolaryngol 1980;90:470-473
3. Blessing R., Mann W., Beck Chl. Wie sinnvoll ist der Erhalt des Nervus accessorius bei der Halsausräumung? Laryng Rhinol Otol 1986;65:403-405
4. Yagnik P.M., Siao Tick Chong P. Spinal accessory nerve injury: a complication of carotid endarterectomy. Muscle Nerve 1996;19:907-909
5. Nahum A.M., Mullally W., Marmor R. A syndrome resulting from radical neck dissection. Arch Otolaryngol. 1961;74:424-428
6. Kuntz A.C., Weymuller E.A. Impact of neck dissection on quality of life. Laryngoscope 1999;109:1334-1338
7. Weisberger E.C. The efferent supply of the trapezius muscle:a neuroanatomic basis for the preservation of shoulder function during neck dissection. Laryngoscope 1987;97:435-445
8. Soo K.C., Guiloff R.J., Oh A., Querci Della Rovere G., Westbury G. Innervation of the trapezius muscle: a study in patients undergoing neck dissections. Head Neck 1990;12:488-495
9. Krause H.R., Bremerich A., Herrmann M. The innervation of the trapezius muscle in connection with radical neck-dissection. J Cran Max Fac Surg. 1991;19:87-89
10. Krause H.R., Kornhuber A., Dempf R. A technique for diagnosing the individual patterns of innervation of the trapezius muscle prior to neck dissection. J Cran Max Fac Surg. 1993;21:102-106
11. Warwick R., Williams P.L. Gray´s Anatomy. 35th edition, Longman Edinburgh 1973:534

12.   Sihler C. Die Muskelspindeln, Kerne und Lage der motorischen Nervenendigungen. Arch Mikroskop
      Anat Entwicklung 1900;56:334-354
13.   Kierner A.C., Zelenka I., Heller S., Burian M. Surgical anatomy of the spainal accessory nerve and the
      trapezius branches of the cervical plexus. Arch Surg. 2000;135:1428-1431
14.   Weitz J.W., Weitz S.C., McElhinney A.J. A technique for preservation of spinal accessory nerve
      function in radical neck dissection. Head Neck Surg. 1982;5:75-78
15.   Niemeyer K., Ludolph A. Zur Bedeutung der subfaszialen Äste des Plexus cervicalis für die motorische
      Innervation des M. trapezius. Dtsch Z Mund Kiefer Gesichts Chir. 1987;11:356-360

316

INTERMITTENT MODIFIED RADICAL NECKDISSECTION AND MINIMAL INVASIVE TUMOR SURGERY DURING COMBINED RADIO/CHEMOTHERAPY OF HEAD AND NECK CANCER.

Georg Mathias Sprinzl, M.D., Arne Wulf Scholtz, M.D., Julia Wimmers-Klick, M.D., Oliver Galvan, M.D., Walter Franz Thumfart, M.D.
Department of Otorhinolaryngology - Head and Neck Surgery, University of Innsbruck, Austria

Key words: neck dissection, head and neck cancer, radio/chemotherapy, minimal invasive tumor surgery .

Correspondence to: Univ. Doz. Dr. med. Georg M. Sprinzl, Universitätsklinik für Hals-, Nasen- und Ohrenheilkunde, Leopold-Franzens-Universität zu Innsbruck, Anichstr. 35, Austria - 6020 Innsbruck, Phone: ++43 / 512 / 504 5204, Fax: ++43 / 512 / 504 67 5204 (e-mail: georg.sprinzl@uibk.ac.at)

INTRODUCTION

Neck dissection remains the standard method of treating cervical metastasis from head and neck squamous cell carcinoma[1]. However, the term neck dissection certainly covers a wide spectrum of differing concepts, controversies and techniques[2].

During the early 1970s, Strong reported that the regional failure following a standard radical neck dissection was as high as 70 % for patients with multiple nodes. With the use of low dose preoperative radiation up to 20 Gray in one week, he was able to reduce the regional failure to approximately 36 %[3,4].

Boysen and others showed in their study that 26 % of the patients had no palpable neck nodes after receiving preoperative radiotherapy. Nevertheless 22 % of the patients with clinically negative neck nodes had pathologically confirmed residual tumor. This study demonstates us that radiation alone cannot sterilize a clinically positive neck[5].

Byers evaluated a treatment protocol consisting of an initial neck dissection followed by definitive radiotherapy. He suggested that a delay greater than 14 days from surgery to the start of radiotherapy reduces survival significantly[6].

317

The cure of locally advanced squamous cell carcinoma of the head and neck is uncommon with radiotherapy alone. The desire for organ preservation in advanced resectable SCCHN and the need for better local therapy for unresectable disease have led to the development of treatment modalities using radiotherapy and concurrent chemotherapy (RT/CCT)[7].

This combination is an attractive strategy because the appropriate drugs may enhance radiation effects and independently contribute to local cytotoxicity. Concurrent treatment may combat tumor repopulation and provide the earliest possible treatment of distant micrometastasis. RT/CCT may be integrated in synchronous or alternating schemes. Most randomized trials of RT/CCT versus radiation alone show superior local control, disease-free survival, and survival with combined modality treatment[8].

In light of recent trends to modify classic treatment modalities[9], we reviewed our experience with radical and modified RND (MRND) with concomitant radiochemotherapy as treatment for N2/N3 neck disease in head and neck squamous cell carcinoma.

PATIENT AND METHODS

Thirty-five patients with squamous cell carcinoma of the head and neck were studied. The treatment consisted of two-cycles of radiation up to 30 Gy administered in 15 conventional fractions over a period of 3 weeks, combined with concomitant administration of mitomycin C on day 1 (10 mg/m2, i.v. bolus) and 5-fluorouracil during the first 4 days of irradiation (1000 mg/m2/24 hours, continuous infusion) in each treatment cycle. After the first cycle tumor resection and/or neck dissection was performed. For the neck dissection we used a modified Morestin´s incision. If tumor resection was estimated reliable preoperatively, the resection was carried out with a surgical CO2-laser system connected to a microscope or with the KTP-laser system which is applied via a fiber. For the resection itself, we used the transoral approach in 18 cases. The median follow up was 24 month. We conducted regular controls after 3, 6, 12, 18 and 24 months.

RESULTS

Surgery at the primary site was performed in 18 patients, and 35 had modified radical neck dissection. Treatment-related mortality was observed in two patients (5,7%). At a median follow-up of 24 months, the 2-year progression-free survival was 64%, locoregional control 92%, and overall survival 55%. Patients with complete clinical response were pathologically tumor free in 59 % before neck dissection. Toxicities included mucositis (grade 3, 35%; grade 4, 16%), neutropenia (grade 4, 28%), and thrombocytopenia (grade 4, 26%). Improved efficacy with RT/CCT is accompanied by increased acute toxicity, which necessitates compromises in the treatment design of most programs. Quality of life declined during treatment but returned from good to excellent by 12 months after treatment.

The following prognostic factors were identified for distant metastasis:
three or more positive nodes, extracapsular spread of malignant tissue, and positive surgical margins in the neck dissection specimen. The influence of distant metastasis on disease-specific survival was evident.

The failure rate increases dramatically in patients with concomitant radiochemotherapy when laryngectomy is required for salvage surgery.

CONCLUSION

At this time, the most effective RT/CCT regimen has not been defined. Chemical modifiers of toxicity are now under investigation in clinical trials and may allow for improved integration of RT/CCT[10].

The combination of radiochomotherapy and MRND is highly effective in controlling neck disease in the absence of persistent or recurrent local disease. In our experience, MRND appears to be as effective as RND in controlling even advanced neck disease which supports preservation of the spinal accessory nerve and the sternocleidomastoid muscle whenever oncologically feasible. Intensive concomitant chemoradiotherapy leads to high locoregional control and survival rates with organ preservation and a reversal of the historical failure pattern. Modified radical neck dissection combined with concomitant chemoradiotherapy is feasible and not associated to higher complication rates. However, laryngectomy after one cycle of combined radiochemotherapy can not be recommended and should be avoided.

Table 1. Patients demographics

Characteristics	Group A (with resection of primary tumor)	Group B (without tumor resection)
Number	18	17
Median age	60	57
Range	49-82	42-75
Sex: male/female	16/2	12/5
Tumor location		
Oral cavity	4	1
Oropharynx	11	9
Nasopharynx	-	1
Hypopharynx	3	5
Larynx	-	1

Table 2. TNM-Classification (n=35)

T	Group A (with resection of primary tumor)	Group B (without tumor resection)
T1	-	
T2	5	4
T3	3	4
T4	10	9
N		
Nx	0	0
N0	0	0
N1	4	2
N2	8	8
N3	6	7
M		
M1	0	0

REFERENCES

1. Vokes EE, Weichselbaum RR, Lippman SM, Hong WK. Head and neck cancer. N Engl J Med 1993; 328(3):184-194.
2. Robbins KT, Medina JE, Wolfe GT, Levine PA, Sessions RB, Pruet CW. Standardizing neck dissection terminology. Official report of the Academy's Committee for Head and Neck Surgery and Oncology. Arch Otolaryngol Head Neck Surg 1991; 117(6):601-605.
3. Strong EW, Henschke UK, Nickson JJ, Frazell EL, Tollefsen HR, Hilaris BS. Preoperative x-ray therapy as an adjunct to radical neck dissection. Cancer 1966; 19(11):1509-1516.
4. Strong EW. Preoperative radiation and radical neck dissection. Surg Clin North Am 1969; 49(2):271-276.
5. Boysen M, Lovdal O, Natvig K, Tausjo J, Jacobsen AB, Evensen JF. Combined radiotherapy and surgery in the treatment of neck node metastases from squamous cell carcinoma of the head and neck. Acta Oncol 1992; 31(4):455-460.
6. Byers RM, Clayman GL, Guillamondequi OM, Peters LJ, Goepfert H. Resection of advanced cervical metastasis prior to definitive radiotherapy for primary squamous carcinomas of the upper aerodigestive tract. Head Neck 1992; 14(2):133-138.
7. Pfister DG, Strong E, Harrison L et al. Larynx preservation with combined chemotherapy and radiation therapy in advanced but resectable head and neck cancer. J Clin Oncol 1991; 9(5):850-859.
8. Clayman GL, Johnson II CJ, Morrison W, Ginsberg L, Lippman SM. The Role of Neck Dissection After Chemoradiotherapy for Oropharyngeal Cancer With Advanced Nodal Disease. Arch Otolaryngol Head Neck Surg 2001; 127(2):135-139.
9. McCaffrey TV. Surgical treatment in head and neck cancer. Curr Opin Oncol 1991; 3(3):519-522.
10. Vacha P, Marx M, Engel A, Richter E, Feyerabend T. Side effects of postoperative radiochemotherapy with amifostine versus radiochemotherapy alone in head and neck tumors. Preliminary results of a prospective randomized trial. Strahlenther Onkol 1999; 175 Suppl 4:18-22.

PROGNOSTIC PARAMETER IN NON-SURGICAL THERAPIES OF ADVANCED SQUAMOUS CELL CARCINOMAS OF THE HEAD AND NECK

T. Wendt (Jena, Germany)

Running title: Prognostic parameter in non-surgical therapies

Key words: Prognostic parameter, radiotherapy, chemoradiation, head and neck cancer

Correspondence to*: Thomas G. Wendt, Professor and Chairman of the Dept. Radiation Oncology, Friedrich-Schiller-University Jena, Bachstrasse 18, D-07743 Jena, Germany, Phone +49 3641 933214, Fax +49 3641 933403, (e-mail: thomas.wendt@med.uni-jena.de)*

The knowledge upon prognostic factors in oncology should enable the physician to taylor diagnostic and therapeutic measurements individually. Furthermore it is of paramount importance when two treatment regimen are tested prospectively to minimize inherent prognostic heterogeneity. In head and neck cancer prognosis depends on local, regional and distant failure or a combination thereof. However these types of failure may not occur independently[26]. Therefore from increased loco-regional tumor control rates a lower frequency of distant metastases can be expected wich will translate into improved disease free survival at least in patients with advanced loco-regional disease with high prevalence of hematogenous spread. In many tumor sites underlying comorbidity compromizes therapeutic endevours and may contribute to low overall survival despite favourable tumor control rates especially in advanced cancers.

 Treatment outcome after radical (that is high total tumor dose, curative intent) radiotherapy alone or combined with any kind of chemotherapy depends on a variety of treatment related and tumor and/or host related factors as well as treatment.

Host related factors
Age at diagnosis has not proven prognostically in a large series comparing patients younger and older than 75 years[28]. Similarly cell kinetics does not differ in the aged compared to younger individuals[8].

Anemia is a common finding in patients with advanced disease despite not bleeding has occured. Although in head and neck cancer the prognostic significance of anemia is less well established compared to gynecologic tumors, recent research point to a correlation between anemia and tissue hypoxia, which may be responsible for decreased radiosensitivity[4].

Tumor related factors
TNM classification and volume of tumor

There is no doubt, that increasing number of tumor category in the TNM classification is correlated with decreased tumor control irrespective of treatment. However high number of T-stage does not necessarily mean higher tumor volume or diameter and the classification of laryngeal and nasopharyngeal tumors does not take into account the size at all. Computerized tomography CT) and ultrasound allows for volumetric estimation or precise tumor diameter measurement. Maximum tumor in cm seems to predict tumor control in laryngeal cancer[30]. Maximum diameter had also an impact on effectivness of hyperfractionation schedule in favour of tumors smaller than 4 cm[10]. Tumor volume measured in CT series seems to influence outcome after both radiotherapy and chemoradiation[16, 21]. The same has been found for patients who were reirradiated due to loco-regional relaps after prior full dose radio-therapy[9].

Beside T-stage and nodal status of the neck is of paramount prognostic significance. It is well accepted that N-stage has a slight prognostic overweight over T-stage. However prognosis does not vary only with N-stage. An increasing number of nodes involved augments the risk of neck failure after neck dissection alone. Beyond neck tumor burden the presence or absence of extracapsular spread (ECS) and the lymphatic vessel invasion have been identified as further risk factors[29]. As outlined below at least the increased risk from presence of ECS can be counteracted by simultaneous chemoradiation[3]. Nevertheless these factors do not only increase neck recurrence rate but also influence the rate of distant metastases[25].

The incidence of distant metastases is not only correlated with these parameters but also with the level of nodes involved. The lower the metastatic node is located at hte neck, the higher the rate of subsequent distant metastases. This has been shown for nasopharyngeal cancer[15], but earlier also for other site of squamous cell carcinoma of the head and neck.

Modern diagnostic imaging also gives information on the structure of lymph nodes. Low density in CT is considered tumor necrosis in both primaries and lymph nodes. In quantitative analysis a correlation between the extent of necrotic lymph node areas in CT and loco-regional control was demonstrated. Patients with greater than one third hypodense lymph node metastases had a significantly (multivariate Cox model) lower local control and survival after radiotherapy or chemoradiation[16].

HISTOLOGY

In squamous cell cancer which constitute more than 95% of all cancers of the oropharynx, the larynx, the hypopharynx and oral cavity degree of cellular differentiation seems to influence locoregional tumor control only marginally. However poorly differentiated tumors showed a significantly higher propensitiy to metastasize (3 versus 18%) and therefore had a significantly poorer survival (58 vs. 76%) compared to well differentiated tumors[30]. Tumors evolving in the nasopharynx show a variety of histologic entities which show different radiocurability. In a series of 378 patients from MD Anderson Hospital undifferentiated cancers have a significantly worse prognosis compared differentiated sqamous cell cancer[15].

TUMORBIOLOGY

Tumor cell proliferation is often characterized by potential tumor doubling time (T_{pot}). The majority of squamous cell carcinoma of the head and neck show T_{pot} measured e.g. by flow cytometry of 5 days or less[11]. These tumors are supposed to proliferate fast and repopulation during a 6 to 7 weeks radiotherapy is considered a major source of local failure. However in a prospective clinical trial short (<4.6 days) and longer T_{pot} (> 4.6 days) measured before radiotherapy did not correlate neither with loco-regional tumor control nor with 5 years survival[7].

Biologic factors to predict treatment results
P53 expression in immunohistological staining seems not to correlate with p53 mutations detected by sequencing in laryngeal cancers[5]. The methodological differences might be a source for diverging results reported recently. However even data obtained with the same method upon correlation between p53 protein (either occasional overexpression in immunohistological staining or intense staining for most cells) and tumor control and disease free survival are conflicting. Some authors find improved survival with increasing positivity, others do not so (table 1).

Other proliferation markers like MIB 1 labelling index, Ki 67 labelling index or proliferating cell nuclear antigen (PCNA) have not proven prognostic after surgery and postoperative radiotherapy[17]. Intratumoral microvessel density (IMD) represented a powerful independent predictive factor for local-regional tumor control after radical irradiation for carcinoma of the oropharynx[1]. High vessel density was correlated with worse prognosis than scarcly vascularization. Since high number of microvessels in a tumor may suggest good oxygenation and consecutively good radiocurability another underlying mechanism for this adverse prognostic effect must be discussed.

Treatment related factors
Prognosis of patients treated with radical radiotherapy alone or chemoradiation largely depends on the tumor remission achieved at the end of treamtent or a short period e.g. six weeks later. To a certain degree rates of complete response do translate into tumor control probability. Therefore treatment protocols designed for increased tumor cell kill by either intensified radiation schemes or the addition of cytotoxic drugs are likely to augment the long term tumor control rates.

Unconventional fractionation
Conventional fractionation still is the standard fractionation scheme for all head and neck cancers.

Modifications have been made in order to exploit normal tissue sparing effect by smaller single doses and thus allowing for higher total doses supposed to be isoeffective as far as late radiation sequelae are concerned, or to increase radiotherapy intensity by increasing weekly dose from 9 to 10 Gy in standard regimen to 12 to 15 Gy or even more. Hyperfractionated radiotherapy increases loco-regional control and disease free survival at 5 years but failed to improve overall survival[14, 19]. A similar advantage observed after accelerated fractionation (similar total radiation dose given in shorter time) was counterbalanced by increasing late toxicity at three years[14]. Very condensed radiotherapy protocols like CHART (three fractions per day, total treatment time 12 days[12]) failed to improve results. Accelerated fractionation seems to be more effective in smaller tumors than in very large ones[10].

Radiochemotherapy

The combination of radiotherapy and chemotherapy resulted in improved long term treatment results. However time and sequencing of chemotherapy proved crucial in a metaanalysis (MACH-HN) perfomed on individual updated data. Concomitant chemoradiation resulted in an 8% increase in 5 years survival, neoadjuvant chemotherapy in an increase of only 2%[31]. Simultaneous chemoradiation has proven to diminish the high risk of loco-regional recurrence in patients with extracapsular spread[3].

Neither drugs nor dosage are currently standardized. Most experience has been accumulated with the combination of 5-fluorouracil and cisplatin introduced by theWayne State Group[2, 22]. Mitomycin C given concomitantly to radiotherapy resulted in improved long term tumor control rates[13, 18]. The additional therapeutic gain obtained by cytotoxic drugs seems to be independant from fractionation schedules empoyed. Simultaneous chemoradiation increases local control and disease free survival rates after both conventionally fractionated and intensified (hyperfractionated) radiotherapy[6, 13, 18, 20, 27, 32].

CONCLUSION

Many tumor and host related prognostic factors have been identified in squamous cell carcinoma of the head and neck. In clinical practice however so far only factors associated with T- and N-stage based on detailed pathologic reports are included in the decision making process. More recently deteted biologic factors need extensive clinical testing in prospective trials.

Type of non-surgical treatment has proven of significant prognostic value. Concurrent chemo-radiation yields better results than radiotherapy alone in advanced cancers. Altered fraction-ation schedules increase loco-regional control but failed so far to augment overall survival.

Table 1: Correlation between p53 gene overexpression and tumor control after radiotherapy or chemoradiation

Grabenbauer	2000	p53 protein IHC	yes
Aebersold	2000	p53 protein IHC	no
Bradford	1999	p53 protein IHC	yes
Kopveld	1998	p53 protein IHC	no
Awwad	1996	p53 protein IHC	no
Koch	1996	p53 DNA sequencing	no

IHC: immunohistolochemistry

324

REFERENCES

1. Aebersold DM, Beer KT, Laissue J, Hug S, Lollar A, Greiner RH, Djonov V Intratumoral microvessel density predicts local treqtment failure of radically irradiated squamous cell cancer of the oropharynx. Int J Radiat Oncol Biol Phys 2000; 48: 17-25

2. Al Sarraf, M., T. F. Pajak, V. A. Marcial, P. Mowry, J. S. Cooper, J. Stetz, J. F. Ensley, E. Velez-Garcia: Concurrent Radiotherapy and Chemotherapy with Cisplatin in inoperable Squamous Cell Carcinoma of the Head and Neck. Cancer 1987; 59: 259-265

3. Bachaud, J.-M., Cohen-Jonathan E, Alzieu C, J-M David, Serrano E, Daly-Schveitzer N Combined postoperative radiotherapy and weekly cisplatin infusion for locally advanced squamous cell carcinoma of the head and neck: Final report of a randomized trial. Int. J. Radiat. Oncol. Biol. Phys. 1996; 36: 999-1004.

4. Becker A, Stadler P, Lavey, Hansgen G, Kuhnt T, Lautenschlager C, Feldmann H-J, Molls M, Dunst J. Severe anemia is associated with poor tumor oxygenation in head and neck squamous cell carcinoma. Int J Radiat Oncol Biol Phys 2000; 46:459-66.

5. Bradford CR, Zhu S, Poore J, Fisher SG, Beals TF, Thoraval D, Hanash SM, Carey TE, Wolf GT p53 mutations as a prognostic marker in advanced laryngeal carcinoma. Department of Verterans Affairs Laryngeal Cancer Cooperative Study Group. Arch Otolarnyngol Head Neck Surg 1997; 123: 605-9.

6. Brizel DM, Albers ME, Fisher SR, Scher RL, Richtsmeier WJ, Hars V, George SL, Huang AT, Prosnith LR Hyperfractionated irradiation with or without concurrent chemotherapy for locally advanced head and neck cancer. NEJM 1998; 338:1798-804

7. Bourhis J, Dendale R, Hill C et al. Potential doubling time and clinical outcome in head and neck squamous cell carcinoma treated with 70 Gy in 7 weeks. Int J Radiat Oncol Biol Phys 1996; 35:471-476

8. Corvò R, Sanguineti G, Vitale V et al In vivo cell kinetics in elderly patients affected by squamous cell carcinoma of the head and neck. Rays 1997; 22 Suppl to nr.1: 69-72

9. De Crevoisier R, Bourhis J, Domenge C, Wibault P, Koscielny S, Lusinchi A, Mamelle G, Janot F, Julieron M, Leridant AM, Marandas P, Armand JP, Schwaab G, Luboinski B, Eschwege F Full-Dose Reirradiation for Unresectable Head and Neck Carcinoma: Expereince at the Gustave-Roussy Institute in a Series of 169 patients. J Clin Oncol 1998; 16: 3556-62.

10. Cummings BJ, Keane TJ, Pintilie M et al. A prospective randomized trial of hyperfractionated versus conventional once daily radiation for advanced squamous cell carcionom of the laryngx and pharynx. Int J Radiat Oncol Biol Phys 1996; 36 Suppl 1: 235

11. Dische S, Saunders MI, Bennett MH, Wilson GD, McNally NJ. Cell proliferation and differentiation in squamous carcinoma . Radiother Oncol 1989; 15: 19-23

12. Dische S, Saunders M, Barrett A, Harvey A, Gibson D, Parmar M A randomised multicentre trial of CHART versus conventional radiotherapy in head and neck cancer. Radiother Oncol 1997; 44: 123-36.

13. Dobrowsky W, Naudé J Continuous hyperfractionated accelerated radiotherapy with/without mitomycin C in head and enck cancers. Radiother Oncol 2000; 57:119-24.

14. Fu KK, Pajak TF, Trotti A, Jones CU, Spencer SA, Phillips TL, Garden AS, Ridge JA, Cooper JS, Ang KK for the RTOG A radiation therapy oncology group (RTOG) phase III randomized study to comapare hyperfractionation and two variants of accelerated fractionation to standard fractionation radiotherapy for head and neck squamous cell carcinomas: First report of RTOG 90003. Int J Radiat Oncol Biol Phys 2000; 48: 7-16.

15. Geara FB, Sanuineti G, Tucker SL, Garden AS, Ang KK, Morrison WH, Peters LJ. Carcinoma of the nasopharynx treated by radiotherapy alone: determinants of distant metastasis and survival. Radiother Oncol 1997; 43:53-61

16. Grabenbauer GG, Steininger H, Meyer M, Fietkau R, Brunner T, Heinkelmann P, Hornung J, Iro H, Spither W, Kirchener T, Sauer R, Distel L Nodal CT density and total tumor volume as prosnostic factors after radiation therapy of stage II/IV head and neck cancer. Radiother Oncol 1998; 47:175-83.

17. Grabenbauer GG, Mühlfriedel Chr, Rödel F, Niedobitek G, Hornung J, Rödel C, Martus P, Iro H, Kirchener T, Steininger H, Sauer R, Weidenbecher M, Distel L Squamous cell carcinoma of the oropharynx: Ki-67 and p53 can identify pateintes at highe risk for local recurrence after surgery and postoperative radiotherapy. Int J Radiat Oncol Biol Phys 2000; 48: 1041-50.

18. Haffty BG, Son YH, Papax R, Sasaki CT, Weissberg JB, Fischer D, Rockwell S, Sartorelli AC, Fischer JJ. Chemotherapy as an adjunct to radiation in the rreatment of squamous cell carcinoma of the head and enck: results of the Yale Mitomycin Randomized Trials. J Clin Oncol 1997; 15: 268-76.

19.   Horiot JC, Le Fur R, N´Guyen T et al. Hyperfactionation versus conventional fractionation in oropharyngeal carcinoma: final analysis of a randomized trial of the EORTC cooperative group of radiotherapy. Radiother Oncol 1992; 25: 231-41.

20.   Jeremic B, Shibamoto Y, Milicic B, Nikolic N, Dagovic A, Aleksandrovic J, Vaskovic Z, Tadic L. Hyperfractionated radiotherapy with or without concurrent low dose daily cis-platin in locally advanced squamous cell carcinoma of the head and neck: a prospective randomized trial. J Clin Oncol 2000; 18: 1458-64.

21.   Johnson, C.R., S.R. Khandelwal, R.K. Schmidt-Ullrich, J. Ravalese III, D.E. Wazer: The influence of quantitative tumor volume measurements on local control in advanced head and neck cancer using concomitant boost accelerated superfractionated irradiation. Int. J. Radiat. Oncol. Biol. Phys 1995: 32; 635 - 641.

22.   Kish JA., Weaver A, Jacobs J, Cummings G, Al-Sarraf M. Cisplatin and 5-fluorouracil infusion in patients with recurrent and disseminated epidermoid cancer of the head and neck. Cancer 1984; 53 : 1819 - 24.

23.   Koch WM, Brennan JA,Zahurak M, Goodman SN, Westra WH, Schwab D, Yoo GH, Lee DJ, Forastiere AA, Sidransky D. p53 mutation and locoregional treatment filaure in head and neck squamous cell carcinoma. J Natl Cancer Inst 1996;88: 1580-6.

24.   Kropveld A, Slootweg PJ, Blankenstein MA, Terhaard CH, Hordijk GJ Ki-67 and p53 in T2 laryngeal cancer. Laryngoscope 1998;108:1548-52.

25.   Leemans, C.R., R. Tiwari, J.J.P. Nauta, I. v.d. Waal, G.B. Snow: Regional lymph node involvement and its significance in the development of distant metastasesin head and neck carcinoma. Cancer, 71 (1993), 452 - 456.

26.   Leibel SA, Scott CB, Muhiuddin M, Marcial VA, Coia LR, Davis LW, Fuks Z The effect of loco-regional control on distant metastatic dissemination in carcinoma of the head and neck: Results of an analysis from the RTOG database. Int J Radiat Oncol Biol Phys 1991; 21: 549-556

27.   Merlano M, Vitale V, Rosso R, Benasso M, Corvo R, Cavallari M, Sanguineti G, Bacigalupo A, Badellino F, Margarino G, Brema F, Pastorino G, Marziano C, Grimaldi A, Scasso F, Sperati G, Pallestrini E, Garaveta G, Accomando E, Cordone G, Comella G, Daponte A, Rubagotti A, Bruzzi DP, Santi L. Treatment of advanced squamous cell carcinoma of the head and neck with alternationg chemotherapy and radiotherapy. N Engl J Med 1992; 327: 1115-1121.

28.   Olmi P, Ausili-Cefaro G; Loreggian L Radiation therapy in the elderly with head and neck cancer. Rays 1997; 22: Suppl. to nr. 1: 77-81

29.   Olsen KD, Caruso M, Foote RL et al. Primary head and neck cancer: Hisotpathologic predictors of recurrence after neck dissection in patients with lymph node involvement. Arch Otolaryngol Head Neck Surg 1994; 120: 1370-74.

30.   Overgaard J, Hansen HS, JØrgensen K, Hansen MH Primary radiotherapy of larynx and pharynx carcinoma-an analysis of some factors influencing local control and survival. Int J Radiat Oncol Biol Phys 1986; 12: 515-21.

31.   Pignon JP, Bourhis J, Domenge C, Designé, on behalf of the MACH-HN Collaborative Group. Chemotherapy added to locoregional treatment for head and neck squamous cell carcinomas: three metaanalyses of updated individual data. The Lancet 2000: 355: 949-55.

32.   Wendt TG, Grabenbauer G, Roedel CM, Thiel H-J, von Lieven H, Rohloff R, Wustrow TPU, Schalhorn A. Simultaneous Radio-Chemotherapy increases local control and survival in locally advanced head and neck cancer. An Analysis of a randomized multicenter study. J Clin Oncol 1998;16: 1318-1324.

IMPROVEMENT OF LOCAL CONTROL IN RADIOTHERAPY TREATMENT OF HEAD AND NECK CANCER

Gerd Straßmann, Rita Engenhart –Cabillic, University of Marburg, Germany

Correspondence to*: Dr. med. Dipl. Ing. Gerd Strassmann, Klinik für Strahlentherapie und Radioonkologie, Baldingerstraße, 35043 Marburg, Phone: 0049 6421 2862522, Fax: 0049 6421/2866426 (E-mail: strassma@med.uni-marburg.de)*

ABSTRACT

Radiochemotherapy in combination with alternated fractionation schedules are improving local control and disease free survival in the treatment of advanced head and neck cancer. The improvement is associated with a higher incidence of acute toxicity.

In contrast, modern treatment techniques like *High Conformal Treatment Planning, CT guided Brachytherapy, Stereotactic Radiotherapy* and *Intensity Modulated Radiotherapy* were presented in this paper. The techniques enables to dose escalation in the tumor region accompanied by the reducion of normal tissue dose to support the improvement.

INTRODUCTION

Due to the improvement of local control in advanced head and neck cancer, disease free survival seems to be dependent. Advances in multimodality therapy are improving local control. Prospective randomized multicenter trials with simultaneously radiochemotherapy including accelerated fractionantion, schedules are suggesting that the impact of chemotherapy in advanced head and neck cancer is improving local control and survival. Three meta analyses have shown, that the success of chemotherapy is highly associated with the time of the application. The RTOG Phase III trial 9003 showed that hyperfractionation and accelerated fractionation with concomitant boost are improving local control, compared to standard fractionation schedules. A strong statistical trend was shown to an improved disease free survival. On the other hand accelerated fractionation schedules, as well as aggressive radiochemotherapy, are causing a higher incidence of acute side effects. They have to be combined with modern radiotherapy techniques, e.g. High Conformal 3D Treatment Planning, CT guided Brachytherapy, Stereotactic Radiotherapy and Intensity Modulated

Therapy for simultaneous prevention to organs at risk (eg. salivery glands, mucosus membranes, mandibles) by lowering the physical dose. However, the concept of multimodality therapy in head and neck cancer has to be reassassed.

Recent advances in combined radiochemotherapy and radiation fractionation

The randomized studies of Wendt et al.[1] and Dobrowsky et al.[2] are comparing accelerated or hyperfractionated simultaneous radiochemotherapy with Radiotherapy used alone. Due to the different schedules the results are not comparable, but every studie contains an arm in which local control and survival is improved, with higher incidence of acute toxicity (see Table 1). The explanation could be the concept of supra-addivity of simultaneus radiochemotherapy which leads not only to an enhanced tumour response and survival, but also to enhanced side effects of the normal tissue. The only study with equal acute toxicity and late toxicity was designed by Budach et al.[3], who decreased the total dose (70.6 Gy) in the radiochemotherapy arm compared with the radiotherapy arm (77.6 Gy) to compensate the additive toxicity of radiation and chemotherapy. With the exception of a study by Staar et al.[4] where the follow-up time was yet to short to allow final conclusions, the results are demonstrating the advantage in local control and survival of radiochemotherapy compared to radiotherapy used alone. Nearly the same impact of radiochemotherapy in the treatment of head and neck cancer is shown by three meta analyses[5-7], in which simultaneous or alternating administration of radiochemotherapy led to an absolute benefit on 5 year survival of about 8%.

The last important revealing randomised trial which was designed to investigate the question of fractionation in the treatment of head and neck cancer was the RTOG 9003 study in which 1113 patients were included. The results of the first report from Karen K. Fu et al.[8] showed that hyperfractionation (1.2 Gy/fraction, twice daily, to 81.6Gy/7weeks) and accelereted fractionation with concomitant boost (1.8 Gy/fraction, daily, plus 1.5 Gy/fraction/day as boost for the last 12 treatment days to 72 Gy/6 weeks) are significantly improving local control compared with standard fractionation (2Gy/fraction/day, to 70Gy/7weeks). Disease free survival was also improved in a statistical trend. The incidence of acute side effects for hyperfractionation and accelerated fractionation was > 50% versus 27% for standard fractionation. There was no significant statistical difference in the incidence of late effects, the most common sites were the pharynx and the salivary glands.

An important conclusion is, that the described recent advances due to altered therapy schedules are also causing a higher incidence of acute side effects in the special patients collective with head and neck cancer. According to this conclusion a higher incidence of therapy interruptions would be obvious if it were ignored.

Recent advances in radiation therapy techniques may compensate the negative effect of aggressive treatment schedules by conserving normal tissue at the same time.

Recent advanced in radiotherapy techniques

An advantage of conforming radiotherapy techniques in case of advanced head and neck cancer like high conformal treatment planning, CT guided brachytherapy, stereotactic radiotherapy and intensity modulated therapy is the prevention of the normal tissue to avoid side effects.

High conformal treatment planning produces a more homogeneus dose distribution for advanced head and neck cancer than the conventional lateral opposed field junction technique. Dose coverage of target volumes is improved, while the organs of risk (e.g. spinal cord) are spared[9].

CT guided Brachytherapy stands for positioning of the catheders under CT control and CT based threedimensional treatment planning[10]. Kolotas et al.[1] described the development, application and evaluation of a fully CT based treatment planning procedure and its clinical evaluation. Especially the implementation of the routinely use of dosevolume histogramms (DVH) implemented in a new implant quality evaluation method (COIN = Conformal Index) revalues Brachytherapy for the comparison with other radiotherapy methods. The power of brachytherapy, is justified with the steep dose fall-off outside the target volume which leads to maximal protection of the soft tissue along with to high conformity (see Figure 1.) The inhomogeneities of the centrifugal dosegradient can be particulary used for central overkill inside the tumour. On the other hand lower dose rate will enhance the capacity of cells to exploit repair and recovery processes, especially from the normal tissue. Recent hardware developments now allow the use of Pulse Dose Rate (PDR) treatment which may offer a therapeutic advantage in terms of late tissue damage as well as acute effects.

Dosimetric implant quality depends to a great extent on needle positioning[12,13]. For the physician using interstitial brachytherapy techniques expert knowledge is required of anatomy and of the radiosensitivity of critical structures, as well as extensive practical experience. Recent advances are navigation systems for Stereotactic Brachytherapy (see Figure 2). They are very useful for tumours where currently it is more difficult than usual to apply the techniques because of many critical structures to consider. Examples are those within the head and neck[14] and the brain[15]. Corresponding to neuro navigation systems the position of the actual needle and their virtual pathway is displayed before and during needle positioning.

Stereotactic external beam irradiation is usually used for intracranial small tumors. Extra precision in target localisation with a stereotactic frame or a noninvasive mask fixation[16] is required. High dose gradients at field edges minimise dose deposition outside the target volume.The volume of tissue beyond the target that receives a significant dose is strongly depended on target size and conformity of the isodose to the target[17]. Chang et al.[18] reportet about the results of a stereotactic radiosurgical boost of (median 12 Gy) following fractionated radiotherapy. 23 patients were achieved at a mean follow up of 21 month. The local control rate was 100%. This interesting study shows that stereotactic radiotherapy is also convertible for nasopharynx carcinoma which is normally adjacent to base of scull as a typical "stereotactic region". The method is also used with varying fractionation schedules for recurrent carcinomas with different response rates[19-21]. Because of the small number of patients, no statistical analysis is reliable, but the feasibility of the method is proved. The main advantages are the prevention of critical structures like the optic chiasma, the optic nerve and the mandible in case of nasopharynx carcinoma. Further studys have to evaluate the transfer of the method to other head and neck regions. In principle, every head and neck tumor can be treated by stereoactic radiotherapy with different safety margin depending on its localisation. Figure 3 shows the typical isodose distribution of stereotactic radiotherapy in the nasopharynx region, and the portal configurations (red lines). Corresponding to IMRT the excellent dosegradient to the normal tissue is visible.

Intensity modulated therapy (IMRT) is a new approach to 3-D treatment planning and conformal therapy optimizes delivery of radiation to irregularly shaped volumes through complex inverse treatment planning and dynamic delivery of radiation. The modulation of the fluence of photon beam profiles leads to a higher conformity of the target volume[22,23]. IMRT has the potential to significantly improve radiotherapy of head and neck cancer by reducing normal tissue dose and simultaneously allowing an escalation of the dose[24,25]. The technique allows the delivery of the dose distribution with concave isodose profiles into isolated areas excluding the surrounding radiosensitive normal tissue. Figure 4 shows a patient with a sinus maxillaris tumour. The sharp dosegradient and the high conformal irregular isodose distribution vis a vis adjacent critical structures in close proximity, like the optic chiasma, optic nerve, mandible, hypophysis or floor of the mouth, is presented. The high precision of the method depends also from exact localisation and repositioning of the patient, respectively as presented in case of stereotactic radiotherapy. Multiple studys are reporting about IMRT-techniques which are sparing the major salivary glands to provide late toxicity[26,27]. Especially the high incidence of xerostomia is decreased.

For patients with inoperable locoregional relapses or new primary after high dose radiotherapy for head and neck cancer, IMRT offers the possibility to perform re-irradiation by encompassing organs at risk with limited remaining radiation.

DISCUSSION

Recent advances in radiochemotherapy and alternated fractionation schedules are combined with higher acute and late toxicity. The most common acute sites for Grade 3 or worse acute effects are the mucous membranes and the pharynx[8]. Prevention and the symptomatic treatment described by Dörr et al.[28], plays particularly in case of higher incidence of the described side effects an important role. The results of a randomised multicenter study with Amifostin as a radioprotector are promising[26] Vacha et al. 1998[27] showed that Amifostine makes a reduction in radiation induced toxicity, on salivery glands and mucositis.

Modern radiotherapy techniques are also helpful in conserving normal tissue with new approaches to 3D treatment planning and conformal therapy. Basically, higher conformity of the dose volume is combined with decreasing dose homogeneity. The opposite effects are restricting the methods. In case of brachytherapy and administration of a concomitant boost the concept of maximal dose homogeneity is changed to particular inhomogeneouse dose-escalation in the macroscopic tumor region. The idea of dose escalation is also implemented in the concept of the established shrinking field technique. The only difference is the time of administration. The RTOG 9003 report presents that accelerated fractionation with concomitant boost seems to be tolerable by the patient as well as hyperfractionation with a higher incidence of acute side effects and equal toxicity levels for late effects. In principle accelerated fractionation with concomitant boost allows homogeneus dose escalation of nearly 200%, which is similar to brachytherapeutic dosage concepts. Furthermore two brachytherapeutic fractions with 3Gy single dose are normally tolerated by the patient. This could be arguments for brachytherapeutic applications. Brachytherapy is still the method with the highest dose gradients to the normal tissue. On the other hand Brachytherapy as well as IMRT is useful in recurrences when extern irradiation is contra-indicated because of previous irradiation.

In summary, due to recent advances the concept of multimodal therapy in head and neck cancer has to be changed, further studies are necessary to define the multimodality.

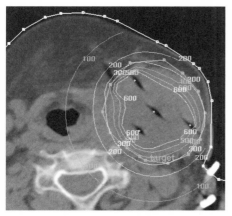

Figure 1. Needle configuration and dose distribution in case of head and neck metastasis. (With kindly permission form Prof. Zamboglou, Offenbach)

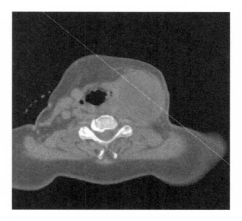

Figure 2. Preview of the needle pathway (yellow line) before positioning. The blue line correspondes to the meassured position of the actual needle.
(With kindly permission form Prof. Zamboglou, Offenbach)

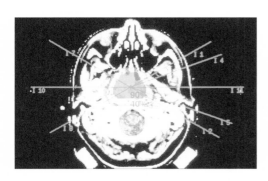

Figure 3. Dose distribution and portal field configuration of fractionated stereotactic radiotherapy treatment in case of nasopharynx carcinoma recurrence.

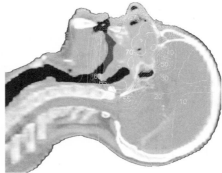

Figure 4. Dose distribution of a typically intensity modulated therapy treatment.

Table 1. Outcome of Simultaneous radiochemotherapy with alterrated fractionation schedules

Author	Patients	Radiochemotherapy schedule	Survival rate	Acute side effects
Wendt et al. 1998[1]	298	Hyperfractionated split course RT with Cisplatin and 5FU/leucovorin vs. Hyperfractionated split course RT	3 yr survival 48% vs. 24%	Grade 3 and 4 mucositis vs. 16%
Dobrowsky et al. 2000[2]	239	Hyperfractionated accelerated radiotherapy with Mitomycin C vs. Standard fractionation	3 yr survival 48% vs. 24%	Grade 3 mucositis 90% vs. 33%
Budach et al. 2000[3]	348	Accelerated hyperfractionated RT(reduced total dose) with Mitomycin C/5FU vs. Accelerated hyperfractionated RT	2 yr survival 61% vs. 45%	Equitoxic levels

REFERENCES

1. Wendt T, Grabenbauer G, Rodel C, Thiel H, Aydin H, Rohloff R, Wustrow T, Iro H, Popella C, Schalhorn A, Simultaneous radiochemotherapy versus radiotherapy alone in advanced head and neck cancer: a randomized multicenter study, J Clin Oncol 1998; 1318-24
2. Dobrowsky W, Jonathan N, Continuous hyperfractionated accelerated radiotherapy with/without mitomycin C in head and neck cancers, Radiother Oncol 57 2000; 119-124
3. Budach V, Haake M, Stuschke M, Stüben G, Jahnke K, Baumann M, Budach W, Sauer R, Wust P, Wernecke K, RTC is more effective than dose escalation in locally advanced H&N-Cancer – Results of a German multicentre randomized trial, Radiother Oncol 2000; 56 (Suppl.1): 45
4. Staar S, Rudat V, Dietz A, et al. Hyperfractionated (HF) Accelerated (ACC) Radiochemotherapy (RCT) versus HF/ACC Radiotherapy (RT) in Advanced Head and Neck (HN) Cancer – A Multicentric Randomized German Trial. Proc Am Soc Clin Oncol, 2000
5. Munro A, An overview of randomised controlled trials of adjuvant chemotherapy in head and Neck cancer. Br J Cancer 1995; 71 (1):83-91
6. El Sayed S, Nelson N, Adjuvant and ajunctive chemotherapy in management of squamous cell carcinoma of head and neck region. A meta analysis of prospective and randomized trials. J Clin Oncol 1996; 14(3):838-47
7. Pignon J, Bourhis J, Domenge C, Designe L, Chemotherapy added to locoregional treatment for head and neck squamous-cell carcinoma: three meta-analyses of updated individual data. MACH-NC Collaborative Group. Meta-Analisys of chemotherapy and radiation therapy for advanced-stage oropharynx carcinoma. J Natl Cancer Inst 1999; 91 (24): 2081-6
8. Fu K, Pajak T, Trotti A, Jones C, Spencer S, Phillips T, Garden A, Ridge J, Cooper J, Ang K, A Radiation Therapy Oncology Group (RTOG) phase III randomized study to compare hyperfractionation radiotherapy and two variants of accelerated fractionation to standard fractionation radiotherapy for head and neck squamous cell carcinomas: first report of RTOG 9003, Int J Radiat Oncol Biol Phys 2000; 48(1):7-16
9. Bratengeier K, Pfreundner L, Flentje M, Radiation techniques for head and neck tumors, Radiother Oncol 56 (2000) 209-220
10. Kovacs G, Hebbinghaus D, Dennert P et al. Conformal treatment planning for interstitial brachytherapy. Strahlenther Onkol 1996; 172: 469-74

11. Kolotas C, Baltas D, Zamboglou N, CT-Based Interstitial HDR Brachytherapy, Strahlenther Onkol 1999, 175: 419-27

12. Jacobs, H. Breast Conserving Therapy: Experience with HDR Afterloading Iridium- 192 Implants. In: Martinez, A.A., Orton, C.G., Mould, R.F, editors. Brachytherapie HDR and LDR. Dearborn Michigan USA. 1st Edition, Veenedaal: Nucletron International B.V. The Netherlands. 1989;251-256.

13. Ezzell, G. Physical principles of treatment planning in interstitial brachytherapy: role of optimisation. In: Zamboglou, N., editor. New Developments in Interstitial Remote Controlled Brachytherapy. 1st Edition, Wien: Zuckschwerdt Verlag. 1997;35-37.

14. Straßmann G, Kolotas C, Heyd R, Walter S, Baltas D, Martin T, Vogt H, Ioannidis G, Sakas G, Zamboglou N, Navigation system for interstitial brachytherapy, Radiother Oncol 2000; 56(1):49-57

15. Auer T, Hensler E, Eichberger P et al. 3D-Navigation for interstitial stereotactic brachytherapy. Strahlenther. Onkol. 1998;174:82-87.

16. Engenhart R, Wowra B, Debus J, Kimmig BN, Hover KH, Lorenz W, Wannenmacher M, The role of high-dose, single-fraction irradiation in small and large intracranial arteriovenous malformations, Int J Radiat Oncol Biol Phys 1994 15;30(3):521-9

17. Clifford K, Chao C, Perez L, Brady W, Stereotactic irradiation , In: Radiation Oncology: Management Decisions, Clifford K, Chao C, Perez L, Brady W (Eds), Lippincott – Raven, Philadelphia 1999, 73-77

18. Chang S, Tate D, Goffinet D, Martin D, Treatment of nasopharyngeal carcinoma: stereotactic radiosurgical boost following fractionated radiotherapy, Stereotact Funct Neurosurg 1999; 73 (1-4):64-7

19. Chua D, Sham J, Hung K, Kwong D, Kwong P, Leung L, Stereotactic radiosurgery as a salvage treatment for locally persistent and recurrent nasopharyngeal carcinoma, Head and Neck 1999; 21(7):620-6

20. Ahn Y, Kim D, Huh S, Baek C, Park K, Fractionated stereotactic radiation therapy for locally recurrent nasopharynx cancer: report of three cases, Head Neck 1999;21(4):338-45

21. Mitsuhashi N, Sakurai H, Katano S, Kurosaki H, Hasegawa M, Akimoto T, Nozaki M, Hayakawa K, Niibe H, Stereotactic radiotherapy for locally recurrent nasopharyngeal carcinoma, Laryngoscope 1999;109(5):805-9

22. Xia P., Fu KK, Wong GW, Akazawa C, Verhey LJ, Comparison of treatment plans involving intensity-modulated radiotherapy for nasopharyngeal carcinoma, Int J Radiat Oncol Biol Phys 2000; 48(2):329-37

23. Nutting C, Dearnaley DP, Webb S, Intensity modulated radiation therapy: a clinical review, Br J Radiol 2000; 73(869):459-69

24. Wu Q, Manning M, Schmidt-Ullrich R, Mohan R, The potential for sparing of parotids and escalation of biologically effective dose with intensity modulated radiation treatments of head and neck cancers: a treatment design study. Int J Radiat Oncol Biol Phys 2000 1; 48(2):329-37

25. The B; Woo S, Buttler E, Intensity modulated radiation therapy (IMRT): a new promising technology in radiation oncology,. Oncologist 1999; 4 (6): 433-42

26. Eisbruch A, Dawson L, Kim H et al. Conformal and intensity modulated irradiation of head and neck cancer: the potential for improved target irradiation, salivary gland function and quality of life. Acta Ortorhinolaryngol Belg 1999; 53(3):271-5

27. Kuppersmith R, Greco S, Teh B, Donovan D, Grant W, Chui J, Cain R, Butler E. Intensity – modulated radiotherapy: first results with this new technology on neoplasms of the head and neck, Ear Nose Throat J 1999; 78(4):238, 241-6, 248

28. Dörr W, Dölling-Jochem I, Baumann M et al., Therapeutische Beeinflussung der radiogenen oralen Mukositis. Strahlenther Onkol 1997; 173:183-92.

29. Strand V, Wannenmacher M, Brizel D, Sauer R et al., Randomized phase III trial of radiation +/- Amifostine in patients with head and neck cancer. Strahlenther onkol 1998; 174

30. Vacha P, Marx M, Engel A, Richter E, Feyerabend T, Side effects of postoperative radiochemotherapy with amifostine versus radiochemotherapy alone in head and neck tumors. Preliminary results of a prospective randomized trial. Strahlenther Onkol 1999; 175 4(2):18-22

TUMOR HYPOXIA AND ANGIOGENESIS
IN HEAD&NECK CANCERS

Juergen Dunst[1], Steffi Pigorsch[1], Peter Stadler[2], Axel Becker[1], Christine Lautenschläger[3], Michael Molls[2]
[1]Dept. of Radiation Oncology, Martin-Luther-University Halle-Wittenberg,
[2]Dept. of Radiation Oncology, Technical University Munich
[3]Depts. of Biostatistics, Martin-Luther-University Halle-Wittenberg

Correspondence to: Prof. Dr. Jürgen Dunst, Dept. of Radiation Oncology, Martin-Luther-University Halle-Wittenberg, Dryanderstrasse 4-7, D-06097 Halle, Germany, Phone: ++ 49 (345) 557-4310, Fax: : ++ 49 (345) 557-4333 (e-mail: juergen.dunst@medizin.uni-halle.de)

INTRODUCTION

Angiogenesis is a complex process involving proliferation, migration and differentiation of endothelial cells[1]. It is regulated by different cytokines of which the most important is vascular endothelial growth factor (VEGF). The expression of VEGF correlates with tumor growth and angiogenesis in experimental tumors[2-6]. The VEGF-protein can be detected immunohistologically in tumors. Quantitative measurement of the VEGF-protein in sera and cell culture supernatants has also been described[7]. Elevated levels of serum-VEGF have been detected in tumor-bearing animals and patients with cancer suggesting that tumors may release relevant amounts of VEGF in the blood circulation.

Tissue hypoxia is the most important stimulus for the up-regulation of VEGF[5, 7]. In this article, we therefore propose the hypothesis that the tumor´s microenvironment represents the main stimulus for angiogenesis.

MATERIALS & METHODS

Patients
From 1998 through 1999, 56 patients with head&neck cancers in whom serum levels of vascular endothelial growth factor (VEGF) were determined underwent additional

335

measurement of tumor oxygenation. Most of the patients had locally advanced disease. Further characteristics are outlined in table 1.

Tumor oxygenation, tumor volume, VEGF-measurements
Tumor oxygenation was measured with the invasive pO_2-histography using the Eppendorf device. According to most investigations in the literature, we classified pO_2-values below 5 mm Hg as hypoxic. Tumor volume was calculated separately at all tumor manifestations (primary tumor and all clinically involved lymph nodes in pretreatment CT-scans) in each individual patient using the ellipsoid formula ($V=1/6$ π x length x width x depth). The total tumor volume was then calculated as the sum of the volumes of all tumor manifestations in each patient. The absolute amount of hypoxic tumor volume was determined as the product of the absolute tumor volume and the relative frequency of hypoxic (< 5 mm Hg) measurements in the pO_2-histography. The concentration of the VEGF-protein ($VEGF_{165}$) in sera was measured with a quantitative immunoassay (Quantikine, R&D Systems, Europe).

RESULTS

Serum levels of VEGF
The serum VEGF levels in the 56 head&neck cancer patients ranged from 102 pg/ml through 1699 pg/ml (median 405 pg/ml, mean 527 ± 396 pg/ml). Elevated serum-VEGF-levels (>700 pg/ml) were found in 14/56 patients (25%).

Association between tumor hypoxia and VEGF
The association between VEGF-levels and various parameters was investigated in univariate analysis in the 56 patients with head&neck cancers (table 1). Serum-levels of VEGF were significantly correlated with hypoxic tumor volume ($R^2=0,63$, $p<0.001$), total tumor volume ($R^2=0,61$, $p<0.001$), hemoglobin levels ($R^2=-0.465$, $p<0.001$), platelet counts ($R^2=0,447$, $p=0.001$) and tumor hypoxia (pO_2-measurements <5mmHg, R^2-0.116, $p=0.043$). There was no correlation with T- and N-category, histological grading, and age.

In a second step, the association of elevated VEGF-levels with the hypoxic tumor volume was investigated for to determine whether tumor volume, tumor hypoxia or both parameters were important factors. In this model, tumor volume was divided in a hypoxic subvolume and an euoxic subvloume based on the oxygenation measurements. The highest correlation was found between the hypoxic tumor volume and VEGF-levels. Tumor volume, the relative frequency of hypoxia, and anemia were also significant factors for increased VEGF-levels. The association between the hypoxic volume and VEGF is further outlined in figure 1. Patients without tumor hypoxia (hypoxic volume = 0) had a mean serum-VEGF of 387 pg/ml (the cut-point of the graph with the y-axis in figure 1) which is nearly identical to the mean of a normal population without cancer. There was a significant linear relationship between the absolute amount of tumor hypoxia (hypoxic volume) and serum-VEGF.

DISCUSSION

It has been well demonstrated in experimental studies that VEGF is up-regulated in response to hypoxia in various tissues[9, 10]. Hypoxia is also a frequent phenomenon in malignant tumors and has been demonstrated to be a major prognostic factor[11-14]. It is therefore reasonable to assume that hypoxia-induced up-regulation of VEGF also occurs in human tumors in vivo. If this is the case, one can expect that the absolute amount of hypoxia within a certain tumor correlates with its angiogenic properties and the amount of VEGF-production.

The spatial distribution of oxygenation and hypoxia in a tumor is heterogeneous. Therefore, investigations of oxygenation require measurement of the oxygen partial pressure (pO_2) at numerous points within the tumor. The current gold-standard for measuring intratumoral hypoxia is the so-called pO_2-histography, an invasive polarographic measurement with needle probes[11]. This technique, however, yields information only on the relative amount of hypoxia (e.g. 30% of all measurements within a tumor reveal pO_2-values in the hypoxic range).

The absolute amount of hypoxia can be quantitified by multiplying the relative amount of hypoxia (pO_2-histography) with the total tumor volume yielding a new parameter, the absolute hypoxic subvolume. Stadler and coworkers have recently shown that this parameter correlates with prognosis in head&neck cancers[14]. In our investigation, the association of various parameters with serum levels of VEGF was determined. The highest correlation was found between the hypoxic tumor volume and serum levels of VEGF. This finding supports the hypothesis that intratumoral hypoxia is a major stimulus for angiogenesis in tumors. The angiogenic switch which has been proposed by Folkman[1] as a main event for tumor progression and metastasis might result from a tumor´s microenvironment that means from conditions which do not directly derive from specific molecular changes in the tumor cells themselves. The micoenvironment of a tumor may therefore represent an independent prognostic factor and a possible target for therapeutic interventions.

Table 1: Patients´ characteristics.

N	56
Measurements	<ul><li>serum-VEGF</li><li>tumor volume</li><li>intratumoral hypoxia (pO_2)</li></ul>
Age	<ul><li>mean: 59 ± 10 years</li><li>range: $37 - 77$ years</li></ul>
Type of disease	<ul><li>squamous cell head & neck cancers</li></ul>
Stages	<ul><li>Localized disease,</li><li>no distant metastases</li></ul>
Hemoglobin levels	<ul><li>mean: 12.7 ± 1.7 g/dl</li><li>range: $9.1 - 16.8$ g/dl</li></ul>

Figure 1: Correlation between the hypoxic tumor volume (with a $pO_2 < 5$mmHg) and serum levels of VEGF, p<0.001.

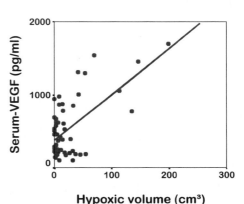

REFERENCES

1. Folkman J: Clinical implications of research on angiogenesis. N Engl J Med 333: 1757-1763, 1995
2. Linderholm B, Tavelin B, Grankvist K et al: Vascular endothelial growth factor is of high prognostic value in node-negative breast carcinoma. J Clin Oncol 16: 3121-3128, 1998
3. Linderholm B, Grankvist K, Wilking N et al: Correlation of vascular endothelial growth factor content with recurrences, survival, and first relapse site in primary node-positive breast carcinoma. J Clin Oncol 18: 1423-1431, 2000
4. Weidner N, Semple JP, Welch WR et al: Tumor angiogenesis and metastasis: correlation in invasive breast carcinoma. New Engl J Med 324: 1-8, 1991
5. Shweiki D, Neeman M, Itin A et al: Vascular endothelial growth factor induced by hypoxia may mediate hypoxia-initiated angiogenesis. Nature 359: 843-845, 1992
6. Plate KH, Breier G, Weich HA et al: Vascular endothelial growth factor is a potential tumour angiogenesis factor in human gliomas in vivo. Nature 359: 845-848, 1992
7. Claffey KP, Brown LF, del Aguila LF et al: Expression of vascular permeability factor/vascular endothelial growth factor by melanoma cells increases tumor growth, angiogenesis, and experimental metastasis. Cancer Res. 172: 172-181, 1996
8. Salven P, Mäenpää H, Orpana A et al: Serum vascular endothelial growth factor is often elevated in disseminated cancer. Clinical Cancer Research 3: 647-651, 1997
9. Chiarotto JA, Hill RP: A quantitative analysis of the reduction in oxygen levels required to induce up-regulation of vascular endothelial growth factor (VEGF) mRNA in cervical cancer lines. Brit J Cancer 80: 1518-1524, 1999
10. Shweiki D, Itin A, Soffer D et al: Vascular endothelial growth factor induced by hypoxia may mediate hypoxia-initiated angiogenesis. Nature 359: 843-845, 1992
11. Vaupel P: Oxygenation of human tumors. Strahlenther Onkol 166: 377-386, 1990
12. Nordsmark M, Bentzen MS, Overgaard J: Measurements of the human tumor oxygenation status by polarographic needle electrode. Acta Oncol 33: 383-389, 1994
13. Becker A, Stadler P, Lavey R et al: Severe anemia is associated with poor tumor oxygenation in head and neck squamous cell carcinoma. Int J Radiat Oncol Biol Phys 46: .., 2000
14. Stadler P, Becker A, Feldmann HJ et al: Influence of the hypoxic subvolume on the survival of patients with head and neck cancer. Int J Radiat Oncol Biol Phys 44: 749-754, 1999
15. Shweiki D, Itin A, Soffer D et al: Vascular endothelial growth factor induced by hypoxia may mediate hypoxia-initiated angiogenesis. Nature 359: 843-845, 1992

ACCELERATED RADIOCHEMOTHERAPY VS. STANDARD RADIOTHERAPY FOR NODAL POSITIVE AND NODAL NEGATIVE POSTOPERATIVE SQUAMOUS CELL CARCINOMA OF THE HEAD AND NECK: A RETROSPECTIVE ANALYSIS

Siefert A.[1], Pöllinger B.[1], Panzer M.[1,] Jund H.[2], Dühmke E.[1]
[1]Klinik für Strahlentherapie und Radioonkologie, Ludwigs-Maximilians-Universität, Munich, Germany
[2]Klinik für Hals-Nasen-Ohren-Kranke, Ludwigs-Maximilians-Universität, Munich, Germany

INTRODUCTION

Postoperative radiotherapy (RT) after surgical resection of squamous cell carcinomas of the head and neck is performed with the intention to eradicate residual disease at the former tumor site and the cervical lymphatic pathways. After combined treatment, earlier retrospective analysis[1-4] found a risk of locoregional failure of 15 - 45%, which varies in relation to risk factors such as histologic type, extension of nodal disease, resection margins, oral cavity as primary tumor site, etc. The randomised study of Peters et al.[5] established a higher risk of recurrence after doses less than 54 Gy. Dose escalation above 63 Gy did not improve the therapeutic ratio. In order to improve the results expecially of high risk patients other modes of treatment intensification have to be tested. Simultaneous chemotherapy with Mitomycin C[6] or Cisplatin[7] resulted in significantly better locoregional control. Recent considerations on tumor biology focus on the time factor[8]. The maximal tumor cell reduction, as achieved by surgery, is hypothesized to be a potent stimulus for tumor cell repopulation. Thus the postoperative setting appears to be characterised by accelerated tumor repopulation and an adequate answer could be an accelerated fractionation scheme as well as an early initiation of RT. A small randomised study[9] found no overall benefit for accelerated postoperative RT, however an advantage for tumors with a high [^{3}H]thymidine labelling index, i.e. for fast growing tumors.

This retrospective study compares the results of accelerated radio(chemo)therapy (aRCT) with those of standard radiotherapy (sRT) in patients treated postoperatively at the same institution during the same period.

MATERIALS AND METHODS

Patients and radio(chemo)therapy
From 1993 to 1996, 229 patients received RT after macroscopically complete resection of advanced tumors of oral cavity/floor of mouth, oropharynx, larynx and hypopharynx. 122 patients were treated with once-daily irradiation with a daily dose of 2.0 Gy five times per week. Tumors originating from or extending to larynx or hypopharynx were irradiated through lateral opposed fields with a 10 degree angle of table rotation to avoid the ipsilateral shoulder (dose calculated at midline). When the tumor had been confined to oropharynx or oral cavity/floor of mouth, RT was performed through lateral portals (dose calculated at midline) and a lower anterior neck field, the latter usually receiving 50.0 Gy in a tissue depth of 3 cm. Within the opposing fields 104 patients (85%) received 60 Gy (or 59.8 Gy) and 18 patients (15%) 62 - 70 Gy. Overall treatment time of 45 days and less is defined as sRT, longer treatment time is addressed as prolonged RT. Whereas most patients were irraditiated through the same portals over the whole course, in 26 cases (21%) total dose was given to shrinking fields (usually after 50 Gy). The spinal cord was excluded after 36.0 Gy.

107 patients received two fractions of 2.1 Gy per day (dose calculated at midline) with a time interval of 6 hours by the same irradiation techniques (b.i.d. RT). Irradiation was given on four days per week (omitting Wednesdays) with a treatment split of 7-14 days after two weeks up to a total dose of 56.7 Gy. First it was supposed that a two weeks break is needed for complete resolution of acute mucositis, but under optimal supportive care mucositis healed more quickly in many patients and the therapy free interval was routinely shortened to one week, resulting in an accelerated course of radiochemotherapy (aRCT), i.e. 56.7 Gy or 64.7 Gy within 35 days or less. 22 (21%) patients received a small volume boost of 4 x 2.0 Gy to the site of the tumor bed during the time of treatment split. On treatment days most patients received simultaneous Cisplatin at a dose of 6 mg/m^2 body surface (57 patients with cumulative dose > 66 mg) or Carboplatin at a dose of 50 mg/m^2 body surface (22 patients with cumulative dose > 550 mg). Chemotherapy was infused over 20-30 minutes immediately before the first RT-fraction in the morning. It was withhold in patients with compromised hearing and renal function, for frailness, multimorbidity, subnormal leuko- and thrombocyte counts and refused consent.

The decision in favor of one of the RT methods was at the discretion of the attending physician responsible for the patient. In the course of the observed period more patients were submitted to accelerated treatment because it was felt that this treatment was more effective. Although there was no randomisation and stratification, the two patient groups are balanced for gender, primary versus secondary treatment, tumor and nodal status, resection margins and short versus prolonged treatment time. The b.i.d. irradiated patients, however, had a significantly longer interval between surgery and start of RT and a trend for more UICC-tumor-stages III-IV. On the other hand there are significantly more tumors with the unfavourable oral cavity/floor of mouth tumor site (p=0.009) and G1-2 grading among the once daily irradiated patients.

Follow-up data were collected from the records of the Radiooncology and/or the Head, Nose and Ear Department. Patients, who did not continue the postherapeutic follow-up program at our institution, were contacted and informations were obtained from their private doctors for Head, Nose and Ear diseases.

RESULTS

Survival

Among all observed patients (n=229), the estimate for 4-year-overall-survival was 65% for all b.i.d. irradiated patients and 54% for all once daily treated patients (log rank p=0.221). By comparing the subgroups of patients with short treatment time, aRCT vs. sRT, there was a trend for better survival after accelerated treatment, but the difference was not significant (log rank p=0.097).

Locoregional control

For the 107 patients treated by b.i.d. RCT the actuarial 4-year-locoregional tumor control (control above clavicles) is 76%. For those 122 patients receiving once daily RT it amounts to 64%. The difference is not significant (log rank p=0.120). Among all patients (n=229) multivariate Cox regression analysis for independent prognostic factors was performed. Potential tumor and patient related variables were screened. The pathological nodal stage emerged as the most powerful prognostic factor. The estimate of 3-year-locoregional tumor control for the different pN-stages was as follows: pN0 84%, pN1 63%, pN2a 85%, pN2b 63%, pN2c 45% and pN3 41%. This allows us to descriminate a low risk group (pN0), a medium risk group (pN1,pN2a-b) and a high risk group (pN2c, pN3).

Among b.i.d. irradiated patients, those who completed their RCT within 35 days (i.e. accelerated treatment, n=65), had a better 4-year-locoregional control than those with longer treatment time, but the difference did not reach significance (log rank p=0.063). Among the patients with once daily RT those with a treatment time of 45 days or less (i.e. sRT, n=72) had a tendency for better locoregional control (log rank p=0.397).

The following analysis includes only those patients of both treatment groups who completed their therapy within 35 days or 45 days respectively. Multivariate Cox regression analysis for treatment related variables could not isolate a significant factor, type of RT treatment was the strongest factor but not significant (p=0.1303). In bilateral comparison, aRCT results in a barely significantly better 4-year-locoregional tumor control than sRT (p=0.047). Most subgroups defined by risk factors profited from aRT. Among the 65 patients receiving aRCT, 4-year-locoregional tumor control was 85% for those with simultaneous Cisplatin, 100% for those with Carboplatin and 83% for those without chemotherapy or low cumulative doses.

Distant metastasis

Multivariate Cox regression analysis identified pN-stage (p=0.0001), hypopharynx as tumor site (p=0.0021) and pN0/pN+ without extracapsular nodal disease versus pN+ with extranodal disease (p=0.0287) as significant predictors for distant metastasis. Within the subgroups of patients with short treatment time 4-year-freedom from distant metastasis was 84% after accelerated treatment and 75% after sRT; the difference is not significant.

Complications

Acute mucositis RTOG II-III was encountered in all observed patients. As there was no standardized prospective recording of acute side effects, this retrospective analysis relies on the remarks written in the records. Those receiving b.i.d. irradiations usually experienced a peak mucosal reaction during the treatment split and again at the end of RT. Those getting standard treatment had maximal mucositis during the last 2-3 weeks of therapy. Acute mucosits RTOG IV was documented for 3 of 107 patients receiving b.i.d. RCT. With intensive support (antibacterial and antimycotic) the therapy-free interval could be shortened without giving up the principle that mucositis should be healed (allowing receding mucositis RTOG I) before continuing treatment.

In this retrospective analysis, dead patients without documentation of complications, or patients alive with extensive local tumor recurrence were excluded (50 of 229 patients) from the evaluation of chronic side effects. Planned laryngectomy was not evaluated as a side effect, whereas the impossibility of regaining larynx function after temporary tracheostomy was addressed as complication. Under grade III toxicity were subsumed according to RTOG: severe laryngeal edema requiring corticosteroides, permanent laryngeal stridor with residual voice function, stenosis allowing only liquid nutrition, chronic severe mucositis, severe fibrosis, skin defect over mandibula metal implantate. As grade IV toxicity were categorized according to RTOG: radioosteonecrosis, stenosis requiring gastric tube feeding, laryngeal necrosis/death by obstruction of airway passage due to laryngeal edema, necrosis of mucosa. The hazard to develop grade III-IV complications after 4 years was 17% for the once daily irradiated patients and 31% for the b.i.d. treated patients, the difference not being significant (log rank, p=0.123). The difference for grade IV toxicity was more pronounced (hazard 4,4% versus 15,7%, log rank test p=0.016).

DISCUSSION

Locoregional tumor control in patients, whose treatment time was up to 45 days for once daily RT, and up to 35 days for b.i.d. RCT, was better than for those patients in each protocol completing therapy within a longer time. Among the twice daily-irradiated patients, the difference of aRCT and prolonged treatment (longer than 35 days) reaches significance (p=0.0509; log rank). By comparing postoperative sRT (60,0 Gy and more in up to six and a half weeks) to RCT of 56.7 Gy or 64.7 Gy over a maximum of five weeks, a significantly better 4-year-locoregional tumor control was found with accelerated fractionation. This benefit does not translate into significant better overall survival.

These observations confirm that treatment time has an important influence on the results of postoperative RT. They are in accordance with the experience of Amdur[1], who found significantly worse disease specific and overall survival for patients receiving postoperative RT in standard fractionation with treatment split.

On the other hand, no significant influence was found neither of the interval between surgery and start of RCT, which varied widely in this retrospective analysis (18 - 277 days, sign. longer for b.i.d. RCT), nor of overall treatment time, defined as interval between surgery and end of RCT (up to 70 days resp. up to 84 days or longer). Other authors[2, 5] report likewise about only a tendency for better tumor control if RT is begun within 6 weeks; in the retrospective analysis of Amdur et al.[1] the time interval was not prognostically relevant. There are, however, two reports about a significant influence of the time (4 resp. 6 weeks) between surgery and RT, both observing collectives of exclusively high risk patients[3, 10]. We observed better locoregional control within the aRCT group although there the mean interval between surgery and initiation of RT had been longer than in the sRT group. Accelerated radiotherapy might be able to compensate for some time elapsed. However, a subgroup of high risk patients (pN2c/3, R1-resection) with particularly long intervals between surgery and RT (mean 58 days in aRCT group vs. 44 days in sRT group) did not profit from aRCT. For high risk patients a long time between surgery and RT might be more detrimental, and limits might exist for this compensation.

Interestingly, high or moderate differentiation of squamous cell carcinoma appeared as a significant adverse factor. The ability to accelerated repopulation might be more developed in well/moderately differentiated tumors than in poorly differentiated ones[11].

Our data reconfirms earlier observations which find tumor features to be strong prognostic factors in postoperative RT. In order to compare different therapeutic approaches or the influence of the time factor, prognostic homogeneity among patient groups is important. Our retrospective data was gained from patient groups which differ somewhat in the distribution of risk factors with a preponderance of tumor site oral cavity/floor of mouth and histologic grading G1-2 in the standard treatment group, but on the other hand among the b.i.d. treated patients a longer interval between surgery and start of RCT.

For patients with high nodal stage, the risk to develop distant metastasis was impressively high (60% after 4-years for pN2c and pN3). Tumor site hypopharynx and extracapsular extension of nodal disease were also predictive of distant metastasis. Whereas the recurrance pattern after primery radio(chemo)therapy for inoperable head and neck tumors is dominated by locoregional failures[12], at least within this subgroup of patients distant metastases became a frequent cause of death. The efficacy of adjuvant chemotherapy to prevent distant metastasis in combination with postoperative RT is not established yet[13, 14].

Severe chronic toxicity was more often encountered after b.i.d.-RCT than after once daily RT (difference not significant), although most patients received a lower total dose than with standard fractionation. Other trials applying accelerated fractionation for head and neck tumors found significantly worse toxicity (overview[10]). We gave b.i.d. single doses of 2.1 Gy in midline eight fractions per week (weekly dose 16.8 Gy) according to a previously developed protocol[15]. As the reaction of late responding tissues is related to the size of dose per fraction, decreasing single dose to 1.8 Gy (nine fractions per week), as meanwhile implemented in our department, might reduce late complications. The fact that the applied accelerated split course RCT causes two "waves" of acute reactions might also contribute to chronic toxicity in the sense that each phase of acute toxicity might be partially transferred into "consequential late effects".

The retrospective data presented support the hypothesis that postoperative aRCT results in tendency for better locoregional control. Further evidence must be expected from a randomized trial with stratification according to risk factors as well as a constant intervall between surgery and initiation of RT. The long-term side effects are more frequent. Therefore other strategies to improve loco-regional control and decrease long-term side effects need to be investigated.

REFERENCES

1.	Amdur RJ, Parsons JT, Mendenhall WM, Million RR, Stringer SP and Cassisi NJ: Postoperative irradiation for squamous cell carcinoma of the head and neck: an analysis of treatment results and complications. Int J Radiat Oncol Biol Phys 1989;17: 25-36.

2.   Parsons JT, Mendenhall WM, Stringer SP, Cassisi N and Million RR: An analysis of factors influencing the outcome of postoperative irradiation for squamous cell carcinoma of the oral cavity. Int J Radiat Oncol Biol Phys 1997;39:137-148.

3.   Trotti A, Klotch D, Endicott J, Ridley M and Cantor A: Postoperative accelerated radiotherapy in high-risk squamous cell carcinoma of the head and neck: long-term results of a prospective trial. Head-Neck 1998; 20(2): 119-23.

4.   Zelefsky MJ, Harrison LB, Fass DE, Armstrong JG, Shan JP and Strong EW: Postoperative radiation therapy for squamous cell carcinomas of the oral cavity and oropharynx: impact of therapy on patients with positive surgical margins. Int J Radiat Oncol Biol Phys 1992;25: 7-21.

5.   Peters LJ, Goepfert H, Ang KK, Byers RM, Maor MH, Guillamondegui O, Morrison WH, Weber RS, Garden AS, Frankenthaler RA, Oswald MJ, Brown BW: Evaluation of the dose for postoperative radiation therapy of head and neck cancer: first report of a prospective randomized trial. Int J Radiat Oncol Biol Phys 1993;26: 3-11.

6.   Haffty BG, Son YH, Sasaki CT, Papac R, Fischer D, Rockwell S, Sartorelli A and Fischer JJ. Mitomycin C as an adjunct to postoperative radiation therapy in squamous cell carcinoma of the head and neck: results from two randomized clinical trials. Int J Radiat Oncol Biol Phys 1993;27:241-250.

7.   Bachaud J-M, David J-M, Boussin G and Daly N: Combined postoperative radiotherpy and weekly cisplatin infusion for locally advanced squamous cell carcinoma of the head and neck: preliminary report of a randomized trial. Int. J Radiat Oncol Biol Phys 1991;20: 43-246.

8.   Peters LJ and Withers RH: Applying radiobiological principles to combined modality treatment of head and neck cancer - the time factor. Int J Radiat Oncol Biol Phys 1997;39:831-836.

9.   Awwad HK, Khafagy Y, Barsoum M, Ezzat S, El-Attar I, Farag H, Akoush H, Meabid H and Zaghloul MS Accelerated versus conventional fractionation in the postoperative irradiation of locally advanced head and neck cancer: influence of tumour proliferation. Radiother Oncol 1992;25:261-266.

10.   Ang KK, Trotti A, Garden A, Foote RL Morrison WH, Geara FB and Peters LJ: Overall time factor in postoperative radiation: Results of a prospective randomised trial. Proceedings of the Fourth International Conference on Head and Neck Cancer. Toronto 1997.

11.   Hansen O, Overgaard J, Hansen HS, Overgaard M, Hoyer M, Jorgensen KE, Bastholt L and Berthelsen A: Importance of overall treatment time for the outcome of radiotherapy of advanced head and neck carcinoma: dependency on tumor differentiation. Radiother Oncol 1997;43:47-51.

12.   Wendt TG, Panzer M, Wustrow TPU, Hartenstein R: Pattern of Failure in Long-Term Survivors after Radio-Chemotherapy for Inoperable Head and Neck Cancer. Onkologie 1996; 19;419-422

13.   Laramore GE, Scott MS, Al-Sarraf M, Haselow RE, Ervin TJ, Wheeler R, Jacobs JR, Schuller DE, Gahbauer RA, Schwade JG and Cmpbell, BH: Adjuvant chemotherapy for resectable squamous cell carcinomas of the head and neck: report on intergroup study 0034. Int J Radiat Oncol Biol Phys 1992;23:705-713.

14.   Jacobs, C and Makuch, R: Efficacy of adjuvant Chemotherapy for patients with resesctable head and neck cancer: a subset analysis of the head and neck contracts program. J Clin Oncol 1990;8:838-847.

15.   Duehmke E, GeibelT, Golms R, Kaiser G, Notter G, Schröder M: Combined modality treatment of advanced head and neck cancer using low dose cisplatinum and accelerated fractionation. Strahlenther Oncol 1988;164:11-16.

344

CARBOPLATIN PLUS VINORELBINE AS PALLIATIVE TREATMENT FOR ADVANCED HEAD AND NECK OR OESOPHAGEAL CARCINOMA IN A SUBSET OF ELDERLY OR POOR PERFORMANCE STATUS (P.S.) PATIENTS

Koussis Haralabos[1], Chiarion-Seleni V.[1], Scola A.[1], Artioli G.[1], Nicoletto MO.[1], Andretta M.[2], Martínez-Monche G.[2], Ruol A.[3], Redi N.[1], Monfardini S.[1]
[1]Oncology dept. University of Padua, Italy
[2]Otorinolaringoiatric dept. University of Padua, Italy
[3]General Surgery IV. University of Padua, Italy

Correspondence to: *Dr. Koussis Haralabos, Divisione di Oncologia Medica, VI° piano Monoblocco, Ospedale Civile di Padova, Via Giustiniani 2 , Padova 35100. Italy, Phone: 0039 049 8212926 (E-mail: gonzalomm@libero.it, koussis@tin.it)*

INTRODUCTION

The aim of this study is to evaluate the efficacy of Carboplatin plus Vinorelbine in the treatment of metastatic or relapsed head and neck / oesophageal cancer after loco- regional treatment (surgery or radiation) or first line chemotherapy in elderly poor performance status patients.

In the Western World, approximately 50% of tumours are diagnosed in patients aged over 65 and represent the second cause of death after cardiovascular diseases.

The life expectancy of subjects aged over 65 is currently about 13 years for males and 17 for females.

Head and neck cancer currently represents approximately 22% of all neoplasms. These tumours mainly affect patients aged over 50, with a median survival of 50% at 5 years.

Oesophageal cancer mainly affects patients aged between 60-70 with an unfortunately poor prognosis and almost always with a global survival of less than one year.

These neoplasms often seem to have the same histology (squamous) and are sensitive to the same drugs.

The choice of treatment for locally advanced head-neck and oesophageal cancer is the association between chemotherapy and radiotherapy followed by surgery when possible [2, 1, 3, 4, 17, 18, 19].

Vinorelbine, a semisynthetic 5'-nor-vinca alkaloid modified in the catharantic ring, is a potent inhibitor of mitotic microtubule polymerization but is less active against axonal microtubules. This may explain the low incidence of severe effects related to Vincristine and Vinblastine that have been observed with Vinorelbine in clinical trials.

In this protocol Vinorelbine and Carbopatin have been used. Vinorelbine belongs to the Vinca Alkaloid-family and is a semi-synthetic derivative of Vinblastine. Vinorelbine is mainly metabolised in the liver and only 16% is eliminated via the kidney. It has a half life of approximately 20-30 hours.

Its activity in different neoplasms i.e. the breast, lung, ovary, head-neck and lymphomas is well known [20, 18, 30, 29, 28, 26, 25, 24, 23, 22, 5].

The dose-limiting toxicity is due to the non-cumulative and irreversible neutropenia. Due to the biochemical properties of this molecule, its toxicity causes hyperestesie, parestesie and constipation. Gastrointestinal toxicity, diarrhoea, vomiting, stomatitis and nausea is less frequent.

A particular type of toxicity of this drug is the diffused, muscular pain that involves both the smooth and the skeletral muscle, and in some cases chest pain, often associated with electrocardiographic alterations similar to an ischemic attack. These side effects lead to the simultaneous administration of Vinorelbine and a pain killer [27, 8].

Carboplatin, well known for its confirmed activity over the past years, is an antiblastic drug similar to Cisplatinum but more stable and less nephro-neurotoxic.

Carboplatin is mainly eliminated via the kidney. Calvert demonstrated that if the creatinine clearance is known, it is possible to individually modify the dose, thus avoiding an over or under dosage phenomena. This is possible by using the Area Under the Curve (AUC) that, considering the glomerular filtration, excludes the body surface from the calculation [16]. The major reported toxicity is haematological with leucopenia and piastrinopenia even with cumulative character, whereas nausea and vomiting are quite uncommon. Otoxicity, nephro-toxicity and neuro-toxicity, are possible but not frequent. We decided to use this schedule JM-8 and Vinorelbine due to the difficulty and often impossibility to treat elderly patients or patients in a poor general condition with the classical association of Cisplatin and 5FU, which are cardio-nephrotoxic.

Table 1.

Age	Gender	Type	Extension
56	F	Epiglottis + tongue	Not assessable
59	M	Inferior lip	Bone metastasis
62	M	Tongue + tonsil + tongue base	Not assessable
69	F	Tongue + oropharynx	T4 N2 M0
59	M	Tonsil	M+ lung
61	M	Oesophagus	Bone metastasis
59	M	Oesophagus	Relapse
61	M	Oesophagus	Relapse
69	F	Oesophagus	Local relapse
58	M	Sinus pyriform	T4 N2b
65	M	Oropharynx	T3 N3
70	F	Salivary gland	Large mass (>10 cm)
75	M	Tongue base + sinus pyriform	M+ lung
82	M	Tongue + tongue base	M+ lung
73	M	Tongue	N+ neck
67	M	Unknown origin	M+
75	M	Oesophagus	Relapse locally
70	M	Oesophagus	T4 N1
72	M	Oesophagus	M+ liver
51	M	Larynx	M+

Table 2. Patients' Characteristics

Number of patients	21
Male	17
Female	4
Median age	66 (range 51-82)
PS (Karnofsky)	80 (range 70-100)
Oesophagus	7
Oro-hypopharynx	9
Salivary glands	2
Larynx	1
Inferior lip	1
Unknown origin	1

Table 5. Results

Number of assessable patients	16
Complete responses	1
Partial responses	7
Disease progression	6
Still on therapy	2

MATERIALS AND METHODS

Patients were eligible if they had histologically confirmed diagnosis of squamous cell carcinoma of the head and neck or of the oesophagus and, with locally advanced disease (T3–T4, every N, M0-M+). Patients were required to have a radiologically, endoscopically and/or clinical assessable disease. Aged over 70 and/or a Performance Status ≤70. All patients presented written consent, and the trial was approved by the Ethical Committee-University

Hospital of Padua. Patients were excluded if they had inadequate bone-marrow reserve, renal, cardiac, hepatic and respiratory alterations or any other important concomitant diseases.

21 patients (17 male and 4 female) with an average age of 66 (51-82yrs) and median performance status of 70% (Karnofsky) (range 70-100) were treated with local or distant metastatic disease from head and neck or oesophageal cancer were treated (table 1 and 2). Eight had previously undergone surgery; five patients had previously received chemotherapy with Cisplatin or chemotherapy and concomitant radiotherapy. Six patients had undergone external radiotherapy, 1 patient photo-dynamic therapy and 1 patient brachytherapy (table 3).

Days 1 and 21, JM-8 AUC 4 were administrated and days 1, 8 and 21 Vinorelbine 25 mg/m^2. 48 courses were achieved (1-4, median courses 2).

Toxicity
18 patients were followed during treatment in order to evaluate the toxicity of the therapy.
Six patients presented haematotoxicity (grade 3-4) which represented the 33,3%. Neurological constipation grade 3 appeared in 3 patients (16,6%). Only 1 (5,5%) patient referred pain (table 4).
There were no deaths related to the toxicity of the treatment.

Table 3. Previous treatment

Chemotherapy	7
Surgery	9
External radiotherapy	7
Brachytherapy	1
Photodynamic therapy	1

Table 4. Toxicity

Evaluated	18
Haematologic (grade 3-4)	6 (33,3%)
Neurological constipation (grade 3)	3 (16,6%)
Pain	1 (5,5%)

RESULTS

Evaluated for response: 16 patients
The following results were seen upon evaluation of response: 1 complete response (CR) and 7 partial responses (PR) (CR+PR = 50%%), 6 disease progressions (37,5%) and 2 patients are still on therapy (12,5%)

CONCLUSION

These preliminary data suggest that this regimen is active in this subset of patients. The toxicity profile was mild.
This study is still in progress.

REFERENCES

1.   Airoldi M., Bumma C., Berletto O. Et al.: Vinorelbine for recurrent adenocarcinoma-like salivary gland malignancies. Eur J Cancer Oral Oncol, 32 B (3): 213-214, 1996.

2.   Ajani J.A.: Current status of new drugs and multidisciplinary approaches in patients with carcinoma of the oesophagus: Chest, Vol. 113 Suppl.1: 112S-119S, 1998,

3.   Ancona E., Ruol A., Castoro C. et al.: First-line chemotherapy improves the resection rate and long–term survial of locally advanced (T4, any N, M0) squamous cell carcinoma of the thoracic esophagus, final report on 163 consecutive patients with 5 year follow-up: Ann of Surg, Vol 226, 6: 714-7223,1997.

4.   Bedenne L., Seitz J.F., Milan C. et al.: Cisplatin, 5-FU, and preoperative radiotherapy in oesophageal epidermoid cancer. Multicenter phase II FFCD 8804 study: Gastroenterol. Clin. Biol.: Vol. 22 No. 3: 273.81, 1998.

5.   Gebbia V., Testa A., Di Gregorio C. et al.: Vinorelbine Plus Cisplatin in Recurrent or Previously Untreated Unresecable Squamous Cell Carcinoma of the Head and Neck. Am J Clin Oncol (CCT) 18(4): 293-296, 1995.

6.   Gridelli C. Perrone F., Monfardini S., et al.: Carboplatin plus Vinorelbine, a new well-tolerated and active regimen for the treatment of extensive-stage small cell lung cancer: a phase II study. Journal of Clinical Oncology. Vol. 16, No 4 (April): 1414-1419, 1998.

7.   Kawashima M., Ikeda H., Yorozu A., et al.: Clinical features of oesophageal cancer in theoctogenarian treated by definitive radiotherapy: a multi-institutional retrospective survey: Jpn J Clin Oncol., Vol 28 No 5: 301-307, 1998.

8.   Kornek G.V., Imperatory L., Casadei V., et al.: Acute tumor pain in patients with head and neck cancer treated with Vinorelbine. J Natl Cancer Inst., 88 (21): 1593, 1996.

9.   Koussis H., Chiarion-Selemi V., Scola A., et al.: Carboplatin plus Vinorelbine in head and neck or oesophageal carcinoma in the elderly or in patients with poor performance status (P.S.): Preliminary report. Annals of Oncology Vol 11, 2000 Suppl 4, Abstract 423 of the 25th ESMO Congress, Hamburg, Germany.

10.   Mattioli R., Imperatori L., Casadei V., et al.: The impact of Vinorelbine in the elderly (aged>70 years) with NSCLC: A preliminary report. Eur J of Cancer, Vol 33, Suppl 8, ECCO, 1997.

11.   Monfardini S. Chabner B.: Joint NCI-EORTC Consensus Meeting on Neoplasia in the elderly. Eur J Cancer, Vol. 27, No 5: 653 654, 1991.

12.   Oliveira J., Geoffrois L., Roland F., et al.: Activity of Navelbine on lesions within previoiuly irradiated fields in patients with metastatic and/or local recurrent squamous cell carcinoma of the Head and Neck (SCHNC): an EORTC-ECSG study. Proceedings of ASCO, Vol 16: 406[a], 1997

13.   Pignon T., Gregor A., Schaake-Koning C., et al.: Age has no impact on acute and late toxicity of curative thoracic radiotherapy. Radiother. Oncol., Vol 46 No 3: 239-248, 1998

14.   Prince P., Hoskin P.J., Hutchinson T., et al.: What is the role of radiation-chemotherapy in the radical non-surgical management of carcinoma of the oesophagus? Upper GI Cancer Working Party of the UK Medical Research Council: BR. J. Cancer, Vol 78 No 4: 504-507, 1998.

15.   Saxman S., Mann B., Canfield V. et al.: A phase II trial of Vinorelbine in patients with recurrent or metastatic squamous cell carcinoma of the head and neck. Am J Clin Oncol, 21 (4): 398-400, 1998.

16.   Shimizu T., Yoshida M., Makishima K.: Importance of AUC of Carboplatin in head and neck cancer. Nippon-Jibinkoka-Gakkai-Kaiho, 101 (3): 259-265,1998

17.   Smith TJ, Ryan LM, Douglass HO., et al.: Combined chemotherapy vs radiotherapy alone for early stage squamous cell carcinoma of the oesophagus: a study of the Eastern Cooperative Oncology Group: Int J Radioat Oncol. Biol. Phys., Vol 42 No 2: 69-276, 1998

18.   Sorio R., Robieux I., Monfardini S., et al.: Pharmacokinetics and tolerance of Vinorelbine in elderly patients with metastatic breast cancer. Eur J of Cancer, Vol. 33, No 2: 301-303, 1997

19.   Stahl M., Vanhoefer U., Stuschke M. Et al.: Pre-operative sequential chemo and radiochemotherapy in locally advanced carcinoma of the lower oesophagus and gastro-oesophageal junction: Eur J Cancer, Vol 34, No 5: 668-673,1998

20.   Tononi A., Panzini I., Oliviero G., et al.: Vinorelbine chemotheapy in non small cell lung cancer. Experience in elderly patients. Eur J of Cancer, Vol 32AA No 10: 1809-1811, 1996

21.   Fleming TR (1982) One sample multiple testing procedure for phase II clinical trails. Biometrics, 38: 143-151

22.   Gebbia V., Testa A., Valenza R., et al.: A pilot Study of Vinorelbine on a weekly schedule in recurrent and /or metastic squamous cell carcinoma of head and neck. Eur J Cancer Vol 29, No 9: 1358-1359, 1993.

23.   Gebbia V., Mantovani G., Agopstata B., Contu A., et al.:Treatment of recurrent and metastatic squamous cell head and neck carcinoma with a combination of Vinorelbine, Cisplatin and 5-Fluoracil: A multicenter phase II trial. Annals of Oncology 6: 987-991, 1995

24.   Testolin A., Recher G., Cristoferi V., Gasparini G.: Vinorelbine in pre-tested advanced head and neck squamous cell carcinoma. A phase II STUDY. Investigational new drugs 12: 231-234, 1994

25.   Koenek V., Scheithauer W., Glaser C., Toth J., et al.: Vinorelbine and Carboplatin in recurrent and/or metatastatic squamous cell carcinoma of head and neck. Oncology 56: 24-27, 1999

26.   Colleoni M., Gaion F., Nelli P., et al.: Vinorelbine in elderly patients with non small-cell lung cancer. Tumori 80: 448-452, 1994

27.   Colleoni M., Gaion F.,Vicario G., et al.: Pain in tumor site after Vinorelbine injection: description of an unexpected side effect. Tumori 81: 194- 196, 1995

28.   Masotti A., Borzellino, Zannini G., et al.: Efficacy and toxicity of Vinorelbine-Carboplatin combination in a treatment of advanced adenocarcinoma or large cell carcinoma of the lung. Tumori 81: 112-116, 1995

29.   Crawford J, O'Rourke MA: Vinorelbin (Navelbine) Carboplatin combination therapy: dose intensification with granulocyte colony-stimulating factor. Sem in Oncol Vol 21, No 5, Suppl 10: 73-8, 1994

30.   Jacoulet P., Breton JL, Westeel V., et al: A phase I study of Vinorelbine and Carboplatin in advanced non small cell lung cancer. Lung Canceer 12: 247-257. 1995

CONCOMITANT CHEMOIRRADIATION
– PACLITAXEL AS RADIATION MODIFIER

Jaakko Pulkkinen, MD, PhD and Reidar Grénman, MD, PhD
Department of Otorhinolaryngology – Head and Neck Surgery, Turku University Central
Hospital, Turku, Finland

Correspondence to: Dr. Grénman at Department of Otorhinolaryngology, PL 52, 20521
Turku, Finland

ABSTRACT

Concomintant chemoirradiation has proven superior to conventional radiotherapy in several
tumour types including head and neck cancer. A significant survival advantage was found
with concomitant chemoirradiation of head and neck cancer in large meta-analysis, whereas
adjuvant or neoadjuvant treatment could not show a similar effect. Several drugs have been
used in this setting. The taxans are good examples showing the theoretical background for this
treatment approach.

Paclitaxel (Taxol®), which belongs to the group of taxans, is an antimicrotubule drug that not
only stabilizes microtubules by inhibiting their dissassembly, but also promotes their
assembly. Head and neck squamous cell cancer (SCC) as well as vulvar SCC cells are in vitro
highly sensitive to paclitaxel, which causes growth inhibition already ad nanomolar
concentrations. The cells are blocked by the drug in the G2-M phase, which is the most
radiosensitive phase of the cell cycle, whereafter they undergo an apoptotic cell death after 6
to 24 hours. The intrinsic radiosensitivity of the SCC cell lines used measured as area under
the survival curve (AUC) varied from 1.4 Gy to 2.9 Gy measured with a 96 well plate
clonogenic assay. An additive effect of radiation and paclitaxel was seen with all cell lines
tested and with all drug concentrations used.

With time-lapse videomicroscopy 2-3 Gy radiation caused only a propagated apoptotic
response in some cell lines. Paclitaxel at 1-5 nM concentration caused int the cell lines studied
a moderate decrease in mitotic frequency and an increase in the apoptotic cell death. After a
24 hour exposure to the same concentration of paclitaxel the same radiation dose caused a
significantly increased apoptosis to mitosis ratio showing the additive cytotoxic effect.

INTRODUCTION

Despite intensive efforts in primary prevention, screening and therapy, long term survival rates for head and neck tumours have not improved significantly over the last 30 years, with overall 5-year survival rate varying between 67% - 75%.[1]

Adjuvant or neo-adjuvant chemotherapy has been used in a large number of clinical studies but little effect on survival has been reported. On the other hand a large meta-analysis summarising the randomised trials between 1965 to 1993 where concomitant chemo-irradiation has been used in head and neck cancer showed a survival benefit.[2] This finding has since been supported by results of several recent reports.[3-6]

Paclitaxel (Taxol®) is a novel drug derived from the bark of the western yew, *Taxus brevifolia*. Paclitaxel promotes microtubule assembly and stabilises microtubules resulting a G2/M block in the cell cycle, which is a different kind of mechanism from those of other chemotherapeutic agents.[7] The clinical antitumour activity of paclitaxel is among the broadest of any agent in our therapeutic armamentarium against cancer.[8] Clinically this drug has shown to be effective in treating human ovarian cancer, breast cancer, lung cancer and head and neck cancer.[8, 9]

Here we describe our findings with pacltaxel alone and in combination with radiation on head and neck squamous cell carcinoma (SCC) *in vitro*. The focus is on the role of apoptosis in laryngeal cancer cells, its effect on radiation response, the chemotherapeutic response of paclitaxel alone and in combination with irradiation. We used a paclitaxel concentration of 10 nM, which is only 1/10-1/120 of the concentration achieved in the patient serum after a single dose of about 200 mg/m^2.

MATERIALS AND METHODS

Cells
Nine head and neck SCC cell lines established in our laboratory were investigated. Information on the origin of the cell lines (primary tumour location, TNM, specimen site, type of lesion, histological grade) and the intrinsic radiosensitivity measured in the 96-well plate clonogenic assay as the area under the survival curve (AUC, corresponding to the mean inactivation dose), SF$_2$ (surviving fraction at 2 Gy), doubling time are listed in Table 1.[10] The cells were maintained by weekly or bi-weekly passages in complete Eagle's minimal essential medium with 2 mM glutamine, 1% nonessential amino acids, 100 U/ml penicillin, 100 µg/ml streptomycin, and 10% fetal bovine serum. All cells were cultured in monolayers in plastic tissue culture dishes (25-cm^2).

Flow cytometry
Flow cytometry measurements of the DNA content in the cultures exposed to paclitaxel and control cultures exposed to paclitaxel and control cultures were taken 24 and 48 h after exposure to paclitaxel. The cells were harvested from the culture flasks by trypsinization; they were then washed and centrifuged, and resuspended in preservative containing equal volumes of citric acid-buffered saline and 96% ethanol.[12] Before flow cytometry the samples were

washed with phosphate-buffered saline, processed and stained with propidium iodine.[13] The samples were analysed with a FACStar flow cytometer (Becton-Dickinson Immunocytometry Systems, Mountain View, CA) as described.[12] A 488 nm argon laser line run at 600 mW was used for fluorescence excitation. A peak width-area analysis to gate out doublets was used. For each histogram 20,000 particles were analysed. MultiCycle software was used to calculate the percentage of cells in different phases of the cell cycle.

Table 1. The charasteristics of head and neck SCC cell lines.

Cell line UT-SCC-	Tumour site	Tumour TNM	Specimen site	Grade	AUC* (Gy)	SF₂†	DT (h)
4	Larynx	T4N0M0	Larynx	G2	1.7±0.02	0.35±0.07	
5	Oral tongue	T1N1M0	Tongue	G2	2.3±0.3	0.45±0.07	44
6B	Supraglottic larynx	T2N1M0	Neck metastasis	G1	2.0±0.1	0.37±0.02	97
8	Supraglottic larynx	T2N0M0	Larynx	G1	1.9±0.1	0.37±0.03	26
9	Glottic larynx	T2N0M0	Neck metastasis	G1	1.4±0.1	0.25±0.03	49
10	Oral tongue	T1N0M0	Tongue	G2	1.9±0.1	0.35±0.04	30
19A	Glottic larynx	T4N0M0	Larynx	G2	1.7±0.1	0.32±0.02	33
19B	Glottic larynx	T4N0M0	Larynx‖	G2	1.7±0.1	0.33±0.08	32
22	Glottic larynx	T1N0M0	Larynx	G1	1.8±0.1	0.30±0.02	
24A	Base of tongue	T2N0M0	Tongue	G2	2.6±0.3	0.52±0.06	30
29	Glottic larynx	T2N0M0	Larynx	G1	1.8±0.1	0.36±0.05	42

*AUC = Area under the survival curve (mean ± standard deviation) referring to mean inactivation dose
†SF₂ = Surviving fraction at 2 Gy (mean ± standard deviation)
DT = Doubling time
‡Reference[11]
‖Persistent disease at primary site after irradiation

Irradiation and clonogenic assay
To measure the intrinsic radiosensitivity of the cell lines, the cells were grown to midlogaritmic phase and fed with fresh medium on the day before the experiments. The 96-well plate clonogenic assay was performed as described earlier.[14] Shortly, the cells were plated into 96-well culture plates and incubated for 24 hours in a cell culture incubator. Irradiation was performed the next day at room temperature using a 4-MV photon beam that delivers a dose rate of 2 Gy/minute (Clinac 4/100, Varian, Calif. USA). After incubation the plates for four weeks, the number of positive wells was counted using a phase-contrast microscope. For the time-lapse video microscopy, the cells were irradiated in culture flasks using 2 Gy and 3 Gy radiation doses.

Time-lapse video microscopy
1-4 days after plating, prior to starting the experiments, the cells were fed with fresh medium. The medium was changed every 96 hours for longer experiments. The culture flask was transferred immediately after irradiation to a 37° C heated stage of an inverted microscope (Nikon, Diaphot, Nikon Corp., Tokyo, Japan) and the filming was started. Cells were viewed using phase-contrast optics at 20x objective magnification coupled to a JVC 3CDD KY-F30

video camera (Victor Company, Tokyo, Japan). An edge of a representative colony was selected for the field to be analysed containing approximately 20 - 60 cells according to the cell size (median 37.5, range 12 - 80). The time-lapse video recording was performed so that two successive pictures were taken at 30 second intervals (Panasonic AG-6720A). The video recorder and the microscope were coupled to a timer (LIBT2, Red Lion, USA) which lit the microscope lamp for five seconds in every 30 seconds in synchrony with the recorder. The culture flask was shielded from ambient room light.

Filming was continued for 96 hours (or for 12 days in four experiments). Subsequently the film was viewed frame by frame on video monitor. The cumulative numbers of premitoses, mitoses, apoptoses and necroses per field were counted at 24-hour intervals. Premitosis was considered to have begun when a cell became round and condensed. Mitosis was considered to have ended with the appearance of cell division. An apoptotic cell death was recorded either when a flat cell condensed rapidly (interphase apoptosis) and died after violent cytoplasmic pulsation and blebbing or an already condensed cell (considered as premitotic) or two daughter cells died simultaneously soon after division (mitotic and post-cytolytic apoptosis correspondingly). Necrosis was characterised by a noncycling cell dying after a rapid swelling and rupture of cell membranes. Every experiment was recorded successfully three to five times (except the 12-day experiments, which were recorded once).

Data analysis
The fraction survival data as a function of radiation dose were fitted by linear quadratic equation $S = \exp(-(\alpha D + \beta D^2))$. The area under the survival curve (AUC) values, corresponding to the mean inactivation dose ($\overline{D}$), were calculated by numerical integration from the fitted survival curve. In addition, the SF_2 was calculated from the fit.[14, 15] To analyse the statistical significance ($P < 0.05$), two-sample t-test was used if not otherwise stated. The P values are two-tailed and Chi square test was used for four-fold table analysis.

RESULTS

The effect of paclitaxel on the cell cycle distribution was studied in seven cell lines. Accumulation of cells in the G2-M-phase was observed in all cultures after 24-h exposure to 10 nM paclitaxel. After 48-h exposure to the drug, the percentage of cells in the G2-M phase was clearly increased in all cell lines in comparison with the control cultures. In cell lines UT-SCC-19A, UT-SCC-19B and UT-SCC-22, paclitaxel had a dramatic effect on the cell cycle distribution: more than 70% of the cells were in the G2-M phase after 24-h exposure to 10 nM paclitaxel (Table 2.).[16]

Table 2. The effect of paclitaxel (10nM) on the cell cycle of the laryngeal squamous cell carcinoma after 24 and 48 h of exposure, measured with flow cytometry.[16]

Cell line	G2/M%			
	Control 24 h	Paclitaxel 24 h	Control 48 h	Paclitaxel 48 h
UT-SCC-4	5.1	13.4	13.2	50.5
UT-SCC-8	5.4	12.4	10.8	24.1
UT-SCC-9	15.6	17.3	26.7	42.5
UT-SCC-19A	18.8	71.7	17.8	72.1
UT-SCC-19B	21.8	75.5	25.3	47.5
UT-SCC-22	14.1.	73.6	10.6	75.4
UT-SCC-29	19.8	47.9	20.0	46.6
Median	15.6	47.9	17.8	47.5
Average	14.4	44.5	17.8	51.2

Time-lapse video microscopy was used to analyse the morphological changes induced by 10 nM paclitaxel in the cultured laryngeal SCC cells. The control cultures of all cell lines showed frequent mitoses. Apoptoses were also seen in the control cultures; they represented 12%-25% of the initial cell number. In the cultures treated with 10 nM paclitaxel the cells rounded up at the same pace as the control cells underwent mitoses. They stayed mitotically arrested for 6-24 h, after which the cells died morphologically by apoptosis i.e. by cellular shrinkage, violent pulsation and blebbing of the plasma membrane during subsequent hour. No mitoses or necroses were observed in the paclitaxel-treated cells. The apoptoses represented 46 – 84% of the initial cell number (Table 3.). In some paclitaxel-treated cultures some of the cells escaped the mitotic arrest without cytokinesis and formed multinucleated cells. These multinucleated cells eventually died very rapidly (in few minutes) showing cell shrinkage, i.e. one of the typical signs for apoptotic cell death.[17]

Table 3. The cumulative number of cells completing mitoses or undergoing apoptoses during 96 h in a medium containing 10 nM paclitaxel. The figures are percentages of the initial cell number and n is the initial cell number.[17]

Cell line	Control culture				10 nM paclitaxel			
	Mitoses (%)	Apoptoses (%)	Time (h) in premitotic phase	N	Mitoses (%)	Apoptoses (%)	Time (h) in premitotic phase	N
UT-SCC-8	142	13	1	31	0	84	24	25
UT-SCC-9	146	12	1	55	0	57	14	45
UT-SCC-19A	240	25	1	20	0	51	16	43
UT-SCC-19B	150	17	1	36	0	46	24	50
UT-SCC-29	65	12	1	40	0	57	6	45

The time-lapse video microscopy was further used to analyse the effect of irradiation and irradiation and paclitaxel concomitantly used. The 2 Gy irradiation decreased the mitotic frequency in three cell lines (AUC 1.4 – 1.7 Gy) but failed to do so in two (AUC 1.8 and 1.9 Gy), when compared to control cultures. The 2 Gy or 3 Gy irradiation did not induce a clear propagated apoptotic response in any of the cell lines studied. Sporadic necrotic cell death was observed after irradiation (Table 4).

5 nM (UT-SCC-8,UT-SCC-9) or 1 nM (UT-SCC-19A, UT-SCC-19B, UT-SCC-29) paclitaxel induced a mild apoptotic response but did not affect the mitotic frequency significantly. The cells that stayed mitotically arrested were doomed to die by apoptosis. The combination of 5 nM or 1 nM (see above) paclitaxel followed by irradiation with 2 Gy inhibited mitotic activity and caused greatly increased apoptotic cell death. The propagated apoptotic response and the inhibitory effect on the mitotic activity were clearly more distinct as time passed by after irradiation (Table 4).[18]

Table 4. The effect of paclitaxel, irradiation and paclitaxel and irradiation concomitantly used on apoptotic and mitotic frequencies in HNSCC cell lines.[18]

Experiment	Apoptoses/n	Mitoses/n	Apoptoses/Mitoses
Control	0.14 (55/399)	1.16 (463/399)	0.12
Irradiation (2Gy)	0.15 (22/147)†	0.77 (113/147)	0.19
Paclitaxel*	0.30 (55/180)	0.85 (153/180)	0.36
Paclitaxel* + Irradiation (2Gy)	0.45 (99/219)†	0.13 (29/219)	3.41

n = Initial cell number
*5 nM paclitaxel for UT-SCC-8 and UT-SCC-9 and 1 nM paclitaxel for UT-SCC-19A, UT-SCC-19B and UT-SCC-29
†Sporadic necroses

DISCUSSION

It has been postulated that paclitaxel might act as a radiosensitiser by inducing a G2-M block, as this phase is known to be a radiosensitive phase of the cell cycle.[19] On the other hand it has been suggested that paclitaxel potentates tumour radioresponse by other mechanisms in addition to blocking the cell cycle in mitosis.[20] Later this drug was reported as having a cytotoxic effect even in radioresistant or chemoresistant cell lines to other drugs by inducing apoptosis through p53-independent mechanism.[21]

In our study paclitaxel and irradiation with 2 Gy concomitantly used induced an increased cell death by apoptosis compared to the treatment involving a single agent. This effect seemed also to be due to other mechanism of action than the premitotic block, namely the cells which where mitotically arrested at the time of irradiation where doomed to die even without irradiation.[17, 18]

The combined effect of paclitaxel and radiation has been reported to be supra-additive or synergistic in some studies,[22-24] though there were other publications indicating that paclitaxel had only an additive effect with irradiation.[25, 26] In our study, an additive effect of paclitaxel and radiation was seen with doses readily achievable in clinical treatment. However, the exposure time of 96 hours to paclitaxel may be longer than can be achieved in head and neck cancer tissue *in vivo* after a single infusion of paclitaxel.
These studies give a good experimental basis for the clinical use of irradiation and paclitaxel concomitantly.

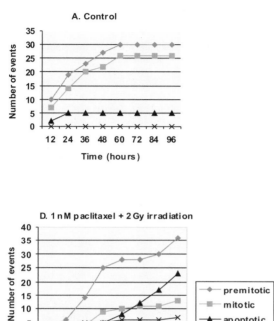

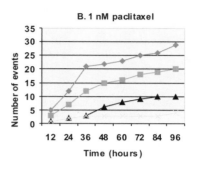

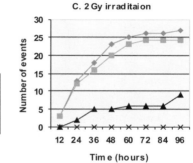

Figure 1. UT-SCC-29 cells followed by time-lapse videomicroscopy. The figure shows the cumulative number of cells per field entering mitosis (premitotic), succesful mitoses, apoptoses and multinucleated cells (mnc) as a function of time. Panel A shows the control culture, panel B the effect of 1 nM paclitaxel, panel C the effect of 2 Gy irradiation and panel D the effect of 1 nM paclitaxel and 2 Gy irradiation concomitantly used. The initial number of cells per field in the beginning of the filming was 40, 29, 23 and 45 respectively. In addition one necrotic cell death was seen in panel D 40 hours after irradiation.[18]

REFERENCES

1. Shah JP, Karnell LH, Hoffman HT, Ariyan S, Brown GS, Fee WE, et al. Patterns of care for cancer of the larynx in the United States. Arch Otolaryngol Head Neck Surg 1997;123:475-483.
2. Pignon JP, Bourhis J, Domenge C. Chemotherapy added to locoregional treatment for head and neck squamous-cell carcinoma: three meta-analyses of updated individual data. Lancet 2000;355:949-955.
3. Munro AJ. An overview of randomised controlled trials of adjuvant chemotherapy in head and neck cancer. Br J Cancer 1995;71:83-91.

4.   Calais G, Alfonsi M, Bardet E, Sire C, Germain T, Bergerot P, et al. Randomised trial of radiation therapy versus concomitant chemotherapy and radiation therapy for advanced-stage oropharynx carcinoma. J Natl Cancer Inst 1999;91(24):2081-2086.

5.   Wendt TG, Grabenbauer GG, Rodel CM, Thiel HJ, Aydin H, Rohloff R, et al. Simultaneous radiochemotherapy versus radiotherapy alone in advanced head and neck cancer: a randomised multicenter study. J Clin Oncol 1998;16(4):1318-1324.

6.   Merlano M, Vitale V, Rosso R, Benasso M, Corvo R, Cavallari M, et al. Treatment of advanced squamous-cell carcinoma of the head and neck with alternating chemotherapy and radiotherapy. N Engl J Med 1992;327(16):1115-1121.

7.   Schiff PB, Horwitz SB. Taxol stabilizes microtubules in mouse fibroblast cells. Proc Natl Acad Sci USA 1980;77:1561-1565.

8.   Rowinsky EK, Donehower RC. Drug therapy: Paclitaxel (Taxol). N Engl J Med 1995;332:1004-1014.

9.   Forastiere AA. Use of paclitaxel (Taxol) in squamous cell carcinoma of the head and neck. Semin Oncol 1993;20:56-60.

10.   Pekkola-Heino K, Jaakkola M, Kulmala J, Grénman R. Comparison of cellular radiosensitivity between different localizations of head and neck squamous cell carcinoma. J Cancer Res Clin Oncol 1995;121:452-456.

11.   Servomaa K, Kiuru A, Grénman R, Pekkola-Heino K, Pulkkinen JO, Rytömaa T. p53 mutations associated with increased sensitivity to ionizing radiation in human head and neck cancer cell lines. Cell Prolif 1996;29:219-230.

12.   Alanen kA, Klemi PJ, Joensuu H, Kujari H, Pekkala E. Comparison of fresh, ethanol-preserved, and paraffin embedded samples in DNA-flow cytometry. Cytometry 1988;10:81-85.

13.   Vindelöv LL, Christensen IJ, Nissen NI. A detergent-trypsin method for the preparation of nuclei for cytometric DNA analysis. Cytometry 1983;3:323-327.

14.   Grénman R, Burk D, Virolainen E, Buick RN, Church J, Schwartz DR, et al. Clonogenic cell assay for anchorage-dependent squamous carcinoma cell lines using limiting dilution. Int J Cancer 1989;44:131-136.

15.   Kulmala J, Rantanen V, Pekkola-Heino K, Tuominen J, Grénman R. Dosimetry of irradiation models. Acta Oncol 1995;34:105-109.

16.   Elomaa L, Joensuu H, Kulmala J, Klemi P, Grénman R. Squamous cell carcinoma of the larynx is highly sensitive to paclitaxel in vitro. Acta Otolaryngol (Stockh) 1995;115:340-344.

17.   Pulkkinen JO, Elomaa L, Joensuu H, Martikainen P, Servomaa K, Grénman R. Paclitaxel-induced apoptotic changes followed by time-lapse video microscopy in cell lines established from head and neck cancer. J Cancer Res Clin Oncol 1996;122:214-218.

18.   Pulkkinen JO, Pekkola-Heino K, Grénman R. Paclitaxel and irradiation induce apoptosis in squamous cell carcinoma cell lines in an additive way. Anticancer Res 1996;16:2923-2930.

19.   Sinclair WK. Cyclic X-ray responses in mammalian cells in vitro. Radiat Res 1968;33:620-643.

20.   Milas L, Hunter NR, Mason KA, Kurdoglu B, Peters LJ. Enhancement of tumor radioresponse of a murine mammary carcinoma by paclitaxel. Cancer Res 1994;54:3506-3510.

21.   Wahl AF. Loss of normal p53 function confers sensitization to Taxol by increasing G2/M arrest and apoptosis. Nature Med 1996;2:72-79.

22.   Choy H, Rodrigues FF, Koester S, Hilsenbeck S, von Hoff DD. Investigation of Taxol as a potential radiation sensitizer. Cancer 1993;71:3774-3778.

23.   Liebmann J, Cook JA, Fisher J, Teague D, Mitchell JB. In vitro studies of Taxol as a radiation sensitizer in human tumor cells. J Natl Cancer Inst 1994;86:441-446.

24.   Saito Y, Mitsuhashi N, Takahashi T, Sakurai H, Nozaki M, Ishikawa H, et al. Cytotoxic effects of paclitaxel (taxol) either alone or in combination with irradiation in two rat yolk sac tumour cell lines with different radiosensitivities in vitro. Int J Radiat Biol 1998;73:225-231.

25.   Minarik L, Hull EJ. Taxol in combination with acute and low dose rate irradiation. Radiother Oncol 1994;32:124-128.

26.   Stromberg JS, Lee YJ, Armour EP, Martinez AA, Corry PM. Lack of radiosensitization after paclitaxel treatment of three human carcinoma cell lines. Cancer 1995;75:2262-2268.

LEIOMYOSARCOMAS IN THE ORAL AND MAXILLOFACIAL REGION
- LOCAL RECURRENCES AND OCCURRENCE OF DISTANT METASTASES -

Dr. Dr. Horst E. Umstadt[1] , Dr. Frank Schmidseder[1] , Prof. Dr. Peter Barth[2]
[1]Departments of Oral and Maxillofacial Surgery (Chairman: Prof. Dr. Dr. Austermann), Philipps-University Marburg
[2]Pathology (Chairman: Prof. Dr. Moll), Philipps-University Marburg

Key words: Leiomyosarcoma, oral cavity, local recurrence, distant metastases, free flap transfer, reconstruction, decision-making.

Correspondence to*: Dr. Dr. Horst E. Umstadt, Klinik für MKG-Chirurgie, Georg Voigt Str. 3, D-35039 Marburg/L., Phone: 06421/2863233, Fax: 06421/2868990 (e-mail: umstadt@mailer.uni-marburg.de)*

ABSTRACT

Leiomyosarcoma (LMS) accounts for approximately 7% of all malignant soft tissue tumors. LMS of the oral cavity are very rare and only about 26 cases have been reported in the pertinent literature. We treated one case of leiomyosarcoma of the cheek. No database for statistical based decision-making concerning leiomyosarcomas of the oral cavity was found in the literature so we used data of 28 cases out of the DÖSAK (German-Austrian-Switzerland Tumorregister) for decision-making to plan surgical procedure. We analyzed percentage of local recurrence and occurrence of distant metastases. We also analyzed clinical and pathohistological lymph-node status as well as recurrence-free survival time.

Results. Local recurrence seems not to correlate with tumor-diameter. Distant metastases seem to be dependent of the tumor-size. The number of the clinical detected lymph-nodes increases parallel to tumor-size but only one lymph-node of 28 patients was positive. The recurrence-free survival-time seems to correlate with the diameter of the primary tumor.

The tumor was resected in a one stage procedure reconstruction. Elective frozen lymph-node sections of the submandibular region nearby the tumor were tumor free, too, so a neck dissection was abandoned.

359

Conclusions. In our case we think prognosis is not too bad because of wide excision of the tumor and freedom of metastases at the time of surgery. An unfavorable aspect has been the advanced size (diameter approx. 5cm) of the tumor. Concerning the literature and our data (DÖSAK) this could mean a high rate of metastases. So the patient has to be consequently re-staged for metastases in short time-intervals. Immediate reconstruction using the bilobed parascapular flap gives the patient a good quality of live independent of the definite longterm-outcome.

INTRODUCTION

Leiomyosarcoma (LMS) is a malignant mesenchymal tumor originating from the smooth muscle cells making up about 7% among all sarcomas[1]. The most common sites are the uterus, the digestive tract, skin and retroperitoneum[2,3]. The occurrence in head and neck has rarely been reported[4], so that incidence of local recurrences and pattern of metastasis is not well known.

Wertheimer-Hatch et al.[5] reported 8 cases of LMS of the cheek in an analysis of all reported cases in the world literature from 1884 to 1996. This location was concerned in 12,7% of all LMS in the oral cavity and pharynx. The prognosis of the lesion depends on local recurrences and occurrence of distant metastasis, mostly regional lymph nodes, the lung and liver[6,7]. On the other side the oral cavity may be the target of metastatic spread[8].

In cases of LMS of the oral cavity and the cheek local recurrence occurs in a range of 19% to 36% of cases; distant metastases are found in 39% of cases[5,7]. Enzinger and Weiss[1] report that clinical behavior and prognosis of LMS depends on the location of the primary. In contrast to retroperitoneal and intraabdominal LMS cutaneous LMS is characterized by a more favorable prognosis. This may in part be due to the fact, that tumors of the skin and subcutaneous tissue are diagnosed more early than deeply seated tumors. However, the histologic aspect of cutaneous and subcutaneous LMS does not significantly differ from retroperiteal and intraabdominal LMS[1-9]. To the best of our knowledge, a total of 26 cases of LMS of the <u>oral</u> region have been reported in the pertinent literature[4]. Decision making for treatment in our case was based on the literature of the last few years and the results of the DÖSAK which based on 28 cases of leiomyosarcomas in the whole <u>oral and maxillofacial</u> region.

CASE REPORT

Case history
A 24 old caucasian woman was visiting since middle of january 2000 two ENT-departments, a ENT in practise, a department for oral and maxillofacial surgery and a oral and maxillofacial surgeon in practise until the diagnosis leiomyosarcomea of the cheek could be made. Only the last colleague could fix the diagnose LMS, he assigned the patient for further therapy at the beginning of march 2000 to us.

Initially the patient was visiting the ENT-department because of pain in the right cheek. An approx. 10x10mm meassuring tumor could be detected by ultrasound in the right cheek. A dental cause of this alteration was excluded by clinical and radiological investigation at the same time by consultation an oral and maxillofacial department.

The patient then changed the treating clinic in the course and imagined in a further clinic; a histological examination yields the diagnosis: Non-specific inflammation. The patient finds since she notices further growth visited a practice for oral and maxillofacial surgery. An only just hen's egg big tumor consists in the right cheek inside at this time. After renewed histological examination the diagnosis leiomyosarcoma was made and the patient was assigned to our clinic.

Preoperative course: Clinical examination shows a hen´s egg big secondary exulcerated tumor inside the right cheek. No suspicious lymph-nodes were detected clinically. The extension of the tumor with a pseudocapsule compets in anterior-posterior direction 4.5 cm in cranial-caudal direction 5.5 cm. The borders of the tumor were located anteriorly 3.5 cm behind the angle of the mouth, caudally they reached the buccal sulcus the distal border reached the ascending ramus of the mandible and cranially the tumor reached the upper sulcus of the vestibule

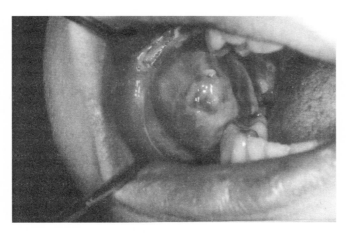

Figure 1. Preoperative clinical situation intraoporally. A hen's egg big secondary exulcerated tumor inside the right cheek.

Staging procedure:
Because of lack of typical clinical and radiological features of LMS, a biopsy was carried out already so we only arranged a reference examination of the specimen by a specialist in smooth muscle tumors.

Ultrasound of the abdominal and retroperitoneal regions presented no signs of a possible primary-tumor in these regions or metastases outgoing from the primary tumor in the cheek. Gynecological examination confirms no signs of primary tumor in this region.
MRI presented a tumor mass of 4x4,5 cm in extension. Axial T2 weighted scans showed isotensic signal behavior like tissue of the parotid gland including small cystic leasions. In T1 weighted scans the tumor is isotensic to muscle tissue and enriches contrast medium. Caudally the tumor mass reaches the alveolar process ventral to the masseter muscle without sharp delimitation. Cranially the tumor reaches the infratemporal fossa and the dorsal border reaches the Mm. pterygoideii.

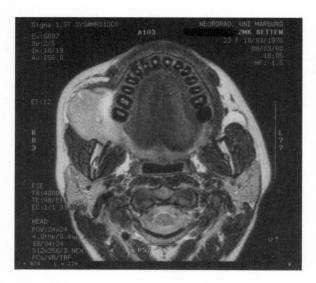

Figure 2. Axial T2 weighted scans showed isotensic signal behavior like tissue of the parotid gland including small cystic lesions.

Because a conventional X-ray is not sufficient for detecting small metastases we performed a CT-examination of the lung. No signs of metastases in this region were detected.

Decision-making for treatment.
Decision-making for treatment of these rare tumor was based on the results of the DÖSAK-register which based on 28 cases of leiomyosarcomas in the oral and maxillofacial region of the last ten years. Further informations for postoperative treatment were extracted out of the current literature which deals with leiomyosarcomas.

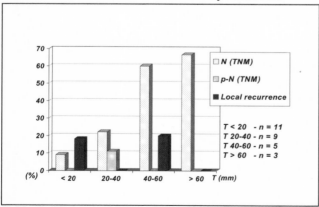

Table 1. 28 cases of leiomyosarcomas in the oral and maxillofacial region out of the DÖSAK-Tumorregister. Correlation of tumorsize, clinical and pathohistological lymph-node status and local recurrence.

First question was if we should do an neck-dissection additionally. Next question was how far the safe distance should be to avoid local recurrence and if local recurrence correlates with the diameter of the tumor.

Table 2. 28 cases of leiomyosarcomas in the oral and maxillofacial region out of the DÖSAK-Tumorregister. Correlation of tumorsize, survival rate, pathohistological lymph-node status, local recurrence and distant metastases.

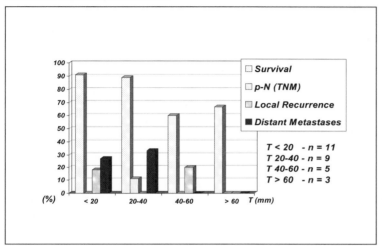

For prognosis our next question was if the occurrence of distant metastases and local recurrence correlates with diameter of the tumor.

Further questions were if postoperative radiotherapy or chemotherapy could improve the prognosis.

Surgical Treatment:

Tumor- resection:

Treatment planning was done with curative intention after exclusion of distant metastases.

The surgical planning includes total resection of the tumor with wide local resection to avoid local recurrence.

The en-bloc-resection includes distally the retromolar region together with the anterior bony border of the ascending ramus of the mandible. Cranilly the dorsolateral border of the maxillary sinus together with the second molar as well as a part of the pterygoid process were resected. Anteroior and caudally the resection border reaches the attached gingiva of lower jaw second molar and the buccal plane 1.5 cm behind the angle of the mouth. After resection of the tumor multiple frozen sections were sent during surgery for histolologic examination of the margins. All margins appeared to be tumor free.

363

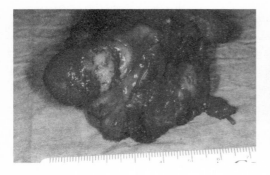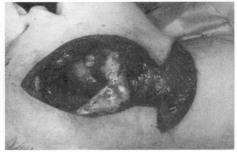

Figure 3. The en-bloc-resection includes the complete transsection (cross-cut) of the cheek.

Figure 4. Continuous defect of the cheek after resection of the tumor

Elective frozen lymph-node sections of the submandibular region nearby the tumor were tumor free, too, so we decided to abandon a supra-omohyoid neck dissection.

Reconstruction:
An immediate reconstruction of the defect was performed using a vascularized bilobed parascapular flap harvested from the left parascapular region. The vessels of the a. and v. circumflexa scapulae were anastomised to the a. and v. facialis.

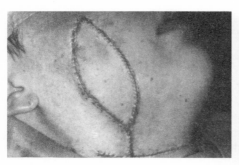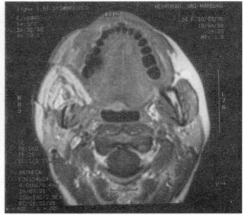

Figure 5. Situation after reconstruction of the defect

Figure 6. MRI six weeks after surgery showing a well perfused bilobed parascapular flap replacing the right cheek.

The extraoral healing was uneventfully. Because of resection of the ductus parotideus we inserted in the main ductus of the parotid gland during reconstruction a soft silicon pipe for drainage of the saliva.

364

Pathological Findings:
Macroscopically the tumor was well defined and showed a fleshy, lobulated cut surface. Ulceration of the covering mucosa and circumscribed tumor necrosis and hemorrhage was present at the site of previous biopsies.

Histologically the tumor was composed of parallely arranged spindle cells of intermediate size forming irregular whorls and broad sheets. A characteristic heringbone or storiform pattern was not observed as well as multinucleated giant cells were not found. The cytoplasm was clear showing few perinuclear vacuoles, PAS stains revealed small amounts of intracytoplasmatic glycogen. The nuclei were enlarged and hyperchromatic, typical and atypical mitoses were abundant. Intercellular collagen was inconspicuous. Immunohistochemically the tumor cells revealed a strong cytoplasmatic reaction with smooth muscle actin, few tumor cells were also weakly positive for desmin. Epithelial and neural markers were not detected by means of immunohistochemistry.

Postoperative treatment:
Most authors[10,11,5] saw no positive effect after postoperative radiation concerning the occurrence of local recurrence or survival time. So we decided not to radiate the patient.
Clinical follow up was done every four weeks. Frequent MRI-scans of the head and neck region for early detection of recurrence and locoregional metastases were carried out. The first MR-scan was taken 12 weeks after tumor-surgery.

13 weeks after resection of the tumor the maxillary sinus was permanently drained and multiple biopsies were taken because of persistent chronically inflammation detected in MRI. Histopathological examination shows no clue for locoregional recurrence.

For detecting distant metastases ultrasound of the liver and CT-scans of the lung had been made every 12 weeks in the first year after surgery.

DISCUSSION

Intraoral soft tissue sarcoma is a rare diagnosis but one of differential diagnosis of intraoral soft tissue growing. Early diagnosis is of great importance and essential for the patients outcome. Risk factors have not been identified for these connective tissue malignancies[12]. Few predisposing or etiological factors are recognized in LMS[13,14]. The sex distribution differs from paper to paper. It seems to be that these tumors are more common in women than men. The significance of this observation is not clear, although growth and proliferation of smooth muscle tissue in women have been noted to coincide with pregnancy as well as estrogenic stimulation[1].
Metastasis of LMS is almost always hematogenous and usually occurs to the lung. Other sites in order of frequency are lymph nodes, liver and skeleton[15,5]. The limited amount of smooth muscle in the oral cavity may account for the low rate of occurrence of LMS in that region[16]. Possible site of origin in our case could be the walls of blood vessels, aberrant hair follicles of erector pili muscles or myoepithelial cells of mucos glands in the cheek.
In the oral cavity, LMS is considered a very aggressive condition with a high rate of local recurrence after surgery between 19%[5] and 35%[7].

Swelling and pain are usually the prominent symptoms in LMS of the oral cavity[5] which can be confirmed in the medical story of our case. In literature (mostly case reports) many patients have a history of dental related to the lesion treatment including often dental extraction. Others suffers first a conservative treatment by their dentist with delay in the diagnosis. One must consider that rapid growth, ulceration and pain not only suggest a malignant process but also a variety of infectious lesions and reactive processes. Reported diagnoses prior to biopsy included: mucous retention cyst, fibroma, advanced chronic peridontitis, fibrous histocytoma, pleomorphic adenoma etc. All in all there is only a little possibility to reach a more precise diagnosis until biopsy and histologic examination. Therefor clinically diagnosis is not easy.

Although recurrences develop in almost 20%-36% of the patients, metastasis are infrequent and seem to correlate with the depth and diameter of the original tumor[3,5]. The high rate of recurrence (60,6%) of 36 superficial LMS reported by Stout and Hill[17] seems to be an indication of inadequacy of the primary treatment in many of these cases. All in all early diagnosis and ablative surgery in an early state of the tumor seems to be the best way to avoid local recurrences and distant metastases. Surgical excision offers the best chances for cure[18]. For primary LMS early wide local excision with adequate clear histologic borders constitutes rational treatment.

LMS is under-recognized in the mouth, often being mistaken for a spindle-celled epithelial neoplasm[9]. The most common histologic variant in the oral cavity is a vascular leiomyoma also known as angiomyoma[5].

Concerning adjuvant therapies it seems to be that for most authors neither radiotherapy nor chemotherapy could improve the outcome of the patients[10,11]. LMS are thought to be resistant to radiotherapy so that combining surgery with adjunctive radiotherapy for the LMS does not influence recurrence or survival[5]. However, postoperative radiotherapy for LMS has been reported by some authors but radiotherapy, when used, is used as an adjuvant and not as definitive treatment in recurrent cases[19]. Only Aydin and Dreyer[20] reported a good response after radiotherapy in a primarily unresectable case.

Immediate reconstruction using a free flap enables the surgeon to make a consequent wide resection. So the reduction of quality of live in these cases will not be significant. The used bilobed parascapular flap gives enough volume for on-feeding the cheek. The inner side of the cheek and the retromolar region could be covered with a epitheliasized surface which is strong enough not to prolapse between the teeth during chewing while the outer side of the flap integrates good concerning color and consistency into the skin of the cheek.

Because of the transsection of a part of the branches of the facial nerve we are planning muscular mounting of the corner of the mouth using temporal muscle one year after primary surgery.
Disadvantage of all soft tissue reconstruction procedures is the fact that recurrences cannot be observed clinically in initial state. Today MRI gives good possibility to control the soft tissue situation in short distances.
The aggressiveness and bad prognosis of LMS in the oral cavity and pharyngs are reflected in data of Wertheimer-Hatch et al.[5]. In the follow-up data of 33 patients 15 were found to be free of disease, and 18 had died, giving an overall 45% survival rate. In our case the prognosis at the long run seems to be good because of wide excision of the tumor and freedom of

metastases at the time of surgery. An unfavorable aspect has been the advanced size (diameter approx. 5 cm) of the tumor at the time of surgery. Concerning the literature this could mean a high rate of metastases (80%). So the patient have to be consequently re-staged for metastases in short time-intervals. Immediate reconstruction using the bilobed parascapular flap gives the patient a good quality of live independent of the definite longterm-outcome.

REFERENCES

1. Enzinger, MF. In: Enzinger MF., Weiss SW., (eds): Soft Tissue Tumors, St. Louis, Mosby, (1988); pp 402-421.
2. Batsakis J.G.. Soft Tissue Tumors of the Head and Neck: Unusual forms In: Batsakis, J.G. (ed): Tumors of the Head and Neck: Clinical and Pathological Considerations Williams & Wilkins, 2. Ed. Baltimore, (1979); pp 350-367.
3. Fields, J.P., Helwig, E.B. Leiomyosarcomas of the Skin and Subcutaneous Tissue Cancer (1981); 47:156-169
4. Moussaoui, O., Menard, P. Leiomyosarcoma of the gingiva. Apropos of a case. Review of the literature Rev Stomatol Chir Maxillofac (1998); Oct;99(3):132-137.
5. Wertheimer-Hatch, L., Hatch, G.F., Hatch, K., Davis, G.B., Blanchard, D.K., Foster, R.S., Skandalakis, J.E. Tumors of the oral cavity and pharynx World J Surg (2000); 24, 395-400.
6. Le Toux, G., Brette, M.D., Arnoux, Y, Pasquiou, P., Besset, G., Monteil, J.P. Bucco-sinusal site of primary leiomyosarcoma Ann Otolaryngol Chir Cervicofac (1995); 112(5): 244-247.
7. Schenberg, M.E., Slootweg, P.J., Koole, R. Leiomyosarcdomas of the oral cavity. Report of four cases and review of the literature. J Craniomaxillofac Surg (1993); 21(8):342-347.
8. Allen, C.M., Neville, B., Damm, D.D., Marsh, W. Leiomyosarcoma metastatic to the oral region. Report of three cases Oral surg Oral Med, Oral Path (1993); 76(6): 752-756.
9. Dry, S. M., Jorgensen, J.L., Fletcher, C.D. Leiomyosarcomas of the oral cavity: an unusual topographic subset easily mistaken for nonmesenchymal tumors Histopathology (2000); Mar;36(3): 210-320.
10. Mohr, C, Schettler, D., Metz, K., Richter, HJ, Schmidt, U. Leiomyosarkome im Kopf-Hals-Bereich Fortschr Kiefer Gesichtschir (1988); 33:20-2
11. Ayad, W., Diekmann, J., Freitag, P., Wierich, W. Leiomyosarkome im Canalis mandibularis Mund Kiefer GesichtsChir (1998); 2:42-43
12. Gorsky, M., Epstein, J.B. Head and Neck and intra-oral soft tissue sarcomas Oral Oncology (1998); 34 (4) 292-296.
13. Jennings, T.A., Peterson, L., Axiotis, C.A., Friedlaender, G. E., Cooke, R.A., Rosai, J. Angiosarcoma associated with foreign body material Cancer (1988); 62: 2436-2444.
14. Goldschmidt, P.R., Goldschmidt, J.D., Lieblich, S.E., Eisenberg, E. Leiomyosarcoma presenting as a mandibular gingival swelling: a case report J Periodontol (1999); 70(1):84-89
15. Barnes, L., Ferlito, A., Soft tissue neoplasmas In: Ferlito A (ed) Neoplasmas of the larynx. 1st edn. Churchill Livingstone, Edinburgh, (1993); pp 265-304.
16. Carter, L.C., Aguirre, A., Boyd, B., DeLacure, M.D. Primary leiomyosarcoma of the mandible in a 7-year-old girl Oral surg Oral Med Oral Path Oral Radiol Endod (1999); 87:477-484.
17. Stout, A.P., Hill, W.T. Leiomyosarcoma of the superficial soft tissues Cancer (1958); 11:844-854.
18. Pandey, M., Thomas, G., Mathew, A., Abraham, E.K., Somanathan, T., Ramadas, K., Iype, E.M., Ahamed, I.M., Sebastian, P., Nair, M.K. Sarcoma of the oral and maxillofacial soft tissue in adults Europ J Surg Oncol (2000); 26: 145-148.
19. Valle, A.A., Kraybill, W.G. Management of soft tissue sarcoma of the extremity in adults J Surg Oncol (1996); 63: 271-279.
20. Aydin, H., Dreyer, T. Leiomyosarcoma of the base of the tongue treated with radiotherapy: a case report Eur J Cancer B Oral Oncol (1994); 30B 85: 351-355.

THE IMPORTANCE OF TELOMERASE ACTIVITY FOR METASTASES IN TUMOR AND TUMOR-FREE RESECTION MARGINS IN HEAD AND NECK CANCERS

Koscielny, S.[1]; Dahse, R.[2]; von Eggeling, F.[2]; Claussen, U.[2]; Beleites, E.[1]; Ernst, G.[2]; Fiedler, W.[3]

[1]ENT-Department
[2]Institute of Human Genetics and Anthropology; Friedrich-Schiller-University Jena, Germany
[3]Molecular Gastroenterological Oncology, Martin-Luther-University Halle

SUMMARY

As in most tumor tissues telomerase is active, reactivation of telomerase seems to be an important step in the carcinogenesis of head and neck cancers. We investigated telomerase activity in tumor tissue from 80 cases and tissue from tumor free resection margins from 69 cases for telomerase activity and its influence on metastatic potential of the tumors. All patients were controlled clinically at least 3 years. Patients with telomerase activity in the tumor tissue and in histological tumor free resection margins developed lymph node metastasis in a higher number compared to patients without metastasis. The prevalent results may indicate that telomerase activity is a possible prognostic marker for the metastatic potential of head and neck cancer. The number of regional recurrences in lymph nodes was higher in patients with telomerase activity in tumor free resection margins. However, patients with telomerase activity in the tumor tissue showed no higher number of regional recurrences. In conclusion, the telomerase activivty could be an indicator for the metastatic potential of head and neck tumors.

INTRODUCTION

Approximately 3 % of all malignant tumors in Germany every year are head and neck cancers (HNC). ENT-surgeons are interested in finding reliable prognostic markers of these tumors to determine the individual prognosis of patients especially regarding the metastatic potential.
Recent studies have shown an association of reactivated telomerase and human cancer. In some kind of tumors (e. g. neuroblastomas) the telomerase activity has proved to be a significant prognostic marker for tumor progression[1-3]Therefore we investigated the clinical

369

implication of telomerase activity as a prognostic and diagnostic marker for metastases in HNC[4-6].

In tumors characterized by a loss of growth control the rate of cell proliferation is increased and the telomeres shorten more rapidly than in adjacent normal tissue. Progressive shortening of the telomeres is an important component of the regulation of cellular senescence as telomeres may function like a mitotic clock limiting the life span of cells. Since telomeres reach a point of critical length telomerase might be reactivated in some cells to stabilize the telomeric repeats. Cells expressing the enzyme telomerase may escape from cellular senescence and possibly gain the ability of indefinite proliferation, i.e. become potentially immortal. The presence of telomerase in most cancer tissues, but not in normal cells and tissues adjacent to tumors, renders the enzyme as a prevalent diagnostic marker for malignant tumors[7, 8].

MATERIAL AND METHODS

Telomerase analysis

Tumor tissue (all cases), normal tissue of the mucous membrane and resection margins (69 cases) were taken from 80 squamous cell carcinomas of the head and neck. Informed consent was obtained from all patients for the use of tissue samples in research.

All tissue probes from the tumors, adjacent surgical margins and the corresponding normal oral mucosa representing the constitutional situation were obtained by surgical resection.

The tissue probes were snap frozen in liquid nitrogen immediately after resection and stored at -80°C. The probes from the resection margins were divided. One part was used for moleculargenetic analysis and the other part for histological investigation to determine the absent of tumor cells. All samples were examined histopathologically.

The Telomerase assay[5] (Telomeric Repeat Amplification Protocol, TRAP) was used in the modification by Fiedler et al.[7]

Localisation and stadium of the tumors

Table 1 and 2 show the tumor localisation and stadium of the investigated head and neck squamous cell carcinomas.

Table 1 Number of tumors and stadium of tumor disease for telomerase analysis in tumor tissue

	I	II	III	IV	total
Oral cavity	2	4	1	4	11
Oropharynx	0	4	2	26	32
Larynx	4	5	6	11	26
Hypopharynx	0	0	2	9	11
Total	6	13	11	50	80

Table 2 Number of tumors and stadium of tumor disease for telomerase analysis in tumor free resection margins

	I	II	III	IV	total
Oral cavity	2	4	1	4	11
Oropharynx	0	3	0	24	27
Larynx	2	4	6	11	23
Hypopharynx	0	0	1	7	8
Total	4	11	8	46	69

RESULTS

Telomerase analysis in tumor tissues and resection margins

The results of the analysis for telomerase activity in tumor tissues and tumor free resection margins are shown in table 3 and 4. We found telomerase activity in 75 % of tumor tissues and in 58 % of tumor free resection margins.

Table 3. Results of telomerase analysis in tumor tissues

telomerase	yes	no	total
Oral cavity	2	9	11
Oropharynx	8	24	32
Larynx	8	18	26
Hypopharynx	2	9	11
Total	20	60	80

Table 4. Results of telomerase analysis in tumor free resection margins

telomerase	yes	no	total
Oral cavity	5	6	11
Oropharynx	15	12	27
Larynx	9	14	23
Hypopharynx	2	6	8
total	31	38	69

Telomerase analysis and lymph node metastases

Patients with telomerase activity in the tumor tissue showed in 58 % lymph node metastases at first diagnosis, however, tumors without telomerase activity developed lymph node metastases in 45 %. Regarding the telomerase status in tumor free resection margins, we detected in 63 % lymph node metastases in patients with telomerase active resection margins and in 48 % in patients without telomerase active resection margins

Tables 5 and 6 show the correlation between telomerase activity and rate of lymph node metastases.

Table 5. Telomerase activity and lymph node metastases in tumor tissues

telomerase	lymph node	no (N0-neck)	yes (pN+-neck)	Total
no		11	9	20
yes		25	35	60
total		36	44	80

Table 6. Telomerase activity and lymph node metastases in tumor free resection margins

telomerase	lymph node	no (N0-neck)	yes (pN+-neck)	Total
No		16	15	31
Yes		14	24	38
Total		30	39	69

Telomerase analysis and regional recurrences

All patients were observed at least 3 years in our tumor dispensaire.
Patients with telomerase activity in tumor tissue developed in 18 % a recurrence in the regional lymph nodes. Patients without telomerase activity showed in 16 % regional recurrences.

Interestingly, patients with telomerase activity in tumor free resection margins developed in a higher number regional recurrences compared to patients without telomerase activity. 27 % of the patients with telomerase-positive resection margins displayed recurrences in regional lymph nodes whereas in telomerase negative resection margins 16 % recurrences occured.
Telomerase activity in tumor tissues and tumor free resection margins did not affect the time of development of an regional recurrence.

CONCLUSIONS

1. As in most tumor tissues telomerase is active, reactivation of telomerase seems to be an important step in the carcinogenesis of head and neck cancers[1-3].

2. Patients with telomerase activity in tumor tissues and tumor free resection margins have a higher number of lymph node metastases at first diagnosis.

3. The number of recurrences in regional lymph nodes is higher in patients with telomerase active tumor free resection margins.

4. Telomerase activity in tumor tissues do not affect the number of and time to regional recurrences

5. Telomerase activity in tumor tissues and tumor free resection margins may be a possible prognostic marker for the metastatic potential of head and neck squamous cell carcinomas. The results of telomerase investigation may help to indicate adjuvant therapies.

372

REFERENCES

1. Kagata HY, Tsukuda M, Mochimatsu I, Kubota A, Furukawa MK, Yasumoto S. Telomerase activity of tumors in the head and neck. Nip Jibiinkoka Gakkai Kaiho 1998;101:205-211
2. Koscielny S, Fiedler W, Dahse R, Claussen U, Beleites E, Ernst G. Telomerase activity as a possible tumor marker in head and neck cancer In: Hrsg: Werner JA, Lippert BM, Rudert, HH: Head and Neck Cancer - Advances in Basic Research. Amsterdam: Elsevier Science B. V; 1996. p 593-598
3. Koscielny S, Fiedler W, Beleites E. Reaktivierung der Telomerase im Rahmen der Kanzerogenese von Plattenepithelkarzinomen im Kopf-Hals-Bereich. HNO 1997;45:277
4. Koscielny S, Fiedler E, Dahse R, Hoffmann SME, Sonntag J, Claussen U, Beleites E. Is telomerase activity a possible marker for the metastasis of head and neck cancer ? Br J Cancer 1998;77:51
5. Kim NW, Platyszek MA, Prowse KR, Harley CB, West MD, Ho PLC, Coviello GM, Wright ME, Weinrich SL, Shay JW. Specific association of human telomerase activity with immortal cells and cancer. Science 1994;266:2011-2015
6. Wright WE, Shay JW. Telomere positional effects and the regulation of cellular senescence. TIG 1992;8:193-197
7. Fiedler W, Dahse R, Schlichter A, Junker H, Kosmehl H, Ernst G, Schubert J, Claussen U. Telomerase activity and telomere length in different areas of Renal Cell Carcinoma. Int J Oncol 1996;9:1227-1232
8. Hahn WC, Stuart SA, Brooks MW, York SG, Eaton E, Kurachi A; Beijersbergen RL, Knoll JH, Meyerson M, Weinberg RA. Inhibition of telomerase limits the growth of human cancer cells. Nat Med 1999;10:1064-1070

PREDICTORS FOR METASTASES IN ADVANCED CARCINOMA OF THE HEAD AND NECK AFTER PRIMARY CHEMORADIOATION

Andreas Dietz, M. D., Heidelberg, Germany

Correspondence to: *Priv. Doz. Dr. Andreas Dietz, M.D. Universitäts-Hals-Nasen-Ohrenklinik, Im Neuenheimer Feld 400, D-69120 Heidelberg, Germany, Phone: 06221/566705, Fax: 06221/566706, (e-mail: Andreas_Dietz@med.uni-heidelberg.de)*

Stage IV in head and neck squamous cell carcinoma is defined by the local tumor extension and the presence of regional or distant metastases. It thereby constitutes a very heterogeneous group with small, infiltrative and lymph node positive cancers as well as bulky tumors. It is common experience that the onset of metastases after primary radiotherapy or radiochemotherapy may be extremely variable and unpredictable.

Apart from well established clinical staging factors like TNM stage, histopathological grading, perineural infiltration and extracapsular spread of neck metastases, numerous cellular molecular factors are currently being assessed for their possible predictive value for outcome of advanced head and neck tumors after primary chemoradiation. This presentation focuses on a trial of our department which was conducted to study the clinical impact of some central predictive factors recently discussed in literature in a homogeneous group of head and neck cancer patients after primary chemoradiation. In detail, the object of this trial was to analyze the prognostic relevance of the tumor cell cycle components (CCC) CDK4, p53, p16INK4a, p21WAF1, Cyclin D1, Ki 67(MIB1), BCL2 and pRb and tumor oxygenation.

METHODS

From 1992 to 1998, 125 patients with squamous cell carcinoma of the oro-. and hypopharynx (98% St. IV, UICC) were treated in two different trials by primary chemoradiation or radiotherapy alone. CCC-expression was analyzed by immuno-histochemistry in pre-therapeutic tumor biopsies. Cervical metastases of 37 patients in this group were evaluated for oxygenation before start of therapy. The oxygen partial pressure in lymph node metastases was determined polarographically with pO_2-Histography (Kimoc 6650, Sigma pO_2-

Histograph, Eppendorf, Hamburg, Germany). As further clinical parameters which are currently discussed as factors of high prognostic relevance, the total tumor volume (TTV) based on tumor extension in the initial CT-scans, pre-therapeutic hemoglobin (Hb) and performance status were monitored. Follow-up was analyzed by detecting time of locoregional control, time of onset of metastases, etc.

RESULTS

Monovariate analysis showed significant prognostic relevance for poor outcome for pathologic over-expression of CDK4, Cyclin D1, p53, high TTV and reduced Hb. In multivariate analysis of the first trial (median follow up: 60 months) CDK4 and TTV showed prognostic significance. Regarding all patients (cutoff: 43 months) only reduced Hb (<median) and high TTV (>median) correlated significantly with poor outcome. The significant results of CDK4 in the first trial could not be confirmed in the second trial.

There was no significant correlation with any of the measured cell cycle components and the onset of metastases after primary chemoradiation. Table 1 shows the prognostic findings for pathologic expression of cell cycle components and onset of metastases after primary chemoradiation in our study sample:

Table 1. Presentation of prognostic trends (p<0,15) "(+)" and significancys (p<0,05) "+" of cell cycle components in the first (A) and second study (B) and both trials together (cutoff 43 months). [Probability of onset of metastases (met.), time of locoregional control (lok.) and survival (surviv.)]

	Study A met.	lok.	surviv.	Study B met.	lok.	surviv.	Study A met.	+ lok.	Study B surviv.
Mib-1 (Ki 67)	-	(+)	-	-	(+)	-	-	(+)	-
P53	-	-	+	-	(+)	(+)*	-	-	-
p21$^{WAF1/CIP1}$	-	-	-	-	-	-	-	-	-
pRb	-	(+)	(+)	-	-	-	-	(+)	(+)
p16^{INK4A}	-	-	-	-	-	-	-	-	-
CDK4	-	+	+	-	-	-	-	-	-
Cyclin D1	-	-	-	(+)	-	-	(+)	-	-
CDK4+Cy. D1	-	-	(+)	(+)	-	-	-	-	-
CDK4+Cy. D1	-	-	-	-	-	-	-	-	-

*trend of pathologic over expression of p53 and survival in study B showed an inverse relation to study A: Over expression of p53 correlates in study B with good and in study A with bad prognosis (statistic non significant)

Only pathological over-expression of Cyclin D1 showed a trend for relevance as a predictor for early onset of metastases. None of the cell cycle components showed significant predictive character for metastases.

Additionally, the degree of tumor oxygenation had no significant predictive character for onset of metastases. Figure 1 shows the probability of survival and onset of metastases depending on oxygenation measurements in our study sample of 37 patients.

Figure 1. Probability of onset of metastases relating to hypoxic fraction lower than pO2: 2.5 mmHg (HF2). The two curves represent data lower and higher than median of HF2 in 37 patients with advanced carcinoma of the head and neck after primary chemoradiation.

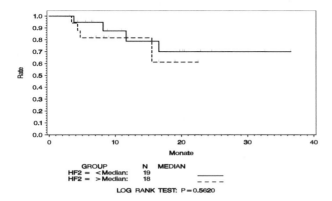

Probability of survival relating to hypoxic fraction lower than pO2: 2.5 mmHg (HF2). The two curves represent data lower and higher than median of HF2 in 37 patients with advanced carcinoma of the head and neck after primary chemoradiation.

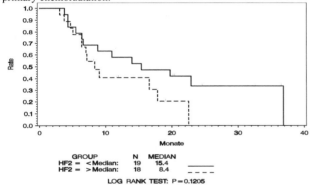

Regarding the data for survival in fig.1 there was a trend for bad prognosis and hypoxia which was not mirrored in onset of metastases.

In our study hemoglobin and total tumor volume was also not predictive for the early onset of metastases. Nevertheless, hemoglobin lower than 13.5 g/dl and total tumor volume more than 66 ml was prognostic with high significance for bad outcome due to reduced time of loco-regional control.

CONCLUSION

Regarding the data of our trial and recent literature, there are no clinically useful predictive factors for the early onset of metastases in advanced squamous cell carcinoma of head and neck after primary chemo-radiation available (Review: Raybaud-Diogène 1997; Wennerberg 1996, Rockwell 1997). Some evident current concepts of biologic behaviour of tumor cells growing to metastases are discussed but they are still not clear enough or confirmed by clinical trials for transposition in diagnostic oncology concepts.

REFERENCES

1.   Raybaud-Diogène H, Fortin A, Marency R, Roy J, Monteil RA, Têtu B. Markers of radioresistence in squamous cell carcinomas of the head and neck: A clinicopathologic and immunohistochemical study. J Clin Oncol 1997;15(3).1030-1038
2.   Wennerberg J: Predicting response to therapy of squamous cell carcinoma of the head and neck (review). Anticancer Res 1996;16.2389-2396
3.   Rockwell S: Oxygen delivery: implications for the biology and therapy of solid tumors. Oncology Research 1997;9.383-390

DISTANT METASTASIS FROM NASOPHARYNGEAL CARCINOMA AT KENYATTA NATIONAL HOSPITAL

H. O. Oburra[1], W. Gachani[1], I. S. Bal[1], M. A. Babu[2]
[1] Ear, Nose and Throat, Head and Neck Surgery, Kenyatta National Hospital, Nairoby, Kenya
[2] Radiotherapy Department of Kenyatta National Hospital, Nairobi, Kenya

ABSTRACT

Background. Poor basic infrastructure, socioeconomic status has been blamed for late presentation of cancer in third world countries. Few studies have been done to define this late presentation precisely and elicit factors associated with it. The aim of this study was to determine the frequency, site and factors associated with distant infraclavicular metastases from nasopharyngeal carcinoma.

Methods. A retrospective review of case notes, radiological and laboratory records of patients presenting with Nasopharyngeal carcinoma at Kenyatta National Hospital between January 1981 and December 1990 were screened for age at presentation, sex incidence, sites and stage of locoregional disease, appearance and location of distant metastasis, histological grading, AJC 1978 staging, treatment and follow up period.

Results. The frequency of distant NPC metastases was 14.6% and 92.3% manifested within 24 months of admission. It was most frequent in the male sex, younger age group and early T1 disease. Bilaterality of the neck nodes had no relevance on metastatic rate. The bone (66.7%) was the most common distant metastatic destination followed by the liver (23.2%). The liver metastasis was associated with shorter follow up period.

Conclusion. Apart from the late presentation of locoregional disease the findings are similar to studies elsewhere. The numbers involved are however inadequate and there is a need to update patient documentation methods and record keeping in Kenyan hospitals to facilitate future research on the same subject.

INTRODUCTION

NPC is the second most frequent head and neck tumour in Kenyatta National Hospital (KNH) Cancer Registry (see table 1).

Table 1. TOP TWENTY CANCERS OF KENYA (1986-1990)

	Cancer	Number cases of
1.	Cervix	500
2.	Non Hodgekin's lymphoma (including Burkitt's lymphoma)	313
3.	Breast	272
4.	Skin	253
5.	Esophagus	239
6.	Nasopharynx	234
7.	Kaposi Sarcoma	154
8.	Eye (primary orbital)	134
9.	Connective tissue	130
10.	Mouth and palate	130
11.	Brain and nervous tissue	125
12.	Bones	104
13.	Hodgekin's lymphoma	100
14.	Stomach	100
15.	Larynx	96
16.	Malignant melanoma	95
17.	Liver	73
18.	Prostate	65
19.	Salivary glands	60
20.	Thyroid	44

Adapted from Cancer registry, Department of Pathology, University of Nairobi

The frequency of distant metastases in NPC amongst various head and neck tumours is known[1, 2]. The implications of this event on management approach and survival are clear. The magnitude of this problem had never been clarified in KNH before this study. In the third world, peculiar problems including shortage of medical facilities and expertise, general ignorance by the lay public on disease processes, lack of basic infrastructure and general poverty may be modulators in disease presentation hence the importance of this study. Various studies have shown delayed presentation of major head and neck cancers to the ENT-HN unit of KNH[3].

Previous claims that distant head and neck cancer metastases below the clavicle were uncommon have been dispelled over the last century[4, 5, 6]. Over the last five decades, there has been a notable increase in NPC patients with distant infraclavicular metastases probably due to effective control of the locoregional disease and improved survival[7]. In this study the frequency, sites and other factors affecting distant infraclavicular metastases in a third world environment are determined.

MATERIALS AND METHODS

Case notes of patients admitted between January 1981 and December 1990, in the Ear Nose and Throat-Head and Neck (ENT-HN) Surgical and the Radiotherapy Units of Kenyatta

380

National Hospital (KNH) with histologically verified NPC were retrieved and screened for evidence of distant metastasis.Bone metastasis had to be radiologically qualified while physical signs, ultrasound and/or laboratory results were the criteria accepted for diagnosis of soft tissue involvement. Those with clinical and/or radiological evidence of distant metastasis were reviewed for age, sex, AJC 1978 stage of locoregional disease and sites of distant infraclavicular metastases. This staging system was used because it was the most reliable operational staging system during the period of patient presentation. The time of presentation during the course of the disease, management modalities and follow up period for different metastatic categories were determined.

RESULTS

A total of 445 patients were presented with NPC during the ten-year period. Of these 333 were males and 112 females. 93.9% had clinically palpable cervical nodes. There was no distant metastasis at presentation. Sixty-five patients (14.6%) developed distant metastasis during the course treatment.The following results are derived from the 65 patients with distant NPC metastasis.

Males were more likely to develop metastasis than females the cumulative risk being 21.1% and 9.9% respectively giving M:F ratio of 4.9:1. Figure 1 shows the age distribution. The younger age groups had more predisposition to distant NPC metastasis.

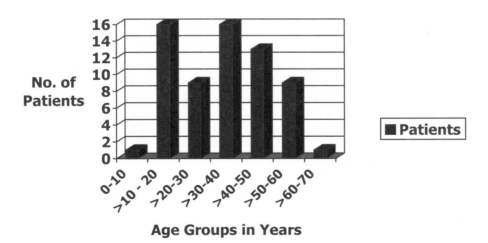

The M:F sex ratio was 4.9:1. WHO Type III was the most frequent histological variant accounting for 89.2% of NPC cases. The incidence of distant NPC was similar among the histological types in the 445 general NPC pool. The highest proportion of patients with distant metastasis was in the T1 stage (table 2).

At presentation of distant metastasis there cervical nodes had regressed in 47.7% persisted in 49.2%, recurred in 3.1% (this has to be compared to 93.3% incidence during the initial presentation of NPC and lack obvious clinically palpable nodes in 6.1 %) there was no obvious clinically palpable node. Bilaterality of the neck disease did not increase to predisposition to distant metastasis (table 3). Controlled primary disease seemed to increase the risk of distant NPC metastasis. Sixty per cent of patients with metastasis had complete control of the primary disease.

Table 2. PRIMARY NPC STAGE VS. DISTANT NPC METASTASIS

Stage	Frequency	%
T1	28	43.1
T2	18	27.7
T3	8	12.3
T4	11	16.9
Total	65	100.0

Table 3 BILATERALITY OF CERVICAL NODES NPC DISTANT MATASTASIS

Nodes	Frequency	%
Unilateral	31	47.7
Bilateral	30	46.2
Not palpable	4	6.1
Total	65	100.0

The vertebral column at the lumbar level was the most frequent distant metastatic destination for the NPC followed by the liver (see table 4). Metastases were frequently characterised by the relevant organ symptoms and signs.

Table 4. INDIVIDUAL ORGAN INVOLVEMENT BY DISTANT NPC METASTASIS

Site	Frequency	%
Lumbar Vertebrae	27	27.3
Liver	23	23.2
Ribs	12	12.1
Pelvis	9	9.1
Femur	7	7.1
Lungs	5	5.1
Thoracic Vertebrae	4	4.1
Sternum	3	3.0
Inguinal Lymph Nodes	2	2.0
Scapula	2	2.0
Sacral Vertebrae	1	1.0
Spleen	1	1.0
Stomach	1	1.0
Tibia	1	1.0
Breast	1	1.0
Total metastatic events	99	100.0

The follow up period seemed to depend on liver involvement. While the average crude follow up period was 4.1 months. Further analysis revealed that it was 5.2 months in those with multiple organ involvement. Of these patients with multiorgan involvement, follow up was

382

6.1 months if the liver was not involved and only 8.8 weeks if the liver was clinically involved. Most patients who did not come back for follow up were noted to be weak on their last visits while others were discharged to health units nearest to their homes for terminal management.

DISCUSSION

The appearance of distant metastases in any malignant disease has profound consequences on the prognosis of the disease and the economics of patient management. NPC is the most frequent head and neck tumour in Kenya. This study is therefore of specific interest to health care providers in third world countries with similar cancer epidemiology and budgetary constraints like Kenya.

Many studies during the last century dispelled previous claims that distant metastases from head and neck cancer are unusual and NPC has been shown to have the most frequent rate of distant infraclavicular metastasis[1, 8, 9]. In this study, all distant metastases appeared within 24 months of treatment and the incidence was found to be 14.9%, a figure comparing favourably with those from reported series elsewhere[10]. Higher incidences of upto 28.1% have been found in other studies[2, 11]. The absence of metastases at presentation is probably a result of the retrospective nature of the study and poor case notes documentation. A recent prospective study in the same hospital showed a 5.8% distant metastases rate at presentation[3]. The same study showed that 96.4% of NPC and laryngeal cancers presented at advanced stage 3 or 4 disease. The higher male predominance in both locoregional and distant metastatic NPC has not been clearly explained.

The low frequency of general NPC patients and those with distant metastases during the fifth and sixth decades is in keeping with the shape of Kenya's population actuarial curves. The high incidence of metastasis in the younger and middle age group however needs to be clarified further by well designed larger population studies. The high preponderance of WHO type 1 is in keeping with the general histological prevalence of NPC and is an expected biological behaviour in all high grade malignant disease. T1 tumours were also shown to have higher incidence of distant NPC metastasis, probably due to better locoregional disease control leading to longer survival and better chances of development of distant metastasis. However, due to numbers involved in this study, no direct correlation between tumour stage and metastasis rate could be shown. Such findings have been documented elsewhere[7]. It is of relevant interest that 60% of patients with NPC metastasis had clinically controlled primary disease and that WHO type 1 are more radiosensitive than the rest of the other types. One would therefore except a situation of good local control and early distant metastasis. The possibility of existence of a significant population of NPC tumour subtype among the WHO type 1 whose biological activity favour early matastasis should also be considered.

Simple bilaterality of cervical nodes without considering the size and level of the nodes did not affect the prognosis of NPC. This finding is expected and is one of the factors that led to harmonisation of UICC and AJC staging of nasopharyngeal carcinoma[12].

There was lack of consistent policy on which treatment regimes for NPC patients were based. However treatment of general NPC patients and those with bony metastases was by radiotherapy. Chemotherapy was left at the discretion of the radiotherapist. This status of affairs underlines the various difficulties that frustrate organised treatment of cancer patients. Erratic supply of the generally expensive chemotherapeutic drugs and long waiting periods for the scarce radiotherapy facility obviously have their contribution to this lack of consistent management strategy.

The average follow up after diagnosis of NPC distant metastases was 4.1 months. As in other cancers, liver involvement was shown to have a negative influence in duration of follow up. In third world countries with no mandatory death registries and where terminal and palliative care facilities are non existent, it is difficult to assess patient survival and management results. Therefore, many cancer management centres have to rely on follow up duration as a crude indicator of survival. This indicator is in turn influenced by distances from the referral hospital, lack of all weather roads, poverty and the patient's trust in alternative medicine. But crude as this indicator may be it is currently the only available pointer of cancer patient survival in many third world countries.

CONCLUSION

Because of the population size the retrospective design of this study, the figures determined from this study could only regarded as rough indicators of the real situation on the ground. There is a need to update the clinical note documentation in our institute, improve the record keeping system and increase the study numbers in order to come to highly significant conclusions.

REFERENCES

1.   Clifford P. Carcinoma of the nasopharynx in Kenya. East Afr Med J 1965; 47:373-396.
2.   Khor TH, Tan BC, Chua EJ, Chia KB. Distant metastases in nasopharyngeal carcinoma. Clin Radiol 1978; 29: 27-30.
3.   Oburra H O. Late presentation of laryngeal and nasopharyngeal cancer in Kenyatta National Hospital. East Afr Med J 1998; 75: 223-226.
4.   Godtfredsen E. Ophthalmologic and neurologic symptoms of nasopharyngeal tumours. Acta Otolaryngologica, suppl.59, 1944.
5.   Teoh TB. Epidermoid carcinoma of the nasopharynx among the Chinese. Journal of Pathology and Bacteriology 1957; 73: 451-463.
6.   Sham JT, Choy D, Choy PHK. Nasopharyngeal carcinoma: The significance of neck node involvement in relation to the pattern of distant failure. British Journal of Radiology 1990; 63: 108-113
7.   Berger DS, Fletcher GH. Distant metastases following local control of squamous cell carcinoma of the nasopharynx, tonsillar fossa and base of the tongue. Radiology 1971; 100: 141-143.
8.   Petrovich S, Kuisk H, Jose l, Barton RT. Advanced cancer of the nasopharynx. Acta Radiologica Oncology 1981; 20: 245-251.
9.   Probert JC, Thompson RW, Bagshaw MA. Patterns of spread of distant metastases in head and neck cancer. Cancer 1974; 33: 127-133.
10.   Papavasiliou CG. Cancer of the nasopharynx: Incidence, clinical course and results of therapy. Clinical Radiology 1972; 25: 409-414.
11.   Chen KY and Fletcher GH. Malignant tumours of the nasopharynx. Radiology 1971; 99: 165-171.
12.   Bears OH, Henson DE, Hutter RVP, Kennedy BJ. American Joint Committee of Cancer: Manual for staging of cancer. 4th Ed 1992. Pp37. I.B. Lippincort Company.

ACTUAL RESULTS OF RADICAL NECK DISSECTION
FOR RECURRENT DISEASE AFTER RADIOTHERAPY

Ebeling , Olaf; Singelmann, Hendrik; Bielefeld, Katja; Volling, Peter
Center for Head and Neck surgery, ENT Diseases Oldenburg, Niedersachsen, Deutschland

Correspondence to: Ltd. Oberarzt Dr. med. Olaf Ebeling, Zentrum f. Hals-Nasen- und Ohrenheilkunde, Kopf- und Halschirurgie, Evangelisches Krankenhaus Oldenburg, Steinweg 13-17, D- 26122 Oldenburg, Tel.: ++49-441.236383, Fax: ++49-0441.9736044

Patients: 22 Patients with clinically recurrence of neck disease after radiotherapy or surgery and radiotherapy irrespective of carotid infiltration
Main outcome measure:Benefit for the patients

Key words: Radical neck dissection, carotid infiltration, Sqamous cell carcinoma of the head and neck, Radiotherapy, Radiochemotherapy

Results: In 18.1% patients died due to a secondary malignancy. Local recurrence occured in 13.6%, a distant metastasis was found in 27%, local control could be achieved in 68.7%, 5 patients are living more than 20 month after surgery.

Conclusions: The outlook for the regarded group remains poor but surgical intervention is potentially curative and includes a high palliative effect with a local control rate of 68%.

INTRODUCTION

Cervical recurrence of head and neck cancers after definitive radiation or surgery and radiotherapy indicates a very poor prognosis. We wanted to examine the benefit of radical surgery partially including carotid resection in this patient group.

PATIENTS AND METHOD

Prior to any decision on the adaquate treatment of their cervical recurrences all patients underwent panendoscopy of the upper aerodigetive tract to exclude local recurrence of the primary tumor and secondary coexisting primaries. All patients underwent CT-scanning and or MRI and angiography of the head and neck region for an exact assesment of the recurrent tumor. Actual we treated 22 patients with recurrent cervical metastasis after radiotherapy (RT)[3], radiochemotherapy (RCT)[4], operation (OP) and RT[15]. Our standard surgical treatment was a radical neck dissection irrespective of carotid infiltration.We performed 4 resections of infiltrated external carotid arteries, 3 interpositions of a saphenous vein graft were necessary, in 2 cases an end-to-end anastomosis of the carotid artery was performed after tumorresection. For skin closure 2 myocutaneus and 1 deltopectoral flap were required, to resect the tumor one hemimandibulectomy and two total and one radical Parotidektomy had to be operated.

RESULTS

Local control could be achieved in 15 patients (68.2%) . 6 patients died of local recurrence of disease (27.2%), 4 died of unrelated secondary malignancy (18%). 5 patients still live more than 20 month, one of them with distant metastasis, the rest disease free. In 3 cases histologically findings showed no complete resection of the cancer, 1 patient still lives with palliative chemotherapy, 2 others died within 5 month after surgery. 18 of 22 were hospitalized for less than 14 days, 3 patients are still living with distant metastasis for more than 12 month. We suspected a carotid infiltration in 14 cases, histological examination confirmed this suspicion in 9 cases. The operative mortality was 0% but there were three postoperative death occuring at day 27,33,41 respectivly. One patient died due to an Addison crisis provoqued by an secondary unrelated nephretic malignancy, the other two were victims of tumor bleeding after incomplete tumor removal. Wound healing complications were registrated in 145 of the procedures.

CONCLUSIONS

Our actual results seems to validate our opinion that radical revision surgery of the neck is not only palliative but may even offer a curative treatment alternative for some patients.

Clearly, however a postoperative mortality of 14% is highly unwelcome but it has to be considered into the counselling for such procedures.Tumor reduction makes no sense! The high rate of proven carotid infiltration shows, that carotid replacement must be an available technique.

The relatively short hospital stay and moderate wound healing complications allow to perform this kind of surgery even in palliative intention.

Table 1

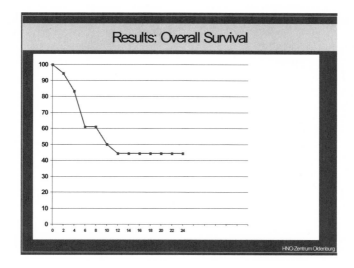

Table 2:

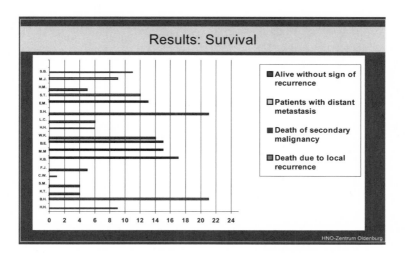

PERISTOMAL RECURRENCES OF LARYNGEAL
AND HYPOPHARYNGEAL CARCINOMA

Hans Edmund Eckel, M.D., Department of Oto-Rhino-Laryngology, University of Cologne, Germany

Correspondence to: *Prof. Dr. Hans Edmund Eckel, Dept. Of Oto-Rhino-Laryngology, University of Cologne, 50924 Koeln Germany, Phone: +49+221-478 4760, Fax: +49+221-478 64 25 (e-mail: hans.eckel@uni-koeln.de)*

Background. Although surgery with or without postoperative radio-therapy is usually considered to provide higher cure rates for laryngeal and hypopharyngeal cancer than any other treatment modality, a small but still significant proportion of patients will eventually present with local or regional treatment failure. Recurrences at the site of the tracheostoma in patients who have previously undergone total laryngectomy for carcinoma of the larynx or hypopharynx represent one typical site of treatment failure and continue to be a major diagnostic and therapeutic challenge in head and neck oncology.[1] These recurrences may occur following incomplete resection of the primary or as a consequence of lymphatic spread of the initial tumor to the lymphatic vessels of the cervical trachea.

However, during the last decades, the ability to reconstruct even extended circular pharyngeal defects by means of advanced and reliable reconstructive surgical techniques has considerably expanded our ability to deal with these lesions and prompt an update on the management of such recurrences.

Incidence

Recurrence rates have remained basically unchanged over time (table 1)[2-7,7-10]. This would indicate that no progress in the prevention of such lesions has been achieved during the last decades, if the indications for total laryngectomy had remained unchanged over time. However, two novel approaches to the treatment of the disease have contributed to the spectrum of therapeutic options during the past two decades: New surgical procedures for organ- and function-sparing resection of laryngeal carcinoma, including novel conventional partial laryngectomies, and transoral laser surgery. These procedures are mostly used for early stage disease and have obviated the need to perform total laryngectomy in many cases. Sequential or concomitant chemotherapy and radiotherapy for organ preservation in advanced stages is another alternative to total laryngectomy that is now widely used for those lesions that are not too far advanced. Therefore, unchanged local recurrence rates following total laryngectomy may well represent an oncological progress, since the percentage of patients with poor prognostic parameters at the time of the initiation of treatment may be higher than only two decades ago.

Risk factors

Some risk factors for stomal recurrences have traditionally been associated with stomal recurrences: Timing of tracheotomy, subglottic extension of the primary, T-Status, N-Status, previous radiation therapy failure, previous conservation surgery failure, and failure to resect the thyroid lobe of the involved side.

Eighty percent of patients with stomal recurrences initially had tumors in the subglottis. Tumor involvement of the subglottis is therefore now believed to be the single most important variable in stomal recurrence of carcinoma (table 2).[2,4-12] Other variables examined and analyzed included primary stage, previous treatment, neck pathologic status, neck treatment, age, sex, postoperative adjunctive therapy, and timing of tracheotomy. Previous conservation laryngeal surgery and preoperative/emergency tracheotomy are not related to stomal recurrence of carcinoma.[12]

The mechanisms that may lead to stomal recurrences include residual primary tumor giving rise to local recurrence, metastatic spread to lymphatic vessels or lymph nodes of the trachea, metastatic spread to lymphatic vessels or lymph nodes of the mediastinum, and implantation of cancer cells during endoscopy or surgical procedures (tracheotomy, laryngectomy). While it was believed for long that metastatic spread to mediastinal lymph nodes was the key to the understanding of these recurrences, it is now clear that metastatic spread to lymphatic vessels or lymph nodes of the trachea may be an even more important mechanism in the etiology of these lesions. Werner and coworkers were able to demonstrate that the laryngeal lymphatic system is in continuity with the lymphatics of the trachea. Lymphatic compartments in the larynx and the trachea cannot be found. They concluded that the continuity of the lymphatic system of the laryngo-tracheal junction may contribute to the understanding of the etiology of stomal recurrences[13,14]

Classification

According to G.A. Sisson[15], stomal recurrences are classified into for types:

Type 1 Localized to superior aspect of stoma. Esophagus, lower trachea, vessels not involved.

Type 2 Localized to superior aspect of stoma with esophageal involvement

Type 3 Lesions originating from inferior aspect of stoma that invade the esophagus and the paratracheal skin, but no other key structures.

Type 4 Lesions invading other key structures than esophagus and paratracheal skin (unresectable)

This classification has meanwhile found general acceptance. It allows for improved treatment planning, prognosticates outcome and allows to compare treatment results.

Management

The pretherapeutic assessment of the patient with suspected stomal recurrence should include a complete history, tracheoscopy and esophagoscopy with biopsies from the suspected recurrence site, CT and/or MRI-imaging of neck and mediastinum. Modern imaging technique now allow for a precise prediction of the extend of the recurrence in the neck and mediastinum, and for a preoperative assessment of pharyngeal and/or esophageal involvement. Distant metastases should be searched for. However, their presence will not necessarily rule out further treatment.

Surgery is usually the only valid option for treatment. Since most patients have initially been treated with radiotherapy alone or with surgery plus postoperative radiotherapy, further irradiation is frequently impossible for the treatment of these relapses, and surgery is the mainstay of recurrence-related treatment. Radiotherapy alone, if feasible at all, has practically never been curative in earlier reports in the literature (0/26 patients with XRT alive after 24 months[5] 0/10 patients with XRT alive after 24 months[7]). It is therefore now apparent that the role of radiotherapy in the management of stomal recurrence is limited to its prevention.[5]

Wide resection of the peristomal skin, along with extended excision of the cervical and thoracic trachea are the basic surgical principals. Involvement of the pharynx or esophagus may require additional microvascular procedures for the reconstruction of an alimentary tract. Except for the small number of patients with limited and small lesions, most recurrences require an interdisciplinary surgical approach, combining the skills of oncologically trained head and neck surgeons, thoracic surgeons, reconstructive surgeons, and anesthesiologists. In such a setting, surgery for peristomal recurrences achieves excellent palliation for a very high percentage of all patients, and long-lasting disease -free survival for a considerable proportion of these. Resection of the recurrence usually requires partial or total pharyngectomy and/or esophagectomy, resection of stoma and cervical trachea, mediastinal dissection an the removal of clavicles and/or manubrium.

Surgical reconstruction frequently includes myocutaneous flaps, gastric pull-up or jejunal free grafts for esophageal reconstruction, myocutaneous flaps and local skin flaps for tracheal reconstruction, and deltopectoral skin flaps, pectoralis major myocutaneous island flap, latissimus dorsi flaps or microvascular radial forearm flaps for external resurfacing.

While the prognosis of patients with stomal recurrence was generally extremely poor before these advanced surgical techniques became routinely available (3/33 (9.1%) patients alive after 24 months[3], 3/14 (21.4%) patients alive after 24 months[4]), recent reports have demonstrated improved survival rates with aggressive surgery for these lesions (45% 2-year survival for types I and II (n=18) and 9% 2-year survival for types III and IV (n=23)[16]; 45% survival at 42 months for selected cases[15].

However, the dismal prognosis of stomal recurrence of carcinoma suggests that management of this condition should focus on prevention rather than on treatment.[12] Among other factors, the following may be effective in reducing the number of peristomal recurrences, although not all of them were statistically significant in a multivariate analysis:[12]

- Avoid tracheotomy prior to laryngectomy,
- Resect tracheotomy track completely,
- Perform hemithyroidectomy with total LE,
- Resect cervical trachea extensively,
- Resect paratracheal lymph nodes,
- Irradiate trachea and paratracheal lymph nodes.

It is unclear to date whether tracheotomy prior to total laryngectomy is an independent risk factor, or whether it is just associated with advanced subglottic primaries who carry a well known high risk for such recurrences in themselves.

Conclusion

Tumor involvement of the subglottis seems to be most important risk factor in stomal recurrence of laryngeal and hypopharyngeal cancer. Treatment should encompass radical surgery whenever feasible. The dismal prognosis of stomal recurrence of carcinoma suggests that management of this condition should focus on prevention. Treatment of patients with tumors of the subglottis should include paratracheal and superior mediastinal lymph node dissection and postoperative radiotherapy to the cervical trachea.

Table 1: Incidence rates of stomal recurrences

Author	Patients with total LE	Patients with stomal recurrence
Stell/van den Broek 1971	196	8 (4.1%)
Myers/Ogura 1979	452	33 (7.3%)
Weisman/Ward 1979	251	14 (5.6%)
Mantravadi/Skolnik 1981	507	26 (5.1%)
Amatsu et al. 1985	340	20 (5.9%)
Rockley et al. 1991	91 (glottic T3N0M0)	12 (13.2%)
Esteban et al. 1993	209	17 (8.1%)
Yokatis et al. 1996	352	21 (6.0%)
Zbären et al. 1996	130	13 (10%)

Table 2: Stomal recurrences and site of primary

REFERENCES

1. Barr GD, Robertson AG, Liu KC. Stomal recurrence: a separate entity? J Surg Oncol 1990; 44:176-179.
2. Stell PM, Broek Pvd. Stomal recurrence after laryngectomy: aetiology and management. J Laryngol Otol 1971; 85:131-140.
3. Myers EM, Ogura JH. Stomal recurrences: a clinicopathological analysis and protocol for future management. Laryngoscope 1979; 89:1121-1128.
4. Weisman RA, Colman M, Ward PH. Stomal recurrence following laryngectomy: a critical evaluation. Ann Otol Rhinol Laryngol 1979; 88:855-860.
5. Mantravadi R, Katz AM, Skolnik EM, Becker S, Freehling DJ, Friedman M. Stomal recurrence. A critical analysis of risk factors. Arch Otolaryngol 1981; 107:735-738.
6. Amatsu M, Makino K, Kinishi M. Stomal recurrence--etiologic factors and prevention. Auris Nasus Larynx 1985; 12:103-110.
7. Rockley TJ, Powell J, Robin PE, Reid AP. Post-laryngectomy stomal recurrence: tumour implantation or paratracheal lymphatic metastasis? Clin Otolaryngol 1991; 16:43-47.
8. Esteban F, Moreno JA, Delgado-Rodriguez M, Mochon A. Risk factors involved in stomal recurrence following laryngectomy. J Laryngol Otol 1993; 107:527-531.
9. Yotakis J, Davris S, Kontozoglou T, Adamopoulos G. Evaluation of risk factors for stomal recurrence after total laryngectomy. Clin Otolaryngol 1996; 21:135-138.
10. Zbaren P, Greiner R, Kengelbacher M. Stoma recurrence after laryngectomy: an analysis of risk factors. Otolaryngol Head Neck Surg 1996; 114:569-575.
11. Leon X, Quer M, Burgues J, Abello P, Vega M, de Andres L. Prevention of stomal recurrence. Head Neck 1996; 18:54-59.
12. Rubin J, Johnson JT, Myers EN. Stomal recurrence after laryngectomy: interrelated risk factor study. Otolaryngol Head Neck Surg 1990; 103:805-812.
13. Duenne AA, Werner JA. Functional anatomy of lymphatic vessels under the aspect of tumor invasion. Recent Results Cancer Res 2000; 157:82-89.
14. Werner JA, Schunke M, Rudert H, Tillmann B. Description and clinical importance of the lymphatics of the vocal fold. Otolaryngol Head Neck Surg 1990; 102:13-19.

15.   Sisson GA, Sr. 1989 Ogura memorial lecture: mediastinal dissection. Laryngoscope 1989; 99:1262-1266.
16.   Gluckman JL, Hamaker RC, Schuller DE, Weissler MC, Charles GA. Surgical salvage for stomal recurrence: a multi-institutional experience. Laryngoscope 1987; 97:1025-1029.

INCIDENCE OF DISTANT METASTASIS AND SECOND PRIMARIES FOLLOWING LOCALLY SUCCESFUL TREATED CARCINOMA OF THE PHARYNX

Jens Büntzel MD[1], Michael Glatzel MD[2]
[1]Department of Otolaryngology, Plastic Surgery, Zentralklinikum Suhl; Germany
[2]Department of Radiotherapy, Zentralklinikum Suhl, Germany

Correspondence to: Jens Büntzel, MD, HNO-Klinik am Zentralklinikum Suhl, Albert-Schweitzer-Str. 2, D-98527 Suhl, Germany

ABSTRACT

Objective. Has an addtional chemotherapy any effect on the incidence of distant metastasis and secondary tumors in patients with advanced cancer of the oro- and hypopharynx ?

Methods. We analyzed the incidence of distant metastasis and secondary cancer in a group of 189 patients with an advanced squamous cell carcinoma of the pharynx according their basic treatment. At the time of diagnosis no patient had a distant metastasis or a second tumor. 156 were in stage IV of UICC, further 33 in stage III. Surgery included laser-resection of the primary tumor and neck dissection of N+ neck. Chemotherapy: * 700 mg/sqm Carboplatin, ** 1050 to 1400 mg/sqm Carboplatin. Radiotherapy:2 Gy single dose, 60 Gy total dose (plus 10 Gy boost for primary radiochemotherapy), daily fractionation.

Results. After a median follow-up of 41 month we observed the following incidences: distant metastases in 10.6 %, and second primary cancers 1.6%. Especially the development of distant metastases was dependent from the usage and the dosage of chemotherapeutic agents.

Conclusion. The presented results suggest an dose-dependent influence of chemotherapy on the development of distant metastasis. No impact was seen on the incidence of secondary cancers.

INTRODUCTION

After multimodal therapies for previously untreated advanced head and neck cancer, 40% - 50% of pa tients develop local or locoregional recurrence, and 20% - 30% develop distant metastases[1-4]. Following single modality treatment because of an early stage (T1/2N0) disease, between 10% and 20% develop local or locoregional recurrence only, and <10% develop distant metastases[2]. The risk of recurrent disease (local, locoregional, distant) decreases substantially two years after completion of local therapy[1, 2]. The risk of secondary primary cancers, however, remains constant about a longer time. It is estimated that the annual incidence of secondray cancers is 4%-6% up to year 8 after succesful local treatment. In the presented paper we will focus our interest to the incidence of distant metastasis as well as seconcary primaries after completion of locally succesful treatment of an advanced pharyngeal cancer. Secondly we will analyze the impact of chemotherapy as a newer part of multimodal treatment on these incidences.

MATERIAL AND METHODS

Primary endpoints of our analysis were two quantities: the incidence of distant metastasis, and the incidence of secondary primaries in patients with advanced pharyngeal cancer. Secondary we were interested in the impact of antineoplastic chemotherapy on these both parameters.

The basic instrument for this investigation was the data base of our patients that were treated between 1991 and 1999 at the departments of radiotherapy and otolaryngology because of a pharyngeal cancer. 189 patients were included. Besides the multimodal treatment approach we had only one further inclusion criterium: at the end of primary treatment the patients had shown no residual tumor.

Following types of basic treatment combinations were differentiated: Group 1: SURGERY PLUS RADIOTHERAPY. This combination was used in the majority of patients between 1991 and 1993. After succesful resection of the primary cancer (lasersurgical technique) a function preserving neck dissection was performed. The adjunctive therapy included only the irradiation. The single radiation dose was 2 Gy, the total dose 60 Gy. No radiosensitizing agent was used. Group 2: SURGERY PLUS RADIOCHEMOTHERAPY. After resection of the tumor a simultaneous radiochemotherapy was performed. In 1992 and 1993 seven patients received the combination of cisplatin and 5-fluorouracil, after 1993 we used carboplatin as the only radiosensitizing agent. Cisplatin was given at week 1 and week 5 of radiotherapy in a dose of 25 mg/m^2 per day about 1 hour (five consecutive days) and 5-fluorouracil in a dose of 600 mg/m^2 per day about 24 hours. Carboplatin was administered in a dose of 70 mg/m^2 about 30 minutes before the daily irradiation. The cumulative doses were 250 mg/m^2 cisplatin and 6.000 mg/m^2 5-fluorouracil or 700 mg/m^2 carboplatin per patient of this group. Group 3: DEFINITIVE SIMULTANEOUS RADIOCHEMOTHERAPY. The radiotherapy included the irradiation of the primary tumor with single doses of 2 Gy up to a total dose of 70 Gy in a daily fractionation. The lymph-node positive neck was irradiated up to 60 Gy, the lymph-node negative neck up to 50 Gy. We had used the combination regimen carboplatin/5-fluorouracil in 31 patients, in further fourteen patients the carboplatin was given alone. The chemotherapy was administered on the days of week 1 and week 5. Carboplatin was given as short infusion before the daaily irradiation (70 mg/m^2) and 5-fluorouracil as prolonged infusion about 24 hours (600 mg/m^2). The resulting cumulative doses were 700 mg/m^2 carboplatin and 6.000 mg/m^2 5-fluorouracil per patient of this group. Group 4: SMALL CAPS INTENSIFIED DEFINITIVE SIMULTANEOUS RADIOCHEMOTHERAPY. No surgery was used in the patients of this group. The radiotherapy was performed as described for group 3 above. Carboplatin was administered as radiosensitizer alone. If the patients were in good general appearance following chemotherapy schedule was choosen: Carboplatin short infusion before the daily radiotherapy in week 1, week 3, week 5 and week 7 of the combined treatment. Amifostine was applicated in a dose of total 500 mg immediately before the platinum derivate (70 mg/m^2 carboplatin per day). The resulting cumulative doses were 1.400 mg/m^2 carboplatin and 20.000 mg amifostine per patient of this group.

SURGERY PLUS RADIOTHERAPY. 45 out of 189 patients were summarized in group 1. The 40 men and 5 woman had a median age of 55.4 years (range 38-77). 15 patients were classified as stage III, 30 patients as stage IV of UICC. Tumor localzations: 25 oropharyngeal cancers, 20 hypopharyngeal cancers (ratio 1,25:1). All patients showed a squamous cell carcinoma of the pharynx. SURGERY PLUS RADIOCHEMOTHERAPY. In group 2 we concluded 68 patients receiving surgery plus simultaneous radiochemotherapy. The 62 men and 6 women had a median age of 56.0 years (range 38-71). 16 patients wer in stage III, the remaining 52 patients in stage IV of UICC. Tumor localizations: 38 oropharyngeal cancers, 30 hypopharyngeal cancers (ratio 1,27:1). DEFINITIVE SIMULTANEOUS RADIOCHEMOTHERAPY. In group 3 we included 45 patients (41 men, 4 women) with a median age of 56.2 years (range 38-78). Only one patient was in stage III, 44 patients were in stage IV UICC. Tumor localizations: 20 oropharyngeal cancers, 25 hypopharyngeal cancers (ratio 1:1,25). Intensified definitive simultaneous radiochemotherapy. Group 4 included 31 patients (28 men, 3 women) with the median age of 55.8 years (range 37-76). One patient was in stage III, the remaining 30 patients stage IV disease. Tumor localizations: 13 oropharyngeal cancers, 18 hypopharyngeal cancers (ratio 1:1,38).

RESULTS

The median follow-up was 41 month (range 21-108 month). Following detailed median observation times were found: group 1 – 80 month, group 2 – 43 month, group 3 – 49 month, group 4 – 24 month.

Distant metastasis: Three patients of group 1 developed metastasis at the lungs (2 cases) and the bone (1 case) after SURGERY PLUS RADIOTHERAPY. Five patients of group 2 had shown metastasis at the lungs (2 cases), the skin (2 cases) and the liver (1 case) after SURGERY PLUS RADIOCHEMOTHERAPY. 10 out of 45 patients of group 3 developed distant metastasis in the lungs (5 cases), the bone (2 cases), the skin (2 cases), and the liver (1 case) AFTER DEFINITIVE SIMULTANEOUS RADIOCHEMOTHERAPY. Only two patients of group 4 developed distant metastasis in the lungs (1 case) and the liver (1 case) after INTENSIFIED DEFINITIVE SIMULTANEOUS RADIOCHEMOTHERAPY.

Summarizing these detailed results the overall incidence of distant metastasis was 20/189 (10,6 %). The differences between the four groups is shown in table 1.

Secondary primaries: We have not observed any patient with secondary primaries in group 1 as well as in group 4. Two out of 68 patients of group 2 developed secondary primaries at the tongue (one case) and the esophagus (one case). One patient of group 3 has been treated because of a secondary primary at the lungs. The overall incidence of secondary primaries was 1,6 % in our population. No real differences were seen between the four groups of basic treatment.

Table 1. Incidence of distant metastasis due to the basic treatment

	Total	Distant metastasis
Surgery + Radiotherapy	45	6,7 %
Surgery + Radiochemotherapy	68	7,4 %
Defintive simultaneous Radiochemotherapy	45	22,2 %
Intensified definitive simultaneous Radiochemotherapy	31	6,5 %

DISCUSSION

In several studies an adjuvant chemotherapy has been reproducibly shown to decrease the rate of distant metastases as the site of first failure indicating clinically measurable systemic anti-cancer activity[1-5]. Concomitant radiochemotherapy protocols continue to be the most promising investigational strategies in head and neck cancer[1, 2]. It is most likely to benefit the patients through a direct interaction between the modalities within the radiation field leading to increased cytotoxicity, and thus improved local and locoregional control, as well as survival[1]. The simultaneous way of application has been shown as the most effective of combined modalities according metaanalysis that were published recently. No information were found in the literature about the influence of addtional simultaneous applicated chemotherapy on the incidence of distant metastases[1]. Our data suggest that the usual dosage of carboplatin, e.g. two cycles split-course application with a cumulative dose of 700 mg/m^2 is not able to decrease the development of distant metastases. At first there was no difference between group1 Surgery plus radiotherapy and group 2 Surgery plus radiochemotherapy at low levels of incidence. This subresult is remarkable because the survival rates for patients with surgery plus adjunctive radiochemotherapy are significant higher than those for surhergy plus radiotherapy alone[1, 2]. At second, there was an incrreasing number of such metastases after definitive simultaneous radiochemotherapy (standard) alone. The observed incidence of 22 % is higher than the reported incidence for advanced stages of disease[2]. But the significant decrease from 22% to 6.5% may be interpreted as a positive impact of intensified chemotherapy dosage on the later development of distant metastases. The follow-up of these patients is at least 21 month, the results should be secured for this patient subpopulation. Of course the intensified doses of carboplatin are not a common and usual way in the combined therapy of advanced head and neck cancer. New combination chemotherapy regimen ans substances will have to show their efficacy in this field too.

No real informations could be received by this study about the incidence of second primary tumors. The overall estimated incidence was less than 2%. One of the reasons seems to be the relatively short follow-up interval. Only if the patients were treated between 1992 and 1993 the time-interval is big enough to get correct informations about this questions. For the first years, the additional chemotherapy had no influence on the development of secondary cancers in our patients.

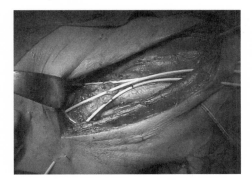

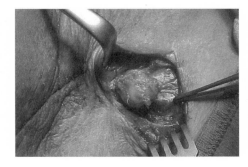

Figure 1. Tumor-infiltrated bulbus caroticum and implanted silicone catheters for interstitial brachytherapy

Figure 2. Fibrosis and iatrogenic subcutaneous metastasis along the posterior catheter

REFERENCES

1. Vokes EE, RR Weichselbaum, SM Lippman, WK Hong: Head and neck cancer. N Engl J Med 328 (1993): 184-194
2. Lippman SM: Chemoprevention of head and neck carcinogenesis. In: ASCO Educational Book spring 1995, pp 117-122
3. Hong WK, SM Lippman, GT Wolf: Recent advances in head and neck cancer – Larynx preservation and cancer chemoprevention. Cancer Res 53 (1994): 5113-5120
4. Hong WK, RH Bromer, DA Amato et al.: Patterns of relapse in locally advanced head and neck cancer patients who achieved complete remission after combined modality therapiy. Cancer 56 (1985): 1242-1245
5. Benner SE, SM Lippman, WK Hong: Chemoprevention of second primary tumours: A model for intervention trials. Eur J Cancer 30A (1994): 727-729
6. Vikram B: Changing patterns of failure in advanced head and neck cancer. Arch Otolaryngol 110 (1984): 564-565
7. Vokes EE, DJ Haraf, RR Weichselbaum, D Brachman: Induction chemotherapy: promises and limitations. Head and Neck Cancer. Vol III. Eds: Johnson JT, MS Didolkar, Excerpta Medica Internat Congress Series 1009, pp 321-326, 1993
8. Forastiere AA: Randomized trials of induction chemotherapy. A critical review. Hem Oncol Clin North Am 5 (1991): 725-736
9. Browman GP: Evidence-based recommendations against neoadjuvant chemotherapy for routine management of patients with squamous cell head and neck cancer. Cancer Invest 12 (1994): 662-671
10. Jacobs C, R Makuch: Efficacy of adjuvant chemotherapy for patients with resectable head and neck cancer. A subset analysis of the Head and Neck Contracts Program. J Clin Oncol 8 (1990): 838-847
11. Schuller DE, B Metch, D Mattox, et al.: Prospective chemotherapy in advanced resectable head and neck cancer. Final report of the Southwest Oncology Group. Laryngoscope 98 (1988):1205-1211
12. Vokes EE, RR Weichselbaum: Chemoradiation for head and neck cancer. Prin Prac Oncol Updates 7 (1993): 1-8
13. Jacobs C: Head and neck cancer in 1994: a change in the standard of care (Editorial) J Natl Cancer Inst 86 (1994): 250-251
14. Vokes EE: Interactions of chemotherapy and radiation. Semin Oncol 20 (1993): 70-79

15.   Vokes EE: Combined modality therapy of advanced head and neck cancer. ASCO Educational Book Spring 1995, pp 123-126

16.   Haffty BG, YH Son, CT Sasaki, et al.: Mitomycin C as an adjunct to postoperative radiation therapy in squamous cell carcinoma of the head and neck: Results from two randomized clinical trials. Int J Radiat Oncol Biol Phys 27 (1993): 241-250

17.   Glatzel, M., J. Büntzel, D. Fröhlich, K. Küttner: Laser-surgical resection and adjunctive concomitant radiochemotherapy in locally advanced head and neck cancer. In: Alvarez Vincent, J.J. (ed.): 1st World Congress on Head and Neck Oncology. Monduzzi, Bologna, 1998, pp 1301-1306

PALIATIVE MEDICINE IN
ADVANCED HEAD AND NECK CANCER PATIENTS

Andreas S. Lübbe, MD., PhD., Associate Professor, Bad Lippspringe, Germany

DEFINITION AND INTRODUCTION

According to the WHO, palliative medicine is the active total care of patients whose disease is not responsive to curative treatment. Control of pain and other symptoms and of psychological, social and spiritual problems is paramount[1]. The goal of palliative care is to achieve the best quality of life for patients and their families. Some aspects of palliative care are also applicable earlier in the course of the illness in conjunction with anticancer treatment. Its purpose then is to relieve symptoms and to enhance quality of life. In this regard, palliative care affirms life and regards dying as a normal process. It neither hastens nor postpones death and provides relief from pain and other distressing symptoms. Palliative care integrates the psychological and the spiritual aspects of care as well as offers a support system to help the family cope during the patient's illness and in their own bereavement.

These ingredients of palliative medicine have to be considered when one recaps the acquired capabilities of cancer cells. They are: self-sufficiency in growth signals, insensitivity to antigrowth signals, evading apoptosis, unlimited proliferation potential, sustained angiogenesis, tissue invasion and metastases. Cancer will be a major cause of human suffering, due to an age effect. The number of new cancer cases is likely to double from 10 to 20 million within the next 20 years, although the world population will only increase by 30%; the mortality rate is expected to remain constant[2]. Traditionally, the focus in the aims of cancer therapy has been the prevention of the disease and the aspect of cure. The fact that life can be prolonged besides the possibility of cure, the importance of rehabilitation, palliation and comfort have received, as a group, far less support and attention[3]. According to currently allocated cancer resources most is spent for active anticancer treatments and not for symptom control. However, cancer management is much more than cure or prolonging life.

Head and neck cancer, as a group, represent roughly 5% of all malignant diseases. Yearly, mortality remains at about 6/100.000 with regional variation and distinct male predilection (4/1). In numbers, roughly 500.000 people die of head and neck cancer every year according to the WHO statistics from 1997[4].

PALLIATIVE TREATMENT OPTIONS

Advanced head and neck cancers can be treated by different means to prolong survival, but also to treat manifest symptoms. Different procedures, such as surgery, radiation, chemotherapy and others, are possible in this regard. In the advanced disease state, combined radio/chemotherapy based on cisplatin and 5-FU are far superior than radiation only in most advanced head and neck carcinomas[5]. Multimodal treatment ought to be implemented whenever possible, depending upon age, WHO performance status, Karnofsky-Index and the overall quality of life framed by proliferation kinetics, patient wish and other social factors. Randomized clinical trials have identified cisplatin, 5-FU and methotrexate as being the substances with highest rates of remission[6, 7]. New substances, such as gemcitabine and paclitacel in conjunction with radiation treatment have also proved to be successful for palliative treatment regiments[8]. Combination therapies have shown efficacy for a cyclophosphamide, adriamycine and cisplatin or cisplatin, vinorelbin alone or in combination with bleomycin[9].

THE DILEMMA OF SYMPTOMS AND THEIR TREATMENT

Since overall survival is limited even by aggressive treatment procedures, symptom control must be primary objective of any treatment. Because of the diversity and variety of individual tumors in the head and neck region, definitive clinical trials are rather uncommon. Palliative therapy of advanced disease has not been subject to a systematic analysis[10]. Tumors of the head and neck produce problems by obstructing hollow organs, by causing neurological impairments (both, sensory and motor) and, perhaps most crucial to the patients, by the destruction of communication - both, expressive and where there is external disfigurement, receptive. Obstructive symptoms, haemorrhage and fistulas are common. Dysphagia can be caused by diverse mechanisms, including compression by local tumor masses, neurological dysfunction, aspiration and post-surgical complications. Because tumors of the head and neck are extremely heterogeneous with regards to macroscopic appearance and in biological behaviour, there are no simple prognostic rules, nor have complex indices been constructed. Unfortunately, even the simplest radical treatment for head and neck cancer, for example radiotherapy for early laryngeal tumors, entails significant distress and discomfort. Radical treatment for some tumors of the head and neck, particularly with surgery and radiation treatment, have to be combined, come close to the limit of acceptability, even if cure can not be guaranteed. It is therefore the principle of palliative treatment that it should not incur significant morbidity. Yet, it is extremely difficult to devise a schedule of radiotherapy that will produce sufficient regression of tumors, to alleviate symptoms from head and neck cancer without producing significant unpleasant local side effects. These considerations have lead many experienced radiotherapists to conclude, that there can be no such thing as palliative radiotherapy for head and neck cancer and that to achieve adequate symptom control, radical doses are required. A similar argument applies to surgery[11].

THE CONCEPT OF DECISION ANALYSIS IN THE TREATMENT OF HEAD AND NECK CANCER SYMPTOMS

Decision analysis offers a repertoire of techniques, which may be useful for the evaluation of complex choices in clinical medicine[12]. It may have a role in providing guidelines for managing groups of patients and in formulating management policies. Quality-adjusted survival can be estimated by multiplying the duration of survival by a quality factor. A quality factor is introduced to take into account any morbidities, experienced by the patients. Ideally, this quality factor should be provided by the patients themselves. Quality-adjusted survival can be used as a measure of utility for each of the defined outcomes in an analysis. For a simple utility assessment, the individual correct decision would be one that results in the greatest number of quality-adjusted life years. For patients that are treated unsuccessfully or left untreated, the quality-adjusted survival must include the impairment of quality, produced by the symptom of the primary tumor. In contrast to any other cancer, the advanced head and neck cancer patients presents an almost intolerable complex situation. When, as in palliative therapy, cancer is already producing symptoms, when treatment itself will inevitably produce further morbidity and when the probability of success is low, then the issue becomes indeed hard to tolerate.

OPPORTUNITY COSTS AND THE ART NOT TO INTERVENE

However, when making decisions in medicine, it is often forgotten, that treatment may deny patients the opportunity to use their time in the ways that they might wish. This phenomenon is known to economists as opportunity cost[13]. Given finite resources, it may be impossible to have both, a holiday abroad and a new car. Either alone can be afforded, but not both. A choice has to be made and, if a holiday abroad is cheaper, then the opportunity cost is the loss of a new car. By using up limited time and energy, attempts to treat patients when cure is impossible will incur their own opportunity cost. Physicians tend to emphasise intervention and the means to improve patient's well being. There is much less concentration on the more difficult art of being able to judge when not to intervene. Pressure from relatives and the society for more practice favour intervention. The patient's own voice is small and often lost.

Parameters such as the probability of cure from radical treatment, survival time for untreated patients, the life expectancy of a cured patient and others can be transferred to lines of threshold to help deciding if radical treatment is preferable or not. The challenge then for the future is to divide palliative regiments with minimal intrinsic morbidity and not only relieve symptoms but also produce modest prolongation of life. Even when cure is impossible, increased survival provided that from the patient's point of view the time is spent usefully, is a goal worth achieving. Simple non-toxic regiments of chemotherapy can therefore improve results in patients treated with radical radiotherapy.

THE "PYRAMID APPROACH" FOR SYMPTOM CONTROL IN ADVANCED CANCER PATIENTS

Together with the WHO, we are now in the process of developing a new model for symptom control. In expansion of the WHO pain ladder, a "pyramid model" has been chosen as a three dimensional approach for symptom control[14]. There are 4 basic approaches for symptom control, procedures with the highest level of evidence come to a top, meta-pyramids can be generated from each side and for the individual patients. Whether one uses one or more types of intervention depends on the stage of the disease, the severity of a symptom, the availability of treatment and whether the clinician is a specialist or a generalist. In this regard, advanced head and neck cancer patients can be tackled for the most common symptoms:

xerostomia, pain, malodorous growths, speech- and communication disorders, swallowing disorders and nutritional sufficiency.

The multidimensional approach takes into consideration symptom severity and quality of life and will be further developed over the next coming years by an international interdisciplinary expert panel under the direction of the WHO.

REFERENCES

1. World Health Organisation. Cancer Pain Relief and Palliative Care. WHO Technical Report Series 804. Geneva. World Health Organisation, 1990
2. Sihova K. Developing a global strategy for Cancer. European J. Cancer 35, pp. 24-31, 1999
3. MacDonald N. A proposed matrix for organisational changes to improve quality of life in oncology. European J. Cancer 31, pp. 18-21, 1995
4. The World Health Report. Geneva, World Health Organisation, 1998
5. Chan AT, Teo PM, Leung TW. The role of chemotherapy in the management of nasopharyngeal carcinoma. Cancer 82, pp. 1003-1012, 1998
6. Voker EE, Athanasiadis I. Chemotherapy for squamous carcinoma of the head and neck: The future is now. Ann Oncol 7, pp. 15-29, 1996
7. Sidvansky D. Molecular biology of head and neck tumors. In: De Vita, Hellmann, Rosenberg (eds.). Principles and practice of oncology. Lippincott-Raven Publishers, Philadelphia, pp 735 ff, 1997
8. Catimel G, Verweij J, Mattijssen V. Doxetacele (Taxotere): An active drug for the treatment of patients with advanced squamous cell carcinoma of the head and neck. Ann Oncol 5, pp 553-537, 1994
9. Wildfang I. Low-dose gemcitabine with radiotherapy in advanced head and neck and thyroid tumors: a phase II study. Proc Am Soc Clin Oncol, 1999
10. Mac Dougall RH, Munro AJ, Wilson JA. Palliation in head and neck cancer. In: Doyle D, Hanks GWC, MacDonald N (eds.). Oxford Textbook of Palliative Medicine. Oxford Medical Publications, Oxford, pp 677-689, 1998.
11. Aird DW, Bihavi J, Smith C. Clinical problems in the continuing care of head and neck cancer patients. Ear, Nose and Throat Journal 62, pp. 10-30, 1983
12. Weistein MC, Fineberg HV, Elstein AS. Clinical Decision Analysis. Philadelphia, WB Saunders, 1980
13. Munro HJ, Sebag-Montefiore D. Opportunity-cost - a neglected aspect of tumor treatment. British J Cancer 65, pp. 309-310, 1992
14. Ahmedzai SA, Lübbe AS, van den Eynden B. A new paradigm for cancer symptom control - the pyramid approach. Lancet Oncology 2001 (in press)

METASTATIC ADENOID CYSTIC CARCINOMAS
OF THE SALIVARY GLANDS

Thomas K. Hoffmann[1,2], Hilmar Balló[1], Theresa L. Whiteside[2,3], Ulrich Hauser[1], Simon Watkins[2], Jonas T. Johnson[3], Carl H. Snyderman[3], Henning Bier[1].

[1]Department of Otorhinolaryngology, Head & Neck Surgery, Heinrich-Heine-University, D-40225 Düsseldorf, Germany.
[2]Pittsburgh Cancer Institute and
[3]Department of Otolaryngology at the University of Pittsburgh, PA 15213, USA.

Running title: metastatic adenoid cystic carcinomas

Key words: salivary gland; adenoid cystic carcinoma; metastasis; cell lines

Acknowledgement: Supported in part by grant D/99/08916 of the Dr. Mildred Scheel Stiftung für Krebsforschung [T.K.H.].

Correspondence to: Thomas K. Hoffmann, M.D., Department of Otorhinolaryngology, Head & Neck Surgery; Heinrich-Heine-University, Moorenstr. 5; D-40225 Düsseldorf; Germany, Phone.: ++49-211-811 7570; Fax: ++49-211-811 8880 (e-mail: t-k-h@web.de)

ABSTRACT

Background. Adenoid cystic carcinomas (ACC) are rare tumors which commonly arise from salivary glands and are characterized by perineural spread as well as a high rate of haematogenic metastasis.

Patients and Results. We present two cases of ACC originating from salivary glands. After surgery (case 1) plus simultaneous radio-chemotherapy (case 2), both patients relapsed with multiple pulmonary metastases after 7 and 41 months, respectively. Metastatic disease was treated with three cycles of adriamycin, cyclophosphamide and cisplatin (case 1) or a combination of 5-FU and methotrexate including leucovorin rescue every two weeks (case 2). A complete remission was achieved in case 1 which was followed by lethal deterioration of disease after 8 months. For case 2, extremely slow progression of metastatic disease was observed over a period of 32 months.

Conclusions. Obviously, both case reports describe different tumor biologies and demonstrate the limited effectiveness of current systemic treatment options for metastatic ACC. In order to explore novel therapeutic strategies we are currently establishing cell lines from ACC (flourescence-microscopically positive for keratin, type IV collagen, fibronectin, laminin and vimentin) which could serve as a basis for future in vitro studies on alternative treatment approaches such as modified chemotherapy regimens or cellular immunotherapy.

INTRODUCTION

Adenoid cystic carcinomas (ACC) are malignant epithelial tumors, which arise from salivary glands of patients at all ages, with a peak incidence in the fourth through sixth decade of life, and at a female to male ratio of 3 : 2. ACC are the fifth most common malignant epithelial tumors of salivary glands behind mucoepidermoid, adenocarcinoma, not otherwise specified (NOS), acinic cell adenocarcinoma, polymorphous low-grade adenocarcinoma[1]. The parotid, submandibular gland and palate are sites of most frequent occurrence and among the intraoral minor salivary glands they are the most common malignant tumor.

ACC are characterized by hardly accessible infiltrative growth with the tendency to spread along nerval structures, and disease progression is marked by numerous local recurrences and considerable protraction. Haematogenic metastasis (40-60%) to lung, brain, bone, liver and skin may appear even many years after aggressive surgical treatment and despite local tumor control[2-7]. True lymphogenous metastases, however, are seen much less frequently, and if they occur they are to be considered unfavorable prognostic indicators. Tumor progression per continuitatem, however, generally ensues lymph node involvement[8,9]. The classification of ACC distinguishes between 3 histological subtypes: tubular, cribiform and solid type with a better prognosis for tubular or cribiform growth pattern as compared to the solid type[3,5,10-15].

Common treatment of ACC is primary surgery and its extent is determined by site and size of the primary tumor. The surgical approach is designed to keep surgical consequences such as mutilation and considerable functional losses in a reasonable proportion to the therapeutic success that can be achieved[16,17]. Although the benefit of postoperative irradiation has been an issue of controversy[3,6-8,10,18-24], adjuvant radiotherapy is generally accepted when residual disease is suspected. Antineoplastic agents employed for chemotherapy of metastatic ACC have included cisplatin, 5-fluorouracil, adriamycin, cyclophosphamide, adriamycin and vincristine.

Here we exemplary describe two typical cases of metastatic ACC demonstrating the broad range of clinical courses associated with this disease. In addition, we present first results of our efforts to establish cell lines of ACC in order to create an adequate in vitro model.

Case Reports

Case 1: A tumor originating from the right submandibular gland was tightly fused with the horizontal ramus of the mandible and extended per continuitatem to the carotid sheath in the mandibular angle. Histology of a biopsy revealed solid type ACC. Imaging showed an isolated cervical lymph node metastasis, and there was no evidence for systemic extension of the tumor (CT-scan of the head & neck region, chest X-ray, bone scintigraphy, ultrasound of abdomen). Treatment consisted of homolateral extended radical neck dissection (external carotid artery and hypoglossal nerve were sacrified) and partial resection of the mandible in the en block tumor excision. The patient was staged T4, N1, Mx, of a solid type ACC demonstrating the most unfavorable prognostic factors except for distant metastases. Seven months later the patient developed cutaneous metastases in the right side of the face, metastatic distension of the manubrium sterni and multiple symptomatic pulmonary metastases. Subsequent treatment consisted of local excision of cutaneous metastases and the initiation of chemotherapy with adriamycin ($60mg/m^2$), cyclophosphamide ($600mg/m^2$, on day 1) and cisplatin ($100 \ mg/m^2$, on day 2). With three therapeutic cycles applied, a complete remission was achieved. However, eight months after systemic chemotherapy, a drastic deterioration of the patient´s condition was noticed. In addition to previous findings, metastasis to liver, kidneys and brain appeared.

Case 2: The patient presented with a tumor arising from small salivary glands of the right soft palate without evidence of regional or distant metastasis (CT-scan of the head & neck, chest X-ray, bone scintigraphy, ultrasound of abdomen). Transoral excision of the tumor including removal of parapharyngeal lymph nodes was performed with the result of a T3, N0, Mx mixed cribiform-tubular ACC. Postoperative radio-chemotherapy consisted of 74Gy in shrinking-field technique including two cycles of cisplatin and 5-FU. The patient relapsed with multiple pulmonary metastases after 41 months. Metastatic disease was treated with a combination of 5-FU ($600 \ mg/m^2$) and methotrexate ($200 \ mg/m^2$) including leucovorin rescue (90 mg) every two weeks. Until today, very slow progression of metastatic disease was observed over a period of 32 months.

Establishment of cell lines: From 4 patients with ACC, tumor tissue was dissected into small pieces which were placed overnight into tissue flasks precoated with fetal calf serum. The following day, culture flasks were carefully floated with medium (D-MEM, 20% fetal calf serum, Glutamine, Penicillin, Streptomycin, Amphotericin B). After 1-2 weeks and weekly thereafter, partial trypsinisation was performed in order to remove outgrowing fibroblasts. After approximately 6-8 months, cell monolayers were characterized by various antibodies. In three out of four cases the outgrowth of epithelial-like cells was demonstrated. Exemplary, the results obtained from a solid type ACC of the ethmoid are shown in Figure 1. The cells are characterized by a very low doubling time (~8 days) and showed no staining activity above background with an anti-fibroblast antibody. The tumor cells were counterstained with an anti-actin antibody (red) and Hoechst 33342 (blue, note: multiple nuclei), and showed positive intracellular staining of keratin, type IV collagen, laminin, vimentin, fibronectin and S-100 (green), all of which are known to be expressed by ACC[1]. At present, however, none of the explants has developed into an established cell line.

CONCLUSIONS

ACC have an undesirable but deserved reputation for persistent and recurrent growth, late onset of metastasis, and very unfavorable course of disease eventually resulting in death of the patients. ACC, in general, have a acceptable 5-year survival rate, however, the 10- to 20-year survival rates are very poor. Typical survival rates are 70% in the 5 years interval, 40% for 15 years and 15% at 25 years. Prognosis depends on stage, primary site (e.g. parotid better than submandibular gland), histology (tubular and cribiform better than solid pattern), certain cell cycle associated proteins (e.g. Ki-67, Kip1) and cell adhesion molecules[3,5,10-13,15,25-27].

Although the two case reports suggest different tumor biologies/tumor-host interactions, they also demonstrate the typical course of ACC as well as the limited effectiveness of current systemic treatment options for metastatic disease. Metastatic ACC are currently treated with various antineoplastic agents but, so far, no rational standard regimen has been established. Reasons are the relatively low frequency of the tumor and the particular course of disease sometimes protracted over decades.

Initial attempts of chemotherapy in ACC were reported by Johnson et al. 1964[28]. Continuous intra-arterial infusion of 5-fluorouracil was observed to induce marked remission of the primary tumor, however, metastasis showed only poor response to the treatment. Later, drugs like adriamycin[29-31] and cisplatin[32-34] could consistently be proved to be active in ACC, and the effect of 5-fluorouracil was confirmed[35-37]. Furthermore, high-dose melphalan[38] and the combination of cyclophosphamide with doxorubicin and cisplatin[39] have shown favorable results and other cisplatin-based chemotherapy protocols described decent response rates[40-43]. Clinical studies of the EORTC Head and Neck Cancer Cooperative Group and Southwest Oncology Group described only modest activity of epirubicin and mitoxantrone, respectively, with response rates of about 10% in patients with advanced, recurrent or metastatic disease[44-46], whereas in another clinical trial partial responses of 20% were obtained in a similar patient population[47]. More recently, two reports described activity for docetaxel[48] and for a combination of gemcitabine plus 5-fluorouracil in ACC[49]. Interestingly, a response of ACC to the oestrogen receptor antagonist tamoxifen has also been described[50]. Since a recent study was unable to detect oestrogen receptors in any of the 27 ACC studied[51], this could be indicative for an alternative mechanism of tamoxifen action in this tumor entity. So far, attempts to establish a widely accepted chemotherapy regimen for ACC have failed. However, the palliative effect of chemotherapy, especially on tumor related pain, is confirmed unanimously[45,52].

Since local recurrence and distant metastasis are common in ACC and currently available treatment options obviously lack efficacy, the improvement of existing or the development of novel strategies is needed. For this reason we are trying to set up an in vitro model of ACC consisting of a panel of established cell lines in order to provide a preclinical test system on alternative approaches such as modified chemotherapy regimens or cellular immunotherapy.

408

Figure 1. Immunofluorescence microscopy of ACC monolayer cells. The tumor cells were counterstained with an anti-actin antibody (red) and Hoechst 33342 (blue, note: multiple nuclei), and showed positive intracellular staining for keratin, type IV collagen, laminin, vimentin, fibronectin and S-100 (green).

Immunofluorescence Microscopy of Adenoid Cystic Carcinoma Monolayer Cells:

Green - FITC-x (Variable); Red - Rhodamin-Phalloidin (Actin Filaments); Blue - Hoechst Dye 33342 (Nucleus)

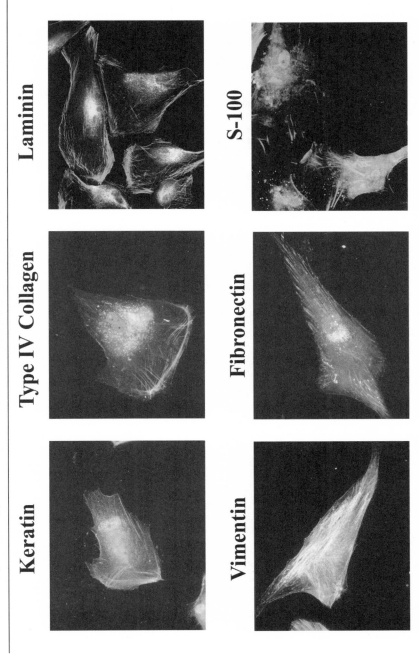

REFERENCES

1.   Ellis GL, Auclair PL. Tumors of the salivary glands. Armed Forces Institute of Pathology 1996; 17:203-216.
2.   Cowie VJ, Pointon RC. Adenoid cystic carcinoma of the salivary glands. Clin Radiol 1984; 35:331-333.
3.   Matsuba HM, Thawley SE, Simpson JR, Levine LA, Mauney M. Adenoid cystic carcinoma of major and minor salivary gland origin. Laryngoscope 1984; 94:1316-1318.
4.   Simpson JR, Thawley SE, Matsuba HM. Adenoid cystic salivary gland carcinoma: treatment with irradiation and surgery. Radiology 1984;151:509-512.
5.   Matsuba HM, Spector GJ, Thawley SE, Simpson JR, Mauney M, Pikul FJ. Adenoid cystic salivary gland carcinoma. A histopathologic review of treatment failure patterns. Cancer 1986;57:519-524.
6.   Shingaki S, Saito R, Kawasaki T, Nakajima T. Adenoid cystic carcinoma of the major and minor salivary glands. A clinicopathological study of 17 cases. J Maxillofac Surg 1986; 14:53-56.
7.   Ampil BO, Misra RP. Factors influencing survival of patients with adenoid cystic carcinoma of the salivary glands. J Oral Maxillofac Surg 1987; 45: 1005-1010.
8.   Conley J, Dingman DL. Adenoid cystic carcinoma in the head and neck (cylindroma). Arch Otolaryngol 1974;100:81-90.
9.   Marsh WL, Allen MS. Adenoid cystic carcinoma; biologic behavior in 38 patients. Cancer 1979;43:1463-1473.
10.   Nascimento AG, Amaral AL, Prado LA, Klingerman J, Silveira TR. Adenoid cystic carcinoma of salivary glands. A study of 6 cases with clinicopathologic correlation. Cancer 1986;57:312-319.
11.   Santucci M, Bondi R. Histologic-prognostic correlations in adenoid cystic carcinoma of major and minor salivary glands of the oral cavity. Tumori 1986;72:293-300.
12.   Hamper K, Lazar F, Dietel M et al. Prognostic factors for adenoid cystic carcinoma of the head and neck: a retrospective evaluation of 96 cases. J Oral Pathol Med 1990;19:101-107.
13.   Spiro RH, Huvos AG. Stage means more than grade in adenoid cystic carcinoma. Am J Surg 1992;164:623-628.
14.   Konno A, Ishikawa K, Numata T, Nagata H, Terada N, Okamoto Y. Analysis of factors affecting long-term treatment results of adenoid cystic carcinoma of the nose and paranasal sinuses. Acta Otolaryngol Suppl (Stockh) 1998;537:67-74.
15.   Fordice J, Kershaw C, El-Naggar A, Goepfert H. Adenoid cystic carcinoma of the head and neck: predictors of morbidity and mortality. Arch Otolaryngol Head Neck Surg 1999;125:149-152.
16.   Marsh WL, Allen MS. Adenoid cystic carcinoma; biologic behavior in 38 patients. Cancer 1979;43:1463-1473.
17.   Bier H. Chemotherapy of adenoid cystic carcinoma. Int J Exp Clin Chem 1989;2:109-112.
18.   Ganzer U. Behandlung und Prognose des adenoidzystischen Karzinoms. Lar Rhinol Otol 1974;53:901-909.
19.   Sur RK, Donde B, Levin V, Pacella J, Kotzen J, Cooper K, Hale M. Adenoid cystic carcinoma of the salivary glands: a review of 10 years. Laryngoscope 1997; 107:1276-1280.
20.   Prokopakis EP, Snyderman CH, Hanna EY, Carrau RL, Carrau RL, Johnson JT, D´Amico F. Risk factors for local recurrence of adenoid cystic carcinoma: the role of postoperative radiation therapy. Am J Otolaryngol 1999;20:281-186.
21.   Kaul R, Hendrickson F, Cohen L, Rosenberg I, Ten Haken R, Awschalow M, Mansell J. Fast neutrons in the treatment of salivary gland tumors. Int Radiot Oncol Biol Phys 1981;7:667-1671.
22.   Wambesie A, Battermann JJ. Review and evolution of clinical results in the EORTC Heavy-Particle Therapy Group. Strahlentherapie 1985;161:746-755.
23.   Krull A, Schwarz R, Heyer D, Brockmann WP, Junker A, Schmidt R, Hubener KH. Results of fast neutron therapy of adenoidcystic carcinomas of the head and neck at the neutron facility Hamburg-Eppendorf. Strahlenther Onkol 1990;166:107-110.
24.   Potter R, Nazaly A, Hemprich A, Haverkamp U, Al-Dandashi C, Hover KH, Loncar I. Neutron radiotherapy in adenoidcystic carcinoma: preliminary experience at the Munster neutron facility. Strahlenther Onkol 1990;166:78-85.
25.   Franchi A, Gallo O, Bocciolini C, Franchi L, Paglierani M, Santucci M. Reduced E-cadherin expression correlates with unfavorable prognosis in adenoid cystic carcinoma of salivary glands of the oral cavity. Am J Clin Pathol 1999; 111:43-50.
26.   Takata T, Kudo Y, Zhao M, Ogawa I, Miyauchi M, Sato S, Cheng J, Nikai H. Reduced expression of p27(Kip1) protein in relation to salivary adenoid cystic carcinoma metastasis. Cancer 1999;86:928-935.

410

27.	Norberg-Spaak L, Dardick I, Ledin T. Adenoid cystic carcinoma: use of cell proliferation, Bcl-2 expression, histologic grade, and clinical stage as predictors of clinical outcome. Head Neck 2000; 22:489-497.

28.	Johnson RO, Lange RD, Kisken WA, Curreri AR. Infusion of 5-fluorouracil in cylindroma treatment. Arch Otololaryngol 1964; 79: 625-627.

29.	Rentschler R, Burgess MA, Byres R. Chemotherapy of malignant major salivary gland neoplasms. Cancer 1977; 40:619-624.

30.	Vermeer RJ, Pinedo HM. Partial remission of advanced adenoid cystic carcinoma obtained with adriamycin. Cancer 1979; 43:1604-1606.

31.	Posner MR, Ervin TJ, Weichselbaum RR, Fabian RL, Miller D. Chemotherapy of advanced salivary gland neoplasms. Cancer 1982; 50:2261-2264.

32.	Schramm VL, Srodes C, Myers EN. Cisplatin therapy for adenoid cystic carcinoma. Arch Otolaryngol 1981; 107:739-741.

33.	Von Scheel J, Kastenbauer ER. Intraaererial therapy of maxillary adenoid cystic carcinoma using cis-platinum. HNO 1981;29:308-311.

34.	Sessions RB, Lehane DE, Smith JH, Bryan RN, Suen JY. Intraarterial cisplatin treatment of adenoid cystic carcinoma. Arch Otolaryngol 1982; 108:221-224.

35.	Horrée WA. Adenoid cystic carcinoma of the maxilla. Arch Otolaryngol 1974;100:469-472.

36.	Tannock IF, Sutherland DJ. Chemotherapy for adenocystic carcinoma. Cancer 1980;46:452-454.

37.	Triozzi PL, Brantley A, Fisher S, Cole TB, Crocker I, Huang AT. 5-fluorouracil, cyclophosphamide, and vincristine for adenoid cystic carcinoma of the head and neck. Cancer 1987;59:887-890.

38.	Slichenmyer WJ, LeMaistre CF, Von Hoff DD. Response of metastatic adenoid cystic carcinoma and Merkel cell tumor to high-dose melphalan with autologous bone marrow transplantation. Invest New Drugs 1992; 10:45-48.

39.	Dreyfuss AI, Clark JR, Fallon BG, Posner MR, Norris CM, Miller D. Cyclophosphamide, doxorubicin, and cisplatin combination chemotherapy for advanced carcinomas of salivary gland origin. Cancer 1987;60:2869-2872.

40.	Gorg C, Gorg K, Pfluger KH, Havemann K, Ganz H, Kleinsasser O. Therapy of adenoid cystic carcinoma with cisplatin, etoposide and vindesine. Onkologie 1988;11:106-108.

41.	Airoldi M, Pedani F, Brando V, Gabriele P, Giordano C. Cisplatin, epirubicin and 5-fluorouracil combination chemotherapy for recurrant carcinoma of the salivary gland. Tumori 1989;75:252-256.

42.	DeHaaen LD, DeMulder PH, Vermorken JB, Schornagel JH, Vermey A, Verweij J. Cisplatin-based chemotherapy in advanced adenoid cystic carcinoma of the head and neck. Head Neck 1992;14:273-277.

43.	Tsukuda M, Kokatsu T, Ito K, Mochimatsu I, Kubota A, Sawaki S. Chemotherapy for recurrent adeno- and adenoidcystic carcinomas in the head and neck. J Cancer Res Clin Oncol 1993;119:756-758.

44.	Mattox DE, Von Hoff DD, Balcerzak SP. Southwest Oncology Group study of mitoxantrone for treatment of patients with advanced adenoid cystic carcinoma of the head and neck. Invest New Drugs 1990;8:105-107.

45.	Vermorken JB, Verweij J, deMulder PH, Cognetti F, Clavel M, Rodenhuis S, Kirkpatrick A, Snow GB. Epirubicin in patients with advanced or recurrent adenoid cystic carcinoma of the head and neck: a phase II study of the EORTC Head and Neck Cancer Cooperative Group. Ann Oncol 1993;4:785-788.

46.	Verweij J, deMulder PH, de Graeff A, Vermorken JB,Wildiers J, Kerger J, Schornagel J, Cognetti F, Kirkpatrick A, Sahmoud T, Lefebvre JL. Phase II study on mitoxantrone in adenoid cystic carcinomas of the head and neck. EORTC Head and Neck Cancer Cooperative Group. Ann Oncol 1996;7:867-869.

47.	Airoldi M, Bumma C, Bertetto O, Gabriele P, Succo G, Pedani F: Vinorelbine treatment of recurrent salivary gland carcinomas. Bull Cancer 1998;85:892-894.

48.	Belli F, Di Lauro L, Zappanico A, Giunta S. Doxetaxel in the treatment of metastatic carcinoma of the salivary glands: report of a case. Clin Ter 1999; 150:77-79.

49.	Rinaldi DA, Lormand NA, Brierre JE, Cole JL, Stagg MP, Fontenot MF, Buller EJ, Rainey JM. A phase I trial of gemcitabine and infusional 5-fluorouracil (5-FU) in patients with refractory solid tumors: Lousiana Oncology Associates protocol no. 1 (LOA-1). Am J Clin Oncol 2000; 23:78-82.

50.	Shadaba A, Gaze MN, Grant HR. The reponse of adenoid cystic carcinoma to tamoxifen. J Laryngol Otol 1997; 111:1186-1189.

51.	Dori S, Trougouboff P, David R, Buchner A. Immunohistochemical evaluation of estrogen and progesterone receptors in adenoid cystic carcinoma of salivary gland origin. Oral Oncol 2000; 36: 450-453.

52. Hill ME, Constenla DO, A´Hern RP, Henk JM, Rhys-Evans P, Breach N, Archer D, Gore ME. Cisplatin and 5-fluorouracil for symptom control in advanced salivary adenoid cystic carcinoma. Oral Oncol 1997; 33:275-278.

METASTASES TO PAROTID REGION

Marcin Szymański, Prof. Dr. Wiesław Gołąbek, Dr. Henryk Siwiec, Witold Olszański
Otolaryngology Department, Medical Academy, Lublin, Poland

Key words: parotid gland, metastases, parotid lymph nodes

Correspondence to: *Marcin Szymański, Otolaryngology Department, Ul. Jaczewskiego 8, 20-090 Lublin, Poland, Phone/Fax: +48 81 742 55 18*

SUMMARY

In a group of 17 patients with metastases to parotid region we assessed the type, origin and extension of a primary tumor. The metastases represented 24% of all the malignant parotid tumors. Most common types of tumor were squamous cell carcinoma (9 cases) and melanoma (3 cases). Ten patients presented with metastases for the first diagnosis and in 7 patients metastases developed as a failure of prior treatment. Treatment results were bad particularly in patients presented with recurrence of the primary tumor.

INTRODUCTION

There are two main routes of lymphatic drainage from the head to neck nodes (Fig. 1). One way is along the facial vein through the submandibular and submental nodes to group II or III of neck nodes. The following areas are drained this way through the superficial lymphatic net of the face: the forehead, the external nose, the eyelids, the lips. The other route collects lymph from the occipital and temporal scalp from the external ear canal and auricle to the peri- or intraparotid nodes and further to group II or III of neck nodes. Also the orbit, the nasal cavity, the pterigo-maxillary fissure, the infratemporal fossa and the palate are drained through the deep lymphatic net to the parotid nodes. Some regions like the nose and palpebra can be drained both routs[1, 2]. Metastases to parotid region are relatively rare, and they can be from regional (supraclavicular) and distant (infraclavicular) primary tumors. The metastases locate much more in the parotid nodes than in parotid parenchyma, which might be invaded by extracapsular spread[1, 3, 4].

The present study reviews a group of patients with metastases to parotid region.

PATIENTS AND METHODS

This study represents an evaluation of 17 patients with metastases to parotid region, treated in our institution in the years 1986-2000. The group included 9 men and 8 women with the age range 19 – 72 years. Patients with primary malignant parotid tumors and lymphomas were excluded from the study. Parotid metastases represented 24% of 69 malignant parotid tumors treated in this period. A retrospective analysis of the type, origin and extension of the primary tumor was performed. Methods of treatment and treatment results were also assessed.

RESULTS AND DISCUSSION

Ten patients presented with a primary tumor and parotid metastases for the first diagnosis and in 7 patients metastases developed with recurrence in the primary site. Two patients had distant metastases from breast cancer diagnosed in one case just before and in the other case 14 years after initial treatment. Fifteen patients had regional metastases from head and neck cancer and they reflected the lymphatic drainage from the primary site.

Regarding pathology, the most frequent type of the primary tumor was squamous cell carcinoma (SCC) and it affected 9 patients. Three patients had buccal cancer, 3 patients maxillary cancer involving the orbit and palpebra, two patients auricle cancer and one patient had uvula cancer. In two patients metastases developed from nasopharyngeal lymphoepithelioma. Three patients had melanoma metastases: one from the nasal cavity, one from the upper alveolar process and one from unknown primary. One patient developed metastases from nasal esthesioneuroblastoma.

In four of 10 patients presented with parotid metastases for the first diagnosis, parotid swelling was the first manifestation of malignancy and this included the following primary tumors: nasal and unknown primary melanoma, uvula cancer and nasopharyngeal lymphoepithelioma. The type and site of the primary tumor, the treatment methods and outcome in this group of patients are shown in Table I. Surgery means excision of the primary tumor (except for nasopharyngeal cancer) and total or subtotal parotidectomy and selective or radical modified neck dissection. The patients with melanoma had surgery only. Other patients had combined treatment apart from two patients who refused surgery. The parotid metastasis in the patient with T1 uvula cancer was larger than 6 cm, in other patients the metastases were smaller than 3 cm.

In seven patients metastases developed as a failure of prior treatment, with recurrence of the primary tumor in 5 patients. The group included three patients with maxillary SCC involving the orbit and palpebra, one patient with the auricle and occipital scalp SCC, one patient with nasopharyngeal lymphoepithelioma, one patient with melanoma of the upper alveolar process and one female with ductal infiltrative breast carcinoma. In 5 patients subtotal parotidectomy with selective neck dissection was performed with adjuvant chemotherapy, two patients refused surgery and received chemotherapy only. Treatment results were very bad, five patients died 1 year and two patients 2 years after the diagnosis of parotid metastases. Treatment outcome in patients presented with parotid metastases for the first diagnosis (Table I) was better but still not good. In the whole group, the facial nerve was sacrificed in two patients who had paralysis before parotidectomy.

414

Metastatic tumors in parotid region represent about 30% of all the parotid malignancies[5, 6]. The majority of parotid metastases (80-90%) originate from head and neck region[3, 5]. Squamous cell carcinoma and malignant melanoma are the most frequent malignancies that metastasize to parotid region[1, 4, 7]. Metastases from cutaneous tumors were widely reported[1, 4, 8], however mucosal tumors of upper airway or digestive tract can also metastasize to parotid region[9].

Metastases from maxillary sinus cancer are not common, but invasion of palpebral skin or the orbit may predispose to parotid or submandibular nodes metastases. Parotid nodes involvement by metastatic nasopharyngeal carcinoma is observed in about 40% of patients with NPC [10]. Parotid gland can also be infiltrated directly by primary lesion from the surrounding skin, the auricle or buccal mucosa.

Metastases from malignant melanoma to the parotid nodes occur in about 20% of patients with melanoma of the head and neck[11]. Secondary involvement of parotid nodes is more often caused by cutaneous than mucosal melanoma. Although our group of patients with melanoma metastases had good outcome of treatment, larger series document poor prognosis for the patients[12].

Carcinoma of the lung, breast and kidneys are the most frequent infraclavicular neoplasms that metastasize to parotid region[7]. Metastases of that kind usually manifest hematogenous dissemination of malignancy and carry poor prognosis. The possibility of metastatic tumor should always be considered when primary parotid lesion has histologic features resembling those of tumors occurring in other parts of the body like melanoma, squamous cell carcinoma, clear cell, undifferentiated carcinoma[5].

In four of 10 patients from our group presented with parotid metastases for the first diagnosis, the parotid tumor was the first manifestation of a malignancy. Franzen et al.[5] reported similar frequency (40%). That has to remind us about precise clinical examination of skin of the head and neck, mucosa of the upper respiratory tract and other parts of the body like chest, abdomen to look for a primary tumor. Fine needle aspiration biopsy and imaging radiology (B sonography, MR) are very useful for diagnosis[3, 13].

It is concluded that parotid metastases present about one fourth of malignant parotid tumors. Patients with parotid metastases had poor prognosis particularly those presenting with a failure of prior treatment.

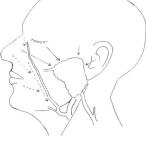

Figure 1. Two routes of lymphatic drainage from the head:
along the facial vein (interrupted arrows) and through the parotid nodes (continuous arrows).

Table 1. Treatment and status of the patients presented with parotid metastases for the first diagnosis.

Patient	Sex	Primary site	Type	Treatment	Status
1	W	Buccal T1N1	SCC	Surgery + RTH	Alive 1y
2	M	Buccal T2N1	SCC	Surgery + RTH	Alive 2y
3	M	Buccal T2N1	SCC	Refused surgery, RTH +CHT	Unknown
4	M	Uvula T1N3	SCC	Refused surgery, RTH +CHT	Alive 1y
5	M	Auricle	SCC	Surgery + RTH	Alive 2y
6	M	Nasal cavity	Melanoma	Surgery	DWD 6y
7	F	Unknown	Melanoma	Surgery	Alive 5y
8	W	Nasopharyx	Lymphoepithelioma	RTH + CHT	DWD 3y
9	W	Nasal cavity	Esthesioneuroblastoma	Surgery + RTH + CHT	DWD 3y
10	W	Breast	Ductal carcinoma	Surgery + RTH + CHT	DWD 6m

SCC - squamous cell carcinoma, RTH- radiotherapy, CHT- chemotherapy, DWD- dead with disease.

REFERENCES

1. Schroeder WA Jr, Stahr WD. Malignant neoplastic disease of the parotid lymph nodes. Laryngoscope 1998;108:1514-9.
2. Kopsch F: Textbook and atlas of human anatomy (German) Vol. II. Leipzig: G. Thieme; 1950.
3. Malata CM, Camilleri IG, McLean NR, Piggott TA, Soames JV. Metastatic tumours of the parotid gland. Br J Oral Maxillofac Surg 1998;36:190-5.
4. Khurana VG, Mentis DH, O'Brien CJ, Hurst TL, Stevens GN, Packham NA. Parotid and neck metastases from cutaneous squamous cell carcinoma of the head and neck. Am J Surg 1995;170:446-50.
5. Franzen A, Pfaltz M. Parotid tumors of non-glandular origin: local and disant metastases in the parotid gland (German). Laryngorhinootologie 1997;76:735-9.
6. Yarington CT Jr. Metastatic malignant disease to the parotid gland. Laryngoscope 1981;91,517-9.
7. Batsakis JG, Bautina E. Metastases to major salivary glands. Ann Otol Rhinol Laryngol 1990;99:501-3.
8. Taylor BW Jr, Brant TA, Mendenhall NP et al. Carcinoma of the skin metastatic to parotid area lymph nodes. Head Neck 1991;13:427-33.
9. Pisani P, Krengli M, Ramponi A, Guglielmetti R, Pia F. Metastases to parotid gland from cancers of the upper airway and digestive tract. Br J Oral Maxillofac Surg 1998;36:54-7.
10. Chong VF, Fan YF. Parotid gland involvement in nasopharyngeal carcinoma. J Comput Assist Tomogr 1999;23:524-8.
11. Schwipper V, Schulze-Osthoff DR. The parotid gland as a filtering station of metastatic head-neck melanoma. Retrospective study of 884 patients (German). Mund Kiefer Gesichtschir 1998;2:242-9.
12. Ollila DW, Foshag LJ, Essner R, Stern SL, Morton DL. Parotid region lymphatic mapping and sentinel lymphadenectomy for cutaneous melanoma. Ann Surg Oncol 1999;6:150-4.
13. Hori A, Yoshida J, Yuichiro H, Mitani K, Takashima S, Kubo T: Pre-operative assessment of metastatic parotid tumors. Auris Nasus Larynx 1998;25:277-283.

TOPOGRAPHY OF CERVICAL LYMPH NODES
IN NEW ZEALAND WHITE RABBITS

Anja-A. Dünne [1], S. Plehn [1], S. Schulz [2], A. Ramaswamy [3], B.M. Lippert [1], J.A. Werner [1]
[1]Department of Otolaryngology, Head and Neck Surgery
[2]Department of Veterinary Services
[3]Department of Pathology of the Philipps-University Marburg, Germany

Keywords: VX2-carcinoma, New Zealand white rabbit, lymph node metastases, HNSCC

ABSTRACT

Background. The value of neck lymph nodes in the treatment concept of head and neck squamous cell carcinoma (HNSCC) is of great importance. A reliable animal model is required to better understand the mechanisms of lymphogenic metastatic spread. The VX2-carcinoma of New Zealand white rabbits is characterized by a lymphogenic metastatic spread. Investigations of the lymphogenic metastatic spread of VX2-carcinomas in New Zealand white rabbits require the exact knowledge of the topography of cervical and facial lymph nodes.

Material and methods. The topography of neck lymph nodes was evaluated from sixteen rabbits macroscopically, histologically and by lymphographic investigations. Additionally the possibility of their surgical removal (neck dissection) was examined.

Results. There are four consistent groups of 12-18 lymph nodes draining the upper aerodigestive tract and the ear of New Zealand white rabbits. Except the paratracheal one, they are easily accessible to surgery.

Conclusion. This investigation encourages the use of induced VX2-carcinomas in New Zealand white rabbits as an animal model to study the lymphogenic metastatic spread of HNSCC. According to these investigations, an improvement of surgical and pharmaceutical treatment of this tumor entity might be possible.

INTRODUCTION

The prognosis of patients suffering from head and neck squamous cell carcinoma (HNSCC) is dependent on the metastatic spread of the tumor, which in the case of this malignancy predominantly occurs in a lymphogenous pattern that predicts the course of the disease. The development of new therapeutical concepts of lymph node metastases requires the exact knowledge of the mechanisms of tumor progression and its accompanying lymphogenic spread utilizing animal models. There are some detailed publications on rats dealing with their lymphatic system[1] and the topography of their lymph nodes[2]. Unfortunately, when investigating the lymphogenic spread of tumors, the rat does not represent a suitable model for human HNSCC, since the induced tumors show hematogenous metastatic spread[3]. In contrast, VX2-carcinomas of New Zealand white rabbits are characterized by lymphogenic metastatic spread similar as observed for human HNSCC. The New Zealand white rabbit is a common experimental model in otolaryngology[4-6]. Furthermore, the VX2 carcinoma in the rabbits ear was used as an experimental model for intraarterial embolization of HNSCC[3]. Investigations of the lymphogenic metastatic spread in HNSCC require the exact knowledge of the topography of cervical and facial lymph nodes. Here it is of special interest to investigate if certain groups of lymph nodes act as a unit, and are involved in the drainage of certain areas of the head and neck region. In this case we would expect the involvement of only certain lymph node groups namely lymph nodes draining from the tumor region to be metastatically affected.

MATERIAL AND METHODS

The lymph node topography of 9 rabbits was evaluated by palpation and preparation as described below. All tissues were also investigated histologically. For complete histological evaluation in 7 rabbits the neck was prepared from the seventh cervical vertebra up to the skull base.

Macroscopical investigations

After ketamine hydrochloride anaesthesia, 3 of the 9 rabbits were killed by T61 injection. In all rabbits a skin incision was performed from the ear to the spine of the scapula and the resulting skin flap was prepared by visualizing the cervical fascia above the trapezius muscle and the respective fascia above the parotid gland. The lymph nodes within the superficial and deeper part of the cervical fascia and below the parotid fascia were identified by means of palpation first and then prepared in the following. To identify the submandibular located lymph nodes we removed the superficial part of the cervical fascia from the mandibular angle and the retractor mandibular muscle. To examine deeper located lymph nodes we lateralized the omotransverse muscle, the cleidomastoid muscle and the cleidocephalus muscle and prepared the perivascular sheath. After examination of adjacent lymph nodes we removed the perivascular sheath. Furthermore we examined the trachea and the prelaryngeal fascia and muscles before removing them for histological evaluation.

Lymphography

After ketamine hydrochloride anaesthesia we performed a lymphography in 6 out of the 9 rabbits. Blue dye (0.35-0.5ml) was injected in the tongue and buccal mucous membrane, as well as the dorsum of the ear. Fifteen minutes later the rabbits were killed by T61 injection and the neck was examined as described above. We documented the lymphatic drainage and the blue colored lymph nodes according to the primary injection site of the dye.

Histology

For complete histological evaluation the rabbits head and neck were fixed for two weeks in 4% formalin. One centimeter broad segments were prepared from the seventh cervical vertebra up to the skull base. We prepared 6-8 µm paraffin sections after radiologically verified decalcification of the specimens in 10% formic acid. Four to twenty histological cuts per paraffin section were generated and stained with Hematoxylin/Eosin.

RESULTS

Macroscopical investigations

New Zealand white rabbits exhibit 12-18 large, clinically veryfied lymph nodes in the head and neck area (table 1). One group is represented by the paratracheal lymph nodes, which are surgically difficult to remove, while there are three groups of lymph nodes in the head and neck region of New Zealand white rabbits, which are easily accessible to surgery, these are the caudal, rostral mandibular and parotid lymph nodes.

Lymphography

Fifteen minutes after injection we isolated the lymph nodes of all four different groups and observed a distinct enrichment of the blue dye at several locations. We found the parotid lymph node to be the first draining lymph node from the skin of the ear since it was the first node to accumulate the dye, followed by the caudal mandibular lymph nodes. Furthermore we found the rostral and caudal mandibular lymph nodes to be the first and secondary draining lymph node stations of the tongue and the buccal mucous membrane.

Histology

We could histologically confirm the affiliation of the examined lymph nodes with the previously characterized four lymph node groups. Both, human lymph nodes and cervical lymph nodes from New Zealand white rabbits are remarkably similar, since they both are enclosed by a fibrous capsule, contain a large number of compact lymphatic follicles in the lymph node periphery and less lymphatic follicles in the centre of the lymph nodes. The examined lymphatic follicles are mainly secondary follicles corresponding to those of human lymph nodes. As observed for humans the examined lymph nodes of the rabbits exhibit a bright, lymph fluid rich center surrounded by a darker lymphocyte wall, which consolidates and widens half-moon like at the closer side of the center.

DISCUSSION

The cervical and facial lymph node topography described in New Zealand white rabbits is similar to those of humans. Possibly, this similarity allows to compare the direction of the lymphogenic metastatic spread and the location of the first draining lymph nodes of primary tumors between these two species. Lymphographic investigations performed in this study demonstrate a constant lymphatic drainage from the oral cavity and the oropharynx to the rostral and caudal mandibular lymph nodes. After blue dye injection into the ear it became obvious, that the parotid lymph node was the first and the caudal mandibular lymph nodes the second stations of the lymphatic drainage from this location. The consistent location and surgical accessibility of the caudal and rostral mandibular as well as the parotid lymph nodes, allow further detailed investigations regarding lymphogenic metastatic spread of induced VX2-carcinomas. The histological pictures of cervical and facial lymph nodes of New Zealand white rabbits are comparable to those observed in humans. Both show similar characteristics regarding the location and type of lymphatic follicles. The observation of lymph fluid in centrally located cavities possibly represents preferential flow through the lymph node and resembles the human sinus.

CONCLUSION

The results presented encourage the use of induced VX2-carcinomas in New Zealand white rabbits as an animal model to study the lymphogenic metastatic spread of HNSCC. Such investigations could lead to an improvement of surgical and pharmaceutical treatment of this cancer.

Table 1. Lymph node topography in New Zealand white rabbits

lymph nodes	location	number	size
parotid lymph node	below the parotid fascia behind the posterior auricular vein in the parotid gland	1	9-10 mm
rostral mandibular lymph nodes	within the range of the lower part of the submandibular gland between the retractor mandibular and the digastric muscle and below the branching of the submental from the linguofacial vein	1-3	1,5-5 mm
caudal mandibular lymph nodes	in the triangle of the external jugular vein into the maxillary and linguofacial vein and between the superficial and the deeper part of the cervical fascia	3	2-3 mm
paratracheal lymph nodes	laterally to the cricoid below the sternothyroid muscle	1-2	3 mm

REFERENCES

1. Werner JA. Untersuchungen zum Lymphgefässsystem der oberen Luft- und Speisewege, Aachen: Shaker, 1995
2. Miotti R. Die Lymphknoten und Lymphgefässe der weissen Ratte (Rattus norvegicus Berkenhout, Epimys norvegicus). Acta Anat 1965;62:489-527
3. van Es RJ, Franssen O, Dullens HF, Bernsen MR, Bosman F, Hennink WE, Slootweg PJ. The VX2 carcinoma in the rabbit ear as an experimental model for intra-arterial embolization of head and neck squamous cell carcinoma with dextran microspheres. Lab Anim 1999;33:175-184
4. Marie JP, Lerosy Y, Dehesdin D, Jin O, Tadié M, Andrieu-Guitrancourt J. Experimental reinnervation of a strap muscle with a few roots of the phrenic nerve in rabbits. Ann Otol Rhinol Laryngol 1999;108:1004-1011
5. Marie JP, Lerosay Y, Dehesdin D, Tadié M, Andrieu-Guitrancourt J. Cervical anatomy of phrenic nerve roots in rabbits. Ann Otol Rhinol Laryngol 1999;108:516-521

6.   Marie JP, Dehesdin D, Ducastelle T, Denant J. Selective reinnervation of the abductor and adductor muscles of the canine larynx after recurrent nerve paralysis. Ann Otol Rhinol Laryngol 1989;98:530-536

ELEVATION OF SERUM MATRIX METALLOPROTEINASE-3 AND -8 ASSOCIATED WITH SQUAMOUS CELL CARCINOMAS OF THE HEAD AND NECK

Sibylle Plehn[1], A.-A. Dünne[1], U. Herz[2], B. M. Lippert[1], H. Renz[2], J. A. Werner[1]

[1]Department of Otolaryngology, Head and Neck Surgery, Philipps-University of Marburg, Germany

[2]Department of Clinical Chemistry and Molecular Diagnostic, Central Laboratory, Philipps-University of Marburg, Germany

Key words: squamous cell carcinomas, head and neck, matrix metalloproteinases, serum markers

Correspondence to: *J.A. Werner, M.D., Professor and Chairman, Dept. of Otolaryngology, Head and Neck Surgery, Philipps-University Marburg, Deutschhausstr. 3, 35037 Marburg, Germany, Phone: + 49 6421 2866478, Fax: + 49 6421 2866367 (e-mail:* *j.a.werner@mailer.uni-marburg.de)*

ABSTRACT

Background. Because an optimal treatment of malignancies according to the individual prognosis of the patients depends on sufficient information about the malignant potency of the primary, search for serum markers is of great interest. We investigated the expression profile of matrix metalloproteinase (MMP)-3, -8 and tissue inhibitor of MMP (TIMP)-1 in pretherapeutic sera of patients with head and neck squamous cell carcinomas (HNSCC).

Methods. Pretherapeutic expression levels of MMP-3, -8 and TIMP-1 were measured in the serum of 74 patients with HNSCC and 74 healthy controls, respectively.

Results. The mean MMP-3 (91.6 ng/ml; $p = 0.001$) and MMP-8 (54.4 ng/ml; $p = 0.003$) serum concentrations in HNSCC patients were significantly higher than the levels in the healthy controls. The serum level of TIMP-1 in HNSCC patients did not show a significant difference compared to the healthy controls.

Conclusions. We conclude that the results of this investigation indicate that elevated serum levels of MMP-3 and MMP-8 have a relevance in HNSCC and could possibly serve as useful tools in cancer diagnostics and monitoring in these patients. Further investigations of a greater group of patients have to show, if there is any correlation towards T-stage, metastases and prognosis.

INTRODUCTION

In most patients with head and neck squamous cell carcinomas (HNSCC) the primary tumor can be removed by surgery or can be treated by radiation therapy depending on its location. The poor prognosis of some of these patients is based on the high lymphogenous metastases frequency of HNSCC[1]. It is assumed that matrix metalloproteinases (MMPs) destroy the integrity of the basement membrane, which is part of the extracellular matrix (ECM), and enable cancer cells to invade normal tissue and facilitate tumor cell dissemination via lymphatics and, during the later stage of disease, blood vessels.

Currently, the most investigations deal with the determination of MMP-mRNA and protein expression in the cancerous tissue or cell lines. In their extensive overview Giambernardi et al. described, among other MMPs, an mRNA expression of MMP-3 and -8 in oral, bone, breast, prostate and colon tumor derived cell lines[2]. For MMP-3 expression in oral SCC biopsies, additionally a positive correlation with prognostic parameters could be shown[3]. Elevated serum levels of MMP-3 and TIMP-1 (tissue inhibitor of MMP) among others were already established in patients with aggressive carcinoma development at locations other than the head and neck region[4, 5].

The optimal treatment should be chosen according to the individual prognosis of the patient. To get further information about the malignant potency of the primary tumor including tumor progression and metastatic spread, it would be useful, to have serum markers in the blood periphery. For this background several groups investigate the relevance of MMPs as potential serum markers[6, 7]. We investigated the expression profile of MMP-3, -8 and TIMP-1 in pretherapeutic sera of patients with HNSCC.

MATERIAL AND METHOD

Sera were obtained from 74 patients with HNSCC just before treatment. Expression levels of MMP-3, -8 and TIMP-1 were measured in the serum of the patients with HNSCC and 74 healthy controls utilizing two site sandwich enzyme immunoassays (BIOTRAK ELISA assays, Amersham Pharmacia Biotech, Little Chalfont, UK).

HNSCC in all patients was diagnosed histologically in surgically resected tissues. According to tumor-node-metastasis (TNM) classification there were 2 patients with Tis, 20 with T1, 19 with T2, 14 with T3 and 19 patients with T4 stage. Furthermore there were 36 patients with N0, 4 with N1 and 34 with N2 neck. Only 3 of the patients showed distant metastasis. As control group healthy volunteers as well as few patients with tinnitus and sudden loss of hearing were testet for MMP serum concentrations.

RESULTS

The mean MMP-3 (91.6 ng/ml; p = 0.001) and MMP-8 (54.4 ng/ml; p = 0.003) serum concentrations in HNSCC patients were significantly higher than the levels in the healthy controls (fig. 1, fig. 2). The serum level of TIMP-1 in HNSCC patients did not show a significant difference compared to the healthy controls.

DISCUSSION

Prognosis of patients suffering from squamous cell carcinomas of the upper aerodigestive tract (HNSCC) is defined to a lesser extent through the size of the primary tumor. It is rather the extent of metastatic disease, which in squamous cell carcinoma predominantly occurs in a lymphogenous pattern that predicts the course of the disease. The extraordinary relevance of lymphogenic metastatic spread with regard to prognosis becomes evident, if the partly drastic reduction of 5-year-survival-rate in cases of histologically confirmed neck node metastases is considered.

The therapy concept of neck lymph nodes depends on the location of the primary and the clinically suspected lymphogenic metastatic spread. Treatment of the neck lymph nodes includes neck dissection or radiochemotherapy according to the treatment concept of the primary.

To avoid overtreatment and functional disorders in cases of advanced metastatic spread and resulting poor prognosis of the patients, it would be desirable to have serum markers indicating the individual malignant potency of the primary and indicating individuals' prognosis. Search for these markers is of potential interest as long as sonography, computed tomography and magnetic resonance imaging represent the actual lymph node status, but cannot give any answers on the malignant potency of the primary, the aggressiveness of the lymphogenic metastatic spread and even not on patients prognosis. One of the most common serum markers is CYFRA 21-1. This marker seems to be of potential importance in cases of distant metastases[8].

Several steps are required to develop malignant tumor cell invasion and metastasis. In the first phase cancer cells have to invade and denaturate the extracellular matrices including the surrounding tissues and vascular basement membranes, which are comprised of various types of collagens and proteoglycans[9, 10]. The matrix metalloproteinases (MMPs), a family of over 20 members of zinc-dependent endopeptidases, are capable of degrading nearly all different components of the extracellular matrix (ECM). Beside these secreted proteinases the matrix degradation also depends on their native tissue inhibitors (TIMPs)[11, 12].

Both in vitro and in vivo investigations have shown that increased expression of MMP-3, -8, and TIMP-1 are associated with several human malignant tumors[2, 13]. Allmost all studies deal with the determination of MMP-mRNA and protein expression in the cancerous tissue or cell lines. In their extensive overview Giambernardi et al. described, among other MMPs, an mRNA expression of MMP-3 and -8 in oral, bone, breast, prostate and colon tumor derived cell lines[2]. For MMP-3 expression in oral SCC biopsies, additionally a positive correlation with prognostic parameters could be shown[3]. While MMP-8 is predominantly produced by neutrophil granulocytes[14, 15], MMP-3 and TIMP-1 can be regulary detected in tumor cells and surrounding stromal cells of HNSCC tissue samples[16, 17].

MMP-3 and -8 are identifiable and quantifiable in normal sera[18, 19]. Changed serum levels of MMP-3 and TIMP-1 among others were already established in patients with aggressive carcinoma development at locations other than the head and neck region[4, 5].

In the present study, we have demonstrated significantly higher serum MMP-3 and -8 concentrations in patients with HNSCC compared to healthy controls. The elevated levels could rank as evidence that these members of the MMP-family play a important role in carcinogenesis of HNSCC.

CONCLUSION

The poor prognosis of patients with HNSCC is mainly influenced by the extent of lymphogenic metastatic spread that predicts the course of the disease. Changed serum concentrations observed in the peripheral blood may serve as useful prognostic molecular markers for malignant potential of malignancies. Because optimal treatment strategy should depend on the individually prognosis of each patient, search for these markers is of potential interest.

To get further information on the patients prognosis, many investigations deal with potential

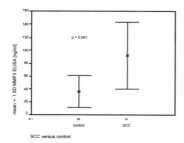

prognostic markers in HNSCC patients. Still, there are no common serum markers, which reflect tumor progression and lymphogenic metastatic spread in clinical routine. Based on the assumption, that the individual treatment modality should be chosen according to the malignant potency of the primary, which predicts patients' prognosis immediatly, research on potential serum marker in the blood periphery is of high interest.

The results of this investigation point towards elevated MMP-3 and MMP-8 serum concentrations as possibly useful tools in cancer diagnostics and monitoring in HNSCC patients. Further investigations of a greater group of patients have to show, if there is any correlation towards T-stage, metastases and prognosis.

Figure 1. Mean MMP-3 serum concentration ± 1 standard deviation of patients with HNSCC vs. healthy controls

Figure 2. Mean MMP-8 serum concentration ± 1 standard deviation of patients with HNSCC vs. healthy controls

426

REFERENCES

1. Werner JA. Aktueller Stand der Versorgung des Lymphabflusses maligner Kopf-Hals Tumoren. Eur Arch Otorhinolaryngol (Suppl I)1997:47-85.

2. Giambernardi TA, Grant GM, Tayler GP et al. Overview of matrix metalloproteinase expression in cultured human cells. Matrix Biol 1998;16:483-96.

3. Kusukawa J, Harada H, Shima I, Sasaguri Y, Kameyama T, Morimatsu M. The significance of epidermal growth factor receptor and matrix metalloproteinase-3 in squamous cell carcinoma of the oral cavity. Eur J Cancer B Oral Oncol 1996;32B:217-221.

4. Ylisirnio S, Hoyhtya M, Turpeenniemi-Hujanen T. Serum matrix metalloproteinase -2, -9 and tissue inhibitors of metalloproteinases -1, -2 in lung cancer - TIMP-1 as a prognostic marker. Anticancer Res 2000;20:1311-6.

5. Gohji K, Fujimotot N, Komiyama T et al. Elevation of serum levels of matrix metalloproteinase-2 and -3 as new predictors of recurrence in patients with urothelial carcinoma. Cancer 1996;78:2379-87.

6. Yoshikawa T, Saitoh M, Tsuburaya A et al. Tissue inhibitor of matrix metalloproteinase-1 in the plasma of patients with gastric carcinoma. A possible marker for serosal invasion and metastasis. Cancer 1999;86:1929-35.

7. Iizasa T, Fujisawa T, Suzuki M et al. Elevated levels of circulating plasma matrix metalloproteinase 9 in non-small cell lung cancer patients. Clin Cancer Res 1999;5:149-153.

8. Niemann AM, Goeroegh T, Gottschlich S, Lippert BM, Werner JA. Cut-off value determination of CYFRA 21-1 for squamous cell carcinomas of the head and neck (SCCHN). Anticancer Res 1997;17:4B:2859-60.

9. Liotta LA, Stetler-Stevenson WG. Metalloproteinases and cancer invasion. Semin Cancer Biol 1990;1:99-106.

10. Fidler IJ. Critical factors in the biology of human cancer metastasis: twenty-eight G.H.A. - Clowes Memorial Award Lecture. Cancer Res 1990;50:6130-8.

11. Liotta LA, Stetler-Stevenson WG, Steeg PS. Cancer invasion and metastasis: positive and negative regulatory elements. Cancer Invest1991;9:543-551.

12. Gomez DE, Alonso DF, Yoshiji H, Thorgeirsson UP. Tissue inhibitors of metalloproteinases: structure, regulation and biological functions. Eur J Cell Biol 1997;74:111-22.

13. Garbett EA, Reed MW, Stephenson TJ, Brown NJ. Proteolysis in human breast cancer. Mol Pathol 2000;53:99-106.

16. Devarajan P, Mookhtiar K, Van Wart H, Berliner N. Structure and expression of the cDNA encoding human neutrophil collagenase. Blood 1991;77:2731-8.

15. Hanemaaijer R, Konttinen YT, Ding Y et al. Matrix metalloproteinase-8 is expressed in rheumatoid synovial fibroblasts and endothelial cells. Regulation by tumor necrosis factor-alpha and doxycycline. J Biol Chem 1997;272:31504-9.

16. Sutinen M, Kainulainen T, Hurskainen T et al. Expression of matrix metalloproteinases (MMP-1 and -2) and their inhibitors (TIMP-1, -2, and -3) in oral lichen planus, dysplasia, squamous cell carcinoma and lymph node metastasis. Br J Cancer 1998;77:2239-45.

17. Kurahara S, Shinohara M, Ikebe T et al. Expression of MMPs, MT-MMP, and TIMPs in squamous cell carcinoma of the oral cavity: correlations with tumor invasion and metastasis. Head Neck 1999;21:627-38.

18. Matsuki H, Fujimoto N, Iwata K, Knauper V, Okada Y, Hayakawa T. A one-step sandwich enzyme immunoassay for human matrix metalloproteinase 8 (neutrophil collagenase) using monoclonal antibodies. Clin Chim Acta 1996;244:129-43.

19. Obata K, Iwata K, Okada Y et al. A one-step sandwich immunoassay for human matrix metalloproteinase 3 (stromelysin-1) using monoclonal antibodies. Clin Chim Acta 1992;211:59-72.

PHOTODYNAMIC DIAGNOSTIC AND THERAPY IN ENT
- TWO CASE REPORTS

D. Thurnher, Formanek M., Burian M. (Vienna, Austria)
Department of Otorhinolaryngology - Head and Neck Surgery Medical School of the University of Vienna

ABSTRACT

Photodynamic therapy (PDT) is a treatment modality using a photosensitizing drug and light to kill cells. The clinical use of PDT requires the presence of a photosensitizing agent, oxygen and light of a specific wavelength which matches the absorption characteristics of the photosensitizer. PDT has been shown to be effective in the treatment of neoplastic diseases. As it is a tissue sparing method the use of PDT is highly attractive in the management of head and neck lesions. First promising results have been reported in the treatment of papillomatosis of the larynx, dysplasia and cancerous lesions of the upper respiratory tract. Moreover, photodynamic diagnosis (PD) may improve the detection of occult or hardly detectable neoplasias.

We will present two cases which reflect the potentials of PD and PDT using 5-Aminolevulinic acid (5-ALA).

INTRODUCTION

Photodynamic therapy is a new and very promising modality for the treatment of premalignant and malignant head and neck disease which offers the following advantages:
1) PDT setting can be used for PD purposes in the same session by using a blue light fountain for the detection of premalignant or malignant areas of the mucosa.

2) Premalignant and malignant conditions arise in mucosa with a large surface area. Beside a clearly visible tumor, satellite lesions, to small to be recognized macroscopically may exist in close vicinity to the main lesion. Thus, the additional treatment of tumor surrounding areas by using an appropriate light applicator may count as a benefit of PDT[1].

3) Classical surgical procedures performed on premalignant lesions, especially if done recurrently, might be associated with significant side effects like increasing scar formation, functional impairment and disfigurement. PDT offers the possibility of repeated treatment without upper mentioned disadvantages.

The clinical use of PDT requires the presence of a photosensitizing agent (which is selectively retained in tumor tissue as distinct from nonmalignant tissue), oxygen and light of a specific wavelength which matches the absorption characteristics of the photosensitizer. As soon as the photosensitizer is activated by the appropriate wavelength of light, it interacts with molecular oxygen to form a toxic, short-lived species known as singlet oxygen. This molecule is thought to mediate cellular death[2].

One frequently used photosensitizing agent is 5-ALA.
5-ALA has already been used to treat a variety of diseases including skin cancer[2], dysplasia and superficial tumors of the esophagus[3] as well as malignancies of the head and neck[4]. We herein present one case of recurrent laryngeal papillomatosis and another case of carcinoma in situ as a recurrency of a tonsillar cancer which had been treated with the aid of 5-ALA.

MATERIAL AND METHODS

In the two cases under consideration we use 5-ALA as the photosensitizing agent, which was administered systemically for PD and PDT[5].

Three hours prior to therapy the patient drinks a preparation of 5-ALA (40mg/kg in 50 ml of water). At the same time the patient gets an infusion of ondensatrone (8mg in 75 ml saline) to prevent nausea. After general anesthesia PD is performed by means of a fluorescent light source (D-light, Storz). Subsequently, a cylindrical or spherical optical diffuser fiber is placed next to the target tissue. Then a 100J/cm2 light dose with a flux of 0,1 W/cm^2 is delivered using a dye module connected to a KTP/532 surgical laser. After the procedure patients remain in a dark room till the evening. Photo documentation is performed 48 hours, 1 week and 4 weeks after PDT.

Case reports
Case 1: A 62 yr. old male suffering from recurrent laryngeal papillomas over the last 15 years. CO2-laser vaporisation of papillomas was performed eight times up to now.

PD showed clear red fluorescence of macro- and microscopically identified papillomas along both vocal cords and within the anterior commissure (Figure 1). Additionally small fluorescent spots could be detected in the area of the epiglottic petiolus. These spots, which would not have been detected without PD have been confirmed histologically as tiny papillomas (Figure 2).

CO2-Laser vaporisation of papillomas (at least of all areas that showed 5-ALA induced fluorescence) was performed, followed by PDT using a cylindrical optical fiber which was inserted into the glottic space via a holding device.

430

Case 2: This case shows a 58 yr. old male suffering from right tonsillar cancer (T2N0). One year after primary radiochemotherapy he developed a local recurrency, which was treated by combined brachy- and chemotherapy. Three years later biopsy of the soft palate revealed a carcinoma in situ.

PD endoscopy showed slightly red fluorescence of the macroscopically visible tumor. Moreover, very faint red areas were seen along the entire right pharyngeal wall. Additional biopsies of these areas revealed grade I and II dysplasia. 48 hours after PDT the tumor as well as the areas along the right pharyngeal wall showed necrosis. Two weeks later the fibrinous sludge was mainly rejected. Four weeks after PDT procedure treated areas presented plain mucosal surface and showed no evidence of neoplasia.

DISCUSSION

Photodynamic diagnosis/therapy (PD/PDT) is a novel therapeutic concept. It is efficient, short acting and, as there is no cumulative toxicity, can be repeated and used with other treatment modalities such as chemo- or radiotherapy.

Furthermore, PD and PDT can be performed in the same session.

As we could demonstrate in case 1 the main advantage of PD as a powerful diagnostic tool is the ability of detecting small incipient papillomas which otherwise fail to be noticed by conventional microscopical detection methods. Therefore the benefit of using PD and PDT in treatment of laryngheal papillomatosis might be twofold: on one hand PD offers the possibility of improved detection of "hidden" papillomas that in turn allows a more accurate removal of papillomas. On the other hand PDT takes effect on the whole irradiated area more or less uniformly. Thus, in contrast to CO2-laser vaporisation papillomas can not escape surgeons notice.

Case 2 demonstrates that PDT has considerable attractions for treating premalignant and malignant lesions of the mouth and the oropharynx[6]. Surprisingly, dysplastic areas in the surrounding of the main lesion showed the same necrotic response to light irradiation although they have not been covered by the actual irradiated area. Probably the light dose in close vicinity to the actual irradiated area was high enough to initiate a photodynamic process in tumor surrounding dysplastic areas. However, the observation that macromorphological hardly detectable satellite lesions can be treated sufficiently seems to be an additional advantage of PDT.

In conclusion, these results support growing evidence that PD using 5-ALA is a save and powerful diagnostic tool in laryngeal papillomatosis[7]. Furthermore the satisfying result in the treatment of highly dysplastic lesions (carcinoma in situ) justifies further PDT-studies in superficial premalignant or malignant lesions of the upper aeordigestive trac

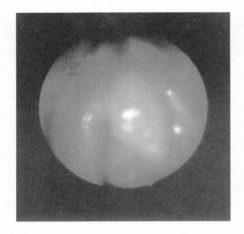 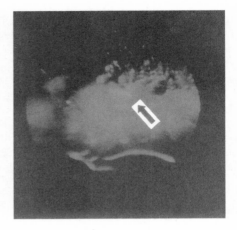

Figure 1. PD showes clear red fluorescence of bulky papillomas in the anterior commissure.

Figure 2. A small fluorescent spot can be detected in the area of the epiglottic petiolus by means of PD. This spot which would not have been detected microscopically has been confirmed histologically as tiny papilloma.

REFERENCES

1. Grant WE, Hopper C, Speight PM, Mac Robert AJ, Brown SG. Photodynamic therapy of malignant and premalignant lesions in patients with "field cancerization" of the oral cavity. J Laryngol Otol 1993; 107:1140-1145
2. Cairnduff F, Stringer MR, Hudson EJ, et al. Superficial photodynamic therapy with topical 5-aminolaevulinic acid for superficial primary and secondary skin cancer. Br J Cancer 1994; 69:605-608
3. Barr H, Sheperd NA, Dix A et al. Eradication of high grade dysplasia in columnar-lined (Barrett's) Oesophagus by photodynamic therapy with endogenously generated protoporphyrins IX. Lancet 1996; 348:584-585
4. Biel MA. Photodynamic therapy and the treatment of neoplastic diseases of the larynx. Laryngoscope 1994; 104:399-403
5. Kennedy JC, Marcus SL, Pottier RH. Photodynamic therapy (PDT) and photodiagnosis (PD) using endogenous photosenzation induced by 5-aminoevulinic acid (ALA): mechanisms and clinical results. J clin Laser Med Surg 1996; 14:289-304
6. Fan KF, Hopper C, Speight PM et al. Photodynamic therapy using 5-aminoevulinic acid for premalignant and malignant lesions of the oral cavity. Cancer 1996; 78:1374-83
7. Leunig A, Betz ChS, Mehlmann M et al. A pilot series demonstrating fluorescence staining of laryngeal papilloma using 5-Aminoevulinic acid. Laryngoscope 2000; 110:1783-85

THE CORRELATION BETWEEN THE ULTRASTRUCTURTAL CHANGES AND THE PRESENCE OF NODAL METASTASES IN ADENOID CYSTIC CARCINOMA

Wojciech Golusinski[1], Wiesława Biczysko[2], Andrzej Marszałek[2], Elzbieta Wasniewska[1], Przemyslaw Majewski[2], Krzysztof Szyfter[3]
[1]Department of Otolaryngology Head and Neck Surgery Karol Marcinkowski University School of Medical Sciences Poznan, Poland
[2]Department of Clinical Pathomorphology, Karol Marcinkowski University School of Medical Sciences Poznan, Poland
[3]Department of Human Genetics Polish Academy of Science Poznan, Poland

Correspondence to: *Wojciech Golusinski, M.D., Ph.D., Department of Otolaryngology Head and Neck Surgery, Przybyszewskiego 49, 60-355 Poznan, Poland*

ABSTRACT

Adenoid cystic carcinoma (ACC) is a malignant tumour characterised by variable histological presentation and types of growth (solid, tubular, glandular). It is still an open question which morphological diagnostic features of ACC can predict the possibility for metastases of the primary tumour into lymph nodes.

The aim of the present study was determination ultrastructural features of the nuclei and cytoplasm of tumour cells and correlation of those observations with the presence of nodal metastases.

Material and method. We studied 34 cases with ACC (15 tubular, 16 glandular and 3 solid) with no nodal involvement and 12 cases (2 tubular, 10 solid) with metastases into regional lymph nodes. For ultrastructural studies we took samples from primary tumours and metastases.

Result. On the electron-microscopic studies we found that the histological type within the primary tumour and metastases differs. In the metastases, the solid pattern was more common, while the typical cribriform one was not found. But in all cases we found a mixture of at least two of three patterns of growth. On ultrastructural level we found that cell nuclei were euchromatic with folded nuclear membrane. Moreover the nucleoli were enlarged and numerous, and segregation of the nucleolar material was observed.

Conclusion. Using electron-microscopic studies we can determine the features of cell de-differentiation and the character of the changes within the nucleoli. This information might be used for the description of the tumour biology.

INTRODUCTION

Adenoid cystic carcinoma (ACC) is one of the most common malignant tumours of salivary glands characterised by variable histological presentation and different patterns of growth (solid, tubular, glandular). Even in one tumour we can observe three different patterns of growth[6]. It was generally regarded that if the predominant pattern of growth within tumour is tubular or cribriform prognosis is better then in solid one[9]. Although there are some publications on the biological behaviour of that tumour, it is still an open question if there is any possibility of predicting ACC metastases into lymph nodes if diagnosis is based on the macro- and microscopically evaluated primary tumour[5,8].

The aim of the present study was determination of ultrastructural features of the nuclei and cytoplasm of tumour cells and correlation of those observations with the presence of nodal metastases.

MATERIAL AND METHODS

We studied 46 cases with ACC. In the studied group there were 73% of women and 27% of men. Patients' age ranged from 26 to 83 years, medium 57 years. Duration of symptoms before surgery lasted from 1 month to 5 years, medium 1,5 year. The tumour size ranged from 1,4 cm to 8 cm, medium 2,8 cm. In all cases tissue samples were taken for routines light microscopic examination. Additionally we performed ultrastructural studies in transmission electron microscope. For ultrastructural studies we took samples from primary tumours and metastases.

RESULTS

In the whole group there were 34 cases (74%) without metastases into lymph nodes and 12 patients (26%) with nodal involvement. In the first group the predominant pattern of growth within the tumour was as follow: glandular (cribriform) in 16 (Fig. 1), tubular in 15 (Fig. 2) and solid in 3 cases (Fig. 3). In patients with involved lymph nodes (Fig. 4) the predominant histological type of ACC was solid in 10 and tubular in 2 cases.

Usually at least two different growth patterns were observed within one tumour. In the area of pseudocyst (pseudolumen) (Fig. 5, 6) there was basement membrane-like material surrounded by numerous fibrilar structures of extracellular matrix (Fig. 5). Lose nests and scant destroyed cells of tumour parenchyma were also observed. In areas of a solid growth, few groups of cells with the features of differentiation into squamous epithelium were found (Fig. 7). In

434

those cells we found bundles of cytokeratins and desmosom-like intercellular junctions were found. In cases with metastases, the solid pattern was more common, while the typical cribriform one was not found. On the electron-microscopic studies we found that the histological type within the primary tumour and metastases differs. If in the solid areas pseudocysts were formed, regional lack of the basement membrane was observed. The cell nuclei were euchromatic with folded nuclear membrane. The nuclei occupied a large area with the cell, and increased N/C ratio was found. Moreover the nucleoli were enlarged and numerous, and segregation of the nucleolar material was observed. Those observations were more typical for cases with nodal involvement.

DISCUSSION

It is general regarded that in ACC even in one tissue specimen two different patterns of growth can be observed. Although it is rather slow growing tumour prognosis of this neoplasm is frequently unpredictable. There were made many attempts for description of the best available prognostic indicators of ACC[3]. Even usage of monoclonal antibodies for evaluation of expression of proliferation antigens such as Ki67 or p53 and proliferating cell nuclear antigen (PCNA) and c-erb-2 oncoprotein and other is insufficient for predicting of tumour biology[4]. Our results and data obtained by others[2,10] indicate that within ACC areas of different proliferative activity can be observed. The following clinical course is probably related to biological behaviour of the less differentiated and the less maturated tumour area. However, several investigators have found no correlation between predominating histological pattern of growth and prognosis[1,5].

In the present study we found that tumour cells within tubular or solid areas had less or even just single ultrastructural features of differentiation toward myoepithelial cells. Those cells had increased N/C ratio and nucleoli were typical for actively proliferating cells. In this study we found that in cribriform ACC lymph nodes were free of metastases on time of surgery. But as it was stressed by other authors[7] metastases in ACC develop slowly and for a long time they can be clinically silent. We have now rather short time of follow up of our patients - usually less than 3 years. It's too early to make generalised conclusions as it was accepted that for ACC recurrences were reported after even more than 5 years. But we think that ACC is a tumour with a very interesting biology, and for describing of its biology several tumour markers should be studied and several different techniques should be used for evaluation of its biology.

CONCLUSION

Using electron-microscopic studies we can determine the features of cell de-differentiation and character of the changes within the nuclei. This information might be used for the description of the tumour biology.

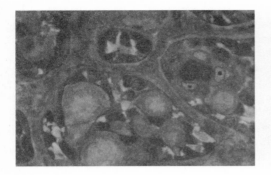
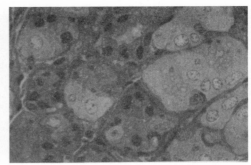

Figure 1. Glandular (cribriform) type of ACC. There are nests of epithelial cells, and numerous pseudocysts are formed. Pseudocysts contain basement-like material and in some of them remnants of tumour cells are present. Semithin section, toluidine blue. Primary magnification 250 x.

Figure 2. Fragment of tumour with a tubular pattern of growth. In some cells of tumour parenchyma vacuolar structures with cell cytoplasm are present. Semithin section, toluidine blue. Primary magnification 250 x.

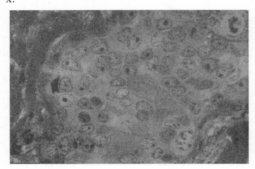
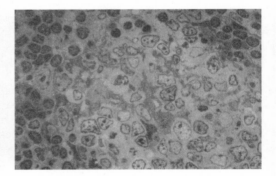

Figure 3. Fragment of ACC with solid pattern of growth with focal deposition of basement membrane-like material. One tumour cell during abnormal mitotic division is visible. The group of cells is surround by stroma containing very numerous collagen fibbers. Semithin section, toluidine blue. Primary magnification 250 x.

Figure 4. Fragment of tumour metastasis into the lymph node from the same case as on Figure 3. The pattern growth is same as in the primary tumour. Semithin section, toluidine blue. Primary magnification 250 x.

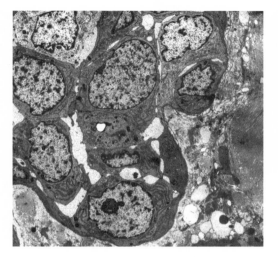

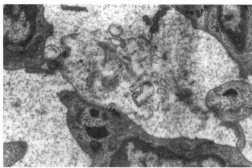

Figure 5. The same case as on the Figure 1. Fragment of tumour with a solid pattern of growth. In the central part of tumour cells nest, one cell with damaged chromatin within nucleus is visible. In the intercellular space a delicate net of proteoglycans is present. At the periphery tumour cells attached to the basement membrane-like structures and numerous bundles of collagen fibrils. Electron micrograph. Magnification 7000 x

Figure 6. In the lumen of pseudocyst proteoglycans and remnants of destroyed cell are present. There are remnants of cellular membranes, polirybosomes and fragments of RER. Electron micrograph. Primary magnification 22.000x.

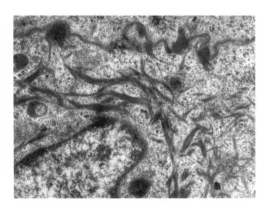

Figure 7. Fragment of ACC with solid pattern of growth. The cells presented on the picture re differentiated toward squamous epithelium. In the cell cytoplasm bundles of cytokeratins are observed. The junctions between cells are of desmosome type. Electron micrograph. Primary magnification 44.000x.

REFERENCES

1.   Cho K.J., Lee S.S., Lee Y.S.: Proliferating cell nuclear antigen and c-erb-2 oncoprotein expression in adenoid cystic carcinomas of the salivary glands. Head Neck 1999, 414-419

2.   Jeng Y.M., Lin C.Y., Hsu H.C.: Expression of the c-kit protein is associated with certain subtypes of salivary gland carcinoma. Cancer Lett 2000, 154, 107-111

3.   Kuhel W.I., Chow H.,Goldwin T.A., Minick C.R., Libby D.M.: Elevated carcinoembryonic antigen levels correlating with disease recurrence in a patient with adenoid cystic carcinoma. Head Neck 1995, 17, 431-436

4.   Lazzaro B., Cleveland D.: P53 and Ki-67 antigen expression in small oral biopsy specimens of salivary gland tumors. Oral Surg Oral Med Oral Tahol Radiol Endod 2000, 89, 613-617

5.   Renehan A., Gleave E.N., Hancock B.D., McGurk M.: Long-term follow-up of over 1000 patients with salivary gland tumours treated in a single centre. Br J Surg 1996, 83, 1750-1754

6.   Seifert G. (Ed.) Histological typing of salivary gland tumors. WHO Classification, Spriger-Verlag Berlin Heidelberg 1991

7.   Spiro R.H.: Distant metastasis in adenoid cystic carcinoma of salivary origin. Am J Surg 1997, 174, 495-498

8.   Sur R.K., Donde B., Levin V., Pacella J., Kotzen J., Cooper K., Hale M.: Adenoid cystic carcinoma of salivary glands: a review of 10 years. Laryngoscope 19997, 107, 1276-1280

9.   Takata T., Kudo Y., Zhao M., Ogawa I., Miyauchi M., Sato S., Cheng J., Nikai H.: Reduced expression of p27Kip1 protein in relation to salivary adenoid cystic carcinoma metastasis. Cancer 1999, 86, 928-935

10.   Yamamoto Y., Itoh T., Saka T., Takahashi H.: Nucleolar organizer regions in adenoid cystic carcinoma of the salivary glands. Eur Arch Otorhinolaryngol 1995, 252, 176-180.

TUMOR-INFILTRATION OF CAROTID ARTERIES – IS THERE AN INDICATION FOR INTERSTITIAL BRACHYTHERAPY WITH 192 IRIDIUM ?

Jens Büntzel, MD[1], Michael Glatzel, MD[2], Dirk Schröder PhD[2], Dietmar Fröhlich MD[2], Klaus Küttner, MD[1]

[1]Department of ORL & Plastic Surgery; Zentralklinikum Suhl, Germany
[2]Department of Radiotherapy, Zentralklinikum Suhl, Germany

Correspondence to: Jens Büntzel, MD, HNO-Klinik am Zentralklinikum, Albert-Schweitzer-Str. 2, D-98527 Suhl, Germany

ABSTRACT

Objective. The non-resectable infiltration of arteria carotis communis by an advanced pretreated squamous cell carcinoma of the head and neck region is commonly a situation with no effective therapeutic possiblity.

Methods. We describe the first experiences with the following management: 1. Neck dissection. With resection of Vena jugularis interna and the majority of tumor. 2. Implantation of silicon-catheders (3 to 5) on the wall of Arteria carotis communis / externa / interna. 3. CT-assisted brachytherapy in the area of vessel-infiltration. The total dose of brachytherapy was 21 Gy, the single dose 1,5 Gy, twice daily application.

Results. Between 1999 and 2000 we treated 10 patients. At the end of brachytherapy no evidence of tumor was registered in 9/10 patients. With a median follow-up of 9 month we have already abserved three patients longer then 12 month without any signs of recurrence. Brachytherapy induced toxicities were mild wound inflammation in 2/10 patients, and fibrosis in 3/10 patients. We observed no bleeding in all patients.

Conclusion. The combination of neck dissection and additional intra- or postoperative brachytherapy offers an effective and safe therapeutic approach also in the case of arterial infiltration by the tumor.

INTRODUCTION

With local control rates between 70 and 80 percent the simultaneous radiochemotherapy remains a defined number of patients with residual tumor. Normally the response of the primary tumor is better than this of the cervical lymph node metastases. So the neck dissection is the most common salvage procedure after definitive radiooncological therapy in the head and neck region. A part of these patients will still show tumors attaching tha carotid arteries, a complete resection of the tumor would be only possible if the artery itself would be resected and a prostethesis would be implanted. Because of their secondary diseases a majority of our patients has absolute contraindications for this kind of vessel surgery. So we have to look for further therapeutic approaches including the remaining radiotherapeutic possibilities.

The interstitial brachytherapy is a well established method in the treatment of recurrent and residual head and neck cancer. Probably we would have the chance to integrate this technique in our multimodal salvage concept, if we are able to implant the silicone catheters already in the intraoperative situation. Tje presented paper should summarize our first experiences with this method regarding the feasibility and safety of such a management.

MATERIAL AND METHODS

If we have found an intraoperative situation with attachement of the tumor to the carotid arteries the following management was performed:

- Implantation of 3-5 silicone catheters (Hentschel) along the carotid artery. Fixation via an absorbable suture.
- Demonstrating of intraoperative situs to the radiooncologist.
- Completion of neck dissection.
- Computertomography assisted planning of target volume for the high dose rate brachytherapy with 192 iridium.
- brachytherapy: twice daily 1.5 Gy single dose, 21 Gy total dose, breaks at week ends and official holidays.
- Removing of silicone catheters after completion of barchytherapy.

All patients were controlled during follow-up visits every 8 weeks. The follow up included a physical examination and an ultrasound of the neck region.

Between 10/1999 and 12/2000 we have treated 10 patients in the described technique. The group included 9 men and one woman with an median age of 59 years (range 39 to 71). All of the patients were treated by an definitive radiochemotherapy with 70 Gy total irradiation dose. We had used carboplatin as radiosensitizer during the basic treatment. The local control rate was 100 % at the primary tumor. All patients had large lymph nodes after completion of the definitive radiochemotherapy. Six patients suffered from an oropharyngeal tumor, further three from a hypopharyngeal cancer and one patient from a tongue cancer.

RESULTS

After the end of interstitial brachtherapy we have observed nin out of ten patients with no evidence of local tumor. In one patient no effect of brachytherapy was seen. After a median follow-up of 9 month (range 3 to 14) we see three cases with complete remissions, further two patients have shown a local controlled tumor, and the remaining 5 patients have suffered from the progredient tumor disease. 5/10 patients are still alive.

During the brachytherapy we have registered only rare acute toxicities. Despite the fact that no rupture of carotid artery occured, we had to treat only two local inflammations in region of the silicone catheters. As late toxicities we found a fibrosis of the sternocleidoid muscle, the subcutaneous tissue and the skin in three patients, a thicker artery wall in ultrasound in four patients, and a iatrogenis distant metastasis in the subcutaneous tissue of our female patient (see case report 1). The metastasis occured at the distal end of the posterior catheter. Probably the brachtherapy dosage was not strong enough to destroy all of the tumor cells and the remaining active tumor cells were moved from the artery wall to the subcutaneous tissue during the removing of the catherter after finishing the radiotherapy.

The following three case histories should demonstrate the potential subgroup of patients as well as the seen results.

Case report 1
Female 50 years old patient. First visit at our department 4-2000. Diagnosis: oropharyngeal cancer left T4 N3 M0. Basic treatment: Definitive radiochemotherapy with 70 Gy total dose, 2 Gy single dose, daily fractionation. 4 cycles carboplatin (weeks 1, 3, 5, and 7) in a weekly dose of 350 mg/m^2 Body surface area. Results: complete regression of the tonsillar tumor, partial remission in both neck regions.

9-2000 follow-up-staging: growing lymph nodes, indication for salvage-neck dissection right-side, date: 10-4-00. Intra-operative a infiltration of the A. carotis communis, and the A. carotis externa was seen. Three silicone catheters were fixed at the infiltrated wall of the carotid arteries. Brachytherapy described above. Se figure 1.

11-2000 functional neck dissection left side. No evidence of tumor at the right side. Beginning fibrosis.

1-2001. Subcutaneous metastasis at the distant end of the posterior catheter. Se figure 2. Resection of the metastasis, adjunctive chemotherapy with doxorubicin/trofosfamide.

Case report 2
Male 63 years old patient. First visit at our department 10-1999. Diagnosis: Supraglottic carcinoma T4 N2a M0. Definitive radiochemotherapy between 10-1999 and 11-1999. 70 Gy total dose, 2 Gy single dose, 3 cycles Carboplatin at weeks 1, 4, and 7 with a weekly dose of 350 mg/m^2 BSA. Complete local remission, incomplete (partial) remission at the lymph node metastasis right side.

12-1999 functional salvage neck dissection with implantation of 3 silicone catheters because of an infiltration of Arteria carotis externa and the skull base. Brachytherapy according the described schedule.

1-2001 disease free situation. Patient is in good general condition. Late toxicities: mild fibrosis, thicker artery wall.

Case report 3
Male 51 years old patient. First visit at our department: 12-1999. Diagnosis: Oropharyngeal cancer left T3 N2b M0. Basic treatment: laser surgical resection of the tumor, functional neck dissection left-side. Adjuvant radiochemotherapy with 60 Gy total dose, 2 Gy single dose, daily fractionation, 2 cycles carboplatin at week 1, and 5 in a weekly dose of 350 mg/m^2 BSA. Complete remission.

10-2000 local recurrence, and new lymph nodes with infiltration of the carotid artery. Salvage Neck dissection (functional) and implantation of four catheters.
1-2001 locoregional controlled disease, local progress. Late toxicities: fibrosis of the skin. The patient died at february 2001 due to the progressive tumor disease.

DISCUSSION

A lot of reports in the world literature since the 1950ies have documented that radiation exposure to the large vessels like the carotid artery will result in damage to the arteries over time[1-3]. This damage has been reproduced by animal models and shown to be identical to the pathoanatomical changes of artherosclerosis[4, 5]. Reported consequences of irradiation-induced changes in the carotid artery included the rupture of the vessel, the thrombosis, a carotid wall thickening, and a progressive artherosclerosis in the irradiated field[6, 7]. A group of papers has described the association between radiotherapy and the damage of carotid arteries in retrospective analysis[8, 9]. The only prospective study was published recently by Muzaffar et al.[10] They found thaat neck irradiation significantly increases the thickness of the carotid wall (intima-media-thickness) during the first year after completion of radiotherapy (external beam) – on avarage, 21 times more than in epidemiologically mathced control volunteers. In conclusion they pointed out that the extension of irradiation fields should carefully reduced in patients with N0 necks.

Despite the discussed problems, a medline research has shown that some study groups have used brachytherapy of the cervical lymph nodes as a feasible technique in patients with advanced disease, especially if the carotid artery in attached by the growing tumor[11, 12]. Fee et al.[13] have analyzed the differences between the application of iodine 125 and 192 iridium. Following their experimental results in 39 healthy dogs they favoured 125 iodine for application in humans because of the lower dose rate delivery of this drug. In their 29 treated patient they have found a local control rate of 76 % and a mean survival of 15 month in the case of primary tumor and 12 month if a recurrent tumor was irradiated. The overall incidence of distant metastasis was 45 %[14]. Their severe complication rate of 11 % is comparable to the experiences we have seen in our smaller group[15]. The results of Chen et al. support these dimension with 21 % major complication rate and 50 % overall complication rate[11].

In conclusion the inproved survival, the high local control rate, and the minimal severe complication rates in these three series makes the intraoperative implantation of 125 iodine or 192 iridium implants to an effective adjunctive treatment to surgery and external beam irridiation if the carotid artery is attached by the tumor. The individual intra-operative decision for indication and the careful planning of target volume and dosage remain the essential preconditions for a succesful treatment in this difficult situation.

The authors thank Mr. Matthias Wackes from the Regional Tumor Center Suhl for his assistance in preparing the figures of this paper.

REFERENCES

1. Thomas E, WD Forbus: Irradiation injury of the aorta and the lung. Arch Pathol 1959; 67: 256-263
2. Levinson SA, MB Close, AX Ehrenfeld, RJ Stoney: Carotid artery occlusive disease following external cervical irradiation. Arch Surg 1973; 107: 395-397
3. Elerding SC, RN Fernandez, JC Grotta et al.: Carotid artery disease following cervical irradiation. Arch Surg 1981; 194: 609-615
4. Aarnoudse MW, HB Lamberts, F Dijk, J Vos, AJ de Vries: Monocytes and radiation induced artheromatosis in rabbits. Virchows Arch 1984; 47: 211-216
5. Smith C, LA Lowenthal: A study of elastic arteries in irradiation in mice of different ages. Proc Soc Exp Biol Med 1950; 75: 859-861
6. Mc Cready RA, GL Hyde, BA Bivins, SS Mattingly, WO Griffen: Radiation-induced arterial injuries. Surgery 1983; 306-312
7. Atkinson JLD, TM Sundt, AJD Dale, TL Cascino, DA Nichols: Radiation-associated atheromatous disease of the cervical carotid artery: report of seven cases and review of the literature. Neurosurgery 1989; 24: 171-178
8. Call GK, PF Bray, RK Wendy: Carotid thrombosis following neck irradiation. Int J Radiat Oncol Biol Phys 1990; 18: 635-640
9. Mc Guirt WF, RS Feehs, G Bond, HL Strickland, WM Kinney: Irradiation induced artherosclerosis: a factor in therapeutic planning. Ann Otol Rhinol Laryngol 1992; 101: 222-228
10. Muzaffar K, SL Collins, N Labropoulos, WH Baker: A prospective study of the effects of irradiation on the carotid artery. Laryngoscope 2000; 110: 1811-1814
11. Chen KY, RM Mohr, CL Silverman: Interstitial iodine 125 in advanced recurrent squamous cell carcinoma of the head and neck with follow-up evaluation of carotid artery by ultrasound. Ann Otol Rhinol Laryngol 1996; 105: 955-961
12. Paryani SB, DR Goffinet, WE Fee, RL Goode, P Levine, ML Hopp: Iodine 125 suture implants in the management of advanced tumours in the neck attached to the carotid artery. J Clin Oncol 1985; 3: 809-812
13. Fee WE, DR Goffinet, D Guthauer, LF Fajardo, C Handen: Safety of 125iodine and 192iridium implants to the canine carotid artery: preliminary report. Laryngoscope 1985; 95: 317-320
14. Fee WE, DR Goffinet, S Paryani, RL Goode, PA Levine, ML Hopp: Intraoperative iodine 125 implants. Their use in large tumors in the neck attached to the carotid artery. Arch Otolaryngol 1983; 109: 727-730
15. Martinez A, DR Goffinet, W Fee, R Goode, RS Cox: 125 iodine implants as an adjuvant to surgery and external beam radiotherapy in the management of locally advanced head and neck cancer. Cancer 1983; 51: 973-979

PITFALLS IN ULTRASOUND DIAGNOSTICS
OF THE SUSPECTED N0 NECK

Ch. Külkens, B.M. Lippert, J.A. Werner (Marburg, Germany)

INTRODUCTION

The prognosis of patients suffering from squamous cell carcinomas of the upper aerodigestive tracts is significantly influenced by the extent of the lymphatic metastasis[16]. In the past the manual palpation was the standard for the staging of the neck and also today it is very often performed routinely as the only method. Because of the low sensitivity and specificity of about 60% to 70% this examination method is generally considered as inexact and thus insufficient[5]. The risk of occult metastasis in the palpably N0 neck is accordingly high if further imaging diagnosis is not made. Among the imaging methods predominantly applied for staging CT scan, MRI and the B-mode sonography (if applicable in connection with the fine-needle aspiration biopsy) are in competition, the latter is considered by several authors as the most sensitive method in the detection of lymph nodes either in the primary staging and in the tumor follow-up[3, 7]. Other examinators classify the mentioned methods as equally[4, 11].

The discussions about the therapy of the palpably N0 neck (elective neck dissection vs. wait-and-see-policy) is thus determined by the sensitivity of the diagnostic methods and here especially the sonography[16]. Despite the sonography it is not possible in most of the cases to detect a neck lymph node metastasis. Here the differential diagnosis between inflammatory and metastatic lymph nodes is often difficult, but it is of crucial for the individual patient. Because of these insecurities some patients are treated in the wrong way (figure 3): In spite of the performance of a wait-and-see-policy often an extreme tumor progress by the occult metastasis can be observed. On the other hand many patients are treated without any obvious reason with elective neck dissection and thus over-treated. At the moment patients are recommended to submit to an elective neck dissection when showing the expected risk of an initial neck lymph node metastasis of more than 15% to 20%, of the primary tumor[8, 14]. The incidence depends on the localization as well as the infiltration depth[15, 16]. The sonography in combination with the fine-needle aspiration biopsy is of great importance in the staging of a palpably N0-neck.

DISCUSSION

A typical pitfall is the exact measuring of the lymph node. Particularly in the region II the exact measurement of the lymph node can be difficult. In addition, different criteria such as size, shape, echo structure and perfusion pattern do not have a standardized definition by which a lymph node can be classified according to its malignant potential[2, 9, 10, 13]. Concerning this subject Van den Brekel at al.[12] also describes additional size criteria for the different neck regions.

The aspiration of cells from the concerned lymph node has also several insecurities (figure 1). Only by sonography it is not possible to detect the actual sentinel lymph node. Besides, in several cases it is also doubtful when using the ultra-sound controlled puncture, whether the lymph node that has to be examined is really hit. Even within the lymph node micro-metastases may be missed in the puncture or necrotic regions are punctured which gives negative the results (figure 2).

The actual cytological examination has also in some of the cases insecurities which can not be neglected in the differential diagnosis.

Additionally, one has to consider that the quality of the results of all three above mentioned techniques (sonography, aspiration and cytological evaluation) strongly depends on the experience of the physican.

Of course the safeness in the wait-and-see-policy is also dependent on the correctly chosen time intervals and on the compliance of the patient.

CONCLUSION

Because of the high quality of the combination of ultra-sound and fine-needle aspiration cytology in comparison to all other diagnostic methods the indication to fine-needle aspiration cytology should be made generously. In case of cytologically doubtful results the latter may be performed repeatedly.

Despite progress in diagnostics with the fine-needle aspiration cytology the therapy management of the N0 neck has furthermore insecurities. Also the sonography in combination with the fine-needle aspiration cytology cannot detect all micro-metastases if those are partly not seen even in the pathologic examination. Decisions concerning the therapeutic approach can only be made on the basis of the additional consideration of statistic frequencies of neck lymph node metastases in dependence on the tumor localization and the stage.

In the future it is crucial to develop standardized criteria for malignancy which are not existing so far. Additionally to technically high-quality ultrasound equipment and well qualified examinators the exact documentation is an essential issue. Only on the basis of those documentation it is possible to control persisting unclear neck lymph nodes sufficiently. If in the course of the four-week control a change in size is obvious, the exstirpation of the neck lymph node in combination with frozen section becomes necessary with definite histological evaluation and according to the result a neck dissection has to be performed.

446

The palpatory N0-neck represents already a so-called pitfall because of the problems of the decision of the right therapy in spite of performed sonography because it harbors insecurities with the remaining risk for the further therapeutic approach.

OUTLOOK

For the future it would be desirable to have an additional safeness to detect the sentinel lymph node by the further development of the lymphoszintigraphy[6, 17] which would make a better aimed fine-needle aspiration cytology possible. Furthermore the diagnosis could be more secure when developing the molecular biological tumor cells detection in the aspirate[1].

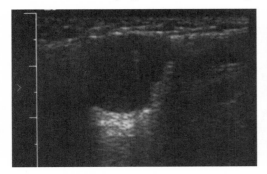 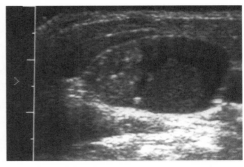

Figure 1: Fine-needle aspiration cytology in a homogenously structured lymph node.

Figure 2: Neck lymph node metastasis with differently structured parts.

Figure 3. In the described schematized treatment concept of the neck the central region is marked with different colors. It is the question of the cutting surface where the clinical N0 neck and palpably not definitely classified neck stage can be evaluated by the sonography. These problems may repeat especially in the wait-and-see-policy in the course of a longer interval with several examinations. The palpably N0 neck represents the highest insecurity in the whole therapy concept beside the palpably doubtful neck stage.

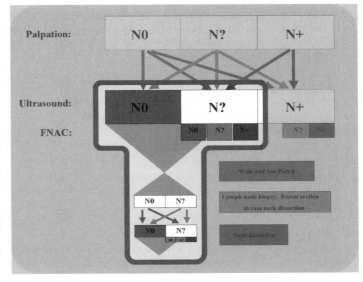

447

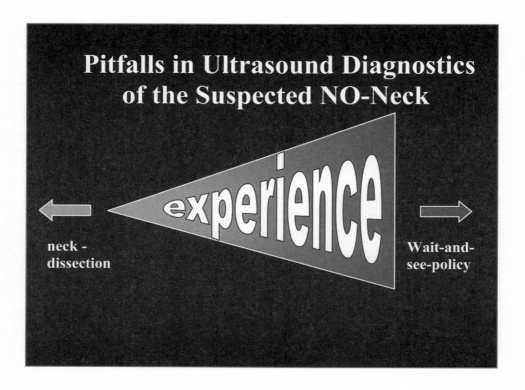

Pitfalls in Ultrasound Diagnostics of the Suspected N0-Neck

neck - dissection

Wait-and-see-policy

REFERENCES

1. Brakenhoff, R.H., Stroomer, J.G., ten Brink, C., de Bree, R., Weima, S.M., Snow, G.B., van Dongen, G.A: Sensitive detection of squamous cells in bone marrow and blood of head and neck cancer patients by E48 reverse transcriptase polimerase chain reaction. Clin Cancer Res 5; 725-732 (1999).
2. Bruneton, J.N., Balu-Maestro, C., Marcy, P.Y., Melia, P., Mouou, M.Y.: Very high frequency (13 MHz) ultrasonographic examination of the normal lymph nodes and thyroid nodules. J. Ultrasound Med 13; 87-90 (1994).
3. Furukawa, M., Kaneko, M., Mochimatsu, I., Sawaki, S., Igari, H., Tsukudu, M.: Comparatative studies of diagnosis with US or CT of the cervical lymph node metastases in head and neck cancer. Nippon Jibiinkoka Gakkai Kaiho 4; 577-586 (1991).
4. Ishii, J., Amagasa, T., Tachibana, T., Shinozuka, K., Shida, S.: US and CT evaluation of cervical lymph node metastasis from oral cancer. J Craniomaxillofac Surg 3; 123-127 (1991).
5. Marinez-Gimeno, C., Rodriguez, E.M., Vila, C.N., Varela, C.L.: Squamous cell carcinoma of the oral cavity: A clinicopathologic scoring system for evaluating risk of cervical lymph node metastasis. Laryngoscope 105; 728-733 (1995).
6. Nieuwenhuis, E.J., Colnot, D.R., Pijpers, H.J., Castelijns, J.A., van Diest, P.J., Brakenhoff, R.H., Snow, G.B., van den Brekel, M.W.: Lymphoscintigraphy and ultrasound-guided fine needle aspiration cytology of sentinel lymph nodes in head and neck cancer patients. Recent Results Cancer Res 157; 206-217 (2000).
7. Quetz, J.U., Rohr, S., Hoffmann, P., Wustrow, P., Mertens, J.: B-image sonography in lymph node staging of the head and neck area. A comparison with palpation, computerized and magnetic resonance tomography. HNO39; 61-63 (1991).
8. Steiner, W., Hommerich, C.P.: Diagnosis and treatment of the N0 neck of carcinomas of the upper aerodigestive tract. Europ Arch Otorhinolaryngol 250; 250-256 (1993).

448

9.   Steinkamp, H.J., Cornehl, M., Hosten,, N., Pegios, W., Vogl, T., Felix, R.: Cervical lymphadenopathy: Ratio of long- to short-axis diameter as a predictor of malignancy. Br J Radiol 68; 266-270 (1995).

10.   Van den Brekel, M.W., Stel, H.V., Castelijns, J.A., Nauta, J.J., van der Waal, I., Valk, J., Meyer, C.J., Snow, G.B.: Cervical lymph node metastasis: Assessment of radiologic criteria, Radiology 177; 379-384 (1990).

11.   Van den Brekel, Castelijns, J.A., M.W., Stel, H.V., Golding, R.P., Meyer, C.J., Snow, G.B.: Modern imaging techniques and ultrasound-guided aspiration cytology for the assessment of neck node metastases: A prospective comparative study. Eur Arch Otorhinolaryngol 250; 11-17 (1993).

12.   Van den Brekel, M.W., Castelijns, J.A., Snow, G.B.: The size of lymph nodes in the neck on sonograms as a radiologic criterion for metastasis : How reliable is it. AJNR Am J Neuroradiol 19; 695-700 (1998).

13.   Vasallo, P., Wernecke, K., Roos, N., Peters, P.E.: Differentiation of benign from malignant superficial lymphadenopathy: The role of high-resolution US. Radiology 183; 215-220 (1992).

14.   Weiss, M.H., Harrison, L.B., Isaacs, R.S.: Use of decision analysis in planning a management strategy for the stages N0 neck. Arch Otolaryngol Head Neck Surg 120; 699-702 (1994).

15.   Werner, J.A.: Untersuchungen zum Lymphgefässsystem der oberen Luft- und Speisewege, Aachen: Shaker, (1995).

16.   Werner, J. A.: Aktueller Stand der Versorgung des Lymphabflusses maligner Kopf-Hals-Tumoren. In Theissing, J. (Hrsg.): Klinik und Therapie in der HNO-Heilkunde, Kopf- und Halschirurgie im Wandel. Verhandlungsbericht Dtsch. Gesellschaft für HNO-Heilkunde, Kopf- und Halschirurgie. Springer, Berlin 1997, S. 47-85.

17.   Werner, J.A., Dünne, A.A., Brandt, D., Ramaswamy, A., Külkens, C., Lippert, B.M., Folz, B.J., Joseph, K., Moll, R.: Studies on significance of sentinel lymphadenectomy in pharyngeal and laryngeal carcinoma, Laryngorhinootologie 78; 663-670 (1999)

INTRAARTERIAL CHEMOTHERAPY OF
LOCALLY ADVANCED HEAD AND NECK CANCER

A. Teymoortash,[1] B. M. Lippert,[1] J. P. Wakat,[2] S. Bien,[2] J. A. Werner[1]
[1]Department of Otolaryngology, Head and Neck Surgery, Philipps University of Marburg, Germany
[2]Department of Neuroradiology, Philipps University of Marburg, Germany

ABSTRACT

Three patients with advanced squamous cell cancer of the head and neck were the subjects for the present study. These patients were previously treated with radiotherapy and/or surgery and have an inoperable progressive residual tumor. After four cycles of regional chemotherapy by intraarterial infusion of high doses of cisplatin all patients showed a significant decrease of tumor size and pain was reduced.

INTRODUCTION

Three modalities of therapy have established roles in the treatment of carcinoma of the head and neck: chemotherapy, radiation therapy, and surgery. In general, smaller lesions are effectively treated either by surgical excision or irradiation whereas more advanced disease (stage III and IV) is best treated with combined surgery and radiation therapy. The prognosis for patients with advanced head and neck cancer treated conventionally is poor and only a small fraction of these patients are cured. Clearly there is a need to change the therapeutic strategy for patients with advanced head and neck cancer with more effective approaches employing non-surgical modalities.

The concept of regional chemotherapy has been applied in head and cancer for more than four decades[1]. According to more recent study results by Robbins et al. a combination of regional chemotherapy by intraarterial infusion of high doses of cisplatin with radiation therapy seems to be an useful approach when planning integrated treatment for locally advanced head and neck cancer[2, 3].

The objective of this study was to determine the effect of intraarterial chemotherapy und tumor response rate in locally progressive, inoperable and previously radiated head and neck cancer.

PATIENTS AND METHODS

Patients characteristics

Three male patients with advanced squamous cell cancer of the head and neck were the subjects for the present study. These patients were previously treated with radiotherapy and/or surgery and have an inoperable progressive residual tumor (Tab. 1).

Patient Nr.	Age (years)	Location	Stage	Previous Therapy
1	47	oral cavity	$T_2N_0M_0$	surgery, radiotherapy 50 Gy, radiotherapy 16 Gy boost
2	65	oropharynx	$T_3N_{2c}M_0$	radiotherapy 60 Gy, neck dissection on both sides, radiotherapy of mastoid area 46 Gy (tumor progression in retroauricular area
3	59	hypopharynx	$T_3N_{2c}M_0$	radiotherapy 66 Gy

Table 1: Pretreatment characteristics of the patients.

All patients were included in the present study because of tumor progression and progredient pain and their urgent request for a further therapy. The patients understood fully the risks and benefits of the study treatment and consented.

Pretreatment evaluation

Patients underwent complete clinical and laboratory evaluations, including haematological studies, hepatic profiles, renal function and general metabolic functions. No serve impairment of cardiopulmonary function was present. Staging of disease was defined by physical examination, panendoscopic examination, biopsy and computed tomography.

Treatment schedules

Patients received pretreatment intravenous hydration with 1 L 0,9% saline solution including Zofran® 8 mg and Novalgin® 2,5 g. Solu-Decortin H® 250 mg was injected before therapy begann.

An angiographic catheter was introduced percutaneously under local anesthesia into the femoral artery, according to the Seldinger technique. The catheter tip was than placed under radiographic control into the external carotid artery. Diagnostic transfemoral carotid arteriography was performed, and the most suitable branch of the artery providing the prevalent blood supply to the tumor was catheterized selectively.

Cisplatin was administered continuously at a dose of 150 mg/m². All patients received intraarterial cisplatin in 500 ml 0.9% saline solution at an infusion velocity of 6 ml/min. A simultaneous intravenous infusion of sodium thiosulfate at a dose of 9 g/m² disolved in 500 ml 0.9% saline solution was also performed. Posttreatment hydration administered intravenously with Zofran® 1 mg/h for 24 hours disolved in 1 L saline solution.

All of the patients should received four cycles of intraarterial chemotherapy, which were administered every four weeks.

Response to therapy was evaluated two weeks after the last drug administration by physical examination, endoscopy and CT scan.

RESULTS

Three transfemoral intraarterial infusions were performed without significant technical complications. Cisplatin treatment was well tolerated by all patients. No instances of gastrointestinal (nausea, vomiting, diarrhoea), renal, cardiac, respiratory or otovestibular toxicity were reported. The measured haematological parameters were without significant changes.

Concerning local toxicity, all patients presented with moderate alopecia. Patient Nr. 1 received the first two chemotherapy cycles in general anaesthesia due to strong pain. In one of the three cases (patient Nr. 3) the treatment was discontinued and he became only three cycles due to deterioration of the general physical condition.

No patients were lost to follow-up. The median overall survival, measured from the beginning of chemotherapy until death was 6.6 months (range 3 to 10 months).

At the end of the chemotherapy all patients showed a significant decrease of tumor size and pain was reduced.

The cause of death was the original cancer in all cases.

DISCUSSION

In recent years, there has been a renewed interest in intraarterial drug delivery in various solid tumors, using modern techniques including implantable catheter systems as well as interventional vascular radiological techniques.

Intraarterial chemotherapy seems a promising strategy in therapy of untreated locally advanced head and neck carcinoma with concurrent radiotherapy due to advantages of high-dose local delivery of drug, minimal procedural complications, low systemic toxicity and high tumor response rate[4].

Cisplatin is the key drug for treating locally head and neck carcinoma, and intravenous injection is the main administration route[5]. However, anti-tumor efficacy is closely related to the drug concentration in the tumor[6]. Intraarterial chemotherapy is an attractive method to achieve a higher drug concentration in the tumor than would be tolerated by the standard intravenous chemotherapy. When cisplatin is used in this manner the perplexing problem of cisplatin resistance may be circumvented by high dose technique. Use of thiosulfate enables the delivery of high intraarterial cisplatin. In covalently binding and neutralizing the relatively low plasma concentration of cisplatin, it reduces cisplatin systemic toxicity without interference with the antitumor activity of the much higher cisplatin concentration within the arterial circulation supplying tumor[7].

Specific indications for the current therapy can not be stated at this point, since we examined a limited number of cases. However, the results of this study seem to be particularly favorable for the symptomatic treatment of patients with inoperable and previously treated head and neck cancer. It helps to reduce tumor pain und bleeding with low treatment morbidity.

CONCLUSION

Selective intraarterial cisplatin therapy can be delivered safely with good efficacy for palliative therapy of locally advanced head and neck cancer untreatable with surgery and radiation therapy.

REFERENCES

1. Klopp CT, Alfort TC, Bateman J. Fractionated intaarterial cancer chemotherapy with methyl bis amine hydrochloride: a preliminary report. Ann Surg 1950; 132: 811-832
2. Fuwa N, Ito Y, Matsumoto A, Kamata M, Kodaira T, Furutani K, Sasaoka M, Kimura Y, Morita K. A combination therapy of continuous superselective intraarterial carboplatin infusion and radiation therapy for locally advanced head and neck carcinoma. Cancer 2000; 89: 2099-2105
3. Regine WF, Valentino J, John W, Storey G, Sloan D, Kenady D, Patel P, Pulmano C, Arnold SM, Mohiuddin M. High-dose intra-arterial cisplatin and concurrent hyperfractionated radiation therapy in patients with locally advanced primary squamous cell carcinoma of the head and neck: report of a phase II study. Head Neck 2000; 22: 543-549
4. Robbins KT, Kumar P, Regine WF, Wong FS, Weir AB, Flick P, Kun LE, Palmer R, Murry T, Fontanesi J, Ferguson R, Thomas R, Hartsell W, Paig CU, Salazar G, Norfleet L, Hanchett CB, Harrington V, Niell HB. Efficacy of targeted supradose cisplatin and concomitant radiation therapy for advanced head and neck cancer: the Memphis experience. Int J Radiat Oncol Biol Phys 1997; 38: 263-271
5. Jacobs C, Lyman G, Velez-Garcia E, Sridhar KS, Knight W, Hochster H, Goodnough LT, Mortimer JE, Einhorn LH, Schacter L. A phase III randomized study comparing cisplatin and fluorouracil as single agents and in combination for advanced squamous cell carcinoma of the head and neck. J Clin Oncol 1992;10:257-263
6. Frei E, Canellos GP. Dose: a critical factor in cancer chemotherapy. Am J Med 1980; 69:585-594
7. Howell SB, Taetle R. Effect of sodium thiosulfate on cis-dichlorodiammineplatinum (II) toxicity and antitumor activity in L1210 leukemia. Cancer Treat Rep 1980; 64:611-616

PARANASAL SINUSES AS A TARGET FOR DISTANT METASTASES

Koscielny, S. Krüger, J.; Bräuer, B., ENT-Department Friedrich-Schiller-University Jena, Germany

SUMMARY

The majority of tumors of the paranasal sinuses are of primary origin. Metastases are very rare. Since there are very few publications on this subject we introduce 4 cases of distant metastases into a paranasal sinus. Three of these were metastases of renal carcinoma, the last case a metastasis of a spindle cell sarcoma.

In all these cases of metastases in paranasal sinuses there was only a palliative treatment possible.

MATERIAL AND METHODS

We investigated the archive of our hospital for all patients which were treated in the university hospital of Jena, Germany for tumors of paranasal sinuses from 1965 until 1998. 142 patients were found in this time period. Most of them had primary tumors of paranasal sinuses. Only four cases were distant metastases. These cases are reviewed. Three patients showed metastases of renal cell carcinoma and one of spindle cell sarcoma.

Renal cell carcinoma[1]

Case 1
- A 73 -year old female presented with a swelling of the left cheek and recurrent epistaxis of the left nose in 1974. The clinical examination showed a tumor mass in the left nose cavity.
- The left maxillary sinus was explored surgically. A bleeding tumor was found and totally excised. Histology revealed a metastasis of a renal cell carcinoma which had been treated surgically six years previously.
- Postoperatively irradiation of left paranasal sinus with 60 Gy was applicated.
- After 5 years a recurrence in left maxillary sinus was observed.
- Further investigation showed haematogenous metastases in the lung, the spine and the pelvis.

• Death occurred from her tumor in the same year.

Case 2
• A 64-year old male with swelling of the right cheek and a displacement of the right eye was seen in 1989. A large tumor was found in the right nose cavity. The CT-Scan showed a bone-destructing tumor in right maxillary sinus.
• Biopsy was obtained through operative exploration. The pathologist found a metastasis of a formerly diagnosed renal cell carcinoma (1984).
• Surgical removal of the tumor was not possible.
• A palliative irradiation of the tumor was done to 45 Gy with partial remission.
• Two years later a occlusion of the right external carotid artery was necessary after recurrent bleeding.
• The patient died after an episode of bleeding in 1994.

Case 3
• 60-year old male presented with a paresis of the abducens nerve as a first symptom.
• The CT-scans showed a bone destructing process in the sphenoid bone with infiltration of the sinus cavernosus.
• In further investigations a tumor of the right kidney was found as possible primary lesion of this process in the sphenoid bone. The histologically investigation of resection specimen after nephrektomie determined this as renal cell carcinoma. The right kidney was resected. The tumor was classified as renal cell carcinoma.
• An endonasal biopsy was taken causing heavy bleeding. The biopsy was found to be a metastasis of the renal cell carcinoma.
• An irradiation with 45 Gy could reached no remission of the tumor.
• A bone scintigram after 3 months showed a progression of the tumor in spine and extremities.
• The patient died 18 months after diagnosis.

Spindle cell sarcoma[2]

• 1994 removement of a spindle cell sarcoma from abdominal wall was done with combined radiation and chemotherapy postoperatively.
• December 1995 a paresis of the right abducens nerve was observed.
• The MRI showed a tumor of sphenoid bone with infiltration of sinus cavernosus (pic. 1), but the in the CT was no bone destruction to see.
• In endonasal surgical exploration a metastasis of spindle cell sarcoma was found.
• A new cycle of chemotherapy was administrated.
• The death was 4 months later because of intracerebral progression.

CONCLUSIONS

Most tumors of paranasal sinuses are primary tumors of this region. Metastases are very rare. In our group were 4 patients with metastases in the paranasal sinuses between 142 tumors in these region. Most of this metastases were from renal cell carcinoma because of the typical histological features of this tumors[4, 5]. The last patient developed a rare metastasis of spindle cell sarcoma in the paranasal sinuses[6, 7].

456

In all cases only palliative treatment was possible.

In diagnosis the combination of CT- and MRI-Scans gave most accurate information about the extension of the tumor and the infiltration to the sinus cavernosus[8].

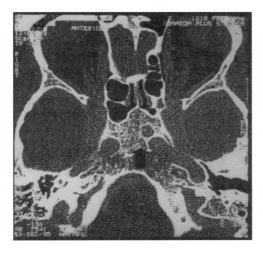 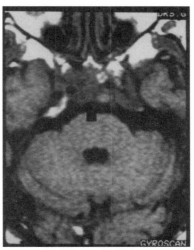

Figure 1. CT-Scan of metastases of spindles cell sarcoma (case 4) in sphenoid bone. No tumor or bone-destructing was detectable.

Figure 2. MRI-Scan of metastases of spindles cell sarcoma (case 4) in sphenoid bone tumor suspectable tissue in sphenoid bone (arrow).

REFERENCES

1. Koscielny S. Die Nasennebenhöhlen als Metastasierungsort des Nierenzellkarzinoms.Laryngo Rhino Otol 1999; 78: 441-445
2. Koscielny S, Gudziol H. Abduzensparese als Erstsymptom maligner Tumoren des Keilbeinkörpers. HNO-aktuell 2000; 8: 5-9
3. Matsumoto Y, Yanahihara N. Renal clear carcinoma metastic to the nose and paranasal sinusses. Laryngoscope 1992;92:1190-1193
4. Menauer F, Issing, WJ. Ungewöhnliche Metastasierung eines Nierenzellkarzinoms Laryngo Rhino Otol 1998;77:525-527
5. Mickel, RA, Zimmermann MC. The sphenoid sinus - a site for metastasis. Otolaryngol Head Neck Surg 1990;102:709-716
6. Miloro M, Quinn PD, Stewart JC. Monophasic spindle cell sarcoma of the Head and Neck: report of two cases and review of the literature. J Oral Maxillofac Surg. 1994;52:309-313
7. Singer S, Baldini EH, Demetri GD, Fletscher JA, Corson JM. Synovial sarcoma: prognostic significance of tumor size, margin of resection and mitotic activity for survival. J Clin Oncol 1996;14: 201-1208
8. Takahashi S, Higano S, Ishii K, Matsumoto K, Shimanuki Y, Ishibashi T, Zuguchi M, Maruoka S, Kayama T, Sakamoto K. CT and MR imaging findings of sphenoidal masses. Nippon Igaku-Hoshasen Gakkai Zasshi 1994;54:751-756

IMPROVED CHEMOSENSITIVITY-PROFILING OF HNSCC: PRELIMINARY RESULTS

Dollner, R.[1], Granzow, C.[2], Dietz, A.[1]
[1]Dept. Otorhinolaryngology, Head and Neck Surgery, University of Heidelberg
[2]German Cancer Research Center, Heidelberg, Germany

INTRODUCTION

To quantify the chemoreactivity of head and neck squamous cell carcinoma (HNSCC) many *in vitro* assays exist[1, 2]. Their general poor reproducibility and reliability could be recently linked to destructive photochemical effects[3, 4], mediated by riboflavin (vitamin B_2), an obligatory component in culture media for mammalian cell cultivation. Since riboflavin acts as a strong photosensitizer, riboflavin-mediated photoreactions are causing cytotoxicity[5], genotoxicity[6] and distort chemosensitivity tests by photodegradation of cytostatic drugs[3]. Elimination of these adverse effects by introducing flavin-protecting conditions[3, 4, 7], led to the development of a miniaturized, colony formation-based *ex vivo* test to quantitate the cytostatic drug response of bronchoscopic lung tumor explants[8]. We adapted this test by including drugs relevant for clinical HNSCC chemotherapy to profile the chemoreactivity of HNSCC specimens.

In the study presented here, we quantitated furthermore the chemoreactivity of i) tumor-free mucosa, ii) primary carcinoma and iii) lymph node metastases simultaneously. This extension of the original protocol[8] has been conducted to characterize the individual disease as a whole.

MATERIALS AND METHODS

Colony formation-based tests were done with eleven surgically removed specimens from five individuals according to the test system approved for lung cancer specimens[8]. In detail, the test setup is characterized as follows:

Flavin-protecting culture methods - Flavin-protecting culture methods were used throughout all experimental steps. For KB-cells as well as for *ex vivo* explants, RPMI 1640 medium w/o riboflavin (Biochrom, Berlin, Germany) was used to protect cells and drugs from photodynamic damage. Media were supplemented with 10 % (v/v) fetal bovine serum

(Integro, Zaandam, Holland). All steps were performed under illumination exclusively with sodium-discharge lamps (SOX), emitting monochromatically at λ = 589 nm (Philips, Marburg, Germany). Since this wavelength cannot excite riboflavin, adverse photoreactions were excluded.

Drugs and test calibration - Cytostatic gradients were calibrated with the 50 percent growth inhibitory concentrations (IC_{50}) for KB-cells: Carboplatin (CP; $IC_{50}=2\mu M$), Cisplatin (Cis; $IC_{50}=200nM$), 5-Fluoruracil (5-FU; $IC_{50}=1,2\mu M$), Mitomycin C (MMC; $IC_{50}=8nM$), Gemcitabine (Gem; $IC_{50}=8,4$ nM), and Docetaxel (DTX; $IC_{50}=280$ pM). Except for drug-free controls, samples were exposed to concentration gradients comprising the 1-, 2-, 4-, 16-, 64- and 256-fold of the respective IC_{50} for each cytostatic drug.

Specimens and chemoreactivity testing - After obtaining local ethics committee approval, specimens were taken from five individuals who gave informed consent (four glottic laryngeal carcinomas, one nasopharyngeal carcinoma; for TNM-stages, see results). Biopsies were obtained from the primary tumors (n=5), tumor-free mucosas (n=4) and from cervical lymph node metastases (n=2) during surgery. The mean wet weight of the harvested specimens was 87,9 mg for the primary tumors (range: 62,3-145 mg), 103,6 mg for tumor-free mucosas (range: 73-123 mg), and 112 and 84 mg for the specimens from cervical lymph node metastases. The biopsies were kept in ice cold medium for max. 6 hours. Following mechanical and enzymatic dissection (collagenase type IV, Sigma, München, Germany), 300 µl aliquots/well of the resulting cell suspension (RPMI 1640 medium w/o riboflavin, 10 % fetal bovine serum, nystatin, gentamycin, G-penicillin, streptomycin) were transferred to 96-well plates coated with extracellular matrix (Pesasel & Lorey, Hanau, Germany). After addition of the cytostatic drugs, plates were incubated for 3 days at 36,5 °C (humidified air, 5% CO_2). Following incubation, test samples were washed twice (PBS) and fixed with methanol for Giemsa-staining and microscopical examination.

Control experiments with KB-cells - Our test protocol could not provide repetitive measurements on a given clinical specimen. Therefore, we performed obligatory parallel standard cytotoxicity tests on KB-cells with the drug solutions and media used previously for testing the biopsies. The KB cell experiments served as internal standards to verify the photochemical and pharmacological integrity of all procedures. The results of all control experiments revealed adequate test conditions (data not shown).

Test evaluation - Following Giemsa-staining, test plates were examined microscopically. Only those tests were considered, where all control wells showed clear epithelial colony-formation. Each test plate (96-wells) included at least 18 control wells. All tests performed with the biopsies from patients with laryngeal carcinoma (n=10) showed sufficient formation of epithelial colonies in the control wells. Samples harvested from the nasopharyngeal carcinoma failed to produce satisfactory growth of control specimens. Therefore, this specimen was excluded from further analysis. Following the concentration gradient for each single drug, all wells were examined for epithelial colony formation. Specimens were considered to respond to a given drug at the highest concentration, where epithelial colony formation could be detected microscopically.

460

RESULTS

With the exception of one preirradiated specimen (nasopharyngeal carcinoma), all explants (10/11) produced epithelial cell colonies within three days. Compared to KB-cells, the chemosensitivity profiles of the clinical specimens showed generally a reduced chemoreactivity, although selective sensitivities could be seen. Individual chemoreactivity varied strongly. The results are summarized in table 1.

Table 1. Chemoreactivity profiles of tumor-free laryngeal mucosa and of primary and metastatic laryngeal carcinomas

Specimen #	Tumor	TNM-Stage	Biopsy site*	Highest drug concentration** where epithelial colony formation was detected					
				5-FU	CP	CIS	MMC	GEM	DTX
#1	Larynx	T3N0M0	Mucosa	16	16	256	256	256	256
			Primary tumor	64	256	256	64	64	256
#2	Larynx	T3N2bM0	Mucosa	256	16	64	256	256	256
			Primary tumor	64	16	64	256	256	16
#3	Larynx	T4N1M0	Mucosa	256	256	16	256	256	256
			Primary tumor	64	256	256	256	256	256
			Lymph node metastases	256	256	256	256	256	256
#4	Larynx	T4N2cM0	Mucosa	256	16	16	256	256	256
			Primary tumor	64	256	256	256	256	256
			Lymph node metastases	256	16	256	256	256	256

* M = Mucosa; T = Primary tumor; N = Lymph node metastasis
** Drug concentrations tested: 1-, 2-, 4-, 16-, 64- and 256-fold of the respective IC_{50} for wild type KB-cells

If one focuses on the chemoreactivity profiles of tumor-free laryngeal mucosa specimens, sensitivity to carboplatin and/or cisplatin can be seen in every preparation. This sensitivity is lost in the corresponding tumor-preparations except for specimen #2, where the sensitivity for CP persists. Interestingly, this CP-sensitivity is accompanied by an additional sensitivity to docetaxel, which had not been detected in the test of the respective tumor-free mucosa.

The lymph node metastasis of #3, exhibited no selective sensitivity, reflecting a phenotype resistant to the drugs tested as it has been found for the respective primary carcinoma. For the lymph node metastasis of specimen #4, a selective sensitivity to CP occurred or recurred, since identical sensitivity could be detected in the respective mucosa preparation but not in the primary carcinoma.

DISCUSSION & CONCLUSIONS

Since riboflavin-mediated photoreactions have precluded reliable *in vitro* chemoreactivity testing so far, we eliminated such reactions from the test system by establishing "flavin-protecting" conditions[2,4,7]. This enabled, for the first time, an *ex vivo* protocol to characterize the chemoreactivity of HNSCC without photooxidative stress.

Using the protocol reported here, explantation of cancerous and tumor-free laryngeal epithelium resulted in prolific colony formation sufficient to perform multiple chemoreactivity tests simultanously. The tests included up to twelve different single cytostatic drugs, or combinations of them, and provided quantitative detection of the respective sensitivity of the tested specimen. Validated by using KB cells as internal standard, our protocol provides reliable quantitation of the individual drug response. In a first attempt, we tested six different cytostatic drugs per specimen. Our results include tests not only from the primary carcinoma, but also from tumor-free mucosa and –in two cases – from lymph node metastases of the respective tumors. The sensitivity patterns from different sites of one patient differed slightly but remarkably and can provide a impression of the chemoreactivity profile of the individual disease as a whole.

The number of specimens tested so far is too low for discussing the clinical and therapeutical implications. Therefore, further tests are needed. However, the following methodical improvements of our protocol could be clearly demonstrated: i) prolific epithelial colony formation (10/11 specimens) and therefore a high feasibility of the test, ii) consistent concentration-dependency of suppressing colony formation for each single cytostatic drug, iii) improved reliability of the protocol validated by obligatory KB control experiments.

As exemplified by the first tests reported here, variations of drug response of HNSCC specimens can be reliably identified by the described *ex vivo* test protocol.

REFERENCES

1. Hoffman RM. In vitro sensitivity assays in Cancer: a review, analysis and prognosis. J Clin Lab Analysis 1991; 5: 133-143
2. Cortazar P, Johnson BE. Review of the efficacy of individualized chemotherapy selected by in vitro drug sensitivity testing in patients with cancer. J Clin Oncol 1999; 17: 1625-1631
3. Granzow C, Kopun M, Kröber T. Riboflavin-mediated photosensitization of vinca alkaloids distorts drug sensitivity assays. Cancer Res 1995; 55: 4837-4843
4. Dollner R, Kopun M, Granzow C. Riboflavin-mediated photoreactions: an unnecessary hazard in mammalian cell cultivation. Eur. J. Cell. Biol. 1995; Abstract no. 55, ECBO-Meeting.
5. Warburg O, Geissler AW, Lorenz S. Wirkung von Riboflavin und Luminoflavin auf wachsende Krebszellen. Z klin. Chem. u. Biochem. 1968; 6: 467-468.
6. Yamamoto F, Nishimura S, Kasai H. Photosensitized formation of 8-hydroxydeoxyguanosine in cellular DNA by riboflavin. Biochem. Biophys. Res. Commun. 1992; 187: 809-813.
7. Granzow C, Kopun-Granzow M, Dollner R, Gros G, Heft I. Riboflavin- und flavinnucleotidfreie Kulturmedien für tierische und menschliche Zellen. German patent no.: 195 12 506, 1996.
8. Granzow C, Becker H, Heuser M, Kopun M. Chemosensitivity profiles of bronchoscopic tumor biopsies. Proc. Amer. Assn. Cancer Res. 1999; 40: Abstract no.1257.

PROGNOSTIC VALUE OF P53 MUTATIONS AND TELOMERASE ACTIVITY IN COMBINED SURGICAL AND RADIATION THERAPY OF CARCINOMAS OF THE PHARYNX AND ORAL CAVITY

Christiane Motsch[1], Regine Schneider-Stock[2], Reinhard Stöcking[1], Albert Roessner[2], Bernd Freigang[1]

[1]Department of E.N.T. Otto-von-Guericke University Magdeburg, Germany, Chairman: Prof. Dr. B. Freigang

[2]Department of Pathology, Chairman: Prof. Dr. A. Roessner

Running title: p53 mutations and telomerase activity in carcinomas of pharynx and oral cavity

Key words: head and neck cancer, pharynx, oral cavity, telomerase activity, p53 mutations

Correspondence to: *Dr. med. Christiane Motsch, Otto-von-Guericke University Magdeburg, Department of E.N.T., Leipziger Straße 44, 39120 Magdeburg, Germany, Phone: 49/391 - 6 71 38 02, Fax: 49/391 - 6 71 38 06*

ABSTRACT

Background. The prognostic significance of p53 mutations and re-activation of telomerase in squamous cell carcinomas has recently been recognized. In this study, we investigated progressive squamous cell carcinomas of the pharynx and the oral cavity for the frequency of both molecular parameters.

Methods. Fresh tumor tissues from 32 cases of squamous cell carcinomas of the pharynx and the oral cavity were investigated. All patients underwent radical surgery with curative intent at the E.N.T.-Clinic, University Magdeburg, Germany, in 1999 and 2000, followed by irradiation. Telomerase activity was determined by using the non-radioactive PCR-based TRAP-assay (ONCOR). Mutations in exons 4 to 8 of the p53 gene were determined using PCR-SSCR-Sequencing analysis.

Results. Telomerase activity was detected in all tumors. We found p53 mutations in 28 % (n=9) of all telomerase positive tumors.

Conclusions. Telomerase activity seems to be a molecular marker for high risk tumors, whereas the specific role of p53 mutations in this scenario still needs to be verified.

INTRODUCTION

Large tumors of the oral cavity and pharynx often require radical and plastic reconstructive surgery to obtain adequate oncological and functional results. Nevertheless, the prognosis of squamous cell carcinomas of the oral cavity, pharynx and larynx at advanced stages of disease is poor, with a 5-year survival rate in approximately 30% to 50 % of the cases.

Although the clinical outcome is influenced by the stage and histopathological grade of the disease at presentation, the TNM system (UICC 1997) and other conventional histo-pathological grading systems (Broders, 1920) are only poor prognostic indicators. Therefore, it is important to recognize those patients who run a high risk of developing metastatic lesions and who will consequently have a poor prognosis.

MATERIALS

The study group consisted of 32 patients (29 males, 3 females, aged 35 - 81 years, median 57,6 years) with histologically confirmed diagnoses of primary squamous cell carcinoma of the pharynx (n=24) and oral cavity (n=8), (Table 1). All the patients underwent radical surgery with curative intent at the Department of E.N.T., University Magdeburg, Germany, in 1999 and 2000, followed by irradiation. In all the cases, we used the radial forearm flap in the reconstructions of the oral cavity and pharynx after the squamous cell carcinomas had been resected. Six patients had stage II disease, three had stage III disease, and 23 had stage IV disease. None of the patients had developed distant metastases at the time of surgery, and no antitumor therapy had been given previously. Five patients died of recurrence during the follow-up period (between 6 and 18 months).

After informed consent had been given, tissue blocks were taken at the time of radical resection of the primary tumor combined with a unilateral or bilateral neck dissection. Tumor tissues were immediately frozen in liquid nitrogen and stored until preparation at -80° C.

METHODS

Telomerase activity was determined by using the non-radioactive PCR-based TRAP-assay (ONCOR). The PCR-products were analyzed on an automated fluorescence sequencer (ALF-Express)[1].
Mutations in exons 4 to 8 of the p53 gene were determined using PCR-SSCP-sequencing analysis[2].

RESULTS

Telomerase activity was detected in all tumors (low activity n=3, high activity n=29, Figure 1).

We found p53 mutations in 28% (n=9) of all telomerase-positive tumors (Table 2, Figures 2-3). Three mutations were missense mutations leading to an exchange of amino acids in the p53 protein (tumors 4, 5, and 8). Three mutations were frameshift mutations caused by deletions or insertions of short DNA sequences (tumors 1, 2, and 7). Three mutations were localized in the intron regions near the splice origins possibly affecting splicing of the p53 mRNA (tumors 3, 6, and 9).

Relationships between T-stage, N-stage, grading, recurrence of tumor, and p53-mutation were not found. Patients with p53 mutation in the tumor tissue were approximately 8 years younger (median age) than patients without p53 mutations.

DISCUSSIONS

Carcinogenesis of the upper aerodigestive tract epithelium is a complex, multi-step process. Telomerase and the tumor suppressor protein p53 are frequently associated with human cancers, and activation of telomerase and inactivation of p53 are involved in cancer cell immortalization[2]. Mutation of the tumor suppressor gene p53 is the most frequent genetic alteration occurring in human tumors. Head and neck carcinomas have also been reported to show a high incidence of p53 alterations both genetically and immunohistochemically, in a range of 26 % to 69 % for mutations and 40 % to 67 % for protein accumulation, with a high concordance rate between the sensitivity of the methods[4].

Telomeres, the ends of chromosomes, consisting of thousands of copies of telomere specific repeats (TT AGGG), are affected by progressive erosion because of the so-called „end-replication problem„. The primary function of telomerase is the synthesis of telomeric DNA, which is the main pathway maintaing telomere length in the human germline and stem cells. Activiation of telomerase is associated with elongation of telomerase and cell immortalization. Telomerase activity has recently been detected in many human cancer tissues[5-7]. However, the fact that it has not been found in the vast majority of normal tissues suggests that telomere stabilization and telomerase activiation play a role in tumorigenesis[8].

Mutirangura et al[9]. detected telomerase activity not only in almost all squamous cell carcinomas of the head and neck (14/16 = 87.5%), but also in 38.5% of premalignant lesions (10/26), such as oral leukoplakias. In leukoplakia, positive activities were more frequently associated with dysplasia (83.3%) rather than with hyperplasia (27.3%). This result may indicate that telomerase is primarily expressed in advanced squamous cell carcinogenesis of the head and neck before a cancer phenotype is fully developed.

We are the first to report telomerase activity in a larger and homogeneous group of advanced tumors of the upper aerodigestive tract. This study revealed a 100 % telomerase positivity in carcinomas of the pharynx and oral cavity, thus confirming the results of Thurnher et al.[10], investigating 16 cases of head and neck squamous cell carcinomas. This is in accordance with the observation of very large tumors showing a very aggressive behavior.

Since the accumulation of genetic alterations in tumor cells, especially in cell cycle regulator genes p53 and Rb, leads to higher proliferation rates, tumor cells reach a critical telomeric length at earlier stages. Enzyme telomerase permits the *de novo* synthesis of telomeric DNA onto chromosomal ends, thus preventing them from senescence or apoptotic death. Our data are in line with this M1/M2 model of cellular senescence and immortalization, according to which telomerase activity is associated with the inactivation of the tumor suppressor gene p53.

Telomerase activity seems to be a molecular marker for high risk tumors, whereas the specific role of p53 mutations in this scenario still needs to be verified.

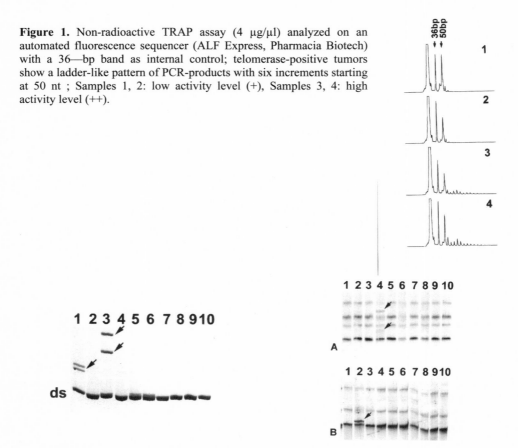

Figure 1. Non-radioactive TRAP assay (4 µg/µl) analyzed on an automated fluorescence sequencer (ALF Express, Pharmacia Biotech) with a 36—bp band as internal control; telomerase-positive tumors show a ladder-like pattern of PCR-products with six increments starting at 50 nt ; Samples 1, 2: low activity level (+), Samples 3, 4: high activity level (++).

Figure 2. PCR control for exon 4 of the p53 gene; arrows mark the heteroduplex structures caused by a deletion (in tumor 2, lane 1) or an insertion (in tumor 3, lane 3). ds: double-stranded exon 4 PCR-product.

Figure 3. SSCP analysis of the p53 gene; abnormal migrated bands are marked by an arrow (A: exon 5 (tumor 4, Table 2); B: exon 7 tumor 9, Table 2).

466

Table 1. Summary of clinicopathology data in progressive squamous cell carcinomas of pharynx and oral cavity

	tumur tissue with p53 mutation n=9	tumor tissue without p53 mutation n=23
<u>age</u> (in years)	52	60
histopathological grading		
G1	0	1
G2	6	14
G3	3	8
staging		
II	0	3
III	3	3
IV	6	17
nodal status		
negative	3	7
positive	6	16

Table 2. Summary of p53 mutations in progressive squamous cell carcinomas of pharynx and oral cavity

Tumor No	Localization	Exon/Codon	Mutation	Aminoacid exchange
1	oropharynx	4	5bp-insertion	frameshift
2	oropharynx	4/75	deletion	frameshift
3	oropharynx	intron 4, 7bp upstream of exon 5 splice origin	insertion A	splicing?
4	hypopharynx	5/175	CGC → CAC	Arg to His
5	hypopharynx	5/168	CAC → CCC	His to Pro
6	oropharynx	intron 5	C → T	?
7	oropharynx	5/177	4bp-deletion	frameshift
8	oral cavity	5/179	CAT → AAT	His to AsN
9	oral cavity	intron 7, 11bp downstream of exon 7 splice origin	A → T	splicing?

REFERENCES

1. Schneider-Stock R, Epplen JT, Walter H et al. Telomeric lengths and telomerase activity in liposarcomas. Mol Carcinog 1999; 24:144-151.
2. Schneider-Stock R, Walter H, Radig K et al. Mdm2 amplification and loss of heterozygosity at Rb and p53 genes: no simultaneous alterations in the oncogenesis of liposarcomas. J Cance Res Clin Oncol 1998; 124:532-540.
3. Li H, Cao Y, Berndt MC, Funder JW, Lin J-P. Molecular interactions between telomerase and the tumor suppressor protein p53 in vitro. Oncogene 1999; 18:6785-6794.
4. Piffko J, Bankfaloi A, Tory K et al. Molecular assessment of p53 abnormalities at the invasive front of oral squamous all carcinomas. Head and Neck 1998; 20:8-15.
5. Mao L, El-Naggar AK, Fan Y-H et al. Telomerase Activity in Head and Neck Squamous Cell Carcinoma and Adjacent Tissues. Cancer Research 1996; 56:5600-5604.
6. Shay JW, Bacchetti S. A survey of telomerase activity in human cancer. Eur J Cancer 1997; 33:787-791.

7. Califano J, Ahrendt SA, Meininger G et al. Detection of Telomerase Activity in Oral Rinses from Head and Neck Squamous Cell Carcinoma Patients. Cancer Research 1996; 56:5720-5722.
8. Meyerson M, Role of telomerase in normal and cancer cells. J Clin Oncol 2000; 18:2626-2634.
9. Mutirangura A, Supiyaphun P, Trirekapan S et al. Telomerase Activity in Oral Leukoplakia and Head and Neck Squamous Cell Carcinoma. Cancer Research 1996; 56:3530-3533.
10. Thurnher D, Knerer B, Formanek M, Kornfehe J. Non-radioactive semiquantitative Testing for Expression Levels of Telomerase Activity in Head and Neck Squamous Cell Carcinomas may be Indicative for Biological Tumour Behaviour. Acta Otolaryngol (Stockh) 1998; 118:423-427.

CYFRA 21-1 AS MARKER FOR DISTANT METASTASES IN HEAD AND NECK CANCER: POSSIBILITIES AND LIMITATIONS

Christiane Kuropkat, M.D.[1], Burkhard M. Lippert, M.D.[1], Harald Renz, M.D.[2], Anna M. Niemann M.D.[1], Jochen A. Werner, M.D.[1]

[1]Department of Otorhinolaryngology, Head and Neck Surgery, Philipps-University of Marburg, Germany

[2]Department of Clinical Chemistry and Molecular Diagnostics, Philipps-University of Marburg, Germany

Running title: Cyfra 21-1 in metastases of head and neck cancer

Key-words: Cyfra 21-1, tumor marker, squamous cell carcinoma, head and neck, metastases

Correspondence to: Christiane Kuropkat, MD, Department of Otorhinolaryngology, Philipps-University of Marburg, Deutschhausstr. 3, D-35037 Marburg, Germany, Phone: ++49-6421-2862850, Fax: ++49-6421-2866367

ABSTRACT

Background. Cyfra 21-1 is a widely accepted tumor marker in non-small-cell lung cancer, whereas in squamous cell carcinoma of the head and neck (SCCHN) it could not been established as routine marker, yet, probably due to the difficulties of finding the appropriate cut-off level.

Method. In this study we investigated retrospectively whether the serum Cyfra 21-1 levels were correlating with the clinical course in 23 patients with SCCHN and proven distant metastases, without determination of a certain cut-off level, by using the antibodies KS 19-1 and BM 19-21 for cytokeratin 19 fragment detection.

Results. There was a wide range of Cyfra 21-1 serum levels at point of primary diagnosis, without correlation with tumor size, lymph node status or time to occurrence of distant metastases. All except one patient did show a clear increase of Cyfra 21-1 when distant metastases were present (1.4 fold to 28.3 fold increase) and in case of local or neck recurrence.

Conclusions. Cyfra 21-1 is neither a suitable screening marker for primary SCCHN, nor for initial detection of distant metastases, but a reliable marker for clinical follow-up and especially detection of distant metastases.

INTRODUCTION

Many efforts have been made so far to find appropriate tumor markers with prognostic significance for clinical follow-up, estimation of prognosis and therapeutic planning in patients with malignant tumors. For patients with squamous cell carcinoma of the head and neck (SCCHN) the most investigated tumor markers are SCC-AG and CEA, but no reliable tumor marker could be established so far for these malignancies[1]. The overall survival for patients with SCCHN did not improve significantly during the last decades and the therapeutic options are often limited. Therefore it is very much desirable to find markers for early detection of disease progression and especially of development of distant metastases. This could e.g. prevent patients from aggressive surgery or radiochemotherapy which often means severe restrictions in their quality of life.

Cyfra 21-1 (cytokeratin fraction 21-1) is a serum-soluble fragment of cytokeratin 19. Cytokeratins are a family of intermediate filament proteins which are part of the cytoplasmic cytoskeleton. They are specific for epithelia and expressed in certain combinations depending on the type of epithelium and degree of differentiation. Cytokeratin 19 is restricted to simple epithelia[2].

Cyfra 21-1 has been used frequently as tumor marker in patients with non-small-cell lung cancer for many years[3]. Elevated serum levels of Cyfra 21-1 have been associated with advanced tumor stage, lymph node metastases and poor prognosis in these patients. For these tumors a cut-off level of 3.3 to 3.6 ng/ml has been established for threshold determination between normal and pathological serum levels. Literature shows that for patients with SCCHN it seems to be difficult to find the appropriate threshold for serum levels of Cyfra 21-1[4]. The serum levels are generally lower than in lung cancer and they often seem to be equivalent to serum levels which are considered to be normal in patients with lung cancer. Therefore Cyfra 21-1 could not been established as a predictive routine tumor marker in SCCHN, yet, despite promising data have been published so far, which show a good potential of Cyfra 21-1 as tumor marker in the follow-up of patients with SCCHN[4-7].

In this study we analysed retrospectively the development of Cyfra 21-1 levels from the point of diagnosis to the first appearance of distant metastases in patients with SCCHN. We investigated whether the serum Cyfra 21-1 levels were correlating with the clinical course of disease for the individual patient without determining a cut-off value for pathological serum levels.

MATERIAL AND METHODS

After informed consent was received, venous blood from patients with histologically proven SCCHN was drawn during routine clinical follow-up. The determination of Cyfra 21-1 serum levels was performed at the Department of Clinical Chemistry and Molecular Diagnostics,

University of Marburg, Germany. The Cyfra 21-1 levels were measured in the serum of the samples by using the EIA Enzymun test kit and the analyzing system ES 300 provided by Boehringer Mannheim, Germany. The cytokeratin 19 fragments were detected by the monoclonal antibodies KS 19-1 and BM 19-21. The antibodies are specific for two different epitopes of cytokeratin 19[3]. Between 1998 and 2000 forty-five patients with clinically proven distant metastases could be identified. Twenty-three of these patients had Cyfra 21-1 serum levels determined regularly. For these patients the development of Cyfra 21-1 serum levels were evaluated retrospectively and compared to the clinical course.

RESULTS

The primary squamous cell carcinomas (SCC) were located at following sites: oropharynx (n = 9), hypopharynx (n = 9), larynx (n = 3), meatus acusticus (n = 1), parotid gland (n = 1). Table 1 demonstrates the tumor size and lymph node status of the disease at the point of primary diagnosis. At this point distant metastases were already present in five patients. The organ manifestation of the metastatic spread was distributed as follows: lung (n = 8), liver (n = 1), bones (n = 1), brain (n = 1), axillary lymph nodes plus neck lymph nodes (n = 1), lung plus local recurrence / neck lymph nodes (n= 4), lung and liver (n = 3), lung and skin (n = 2), lung and bones (n = 2).

Our data show a wide range of Cyfra 21-1 serum levels at point of diagnosis from 0.2 to 55.0 ng/ml, with a mean of 4.98 ($\pm$ 11.55) ng/ml and a median of 1.4 ng/ml. If patients with distant metastases at point of diagnosis were not considered in the analysis the range of Cyfra 21-1 serum levels was from 0.2 to 5.4 ng/ml with a mean of 1.7 ($\pm$1.44) ng/ml and a median of 1.3 ng/ml. Neither a correlation between Cyfra 21-1 serum levels and T-status (r = 0.19), nor between Cyfra 21-1 levels and N-status (r = 0.3) of the primary tumor could be found. There was no correlation between Cyfra 21-1 level and time to occurrence of distant metastases. A decrease of Cyfra 21-1 levels after surgery or during combined radio- and chemotherapy could be observed in 14 patients (60.9%). In these patients the average decrease of Cyfra 21-1 serum levels ranged from 11.2% to 86% with a mean of 50.2% ($\pm$21.4) and a median of 51.5%. The Cyfra levels at the point of presence of distant metastases ranged from 0.42 ng/ml to 55 ng/ml, with a mean of 7.15 ($\pm$ 11.6) ng/ml and a median of 3.5 ng/ml. Excluding the patients with distant metastases at time of diagnosis the Cyfra 21-1 levels ranged from 0,42 ng/ml to 19.8 ng/ml with a mean of 4.5 (+4.67) ng/ml and a median of 3.05. The increase of the Cyfra 21-1 serum levels at the point of distant metastases compared to the Cyfra level after end of therapy, or, if Cyfra level did not decrease during therapy, compared to the Cyfra 21-1 level at the point of diagnosis ranged from a 1.4-fold increase as a minimum to 28.3-fold increase as a maximum. Only one patient had no increase of Cyfra 21-1 after detection of distant metastases up to this point. The mean was a 6.5-fold increase ($\pm$ 6.9) of the Cyfra 21-1 serum level at the presence of distant metastases, the median was a 3.3-fold increase. Additionally, an increase of Cyfra 21-1 could be observed in case of local recurrence (data not shown). Figure 1 and 2 are demonstrating examples of the development of the Cyfra 21-1 serum level in the individual patient during the clinical course.

DISCUSSION

Our data suggest that Cyfra 21-1 does not seem to be a suitable prognostic marker at the point of primary diagnosis, since there was a wide range of Cyfra 21-1 serum levels at the point of primary diagnosis and all of these patients developed distant metastases. Additionally, we could observe that patients with benign as well as malignant diseases of the salivary glands had comparatively high Cyfra 21-1 levels (data not shown). There was no correlation with tumor size or lymph node status, nor with time to occurrence of distant metastases, although in three of the five patients where distant metastases were already present at time of diagnosis the Cyfra 21-1 serum levels were extraordinary high. The lack of correlation with tumor size and lymph node status might be due to the small number of patients investigated, especially because this correlation could be demonstrated in previous publications[6,7]. Since distant metastases are not very frequent in SCCHN, we could only investigate a limited number of patients and therefore the options of statistical analysis were limited. But looking at the individual patient, all except one did show a clear increase of the Cyfra 21-1 serum level at the point of distant metastases compared to the level at primary diagnosis. Therefore Cyfra 21-1 is of prognostic value in the individual patient what clinical course is concerned, if not a certain cut-off level is determined but the individual development of the Cyfra 21-1 serum level is observed. The majority of patients had a decrease of Cyfra 21-1 serum levels after surgery and especially after combined radiochemotherapy and an increase in case of local recurrence, neck recurrence and/or distant metastases. In Conclusion, Cyfra 21-1 is neither a suitable screening marker for primary head and neck tumors, nor for initial detection of metastases in these patients. But our results encourage the observation that the development of Cyfra 21-1 serum levels in the individual patient is of good prognostic potential in the clinical follow-up to predict disease progression. Maass et al.[8] already demonstrated the potential of Cyfra 21-1 as a serological marker in the follow-up of patients with SCCHN. They recommended the performance of staging procedures if the threshold of 3.3 ng/ml is exceeded, since this is the accepted threshold for lung cancer and lung metastases are the most frequent ones in head and neck cancer. In contrast, we recommend the performance of staging procedures if the Cyfra 21-1 serum level is clearly increasing in the individual patient without determination of a cut-off level.

Table 1
Distribution of tumor size and lymph node status at point of primary diagnosis according to

	T_1	T_2	T_3	T_4
N_0	1	2	2	1
N_1	0	1	1	0
N_2	2	5	3	4
N_3	0	0	0	1

the TNM-classification (UICC, 1997) in 23 patient with squamous cell carcinoma of the head

REFERENCES

1. Goumas PD, Mastronikolis NS, Mastorakou AN, Vassilakos PJ, Nikiforidis GC. Evaluation of TATI and Cyfra 21-1 in patients with head and neck squamous cell carcinoma. ORL J Otolaryngol Relat Spec 1997;59(2):106-114.
2. Osborn M, Weber K. Intermediate filaments: Cell-type-specific markers in differentiation and pathology. Cell 1982;31:303-306.
3. Pujol JL, Grenier J, Daures JP, Pujol H, Michel FB. Serum fragment of cytoceratin subunit 19 measured by CYFRA 21-1 immunoradiometric assay as a marker of lung cancer. Cancer Res 1993;53:61-66.
4. Niemann AM, Görögh T, Gottschlich S, Lippert BM, Werner JA. Cuf-off value determination of CYFRA 21-1 for squamous cell carcinomas of the head and neck (SCCHN). Anticancer Res 1997;17:2859-2860.
5. Bongers V, Braakhuis BJM, Snow GB. Circulating fragments of cytokeratin 19 in patients with head and neck squamous cell carcinoma. Clin Otolaryngol 1995;20:479-482.
6. Doweck I, Barak M, Greenberg E, et al. Cyfra 21-1. A new potential tumor marker for squamous cell carcinoma of head and neck. Arch Otolaryngol Head Neck Surg 1995;121:177-181.
7. Niemann AM, Paulsen JI, Lippert BM, et al. Cyfra 21-1 in patients with head and neck cancer. In: Werner JA, Lippert BM, Rudert HH, editors. Head and neck cancer: Advances in basic research. Amsterdam: Elsevier; 1996. p 529-537.
8. Maass JD, Hoffmann-Fazel A, Görögh T, et al. Cyfra 21-1: a serological help for detection of distant metastases in head and neck cancer. Anticancer Res 2000;20(3B):2241-2243.

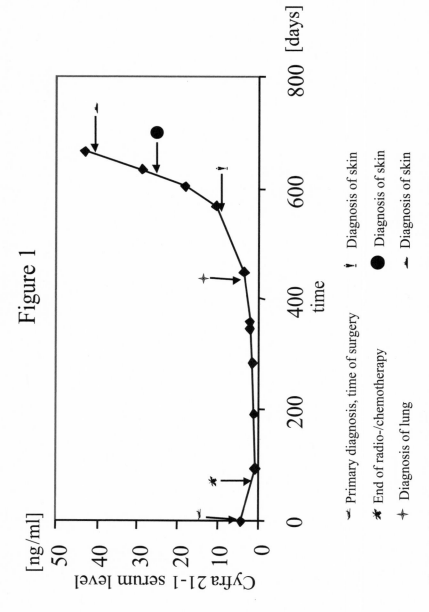

Figure 1

Figure 1: Cyfra 21-1 serum level during the clinical course of a patient with a $T_2N_2M_1$ sqamous cell carcinoma of the oropharynx. The Cyfra 21-1 level decreases after therapy and shows a clear increase when distant metastases are present.

Figure 2

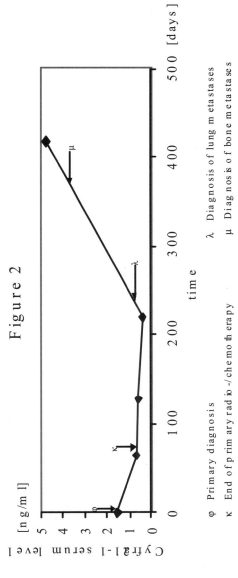

Figure 2: Cyfra 21-1 serum level during the clinical course of a patient with a $T_3N_2M_1$ squamous cell carcinoma of the oropharynx. In contrast to the first patient the Cyfra 21-1 serum level was low at the point of primary diagnosis. Nevertheless, a decrease of Cyfra 21-1 after therapy could be observed as well as a clear increase when distant metastases were present.

SURGICALLY TREATED PATIENTS WITH LARYNGEAL CARCINOMA IN THE ENT DEPARTMENT OF MEDICAL FACULTY, SOFIA, DURING THE PERIOD 1995 – 2000

K. Popov, D. Konov, Department of Otorhinolaryngology, Medical University, Sofia, Bulgaria

ABSTRACT

There are 1134 patients analyzed with primary diagnosed laryngeal carcinoma, who had been operated in Ist ENT Clinic, ORL Department, Medical University-Sofia for 5 years period. Patients are classified according to their age, assessing the extent of the primary tumor (T), localization, type of operation and tumor's histologic appearance.

Most affected (39%) are the patients in their sixties (50-59), more of them are with glottic localization – 68%, the ratio between the laryngectomies and laryngeal resections is 2.2/1. The most common tumor variant is well differentiated – 58.2%. There is a alarming tendency for increasing the number of patients with advanced stage of tumor development (T3 – 36.3% и T4 – 34.9%).

The study shows that there is a reserves in the field of prevention and early discovering of laryngeal carcinoma.

The personal records of 1134 patients with primary diagnosed laryngeal carcinoma, who underwent surgical treatment in Ist ENT Clinic, ORL Department, Medical University-Sofia for a 5 years period are analyzed. The patients operated in 1995 are 232, in 1996 – 241, in 1997 – 221, in 1998 – 225 and in 1999 – 215. Among them there are 39 women – 3.4%. The patients are reviewed in accordance to their age, assessing the extent of primary tumor - T (TNM classification), localization of primary tumor, type of surgical intervention and histologic appearance. A comparison with our similar study from 1997 – 1998 (Popov K., V. Golemanov, U. Heirat – "Age related features of laryngeal carcinoma treatment") is made.

Age distribution shows prevalence of patients in the 6th decade (50-59 years) – 442, or 39% and in the 7th decade (60-69 years) – 327 (28.8%). /fig.1/.

477

With the advance of age the percentage of patients in T1-2 lesion decreases (overall count 327, or 28.8%) (fig.2) and respectively the percentage with T3 lesion increases (overall count 484, or 36.3%) (fig.3).

Patients with T4 lesion constitute a relatively constant percent in the 5th, 6th and 7th decade – about 34.9% (396 patients) (fig.4).

The distribution of patients based on localization of primary tumor showed glottic localization in 68% (771 patients), supraglottic - in 27% (307 patients) and subglottic – in nearly 5% (56 patients). The ratio glottic:supraglottic cancer is 2.5: 1. (fig.5).

Laryngectomized are 56.2% (637 patients). 10.3% (117 patients) underwent laryngectomy with unilateral radical neck dissection (the so-called monoblock operation). Laryngeal resections are made in 340 cases (30% - 23.9% - vertical and 6.1% - horizontal type). 3.6% (40 inoperable patients) underwent only tracheotomy. Fig. 6 shows age distribution of patients and the corresponding type of operation.

With age advance the percentage of patients with laryngectomy decrease while the patients with resection decrease. The decreasing number of resections among the elderly can be explained not only with the decrease of patients with T1-2 lesion, but also with age related functional changes in respiratory system. With the years increases the number of patients, classified as inoperable, who just underwent tracheotomy. Relatively constant among the decades stays the number of patients, who underwent monoblock operation – about 10% (for the 5th decade – 9.5%, for the 6th decade – 11.8%, for the 7th – 8% and for the 8th – 9.1%.

Histologic appearance (grading) of the extirpated tumors were also analyzed. They were divided into 3 main groups – well differentiated, moderately differentiated and poorly differentiated. The 4th group consisted of rare carcinomas (verucous, adenocystic, basaloidocellular etc.). Fig.7 shows age distribution of the 3 groups.

In general well-differentiated carcinoma was found in 31.4% of patients, moderately differentiated - in 58.2% and poorly differentiated – in 8.1%. The concept that with the advance of age the percentage of patients with well-differentiated cancer increases and for greater malignancy during earlier decades of life was not confirmed by our analysis. In the group of rare carcinomas fell only 2.3% of the cases, and no age differences were found.

The data from this study, compared to those from 1987-1988 (200 patients were analyzed) showed the following differences. Laryngeal carcinoma most often affects the age 50-59 years, but a tendency for "rejuvenation" of the disease is observed. An alarming tendency for admission and operation of patients in advanced stage is also visible. In 1987-88 patients with T4 lesion were 22.5% and in this study they are 34.9%

The results are representative for our country. In the Oncologic Clinic of Sofia ORL Department are operated more than one half of patients with primary diagnosed laryngeal carcinomas in Bulgaria (on the average 400 cases per year). Our study showed that there are reserves in the prophylaxis, early diagnosis and treatment of patients with laryngeal carcinoma.

Figure 1. Age distribution of patients (in decades)

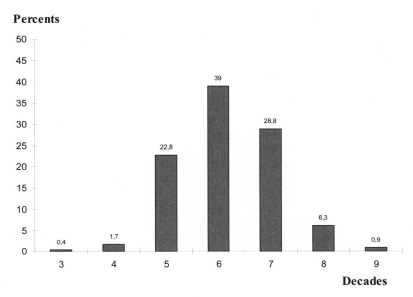

Figure 2. Age distribution of patients (in decades) with T1-2 lesions in %

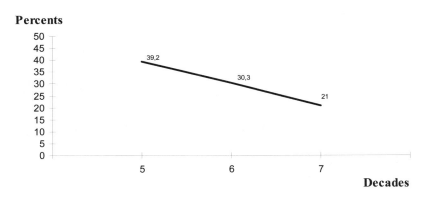

479

Figure 3. Age distribution of patients (in decades) with T3 lesions in %

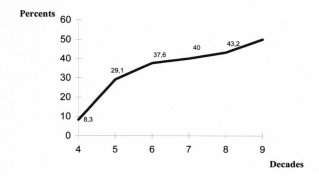

Figure 4. Age distribution of patients (in decades) with T4 lesions in %

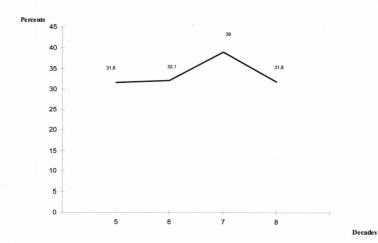

Figure 5. Tumor localization

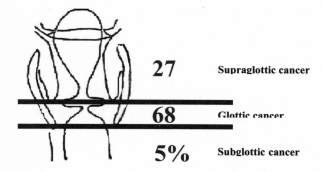

480

Figure 6. Age distribution of patients according to the type of operation

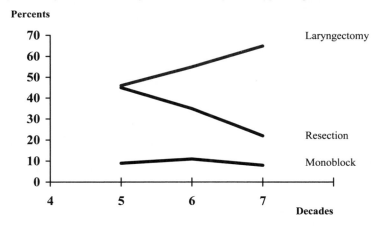

Figure 7. Correlation between age (in decades) and tumor histologic appearance

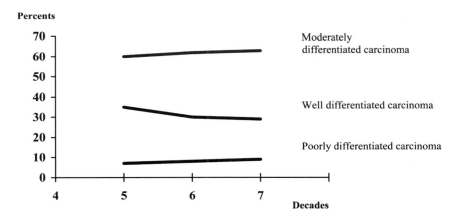

VASCULAR ENDOTHELIAL GROWTH FACTOR RECEPTOR 3 (VEGFR3) AND VEGF-C EXPRESSION IN SQUAMOUS CELL CARCINOMAS OF THE HEAD AND NECK

C. Neuchrist[1], B.M. Erovic[1], A. Handisurya[2], M.B. Fischer[3], G.E. Steiner[2], D. Hollemann[1], C. Gedlicka[1], K. Alitalo[4] and M. Burian[1]

[1]Department of Otorhinolaryngology, University of Vienna, Austria
[2]Department of Urology University of Vienna, Austria
[3]Department for Transfusion Medicine, University of Vienna, Austria
[4]Molecular/Cancer Biology Laboratory Haartmann Institute, University of Helsinki

Running title: VEG-C and VEGFR3 in head and neck cancer

Key words: HNSCC, VEGF-C, flt4, microvessel, lymphangiogenesis, tumor

Acknowledgements: We would like to thank Mrs M.Peterlik for her excellent technical assistance.

Correspondence to: *Dr. Csilla Neuchrist, Univ. Klinik fuer Hals- Nasen und Ohrenheilkunde, Allgemeines Krankenhaus der Stadt Wien, Waehringer Guertel 18-20, 1090 Wien, Austria (e-mail: csilla.neuchrist@univie.ac.at)*

Abbreviations: VEGF: vascular endothelial growth factor; VEGFR: vascular endothelial growth factor receptor; HNSCC: head and neck squamous cell carcinoma

SUMMARY

VEGF proteins and their receptors are central components in tumor induced neoangiogenesis. Recently, a third VEGF receptor based on its expression on lymphatic vessels, VEGFR3, has been described. It binds VEGF-C and VEGF-D, and seems also important during blood vessel development. Preferentially metastasising into regional lymphnodes, HNSCC is a useful model to study the involvement of VEGFR3 and its ligand VEGF-C in tumor induced lymphangioangiogenesis. Therefore we investigated the expression and distribution of the lymphangiogenic factor VEGF-C and it's receptor VEGFR3 in HNSCC cultured cell lines (n=4) and HNSCC specimens by RT-PCR (n=6), western blot (n=6) and immunohistochemistry (n=16). VEGF-C mRNA was markedly expressed in 3 of the 4 HNSCC cell lines (SCC9, SCC25, LFFR), weakly expressed in the JPPA cell line and markedly in all 6 HNSCC tumor specimens. For VEGFR3, message was found in the JPPA and SCC25 but only small amounts in SCC9 and LFFR cell lines. A strong VEGFR3 mRNA signal was recognised in all 6 patients` tumor specimens. Protein expression of VEGFR3 at 210 kD was found to be modest in JPPA and SCC9 and hardly detectable in SCC25 and LFFR cell lines compared to the positive control cell line HUVEC. All 6 HNSCC biopsies displayed strong VEGFR3 protein bands. Immunohistochemistry in 16 HNSCC patients revealed VEGF-C positive tumor cells in the majority of tumor specimens. VEGFR3 immunoreactivity (IR) was specified on numerous endothelial cells of lymphatic and vascular vessels within the tumor stroma. VEGFR3 positive vessels appeared partially double positive with CD34 indicating a common origin of blood and lymphatic vessels. Isolated VEGFR3 positive endothelial cells also coexpressed VEGFR2. HNSCC tumor cells showed only minor VEGFR3 IR. The broad expression of VEGF-C and VEGFR3 in HNSCC suggests massive lymphangiogenesis in these malignomas, involvement in vascular angiogenesis and implicates inhibitors of lymphangiogenesis as a possible therapeutic option.

INTRODUCTION

Tumor growth and spreading is virtually impossible without neoangiogenesis, a process which is controlled by several angiogenic factors and cooperating molecules[1]. Central regulators of angiogenesis and lymphangiogenesis are members of the vascular endothelial growth factor family. Five genes encoding VEGF-like proteins have been identified which generate different isoforms by alternative splicing mechanisms. VEGF proteins are produced primarily by tumor cells, macrophages and keratinocytes[2] recognising tyrosine kinase receptors (VEGFR1,2,3) and accessory receptors. VEGF expression is stimulated primarily by hypoxia-dependent mechanisms and receptor binding finally results in increased microvessel density (MVD) - a clinical correlate for neoangiogenesis. Upregulated VEGF protein expression by tumor cells and macrophages has already been reported in HNSCC[3,4] and in other cancers[5]. VEGFR 1 and 2 have also been described on HNSCC and are predominantly expressed on endothelial cells[3,6,7]. VEGFR1 binds VEGF, PlGF and VEGF B and in first line is responsible for reassembly of endothelial cells and functions in some way as a decoy receptor[3]. VEGFR2, ligand for VEGF, VEGF-C and D, is involved in endothelial cell mitosis, vasculogenesis and neoangiogenesis[9]. The most recently discovered VEGFR3 binds VEGF-C and D and has originally been described to be a predominantly lymphatic endothelial marker where it is assumed to take part in permeability functions and transport of lymphatic fluid[10]. However, in certain stages of embryonic development VEGFR3 is coexpressed with the other VEGF receptors[11-13] indicating a common origin of lymph- and blood vessels during embryonic development. Tumor transformation or inflammation probably in a similar way induce upregulation of VEGFR3 with consecutive blood and lymph vessel sprouting[13]. This would assign VEGFR3 a role as a global neoangiogenic marker. Particularly head and neck cancer metastasise initially into regional lymphnodes rather than into the periphery. This clinical feature favours HNSCC for investigating the lymphangiogenic factor VEGF-C and its receptor VEGFR3, which could turn out as an indicator for lymphangiogenesis, lymphatic metastasation and as an additional microvessel marker. In this study we investigated the expression patterns of VEGFR3/VEGF-C in 4 HNSCC cell lines and 16 tumor specimens. We found a strong upregulation of the VEGF-C protein in tumor cells as well as of VEGFR 3 on microvascular and lymphatic vessels. Further specification of VEGFR3+ endothelial cells by double immunolabelling with CD34 and VEGFR2 identified a population of undetermined microvessels.

MATERIAL AND METHODS

Cell Culture, Patients and reagents
JPPA (laryngeal carcinoma cell line), LFFR (tonsil carcinoma), SCC9 (tongue carcinoma) and the SCC25 (hypopharyngeal carcinoma) cell lines represented HNSCC cell lines, as control cell lines served HELA (cervix carcinoma), HaCat (human immortalised keratinocytes) and HUVEC (fresh human umbilical venous endothelial cells). 16 HNSCC tumor specimens were (clinical data see table 1) snap frozen in OCT embedding media and stored at −80°C. Six biopsies were used for examination by RT-PCR and immunoblotting.

Antibodies
Polyclonal antibodies specific for VEGFR3 (goat a-human-flt-4, R&D), and VEGF-C (rabbit a-human VEGF-C, Zymed), mAb a-CD34-FITC (mIgG, Serotec), mAb a-flt-4 (VEGFR3, mIgG1) a kind gift from Dr. K.Alitalo (Helsinki, Finland) and mAb a-flk-1 (VEGFR2; mIgG1, 2.5 □g/ml), a kind gift from Dr. P. Rockwell (ImClone USA). Isotype controls consisted of irrelevant mouse IgG1 (Dako, Denmark) and whole goat serum (Vector Lab.USA)

Immunoblotting
Membrane protein fractions were prepared from squamous cell carcinomas of the head and neck (HNSCC). Protein lysates were analysed through a 7,5 % polyacrylamide gel and transferred onto nitro-cellulose membranes (Bio-Rad, Hercules, California). The polyclonal goat-a-human flt-4 antibody (1:1000), and whole goat-serum as control were used as primary antibodies and the ECL-kit (Amersham Pharmacia Biotech) as detection system.

Reverse Transcription Polymerase Chain Reaction (RT-PCR)
RNA preparation from cell lines and tumor biopsies were performed as described previously [Chomczynski, 1987 #269]. Amounts of cDNA of VEGF-C[14], primer sequence: 5′-GAGGCTGGCAACATAACA-GAG-3, Rw: 5′-CCTTGAGAGAGAGG CACTGT-3 and VEGFR3[15] primer sequence: 5′-CACTCCCGCCATACGCCACATCAT POS:3441, Rw: 5′-CTGCTCTCTATCZGCTCAAACTCC POS 3867 were adjusted by 20 cycles using intron spanning primers specific for beta actin (Clontech Laboratories Inc., Palo Alto, CA 94303-4230, USA):primer sequence: Fw: 5` ATCTGGCACCACACCTTCTACAATGAGCTG CG-3', Rw: 5'-CGTCATACTCCTGCTT GCTGATCCACATCTGC-3'.

RT-PCR was performed by a initial heating step at 94°C for 3 minutes, and 30 PCR cycles. Amplification products were separated on a 1.5% agarose gel and visualised by ethidium bromide staining. All RT-PCR assays were conducted as three independent runs in order to confirm the results obtained. As positive control cDNA from human umbilical vein endothelial cells was used.

Immunohistochemistry

5 □m – thick frozen sections of HNSCC tumour specimens were cut, mounted onto poly-L-lysine-coated slides, fixed in ice cold acetone for 10 min and stored at –80°C. For immunohistochemistry sections were additionally fixed in 4% PFA for 10 min. Blocking of unspecific Fc binding was achieved with TBS/10% human serum/5%. MAb a-VEGFR3 (2 □g/ml)[12] was incubated over night at 4°C, consecutively incubated with rabbit anti-mouse IgG (1:50, 1h, RT, Dako), APAAP (1:50, 1h, RT, Dako) and final visualisation with fast blue. Levamisole was used to inhibit endogeneous alkaline phosphatase activity, nuclear staining was done with nuclear fast red.

Double immunolabelling

After blocking unspecific Ab binding, first mAb (unconjugated flt-4, 2 □g/ml) was administered as described above. Incubation with second Ab (rabbit anti-mouse IgG Ab, Dako, 1:50, 1h, RT) was combined with blocking of endogenous peroxidase (10mg glucose/ml TBS; 2mg glucoseoxidase/ml TBS; 1:1) Finally PAP complex (DAKO, 1:50, 1h, RT) was applied, peroxidase was visualised with DAB. After washing in TBS procedure was continued by incubation with the second antibodies (a-VEGFR2-biotinylated 1:100; a-CD34-FITC 1:70) at 4°C over night. In the next step streptavidin-AP (1:200, Dako) and sheep a-FITC-Fab fragments-AP (1:500, Boehringer Mannheim), respectively were applied. Development of alkaline phosphatase was performed with fast blue (as described above) and nuclear staining with methyl-greene.

RESULTS

VEGF-C and VEGFR3 mRNA expression in cultured HNSCC and tumor tissues (table1): VEGF-C mRNA formed a specific band at 324 bp and could be assessed in 3 HNSCC cultured cell lines (SCC9, SCC25, LFFR) and in all 6 tumor specimens. However, 1 HNSCC cell line (JPPA) was found to express just small amounts of VEGF-C mRNA. In control cell lines HUVEC and HACAT showed strong VEGF-C mRNA message whereas the HELA cell line remained negative. Out of 4 HNSCC cell lines JPPA and SCC25 displayed a bright band corresponding to the predicted size of 450 bp of VEGFR3. In SCC9 and LFFR just a very faint VEGFR3 mRNA signal could be detected. The control cell line HUVEC showed a clear VEGFR3 mRNA signal whereas in the HACAT and HELA cell lines signal was weak. In contrast, in all 6 HNSCC tissue samples VEGFR3 message was found (table 1).

VEGFR-3 protein expression in cultured HNSCC and tumor tissue (table 1): As the total amount of mRNA is not always translated into the respective protein, the presence of VEGFR3 protein was detected by western blotting. In cultured HNSCC cell lines (table 1) the polyclonal anti-VEGFR3 antibody yielded a specific, albeit weak band at 210 kD for the SCC9, JPPA and HACAT cell lines. No VEGFR3 band was seen in LFFR. The control cell lines HUVEC and HELA revealed a distinct VEGFR-3 specific protein signal whereas HACAT cells expressed weakly VEGFR-3. Immunoblotting for VEGFR-3 in all 6 HNSCC tissue samples showed strong VEGFR-3 specific bands.

In situ distribution of VEGF-C and VEGFR3 in tumor tissue: a-VEGF-C antibody stained 70% of tumor cells in most patients examined (fig.1c). MAb a-VEGFR3 clearly labelled numerous vessels around tumor formations (table 1, fig.1a). In contrast only few VEGFR3+

vessels were found in the wall of a lateral cyst of the neck or in normal mucosa. VEGFR3+ vessels included lymphatic vessels defined by flat lined endothelium lacking any further smooth muscle cell covering, as well as vascular microvessels containing erythrocytes and other cells (fig.1b). In some specimens huge tumor formations could be observed in bloated lymph vessels. VEGFR3 IR varied considerably on endothelial cells but was particularly strong in small vessels with narrow lumen and prominent rounded nuclei in the respective endothelial cells. In 6 cases we used double immunostaining to define a coexpression of VEGFR3 with CD34 or VEGFR2 on endothelial cells. In approximately 20% we found equally labelled VEGFR3+/CD34+ vessels which belong to the above mentioned small vessels. In addition lymphatic, VEGFR3+ vessels with weak coexpression of CD34 were detected. Reversely, many CD34+ vessels showed faint VEGFR3 IR. In general baseline expression of VEGFR3 in mature lymphatic vessels of tumor tissue appeared constantly high in contrast to varying VEGFR3 IR on endothelial cells of tumor microvessels.

DISCUSSION

VEGFR3 staining on different shaped vessels suggests involvement of the receptor not only in tumor lymphangiogenesis but also in blood vessel neoangiogenesis, confirmed by coexpression of VEGFR3 with the blood vessel marker CD34. This observation implicates significance of VEGF-C and VEGFR3 in tumor dependant angiogenesis, tumor growth and metastasation[16]. In HNSCCs evidence of angiogenesis has been provided[3,4,6,7,17-21]. Nobody so far featured details about lymphangiogenesis in HNSCC, tumours which commonly generate lymphatic metastasation. Coexpression of the blood vessel marker CD34 points at the induction of an undetermined precursor vasculature for neoangiogenesis of lymphatic and blood vessels. This thesis fits to results published recently in breast carcinomas, in which VEGFR3 and PAL-E (also a conventional blood vessel marker) coexpression has been described on tumor vessels in a similar fashion[13]. These presumptive precursor vessels are small vessels with narrow lumen, occasionally containing blood cells and they show rounded endothelial cell nuclei in contrast to the flattened endothelium by typical lymphatic vessels. With ongoing specialisation the vessel specific protein (VEGFR3 or CD34) is kept upregulated whereas the respective other protein ceases. Our findings also agree with the concepts proposing neovascularization[7,22] and remodelling of the preexisting vascular system for the purpose of neoangiogenesis during tumor growth. The destabilisation of preexisting vessels by paracrine influences elaborated by the tumor[23] and the simultaneously available angiogenic factors mimic an early embryonic situation, leading to upregulation of the respective growth receptors and finally to angiogenesis.

We conclude from our data that similar processes take place in HNSCC and other tumors, reupregulate endothelial VEGFR3 as well as probably other growth factors and lead endothelial cells to reenter the cell cycle for mitosis and sprouting. In contrary, the preexisting number of mature, lymphatic vessels stays more or less unchanged, at most increasing their intensity of VEGFR3 IR. So only VEGFR3+ microvessels would represent the angiogenic active cells. Apart from the small number of patients (n=16) this might be an explanation for the missing correlation of VEGFR3 expression and clinical parameters like tumor mass, nodal status, histological grading, tumor relapse or overall survival. Maybe for the same reasons, other studies dealing with VEGFR3 expression in colon, thyroid and gastric carcinomas could not find a correlation to clinical parameters either, despite a larger number of tumor patients has been examined[24-26].

Another explanation for the missing correlation of VEGFR3 to clinical data could be given by the existence of different isoforms of VEGFR3: two isoforms of VEGFR3 have been described[27] which encode a short and a long form for the receptor and differ in their cytoplasmic tyrosine kinase catalytic domain. Modification of signals transduced by the two VEGFR3 isoforms seems likely: functional assays revealed that only the long form of VEGFR3 was able to induce cell growth[28]. Therefor it seems necessary to consider the different VEGFR3 isoforms when correlating receptor expression to clinical parameters. However, results considering the functions of VEGFR3 splice variants still await further clarification[29].

The question of whether tumor cells themselves express VEGFR3 was of additional interest because one could expect an VEGFC driven autocrine growth loop like it is the case for VEGF/VEGFR2. In this study tumor cells in culture and in situ showed only minor VEGFR3 expression. Similar results have been gained in breast cancer and gastric carcinoma in which [13,26] tumor cells remained negative for VEGFR3. In contrast, upregulated VEGFR3 expression was described in mesotheliomas and teratocarcinomas, which was linked to increasing dedifferentiation[25,27]. HNSCCs in this study were mostly classified as well to medium differentiated (G2), which could explain the rare VEGFR3 IR on tumor cells.

Our observations describe upregulation of VEGF-C and VEGFR3 in HNSCC and confirm the putative important role of VEGF-C and VEGFR3 in neoangiogenesis of malignomas. Due to our results it is likely that upregulated VEGF-C and VEGFR3 contribute to the predilection for lymphatic metastasasion in HNSCC. Detailed knowledge about specific angiogenic features of carcinomas are certainly a prerequisite for the development of new antiangiogenic strategies which can then be adjusted to the different types of malignomas. VEGFR3 expression on tumor microvessels could confer prognostic and even therapeutical qualities to this receptor when using a-VEGFR3 mAbs or inhibiting compounds[30].

Table 1. Results of RT-PCR and immunoblotting for VEGF-C and VEGFR-3 in 4 HNSCC cell lines, 3 control cell lines and 6 HNSCC specimens.

Tissue	VEGF-C mRNA	VEGFR-3 mRNA	VEGFR-3 immunoblotting
JPPA (larynx ca)	(+)	(++)	(+)
SCC9 (tongue ca)	(+++)	(+)	(+)
SCC25 (hypopharyngeal ca)	(+++)	(+++)	(++)
LFFR (tonsillar ca)	(+++)	(+)	(-)
HELA (cervix ca)	(-)	(+)	(++)
HACAT (keratinocytes)	(+++)	(++)	(+)
HUVEC	(+++)	(+++)	(++)
Pat 1	(+++)	(+++)	(+++)
Pat 2	(+++)	(+++)	(+++)
Pat 3	(+++)	(+++)	(+++)
Pat 4	(+++)	(+++)	(+++)
Pat 5	(+++)	(+++)	(+++)
Pat 6	(+++)	(+++)	(+++)

Table 2. Clinical data of patients included in this study. VEGFR3 is represented by numbers of VEGFR3 positive vessels counted per mm^2.

pat. No	age	diagnosis	histological grading	staging	VEGFR3
1	65	hypopharynx ca	3	T2N2bMx	145
2	64	glottic ca	2	T2N1Mx	122
3	64	supragottic ca	2	T3N0Mx	226
4	53	glottic ca	3	T3N2bMx	299
5	61	tonsil ca	2	T1N2Mx	200
6	68	supraglottic ca	2	T2N2bMx	219
7	51	hypopharyngeal ca	2	T3N1Mx	230
8	69	tonsillar ca	2	T3NxMx	219
9	50	supraglotticca	2	T2N2Mx	320
10	73	glottic ca	2	T3N0Mx	48
11	44	supraglottic ca	2	T4N0Mx	108
12	85	sinus ca	2	T4N0Mx	84
13	71	supragottic ca	3	T4N2Mx	265
14	60	supraglottic ca	2	T2N0Mx	320
16	70	r-glottic ca	2	Rt2N2M1	153
17	70	lateral cyst of the neck			neg
10	73	peritumoral mucosa			48

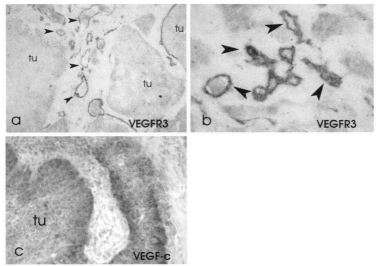

Figure 1. Immunohistochemistry in frozen sections of HNSCC biopsies, mAb a-VEGFR3 and rabbit a-VEGF-C, using APAAP system and fast blue as substrate, counterstaining was done with nuclear fast red. a) x 100; between HNSCC tumor formations (tu) mAb a-VEGFR3 stains the endothelium of multiple vessels, including large lymphatic like (arrowheads) and small microvessel like endothelial cells. In some cases vessels are strechted along the tumor border and seem to form rim-like structures around the tumor nodule. Tumor cells at the outer border of the tumor nodules express weakly VEGFR3. b) High power view (x 400) of VEGFR3-IR in small vessels, which in some cases contain cells c) x 200; HNSCC expressing VEGF-C in particular at the outer edge of tumor formations.

REFERENCES

1. Petruzzelli GJ. The biology of tumor invasion, angiogenesis and lymph node metastasis. ORL J Otorhinolaryngol Relat Spec 2000;62:178-85
2. Frelin C, Ladoux A, D'Angelo G. Vascular endothelial growth factors and angiogenesis. Ann Endocrinol Paris 2000;61:70-4.
3. Denhart BC, Guidi AJ, Tognazzi K, Dvorak HF, Brown LF. Vascular permeability factor/vascular endothelial growth factor and its receptors in oral and laryngeal squamous cell carcinoma and dysplasia. Lab Invest 1997;77:659-64.
4. Neuchrist C, Quint C, Pammer A, Burian M. Vascular endothelial growth factor (VEGF) and microvessel density in squamous cell carcinomas of the larynx: an immunohistochemical study. Acta Otolaryngol 1999;119:732-8.
5. Claffey KP, Robinson GS. Regulation of VEGF/VPF expression in tumor cells: consequences for tumor growth and metastasis. Cancer Metastasis Rev 1996;15:165-76.
6. Herold-Mende C, Andl T, Laemmler F, Reisser C, Mueller MM. [Functional expression of vascular endothelial growth factor receptor Flt-1 on squamous cell carcinoma of the head and neck]. Hno 1999;47:706-11.
7. Neuchrist C, Erovic B, Handisurya A, et al. VEGFR2 (Vascular endothelial growth factor receptor 2) expression in squamous cell carcinomas of the head and neck. Laryngoscope accepted 2001.
8. Fong GH, Rossant J, Gertsenstein M, Breitman ML. Role of the Flt-1 receptor tyrosine kinase in regulating the assembly of vascular endothelium. Nature 1995;376:66-70.
9. Shalaby F, Ho J, Stanford WL, et al. A requirement for Flk1 in primitive and definitive hematopoiesis and vasculogenesis. Cell 1997;89:981-90.
10. Kaipainen A, Korhonen J, Mustonen T, et al. Expression of the fms-like tyrosine kinase 4 gene becomes restricted to lymphatic endothelium during development. Proc Natl Acad Sci U S A 1995;92:3566-70.
11. Lymboussaki A, Olofsson B, Eriksson U, Alitalo K. Vascular endothelial growth factor (VEGF) and VEGF-C show overlapping binding sites in embryonic endothelia and distinct sites in differentiated adult endothelia. Circ Res 1999;85:992-9.
12. Partanen TA, Alitalo K, Miettinen M. Lack of lymphatic vascular specificity of vascular endothelial growth factor receptor 3 in 185 vascular tumors. Cancer 1999;86:2406-12.
13. Valtola R, Salven P, Heikkila P, et al. VEGFR-3 and its ligand VEGF-C are associated with angiogenesis in breast cancer. Am J Pathol 1999;154:1381-90.
14. Andre T, Kotelevets L, Vaillant JC, et al. Vegf, Vegf-B, Vegf-C and their receptors KDR, FLT-1 and FLT-4 during the neoplastic progression of human colonic mucosa. Int J Cancer 2000;86:174-81.
15. Kociok N, Heppekausen H, Schraermeyer U, et al. The mRNA expression of cytokines and their receptors in cultured iris pigment epithelial cells: a comparison with retinal pigment epithelial cells. Exp Eye Res 1998;67:237-50.
16. Weidner N. angiogenesis as apredictor of clinical outcome in cancer patients. Human Pathology 2000;31:403-5.
17. Williams JK, Carlson GW, Cohen C, Derose PB, Hunter S, Jurkiewicz MJ. Tumor angiogenesis as a prognostic factor in oral cavity tumors. Am J Surg 1994;168:373-80.
18. Salven P, Heikkila P, Anttonen A, Kajanti M, Joensuu H. Vascular endothelial growth factor in squamous cell head and neck carcinoma: expression and prognostic significance. Mod Pathol 1997;10:1128-33.
19. Quint C, Neuchrist C, Breitschopf H, Pammer J, Burian M. Expression of basic fibroblast growth factor in squamous cell carcinomas of the larynx - examination by in situ hybridization. Onkologie 1999;22:41-6.
20. Janot F, el-Naggar AK, Morrison RS, Liu TJ, Taylor DL, Clayman GL. Expression of basic fibroblast growth factor in squamous cell carcinoma of the head and neck is associated with degree of histologic differentiation. Int J Cancer 1995;64:117-23.
21. Eisma RJ, Spiro JD, Kreutzer DL. Role of angiogenic factors: coexpression of interleukin-8 and vascular endothelial growth factor in patients with head and neck squamous carcinoma. Laryngoscope 1999;109:687-93.
22. Kappel A, Ronicke V, Damert A, Flamme I, Risau W, Breier G. Identification of vascular endothelial growth factor (VEGF) receptor-2 (Flk-1) promoter/enhancer sequences sufficient for angioblast and endothelial cell-specific transcription in transgenic mice. Blood 1999;93:4284-92.

490

23. Yancopoulos GD, Davis S, Gale NW, Rudge JS, Wiegand SJ, Holash J. Vascular-specific growth factors and blood vessel formation. Nature 2000;407:242-8.

24. Jacquemier J, Mathoulin-Portier MP, Valtola R, et al. Prognosis of breast-carcinoma lymphagenesis evaluated by immunohistochemical investigation of vascular-endothelial-growth-factor receptor 3. Int J Cancer 2000;89:69-73.

25. Ohta Y, Shridhar V, Bright RK, et al. VEGF and VEGF type C play an important role in angiogenesis and lymphangiogenesis in human malignant mesothelioma tumours. Br J Cancer 1999;81:54-61.

26. Yonemura Y, Endo Y, Fujita H, et al. Role of vascular endothelial growth factor C expression in the development of lymph node metastasis in gastric cancer. Clin Cancer Res 1999;5:1823-9.

27. Pajusola K, Aprelikova O, Korhonen J, et al. FLT4 receptor tyrosine kinase contains seven immunoglobulin-like loops and is expressed in multiple human tissues and cell lines [published erratum appears in Cancer Res 1993 Aug 15;53(16):3845]. Cancer Res 1992;52:5738-43.

28. Borg JP, deLapeyriere O, Noguchi T, Rottapel R, Dubreuil P, Birnbaum D. Biochemical characterization of two isoforms of FLT4, a VEGF receptor-related tyrosine kinase. Oncogene 1995;10:973-84.

29. Shushanov S, Bronstein M, Adelaide J, et al. VEGFc and VEGFR3 expression in human thyroid pathologies. Int J Cancer 2000;86:47-52.

30. Kubo H, Fujiwara T, Jussila L, et al. Involvement of vascular endothelial growth factor receptor-3 in maintenance of integrity of endothelial cell lining during tumor angiogenesis. Blood 2000;96:546-53.

CHOSEN TUMOUR INDICATOR OF NODAL METASTASES APPEARANCE IN PATIENTS WITH LARYNGEAL CANCER

Maciej Gryczyński MD PhD, Józef Kobos MD PhD, Hanna Niewiadomska MD PhD, Wioletta Pietruszewska MD
Department of Otolaryngology, Medical University of Lodz, Lodz, Poland

This study was supported by grant N°502-11-472(55) from Medical University of Lodz

Key words: angiogenesis, Nm23 protein, CD44, laryngeal cancer

Correspondence to: *Dr. Wioletta Pietruszewska, Department of Otolaryngology, Medical University of Lodz, 22 Kopcińskiego str., 90-153 Lodz, Poland, Phone: (+4842) 678 57 85, Fax: (+4842) 678 11 76 (E-mail: vimp@friko2.onet.pl)*

ABSTRACT

One of the most important factors in prognosis of the patients with laryngeal cancer is evidence of neck lymph nodes metastases. The nm23 gene has been implicated as suppressor gene involved in the control of metastatic process of neoplastic cells. The process of tumour angiogenesis is another one, which is required for the growth and progression of solid tumour and correlate with metastases. Moreover, the integral membrane glycoprotein CD44, which has diverse functions in cell-cell and cell-substrate interactions, is assumed to play a critical role in the malignant progression of many human tumours. Paraffin-embedded tissue sections from 89 patients with laryngeal cancer were stained with a monoclonal antibody raised against CD34 antigen as angiogenesis marker, against Nm23 protein and against CD44 antigen. Measuring the density of the microvasculature in tumour was investigated. We found significant correlation between intensity of angiogenesis and pT (p=0,04), nodal metastases (p=0,04), histological grading (p=0,02) and survival (p=0,01). Reduced expression of nm23 protein and CD44 adhesion molecule were observed in patients with positive nodal status and appearance of local recurrences. We found significant correlation between nm23 protein expression and nodal metastasis (p=0.02, chi(2)), and between CD44 antigen expression and pT (p=0.03) and Nm23 protein expression (p=0.04). However, no significant differences in survival of our patients based on nm23 and CD44 expression could be shown with the Kaplan-Meier analysis. We did not observed any differences between expression of Nm23 protein in laryngeal cancer cells and local recurrences and histological grading. Evaluation of angiogenesis and Nm23 protein allow to asses the aggressiveness of tumour cells and can help to predict the risk of nodal metastases appearance and may be crucial in the choice of a more aggressive management of the disease in patients with squamous cell carcinoma of the larynx. Moreover, neovascularisation may be an independent prognostic factor in patients with laryngeal cancer. Evaluation of CD44 expression needs further investigation in laryngeal cancer.

INTRODUCTION

One of the most important factors in prognosis of the patients with laryngeal cancer is evidence of neck lymph nodes metastases. The development of a tumour and its progression to a metastatic phenotype involves a serious of genetic events with abnormal activation of oncogenes or inactivation of tumour supressor genes and others genes connected with proliferation, apoptosis or angiogenesis. The Nm23 gene has its two homologues designated as Nm23-H1 and Nm23-H2 and it has been implicated as suppressor gene involved in the control of metastatic process of neoplastic cells. It encodes a 17-kilodalton cytoplasmic and nuclear protein that reduced level was found in many tumours including breast, lung, colorectal and gallbladder[1].

The process of tumour angiogenesis is required for the growth and progression of solid tumours, which are limited to 2-3 mm3 volume in avascular condition, and correlate with metastasis in many types of cancers[2-6]. Neovascularisation requires the cooperation of a variety of molecules that regulate processes such as extacellular matrix remodeling, invasion, migration and proliferation. One of the adhesion molecules is the integral membrane glykoprotein CD44, which is responsible for interaction of cells with them and with extracellular matrix and is assumed to play a critical role in the malignant progression of many human tumours[7]. The role of antigens CD44 and Nm23 in head and neck squamous cell carcinoma (HNSCC) are still unclear. The aim of this study was the evaluation of angiogenesis, Nm23 protein and adhesion molecule CD44 expression in patients with laryngeal cancer and investigation of their role in progression of this tumour.

MATERIAL AND METHODS

The group of 89 patients with laryngeal cancer, surgically treated with minimum 5 years observation after laryngectomies, was multivariously analysed. In this group there were 84 men (94,4%) and 5 women (5,6%) at ages from 37 to 77 (mean – 57,1). We assessed cancer grading and clinical stage of cancer according to UICC (1991).

Paraffin - embedded tissue sections from each case were stained with a monoclonal antibody raised against CD34 antigen (mouse monoclonal antibody endothelial cell marker, Novocastra, NCL-END, 1:25), agaits Nm23 protein (mouse monoclonal antibody, Novocastra, NCL-nm-2, 1:100) and against CD44 antigen (H-CAM, mouse monoclonal antbody, Novocastra, NCL-CD44-2, 1:40) using a peroxidase labelled streptavidin - biotin kit in standard immunohistochrmistry techniques[8].

Measuring the density of the microvasculature in and around tumours (in the "hot spot") under the light microscope (x200) has been investigated, based on the criteria of Weidner et al.[5]. Microvessel density (MVD) was scored independently by two observers. Five to ten scores were multiplied to obtain a numerical value. Endothelial cells, which could be separated from tumour cells and connective tissues were taken into consideration. Vessels on the border of the tumour and normal tissue were excluded from evaluation.

For Nm23 and CD44 immunostaining assays, a semiquantitative score of proportion of stained cells was performed. The cases with percentage from 0% to 30% were treated as negative, and above 30% cancer cells with present reaction - as positive.

The results of each individual factor examined were compared with T and N stage, histologic grading and overall survival. The results were statistically transformed (Chi-square test with Yates' correction, Mann-Whitney test). The Kaplan and Meier model was used for overall survival curves (for MVD median value was considered). Only p value of less than 0,05 were considered significant.

RESULTS

Characteristic of 89 patients analysed in this study is presented in Table I.

Table 1. Characteristic of group of patients with laryngeal cancer (N=89).

Variable	N (%)
Age: <65 year	70 (78,7%)
>65 year	19 (21,3%)
Sex: Female	5 (5,6%)
Male	84 (94,4%)
Localisation : supraglottic	51 (57,3%)
glottic	38 (42,7%)
Tumor size: T1-T2	9 (10,1%)
T3	47 (52,8%)
T4	33 (37,1%)
N status: N 0	59 (66,3%)
N 1-3	30 (33,7%)
Distant metastases: M0	88 (98,8%)
M1	1 (1,1%)
Recurrences of cancer	13 (14,6%)
No recurrences	76 (85,4%)
Histologic grading: G1	21 (23,6%)
G2	59 (66,3%)
G3	9 (10,1%)
Expression of Nm23 protein:	
Negative (<30% of positive cells)	32 (36%)
Positive (≥30% of positive cells)	57 (64%)
Expression of CD44 protein:	
Negative (<30% of positive cells)	42 (47%)
Positive (≥30% of positive cells)	47 (53%)
Average MVD: 46 (median 39, SD 18)	

Expression of CD34 we found in all cases. We found statistically significant correlation between MVD and tumour size (p=0,04), nodal metastases (p=0,04), histologic grading (p=0.02) and overall survival of the patients (p=0.01) (table II). We did not observed any correlation between MMD and local recurrences (p>0,05).

Table 2. The Kaplan-Meier survival curves of 89 patients with laryngeal cancer with regard to the median microvessel density (log-rank test, p<0.05).

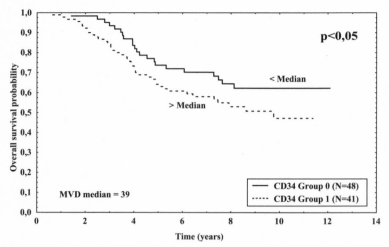

Strong and moderate expression of CD44 adhesion molecule was observed as intense cytoplasmic immunostaining. Expression of Nm23 protein was seen as cytoplasmic and occasionally nuclear immunostaining diffusely distributed in cancer cells. Reduced expression of Nm23 and CD44 was observed in patients with positive nodal status and appearance of local recurrences. We found significant correlation between Nm23 protein expression and nodal metastases (p=0,02), but we did not observed any significant differences assessing CD44 and pN (table III). However we found correlation between CD44 expression and pT (p=0,03) and positive expression correlated with more extensive tumour growth. We could not notice any significant differences between expression of mentioned markers and histologic grading, and recurrences (p>0,05). We found significant correlation between expression of Nm23 and CD44 (p=0,04). However no significant differences in survival of our patients based on Nm23 and CD44 expression could be shown with the Kaplan – Meier analysis.

Table 3. Comparison of Nm23 protein and CD44 antigen expression of primary tumours with nodal metastases appearance in patients with laryngeal cancer (N=89).

Feature	Nm23 protein expression		CD44 adhesion molecule expression	
	Negative	Positive	Negative	Positive
Negative nodal status (N0)	19 (32,2%)	40 (67,8%)	27 (45,8)	32 (54,2%)
Positive nodal status (N1-N3)	13 (43,3)	17 (56,7%)	15 (50%)	15 (50%)
Total	32	57	42	47

DISCUSSION

Lymph node metastasis is the single greatest predictor of recurrences in laryngeal cancer. The number of microvessels is one of the most examined parameters for neovascularisation and due to the postulated importance of angiogenesis in tumour growth and progression affecting in metastases, it is intensively examined in many solid tumours[5, 6]. The evaluation of tumour angiogenesis has been proposed to be an independent prognostic marker of some solid tumours (breast cancer, prostate cancer, lung cancer, head and neck cancer): it has been demonstrated that an intense vascular proliferation correlates with the aggressiveness of the neoplastic disease[2-5]. Data for HNSSC are still controversial. In our study tumour size, positive N status and patients' overall survival were correlated with angiogenesis in laryngeal cancer and it is similar to other authors results[9]. However, recently published investigation of Burian et al.[10] are in contrast with mentioned above and do not find microvessel count predictive of the patient's survival. Murray et al.[11] emphases that significance of angiogenesis may be used as an independent prognostic indicator in patients who are at higher risk for metastases and require adjuvant therapy.

Some genes may be involved in suppressing metastatic or aggressive tumour behaviour and to assess the aggressiveness of tumour cells and their metastatic potential many genes and its products are estimated. Expression of Nm23 protein is associate with a less aggressive phenotype of many tumours with also laryngeal cancer[1, 12-14]. Our study on expression of Nm23 protein confirms it. Although, in recent study[15] it was stated that increased, but not decreased, activity of NM23 is associated with poorer prognosis. It is difficult to say what is the reason of these results. Many discrepancies are also connected with CD44 antigen, but it seems to be obvious that Nm23 and CD44 genes are involved in progression of HNSCC[12-15]. Many studies indicate that those markers could help in the assessment of the biology of laryngeal cancer cells, but relating to our researches, only Nm23 protein might be a metastasis suppressor factor and may be useful for predicting metastases in squamous cell carcinoma of the larynx.

CONCLUSIONS

Evaluation of angiogenesis and Nm23 protein allow to asses the aggressiveness of tumour cells and can help to predict the risk of nodal metastases appearance and may be crucial in the choice of a more aggressive management of the disease in patients with squamous cell carcinoma of the larynx. Moreover, neovascularisation may be an independent prognostic factor in patients with laryngeal cancer. Expression of CD44 needs further investigation in laryngeal cancer.

REFERENCES

1.   Haut M., Steeg PS, Wilsom JKV, Markowitz SD. Induction of nm23 gene expression in human colonic neoplasms and equal expression in colon tumours of high and low metastatic potencial. J Natl Cancer Inst 1991; 83; 712-716.
2.   Bosari S, Lee AKC, DeLellis RA et al. Microvessel quantification and prognosis in invasise breast carcinoma. Hum Pathol 1992; 23; 755-61.
3.   Brawer M.K, Deering RE, Brown M et al. Predictors of pathological stage in prostatic carcinoma. Cancer 1994;3;678-87.

4. Gasparini G, Weidner N, Maluta S. Intratumoral microvessel density and p53 protein correlation with metastasis in head-and-neck carcinoma. Int J Cancer 1993; 55; 739-744.
5. Weidner N, Folkman J, Pozza F et al. Tumor angiogenesis: a new significant and independent prognostic indicator in early- stage breast carcinoma. J Natl Cancer Inst 1992; 84; 1875-1887.
6. Folkman J: The role of angiogenesis in tumor growth. Semin. Cancer Biol. 1992, 3, 65-71.
7. Matsumura Y, Tarin D. Significance of CD44 gene products for cancer diagnosis and disease evaluation. Lancet 1992; 340; 1053-58.
8. Hsu SM, Raine L, Fanger H. Use of avidin-biotin-peroxidase complex (ABC) in immunoperoxidase techniques. J Histochem Cytochem 1981; 29; 577-80.
9. Beatrice F, Cammarota R., Giordano C et al. Angiogenesis: prognostic significance in laryngeal cancer. Anticancer Res 1998; 18 (6B); 4737-40.
10. Burian M, Quint Ch, Neuchrist C. Angiogenesis factors in laryngeal carcinomas: do they have prognostic relevance? 1999, Acta Otolaryngol (Stockh) 1999; 119; 289-292.
11. Murray JD, Carlson GW et al. Tumor angiogenesis as a prognostic factor in laryngeal cancer. Am J Surg 1997; 174(5); 523-6.
12. Spafford MF, Koeppe J, Pan Z, Archer PG, Meyers AD, Franklin WA. Correlation of tumor markers p53, bcl-2, CD34, CD44H, CD44v6, and Ki-67 with survival and metastasis in laryngeal squamous cell carcionoma. Arch. Otolaryngol Head Neck Surg 1996;122(6); 627-32.
13. Gunduz M, Ayhan A, Gullu I et al. nm23 Protein expression in larynx cancer and the relationship with metastasis. Eur J Cancer 1997; 33(14); 2338-41.
14. Lee CS, Redshaw A, Boag G: nm23-H1 protein immunoreactivity in laryngeal cancer. Cancer 1996; 1; 77(11); 2246-50.
15. Pavelic K, Kapitanovic S, Radosevic S et al. Increased Activity of nm23-H1 Gene in Squamous Cell Carcinoma of the Head and Neck is Associated with Advanced Disease and Poor Prognosis. J Molecular Med 2000; 78; 111-118.

498

INHIBITION OF ANTITUMOR TNFALPHA ACTIVITY
BY SOLUBLE RECEPTORS IN SQUAMOUS CELL CARCINOMAS
OF THE HEAD AND NECK

Ch. Gwosdz, T. Hoffmann, H. Bier
Dept. of ORL / Head & Neck Surgery, Heinrich-Heine-University, Duesseldorf, Germany

Key words: TNFalpha, soluble Tumor Necrosis Factor Receptor, Squamous cell carcinoma

Correspondence to*: Ch. Gwosdz, Heinrich-Heine-University, Duesseldorf, Moorenstrasse 5, 40225 Duesseldorf, Germany*

ABSTRACT

Tumor necrosis factor (TNFα) alpha mediates a wide range of biologic responses, including immunological, antiproliferative, and cytotoxic effects. Secretion of sTNFR by target cells has been found to be a potent mechanism for the modulation and inhibition of this pleiotropic cytokine. In 10 established cell lines of squamous cell carcinomas of the head and neck (SCCHN) we determined a) the anti-tumor activity of TNF alpha (MTT-assay), b) the amount of sTNFRI and II in culture supernatents (sandwich immunoassay), and c) the expression of membrane bound mTNFRI and II (immunohistochemistry). In vitro exposure to TNF alpha caused dose dependent growth inhibition in all cell lines tested. Furthermore, all cell lines showed production of both sTNFR's, however, the antitumor effect of TNF alpha displays a strong correlation with sTNFRI only. High levels of this receptor were found in the supernatent of TNF alpha-resistant cell lines, whereas low concentrations characterized the sensitive ones. There were no correlations between the degree of mTNFR expression and either TNF alpha activity or amount of sTNFRI and II. These results suggest that the release of sTNFRI may confer resistance to antitumor effects of TNF alpha in SCCHN.

INTRODUCTION

Tumor Necrosis Factor Alpha (TNFα) is a polypeptide cytokine with a variety of in vivo and in vitro effects. TNFα was first identified in the serum of mice challenged with endotoxin after BCG innoculation[1]. Infusion of serum containing TNFα into untreaded mice induced hemorrhagic necrosis of transplanted subcutaneous tumors. In further investigations TNFα

499

exerts a broad spectrum of bioactivities including inflammation, cellular proliferation and various immunolregulatory and antiviral responses and is the name giving memeber of a growing cytokine family including e.g. Fas/Apo-1 ligand, as well as TRAIL/Apo-2, CD30L and CD40L[2] [3]. TNFα, like most memebers of this ligand family are expressed as type II transmembrane proteins, soluble ligands are released from the producer cells by proteolytic cleavage. The soluble form of TNFα as well as the transmembrane TNFα bind to two homologous membrane receptors, TNF-R1 and TNF-R2. TNF-R1 is a 55 kDa ubiquitously expressed transmembrane proteine, whereas TNF-R2 (75 kDa transmembrane proteine) is found predominantly on hemopoetic and endothelial cells[4]. There exist also a soluble form of both receptor. This sTNF-R1 and –R2 was originaly identified in the urine of febrile[1] and renal failure[2] patients. After purification, cloning and sequencing its cDNA[3-5] it revealed as the extracelular domain of mTNF-Rs[6], resulted from a proteolytic cleavage event which librates the extracelular domain from the transmembrane and intracellular domain. Typical TNFα-related effects, including cytotoxitity and induction of apoptos could be linked to TNF-R1[7]. Therefore it shows a higher affinity to TNFα than sTNF-R2[8].

The effects of TNF α are not well understood. Direct cytotoxicity and apoptosis is apparently mediated by specific binding to hihg affinity cell surface receptors. However the presence of cell surface receptors is not a sufficient explanation for different cytotoxity since normal cells and TNFα-reistant cells also have high specifity cell surfce receptors. Furthermore all different cell responses are mediated by only two receptors. Therefore it follows that regulatory mechanisms exist to modulate ist activity. sTNF-R1 is a good candidate involved in such mechanisms. Recent studies showed sTNF-R1 as naturally occuring blocking factor for TNFα. The soluble form of TNF-R1 retains the ability to bind TNFα with high affinity and, inhibit the binding of TNF to mTNF-R1 on the cell surface. The levels of sTNF-R1 are increased in sepsis/endotoxemia[9], meningitis[10], autommimune rejection[11], human immunodeficiency virus infection[12] and also in tumor bearing hosts[13-17]. sTNF-R1 is spontaneously produced in culture[18, 19]. sTNF-R1 serum levels are elevated in tumor bearing hosts during advanced stages of disease and increase during remission[17, 18, 20]. It was shown that sTNF-R1 protect transformed cells in vitro from cytotoxic effects of TNFα and from cytolysis mediated by Natural killer cells[20] and in mouse model was demonstrated that secretion of soluble receptor by tumor cells enhance their tumorigenecity and that this benifit is abrogated by antibodies which neutralize the binding of sTNF-R1 to TNFα[21].

The aim of this studie was to demonstrate that squamous cell carcinomas of the had and neck produce sTNF-R1 and that this production correlates to TNFα induced growth inhibition in cell culture.

MATERIAL AND METHODS

Cell lines: In all our experiments we used 10 established cell lines of squamous cell carcinomas of the head and neck (SCCHN): UM-SCC 10A, 10B, 11B, 14A, 14C, 17A and 22B, Hlac 79, 8029 NA and DDP.

Receptors: The membrane bound TNF-R1 and -R2 were determined by immunohistochemistry (primary antibody: Anti-human tumour necrosis factor binding protein 1 / 2 detection antibody, R&D, Wiesbaden, Germany), the amount of soluble forms was

500

measured in culture supernatant by an sandwich immunoassay (h-Tumour Necrosis Factor Receptor I/II ELISA, Boeringer,Mannheim, Germany)

Anti-Tumour activity of TNFα: To determine the anti-tumour activity of TNFα we used the colorimetric MTT-Assay: Day 0 cell seeding (6000 cells / 200 µl medium / well), day 3 change of medium by addition of TNFα / controls, Day 6, 7, 8, and 9 MTT-Assay.

Amount of TNFα: To measure the amount of TNFα an enzyme immunoassay was used for the quantification of TNFα in culture supernatants (h-Tumour Necrosis Factor α ELISA, Oncogen Science, Uniondale, USA).

RESULTS

Cytotoxicity assay: All cell lines were incubated with increasing consentrations of TNFα for 3 to 6 days. After exposure to TNFα dose dependent inhibition of tumor cell proliferation becam evident in all cell lines tested. In 3 out of 8 responsive cell lines, only minor growth inhibitory effects were observed, the maximum reduction of cell viability not exceeding 30% of the control. In 4 cell lines more pronounced growthh inhibitory effects were observed, resulting in a reduction of cell viability to 54% ± (8029 DDP), 60% ± (8029 NA), 48% ± (UM-SCC 10A) and 51% ± (UM-SCC 22B). Two cell lines showed growth inhibitory effects less than 20% and were defined as resistant.

Production of Tumor Necrosis Factor Receptors and TNFα: In all cell lines production of both sTNF-R and both mTNF-R could be observed. The concentration of sTNF-R1 in supernatant was between 69 and 394 pg / 0,2 ml(Graph and Table 1), with a mean concentration of 151 pg / 0,2 ml and between 1 and 20 pg / 0,2 ml supernatent for sTNF-R2 (mean concentration 6 pg / 0,2 ml). UM-SCC 10A and 22B showed the lowest expression of sTNF-R1 (69 pg / 0,2 ml supernatant), UM-SCC 11B (394 pg / 0,2 ml supernatant) and UM-SCC 14C (214 pg / 0,2 ml supernatant) the highest expresson of sTNF-R1. In all other cell lines the expresion of sTNF-R1 was between 97 and 176 pg / 0,2 ml supernatant. mTNF-R1 and –R2 and TNFα were expressed by all cell lines (pictures of immunohistochemistry not shown). The concentration of TNFα was between 0.2 pg / 0,2 ml and 38.5 pg / 0.2 ml supernatant.

However, the antiproliferative effect of the cytokine displays a strong correlation with sTNF-R1 only. High levels of this receptor were found in the supernatant of TNFα-resistant cell lines, whereas low concentrations characterised the sensitive ones (graph and table 1). There were no correlations between the degree of mTNFR expression and either TNFα activity or amount of sTNF-R2.

DISCUSSION

TNF-R1 is the mediator of TNFα induced cytotoxity and apoptosis. The soluble form of TNF-Receptor 1 was originally identified in the urine of febrile and renal failure patients. Because of ist capability to modulate a variety of immune reactions this naturally occuring

TNFα blocking factor may have a significant impact on the host response to inflammatory and malignant diseases.

In the present investigation, all human squamous carcinoma cell lines of the head and neck produced sTNF-R1. Furthermore, we were able to demonstrate a correlation between sTNF-R1 expression and TNFα-sensitivity. Therefore, we hypothesize that in this experimental system sTNF-R1 can block TNFα activity.

In vitro, malignant cell lines have been shown to produce higher amounts of sTNF-R1 in comparison with their respective benign precursors. In vivo, increased sTNF-R1 serum levels have been reported in tumour bearing hosts which decline after successful tumor therapy. Hence, the limited benefit of TNFα-based treatment strategies may be due to increased levels of sTNF-R. However, in the cell line panel tested, we found no correlation between the amount of endogenous TNFα-production and sTNF-R1 concentration.

These findings suggest that sTNF-R1 may protect malignant cells from the cytotoxic effects of TNFα.

Graph and Table 1: Correlation of maximum growth inhibition by TNFα and sTNF-R1 expression

Cell lines	10A	22B	DDP	NA	10B	Hlac	14A	17A	14C	11B
Maximum growth inhibition in %	42	49	46	60	70	71	75	76	81	84
sTNF-R1 expression in pg/0,2ml	69	69	135	136	176	112	97	109	214	394

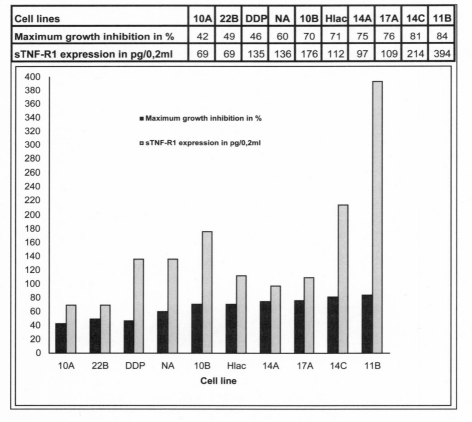

REFERENCES

1. Carswell, E.A., Old L.J., Kassel R.L., Green S., Fiore N. and Williamson B.: An endotoxin induced serum factor that causes necrosis of tumors. Proc. Natl. Acad. Sci. USA 72: 3666-3370 (1975)
2. Smith C.A., Farrah T. and Goodwin R.G.: The TNF receptor superfamily of cellular and viral proteins, activation, constimulation and death. Cell 76: 959 (1994)
3. Pitti R.M., Marsters S., Ruppert S., Donahue C.J., Moore A. and Ashkenazi A.: Induction of apoptosis by Apo-2 ligand, a new member of the tumor necrosis factor caytokine family. J. Biol. Chem. 271: 12687 (1996)
4. Adolf R.A., Grell M., Scheurich P.: Tumor necrosis factor. In: Epidermal Growth factors and cytokines. T.A. Luger and T. Schwrz, eds. Marcel Dekker Inc., New York p63 (1994)
5. Purification and biologic characterization of a specific tumor necrosis factor alpha inhibitor. J Biol Chem 1989 Jul 15;264(20):11966-73 (ISSN: 0021-9258) Seckinger P; Isaaz S; Dayer JM
6. Seckinger P; Isaaz S; Dayer JM, A human inhibitor of tumor necrosis factor alpha. J Exp Med 1988 Apr 1;167(4):1511-6
7. Schall TJ; Lewis M; Koller KJ; Lee A; Rice GC; Wong GH; Gatanaga T; Granger GA; Lentz R; Raab H; et al., Molecular cloning and expression of a receptor for human tumor necrosis factor. Cell 1990 Apr 20;61(2):361-70
8. Olsson I; Lantz M; Nilsson E; Peetre C; Thysell H; Grubb A; Adolf G, Isolation and characterization of a tumor necrosis factor binding protein from urine. Eur J Haematol 1989 Mar;42(3):270-5
9. Engelmann H; Aderka D; Rubinstein M; Rotman D; Wallach D, A tumor necrosis factor-binding protein purified to homogeneity from human urine protects cells from tumor necrosis factor toxicity. J Biol Chem 1989 Jul 15;264(20):11974-80
10. Loetscher H; Pan YC; Lahm HW; Gentz R; Brockhaus M; Tabuchi H; Lesslauer W, Molecular cloning and expression of the human 55 kd tumor necrosis factor receptor. Cell 1990 Apr 20;61(2):351-9
11. Shapiro L; Clark BD; Orencole SF; Poutsiaka DD; Granowitz EV; Dinarello CA, Detection of tumor necrosis factor soluble receptor p55 in blood samples from healthy and endotoxemic humans. J Infect Dis 1993 Jun;167(6):1344-50
12. Cerebrospinal fluid concentrations of soluble tumor necrosis factor receptor in bacterial and aseptic meningitis. Neurology 1996 Mar;46(3):837-8
13. Correlation between serum levels of soluble tumor necrosis factor receptor and disease activity in systemic lupus erythematosus. Arthritis Rheum 1993 Aug;36(8):1111-20
14. Kalinkovich A; Engelmann H; Harpaz N; Burstein R; Barak V; Kalickman I; Wallach D; Bentwich Z, Elevated serum levels of soluble tumour necrosis factor receptors (sTNF-R) in patients with HIV infection. Clin Exp Immunol 1992 Sep;89(3):351-5
15. Aderka D; Englemann H; Hornik V; Skornick Y; Levo Y; Wallach D; Kushtai G Increased serum levels of soluble receptors for tumor necrosis factor in cancer patients. Cancer Res 1991 Oct 15;51(20):5602-7
16. Kalmanti M; Karamolengou K; Dimitriou H; Tosca A; Vlachonikolis I; Peraki M; Georgoulias V; Kalmantis T Serum levels of tumor necrosis factor and soluble interleukin 2 receptor as markers of disease activity and prognosis in childhood leukemia and lymphoma. Int J Hematol 1993 Apr;57(2):147-52
17. Elsasser-Beile U; Gallati H; Weber W; Wild ED; Schulte Monting J; von Kleist S Increased plasma concentrations for type I and II tumor necrosis factor receptors and IL-2 receptors in cancer patients. Tumour Biol 1994;15(1):17-24
18. Gadducci A; Ferdeghini M; Fanucchi A; Annicchiarico C; Prato B; Prontera C; Facchini V; Genazzani AR Serum levels of soluble receptors for tumor necrosis factor (p55 and p75 sTNFr) in endometrial cancer. Anticancer Res 1996 Sep-Oct;16(5B):3125-8
19. Digel W; Porzsolt F; Schmid M; Herrmann F; Lesslauer W; Brockhaus M. High levels of circulating soluble receptors for tumor necrosis factor in hairy cell leukemia and type B chronic lymphocytic leukemia. J Clin Invest 1992 May;89(5):1690-3
20. Adolf GR; Apfler I A monoclonal antibody-based enzyme immunoassay for quantitation of human tumor necrosis factor binding protein I, a soluble fragment of the 60 kDa TNF receptor, in biological fluids. J Immunol Methods 1991 Sep 20;143(1):127-36
21. Neuner P; Klosner G; Pourmojib M; Trautinger F; Knobler R Selective release of tumor necrosis factor binding protein II by malignant human epidermal cells reveals protection from tumor necrosis factor alpha-mediated cytotoxicity. Cancer Res 1994 Nov 15;54(22):6001-5

22.   Selinsky CL; Boroughs KL; Halsey WA Jr; Howell MD Multifaceted inhibition of anti-tumour immune mechanisms by soluble tumour necrosis factor receptor type I. Immunology 1998 May;94(1):88-93

23.   Selinsky CL; Howell MD, Soluble tumor necrosis factor receptor type I enhances tumor development and persistence in vivo. Cell Immunol 2000 Mar 15;200(2):81-7

EARLY OUTCOMES FROM SELECTIVE NECK DISSECTION AND MODIFIED NECK DISSECTION TYPE III IN THE TREATMENT OF PATIENTS WITH LARYNGEAL CANCER

Ilia P. Yovchev M.D. Ph.D. Associated Professor, Spas S. Konsulov M.D. Assistant Professor, Dimitar D. Pazardzhikliev, Resident, Department of Otorhinolaryngology at the Higher Medical Institute Plovdiv, Bulgaria

Key words: cancer, larynx, metastases, neck, dissection.

Correspondence to: *Dimitar D. Pazardzhikliev, Bulgaria, Plovdiv 4000, Joseph Schniter 8a str., Phone: + 359 88 51 53 24*

ABSTRACT

Background. Radical neck dissection is the procedure according to which all other techniques for treating the clinically positive neck in cases with carcinomas of the head and neck are judged. It is associated with major functional and cosmetic defects. This urged introduction of more conservative procedures. The reported good results of these techniques encouraged us to introduce the modified radical neck dissections (MND) and the selective neck dissections (SND) in our practice.

Materials and Methods. 14 patients were observed prospectively: 8 patients T3 N0 M0; four – T3 N1 M0 and two – T3 N2 M0. In cases with N0 en bloc laryngectomy and SND were performed and in cases with N+ - en bloc laryngectomy and MND type III.

Results. By now the patients were followed up for an year, no regional recurrences were observed.

Conclusions. In carefully selected patients MND and SND are effective and oncologically sound procedures.

INTRODUCTION

The lymph nodes are lymphatic organs on the way of the lymphatic vessels. There are about 130 lymph nodes on each side of the neck. They are described in certain groups or chains. The Memorial Sloan-Kattering Cancer Center offered the following classification:

Level I – the lymph nodes in the submandibular and submental spaces
Level II – superior jugular level
Level III – middle jugular level
Level IV – inferior jugular level
Level V – the posterior triangle of the neck
And later a sixth level was added which is the anterior compartment.

The treatment of the cervical lymph node metastases is one of the unsolved and controversial problems concerning laryngeal cancer. Most of the head and neck surgeons assume Dr George Crile to be the father of the therapeutic neck dissection. In his manuscript from 1906 he described the principles and the controversies concerning the lymph dissection in cases of primary carcinomas of the upper aerodigestive tract[1].

Many of the head and neck surgeons began advocating and popularizing the conservative (functional) neck dissections since the radical neck dissection(RND) was associated with significant functional and cosmetic defects and demanded removing the structures of the neck even in cases with limited or no neck disease[2-4].

The modern trends in the surgical treatment of neck metastases, which include: precise staging of the neck, removing the endangered by metastatic involvement lymphatic nodes on certain levels, preservation of all structures of the neck, and avoiding of functional and cosmetic defects in cases of RND, resulted in the introduction of the functional neck dissection. Originally, authors were sceptical about the latter, but the practice proved it to be reliable and effective.[5]

We have a broader understanding of the term functional neck dissection and include in it both the Modified neck dissection type III and all kinds of selective neck dissections: suprahyoid, supraomohyoid, extended supraomohyoid, postero-lateral, lateral and antero-lateral (table 1).

Type of dissection	Levels removed	Structures preserved
Modified radical neck dissection type III	I,II,III,IV,V,VI	m.SCM; VJI; n.accessorius
Suprahyoid	I	m.SCM; VJI; n.accessorius
Supraomohyoid	I,II,III	m.SCM; VJI; n.accessorius
Extended supraomohyoid	I,II,III,IV	m.SCM; VJI; n.accessorius
Postero-lateral	II,III,IV,V	m.SCM; VJI; n.accessorius
Lateral	II,III,IV	m.SCM; VJI; n.accessorius
Antero-lateral	II,III,IV,VI	m.SCM; VJI; n.accessorius

Table 1

OBJECT

The main object of MND III and SND is the removal of the lymphatic nodes endangered by metastases in patients with laryngeal cancer. The main principle on which they are based states that laryngeal cancer has a predictable pattern of metastasizing, depending on the localization of the primary tumor.[6, 7]

TASK

1. To preserve the cranial nerves (n.accessorius, n.hypoglossus) by means of intraoperative regional monitoring employing the equipment of Magstim Company Limited, Wales, UK
2. To preserve the remaining structures of the neck: v. jugularis int., m. sternocleidomastoideus, which are removed by the classic RND.

MATERIAL AND METHODS

14 patients with laryngeal cancer underwent functional neck dissections in the ENT department of HMI Plovdiv until October 2000. They were staged as follows: 8 patients T3 N0 M0; four – T3 N1 M0 and two – T3 N2 M0. All of the patients had glottic localization of the primary. The N stage was pathologically identified. The following surgical techniques were applied: in cases with N0 – en bloc laryngectomy and selective neck dissection and in cases with N+ - en bloc laryngectomy and modified neck dissection type III (table 2).

Nodal staging	Patients	Technique applied
N0	8	Selective neck dissection
N1	4	Modified neck dissection type III
N2	2	Modified neck dissection type III
N3	0	—
Total	14	

Table 2

RESULTS

The patients subjected to these surgical techniques were followed up for a period of one year, during which no local recurrences were observed.

DISCUSSION

The enhanced knowledge on the draining of lymph nodes, the identification of the fascial spaces, which divide the lymphatic structures of the neck from the structures which are removed in RND, as well as the improved knowledge of the benefit of the radiotherapy additionally supported the use of the SND in the treatment of cervical metastases.[8] In case of negative neck status only the lymphatic nodes on certain levels endangered from metastases are removed.[9] The surgical treatment of cases with positive neck status still remains ambiguous. The broader indications of this operation and the incorporation of N+cases seems logic, because in the absence of factors destroying the fascial spaces or disrupting the lymphatic flow, such as massive adenopathy or major extracapsular spread, the principles on which it is based remain valid.[10, 11] In those cases we applied MND type III.

CONCLUSION

We presented our modest experience with 14 patients with negative and positive cervical lymph node status classified as N0 N1 N2, having undergone SND and MND type III. In the one-year-long follow-up no neck recurrences were observed. The results of our research imply that the application of SND in cases of negative neck status as an elective procedure and the prudent broadening of its indications to include cases with clinical and histological evidence of metastatic disease seems reasonable.

REFERENCES

1. Harold C. Pillsburry III, Madison Clark; A Rationale for Therapy of the N0 Neck. The Laryngoscope 1997; 107:1294-1315.
2. Bocca E. Pignatoro O. A Conservation Technique in Radical Neck Dissection. Ann Otol Rhinol Laryngol. 1976; 76: 975-987
3. J.R. Saunders Jr, R.M. Hirata, D.A. Jaques. Considering the Spinal Accessory Nerve in Head and Neck Surgery. The American Journal of Surgery 1985; 150:491-494
4. Byers RM, Wolf PF, Ballantyne AJ. Rationale for Elective Modified Neck Dissectioon. Head Neck Surg.1988: 160- 167
5. O. Kleinsasser Tumors of the Larynx and Hypopharynx Georg Thiem Verlag Stuttgart – New York 1988. 220p.
6. A. Ferlito, A. Rinaldo. Level I Dissection for Laryngeal and Hypopharyngeal Cancer: Is It Indicated?.The Journal of Laryngology and Otology. 1988; 112:438-440
7. B.J. Davidson, V. Kulkarny, M.D. Delacure, J.P. Shah. Posterior Triangle Metastases of Squamous Cell Carcinoma of the upper Aerodigestive Tract. The American Journal of Surgery 1993; 166: 395-398
8. N.W. Pearlman,F.B. Johnson, R.C. Kennaugh. Modified Radical Neck Dissection and poostoperative Radiotherrapy in Squamous Cell Head and Neck Cancer. The American Journal of Surgery 1985; 150:488-490
9. J.Kligerman, L.O. Olivato, R.A. Lima et al. Elective Neck Dissection in the Treatment of T3/T4 N0 Squamous Cell Carcinoma of the Larynx. The American Journal of Surgery 1995; 170:436-439
10. Sean J. Traaynor, James I. Cohen, Jason Gray, Peter Andersen, Edwin C. Everts. Selective Neck Dissection and the Management of the Node-positive Neck. The American Journal of Surgery 1996; 172:654-657
11. A. Ferlito, A. Rinaldo. Selective Lateral Neck Dissection for Laryngeal Cancer with Limited Metastatic

RADIOIMMUNOTHERAPY IN SQUAMOUS CELL CARCINOMA OF THE HEAD AND NECK

Pontus K.E. Börjesson, David R. Colnot, Remco de Bree, Gordon B. Snow, Guus A.M.S. van Dongen
Department of Otolaryngology, Head and Neck Surgery, Vrije Universiteit Medical Center, P.O. Box 7057, 1007 MB Amsterdam, The Netherlands

Correspondence to: *G. A. M. S. van Dongen, Vrije Universiteit Medical Center, P. O. Box 7057, 1007 MB Amsterdam, The Netherlands, Phone: +31-20 444 3690, Fax: +31-20 444 3688, e-mail:* <u>*gams.vandongen@azvu.nl*</u>

ABSTRACT

The purpose of this paper is to review the possibilities and limitations of monoclonal antibodies (MAbs) and radionuclides for the use in radioimmunotherapy (RIT) in patients with a squamous cell carcinoma of the head and neck (HNSCC). Results of pre-clinical and clinical RIT studies are provided. So far, there is no effective systemic adjuvant treatment available for patients with HNSCC. With a high rate of locoregional recurrence and distant metastasis, possibly arising from minimal residual disease and disseminated tumor cells, the development of RIT for HNSCC-patients at risk seems justified. After initial difficulties in developing a MAb selective for HNSCC, the CD44v6-specific MAb U36 was chosen as the best candidate for clinical RIT studies. A phase I RIT study revealed that this MAb when labeled with the radionuclide rhenium-186 (^{186}Re), was safe, showed excellent tumor targeting and reached tumoricidal doses at the maximum tolerated dose (MTD) level of 27 mCi/m^2. Myelotoxicity was the only toxicity observed. In a second trial, further dose escalation of ^{186}Re-labeled MAb U36 was aimed by counteracting myelotoxicity. To this end, patients received G-CSF during 5 consecutive days. Subsequently, 1 litre of the G-CSF-primed blood was collected and stored unprocessed at 4°C until re-infusion 72 hours after the start of RIT. By doing so, the MTD could be enhanced to 54 mCi/m^2 while no dose limiting myelotoxicity was observed. However, as MAb U36 appeared to be immunogenic, even after chimerization to a murine/human construct, it was replaced by another CD44v6-specific MAb, the humanized MAb BIWA 4. Results from an ongoing phase I trial confirm the potential of ^{186}Re-labeled MAb BIWA 4 for targeting HNSCC. Although RIT of HNSCC is in an early phase of development, substantial progress has been made. Even if it has not shown the same spectacular results in HNSCC as observed in hematological malignancies, tumoricidal effects have especially been seen in small tumors, indicating that it may have a role especially for eradication of minimal disease remaining after surgery and/or radiotherapy.

INTRODUCTION

Squamous cell carcinoma of the head and neck (HNSCC) is by far the most common type of all malignancies of the head and neck and has a worldwide incidence of more than 500,000 cases each year. It accounts for approximately 5% of all malignancies in northwestern Europe and the USA[1]. Early stages (Stage I/II) of HNSCC generally have a good prognosis after surgery or radiotherapy. Unfortunately, this does not hold true for advanced stages (Stage III/IV). It is of importance to note that approximately two-thirds of all HNSCC patients present with advanced stage disease.

Despite improvements in locoregional treatment modalities used in advanced HNSCC, the rate of locoregional recurrence is more than 50% and approximately 25% of these patients develop distant metastases while autopsy studies have shown incidences up to 57%[2-5].

In particular patients with multiple lymph node metastases are at risk for locoregional recurrence and distant metastases[6,7]. It is plausible that after surgery and radiotherapy, many patients with advanced HNSCC harbor histologically undetectable disease, also called minimal residual disease causing locoregional failure, and/or disseminated tumor cells in other parts of the body resulting in distant metastasis. The role of adjuvant chemotherapy for this group of patients has proven to be limited. Responses have been seen but the impact on survival has been disappointing and its role is mainly restricted to palliative treatment of HNSCC[8].

In order to decrease the incidence of locoregional failure and distant relapse in HNSCC, development of an effective adjuvant systemic treatment is needed. Targeting of radionuclides selectively to HNSCC by use of monoclonal antibodies (MAbs) might contribute to a more effective therapy for advanced stage disease. Bearing in mind that HNSCC has a relatively high intrinsic radiosensitivity compared to other solid tumors, this fairly new systemic therapeutic modality, also called radioimmunotherapy (RIT), can become a realistic option[9]. With this paper we intend to give a brief review of the experiences and achievements with RIT in HNSCC so far.

POSSIBILITIES AND LIMITATIONS OF MONOCLONAL ANTIBODIES

With the introduction of the hybridoma technology by Köhler and Milstein in 1975 it became possible to produce MAbs directed against practically any type of tumor-associated antigen and to investigate the potential of MAbs to target and eradicate tumors[10]. A MAb may have intrinsic potential to trigger selective tumor cell death by mediation of immunological effector mechanisms or to block receptors associated with tumor cell growth. Besides that, a MAb can also be applied as a vector for the selective delivery of radionuclides, toxins and chemotherapeutic agents to tumor cells.

The choice for coupling radionuclides to tumor-selective MAbs has several potential benefits. It is understandable that selective delivery of radionuclides to the surface of a tumor cell may eradicate that particular cell. Besides that, a so called "cross-fire" effect occurs, meaning that these MAbs also deliver radiation to adjacent tumor cells whether targeted or not.

510

To date, most successes in the field of RIT have been achieved in patients with hematologic malignancies, such as non-Hodgkin's lymphomas (NHL) and leukemias, where high rates of partial and complete responses have been observed. In the treatment of B-cell NHL, most experience has been gained with iodine-131- (^{131}I) and yttrium-90- (^{90}Y) labeled MAbs such as ibritumomab, rituximab and tositumomab, which are all directed against the CD20 antigen. The two major approaches used in NHL are non-myeloablative- respectively myeloablative RIT. In selected clinical trials using non-myeloablative RIT, overall response rates between 67% and 79%, with complete response rates between 26% and 50%, have been observed[11-13]. However, it appears that the best results can be achieved with a myeloablative dose. In a trial conducted by Press et al. in 21 relapsed B-cell NHL patients, an overall response rate of 86% and a complete response rate of 81% was achieved using ^{131}I-labeled tositumomab[14]. These successes can be explained by the high intrinsic radiosensitivity of these tumor cells and by the fact that radiolabeled MAbs can easily be delivered to blood, bone marrow and spleen, where these tumor cells often are localized.

Although research in RIT of solid tumors including HNSCC has shown progress during the last decade, the encouraging response rates as seen in hematological malignancies have not been reached yet. This is likely due to tumor heterogeneity, the lower intrinsic radiosensitivity and poor MAb penetration in large solid tumors. De Bree et al. reported tumor volume to be the single most important factor for MAb uptake in HNSCC tumors[15]. In line with these findings, clinical RIT trials for the treatment of breast-, ovarian- and colorectal cancers have shown a general trend of increasing chance of tumor control for smaller sized tumors[16-19].

Besides the low overall tumor uptake in large tumors, the other obstacle in the use of MAbs is immunogenicity. Murine MAbs (mMAbs) as frequently used in RIT often cause immunogenicity with the formation of human anti-mouse antibodies (HAMA's). Although the rate of occurrence of HAMA responses may differ between MAbs, approximately 40% to 50% of all patients develop HAMA's after a single administration while after multiple administrations this percentage can be as high as 90%[20-22]. It is of great importance that HAMA formation is eliminated, in order to prevent allergic reactions and rapid clearance of the radioimmunoconjugate from the blood. In addition it is needed to facilitate repeated RIT dosing.

The development and the use of chimeric (mouse/human) MAbs in general has decreased the rate of immunogenicity, but sometimes inadequately, with the formation of human anti-chimeric antibodies (HACA's). The engineering of humanized MAbs, being almost completely human apart from a small part of the antigen-binding sites became the next approach to deal with this problem. In several studies, humanized MAbs (hMAbs) showed excellent tumor targeting in combination with low immunogenicity. It seems that their introduction can solve the problem of HAMA's and HACA's and make RIT more safe and effective[23-25].

511

MONOCLONAL ANTIBODIES FOR RADIOIMMUNOTHERAPY OF HEAD AND NECK CANCER

The ideal characteristics for a MAb to be used in RIT are reactivity with an antigen which is abundantly expressed on the surface of all tumor cells and which is not expressed in any normal tissues. Preferably, a MAb should also have good retention in tumors. As discussed earlier, to prevent the induction of HAMA's, chimeric or preferably humanized MAbs should be used.

To date, this ideal MAb has yet to be developed for HNSCC or any other type of malignancy. In the beginning of the past decade the first HNSCC-selective MAbs were developed at our department[26-28]. After extensive immunohistochemical screening on large panels of HNSCC and normal tissues and after biodistribution studies in HNSCC-bearing nude mice, two IgG MAbs designated E48 and U36 were selected for further studies in patients with HNSCC[28-31]. MAb E48 recognizes a 16-22 kDa surface antigen, apparently involved in cell-cell adhesion[32,33], whereas MAb U36 recognizes the v6 domain of the 200 kDa squamous cell specific CD44 splice variant epican[34].

Radioimmunoscintigraphy (RIS) and biodistribution studies performed with ^{99m}Tc-labeled MAb E48 and MAb U36 respectively, showed tolerability in all patients and high and selective tumor uptake for both Mabs[35-38]. Eventually, differences in antigen expression in HNSCC, were deciding in the final selection. A high and homogenous expression of the U36-defined antigen (CD44v6) was found in 96% of HNSCC compared with only 70% for the E48 antigen, giving MAb U36 priority above MAb E48 for use in further development of RIT[38]. Expression of the CD44v6-antigen has also been observed for a variety of other carcinomas such as lung, esophagus, cervix, breast, colon, skin and stomach. In normal tissues, expression of CD44v6 was observed in skin (keratinocytes), tonsils (epithelium), and uterus (cervix). Lower expression was detected in breast (ducts/lobuli), duodenum (Brunner's glands), lung (pneumocytes/bronchial epithelium), prostate (myoepithelium), pancreas (ducts), urinary bladder (epithelium) and ureter (epithelium)[28,39,40].

RADIONUCLIDES FOR RIT

When selecting a radionuclide for RIT, the ideal situation is a durable, homogenous dose distribution in the tumor with a low exposure of normal tissue. The type of energy emitted, the path length and the physical half-life of the radionuclide together with the biological half-life of the antibody determine the antitumor effect, but also the toxic effects.

To date, beta-energy emitters are the most widely used radionuclides in RIT. Beta-emitters are most suitable for use in RIT because they deliver their energy in the form of ß-particles within a small radius from their origin. This radius, also called path length is for most of these beta-emitters 0.5 to several millimeters.

[131]I is the most widely used radionuclide in clinical RIT studies. Although its physical half-life of 8.1 days is suitable for RIT, the disadvantages such as a relatively low energy beta-emission, dehalogenation of the ^{131}I-labeled conjugates, necessity to prevent uptake of detached ^{131}I by the thyroid and a high percentage of toxic high energy gamma-emission make ^{131}I less attractive in RIT.

Another frequently used radionuclide is ^{90}Y, a pure beta-emitter with a physical half-life of 2.5 days, which is suitable for RIT. A disadvantage is its high beta-energy, which results in a path length too long for optimal RIT of minimal residual disease. These properties could also cause an unnecessary high radiation exposure of normal tissues. ^{90}Y does not emit gamma-radiation and can therefore not be imaged and monitored after administration. In case of instability of the antibody-chelate-radionuclide complex, released ^{90}Y can be sequestered in organs like bone marrow, spleen and liver and cause severe toxicity[41,42].

For RIT, rhenium-186 (^{186}Re) seems a more suitable radionuclide[43,44]. Its beta-energy, half-life of 3.7 days and path length of 1,8 millimeter all seem to be favorable for RIT of minimal residual disease. Furthermore, ^{186}Re decays for 9% by gamma-emission which is enough as far as imaging is concerned and which is low with respect to environmental safety[45,46]. For ^{186}Re the optimal tumor size for curability was calculated to be in a range from 7 to 12 millimeter[47].

Although not therapeutically applicable, ^{99m}Tc a widely used radionuclide in diagnostic studies, can play an important part in RIT. It belongs to the same group in the periodic table of elements as ^{186}Re and can therefore be coupled to MAbs using similar chemistry. Both radionuclides also have comparable energies of their gamma-emission. These similarities make it possible to select ^{186}Re-MAb RIT candidates by using less toxic ^{99m}Tc-MAb conjugates in a RIS "scouting procedure" to confirm tumor-targeting. To be the ideal "matched pair" for combined RIS-RIT studies, the biodistribution of the ^{99m}Tc- and ^{186}Re-MAb conjugates must be similar.

However, before ^{186}Re and ^{99m}Tc could be utilized in clinical studies, their coupling to MAbs had to be improved. Direct labeling methods with these radionuclides have shown to create radioimmunoconjugates with a poor in vivo stability and a limited number of coupled radionuclide atoms. Visser et al. developed an indirect labeling method, using the MAG3 chelate as a linker between the radionuclide and its MAb. This method enabled the production of stable radioimmunoconjugates with a high number of radionuclide-MAG3 groups[48].

PRE-CLINICAL RIT STUDIES

In pre-clinical RIT studies, nude mice bearing HNSCC xenografts were treated with ^{186}Re-labeled MAbs E48 and U36[30,31]. Both MAbs showed promising therapeutical results. After a single dose of 600 µCi ^{186}Re-labeled MAb E48, 100% complete remissions were seen of all tumors up to 75mm^3. After a single dose of 500 µCi ^{186}Re-labeled MAb U36, all tumors of the size 102 ± 15 mm^3 also regressed completely. These results indicate that ^{186}Re-labeled MAbs could have the potential to eradicate minimal residual disease and disseminated tumor cells in HNSCC patients.

RESULTS OF A PHASE I RIT DOSE ESCALATION STUDY OF ^{186}RE-LABELED CHIMERIC MAB U36 IN PATIENTS WITH HNSCC

The main purpose of this study conducted at our department by Colnot et al. was to determine the safety, maximum tolerated dose (MTD) through dose escalation, pharmacokinetics, dosimetry, immunogenicity and therapeutic potential of ^{186}Re-labeled chimeric MAb (cMAb) U36 in patients with HNSCC. Also, the potential of using ^{99m}Tc-labeled cMAb U36 as a "scouting procedure" for the selection of RIT candidates was evaluated[49].

Thirteen patients with recurrent or metastatic HNSCC were given 740MBq (20mCi) ^{99m}Tc-labeled cMAb U36 followed 1 week later by a single dose of cMAb U36 labeled with escalating doses of ^{186}Re. All patients tolerated the administration and nuclear imaging showed excellent tumor targeting for both conjugates in all patients. Myelotoxicity was the only toxicity encountered. Dose limiting toxicity in the form of grade 4 myelotoxicity occurred in 2 patients treated with 1.5 GBq/m^2 (41mCi/m^2). One of these patients, developed grade 4 thrombocytopenia and leukocytopenia 4 weeks after RIT and died from an opportunistic lung infection shortly thereafter. At the MTD established at 1.0 GBq/m^2 (27 mCi/m^2), grade 3 thrombocytopenia occurred in 1 patient. One patient treated at the MTD level showed stable disease during 6 months after treatment. The 2 patients who developed dose limiting myelotoxicity showed tumor regression, although of short duration.

Analysis of pharmacokinetics showed variation between patients treated at the same dose level. Furthermore, the fact that the pharmacokinetic behavior of the two conjugates appeared to be similar, indicates that a biodistribution study with ^{99m}Tc-labeled MAbs can be used to predict the biodistribution of ^{186}Re-labeled MAbs in individual patients.

This study showed us that tumoricidal doses can be reached with RIT in HNSCC patients.

RESULTS OF A HIGH-DOSE RIT STUDY OF ^{186}RE-LABELED CHIMERIC MAB U36 WITH RE-INFUSION OF UNPROCESSED, G-CSF-PRIMED WHOLE BLOOD IN PATIENTS WITH HNSCC

In the previously described phase I dose escalation study with ^{186}Re-labeled cMAb U36, dose limiting grade 4 myelotoxicity was observed at 41 mCi/m2, and the MTD was established at 27 mCi/m2. In a second trial, Colnot et al. aimed for further dose escalation by counteracting myelotoxicity. To this end, patients received granulocyte-colony-stimulating factor (G-CSF) during 5 consecutive days, in order to mobilize stem cells from the bone marrow to the peripheral blood. Subsequently, 1 litre of the G-CSF-primed blood was collected and stored unprocessed at 4°C until re-infusion 72 hours after the start of RIT. By doing so, the MTD could be enhanced to 54 mCi/m^2.while no dose limiting myelotoxicity was observed[50]. This relatively simple and inexpensive method had been used in previous studies for shortening the pancytopenic period in patients receiving high dose chemotherapy.

The procedure proved to be safe and was well tolerated in all patients. No patients developed dose limiting toxicity, while hematologic toxicity did not exceed grade 3. In one of the patients treated with 41 mCi/m^2, one of the diagnosed pulmonary metastases showed a decrease in size while the other pulmonary metastases remained stable for 6 months. It could be concluded that the use of G-CSF-primed whole blood, reduces the myelotoxicity and

514

therefore allows further dose escalation of [186]Re-labeled cMAb U36 above the MTD of 27 mCi/m^2 as established in the prior phase I study.

DEVELOPMENT OF NON-IMMUNOGENIC MABS FOR RIT

Since cMAb U36 appeared to be immunogenic in ± 40% of the HNSCC patients, a switch was preferred to a non-immunogenic MAb allowing for multiple dosing in future studies of RIT in HNSCC patients.

Parallel to the achievements at our department, another research group had developed a panel of MAbs, which were also directed against the v6 region of CD44[39]. This group had selected the high affinity murine MAb BIWA 1 as the best candidate for HNSCC targeting and initial biodistribution studies in HNSCC patients confirmed its potential[51]. Besides that they had constructed, 1 chimeric and 2 humanized derivatives of BIWA 1[51]. Finally, one of the humanized MAbs named BIWA 4 was selected for further studies. In hMAb BIWA 4 we seem to have found the non-immunogenic MAb we were searching for, since administration of [186]Re-BIWA 4 to 27 HNSCC patients, 9 lung cancer patients (non-small cell) and 9 breast cancer patients, did not result in any HAHA response. Results of these ongoing phase I trials will become available shortly.

FUTURE DEVELOPMENT OF RIT IN HNSCC

So far, phase I RIT studies in HNSCC have shown promising results. No complete responses have been obtained, but the observed cases with stable disease and even tumor regressions show that tumoricidal doses can be reached even in large tumors. Bearing in mind that RIT is needed for eradication of minimal residual HNSCC, and that MAb uptake levels are much higher in small-sized tumors, further development seems justified[15].

REFERENCES

1. Landis S.H., Murray T., Bolden S, and Wingo P. A. Cancer statistics 1998. CA Cancer J. Clin. 48: 6-29, 1998.
2. Vokes E.E., Weichselbaum R.R., Lippman S.M. and Hong W.K. Head and neck cancer. N. Engl. J. Med. 328: 184-193, 1993.
3. Dennington M.L., Carter D.R. and Meijers A.D. Distant metastases in head and neck carcinoma. Laryngoscope 90:196-201, 1980
4. Zbären P. and Lehmann W. Frequency and sites of distant metastases in head and neck squamous cell carcinoma. An analysis of 101 cases at autopsy. Arch. Otolaryngol. Head Neck Surg. 113:762-764, 1987
5. Nishijima W., Takoda S., Tokita N., Takayama S. and Sakura M. Analyses of distant metastases in squamous cell carcinoma of the head and neck and lesions above the clavicle at autopsy. Arch. Otolaryngol. Head Neck Surg. 119:65-68, 1993
6. Leemans C.R., Tiwari R.M. , Nauta J.J.P., Van der Waal I. and Snow G.B. Recurrence at the primary site in head and neck cancer and the significance of neck lymph node metastases as a prognostic factor. Cancer (Phila.) 73: 187-190, 1993
7. Leemans C.R., Tiwari R.M. , Nauta J.J.P., Van der Waal I. and Snow G.B. Regional lymph node involvement and its significance in the development of distant metastases in head and neck cancer. Cancer (Phila.) 71: 452-456, 1992
8. Stell P.M, Rawson N.S.B.: Adjuvant therapy in head and neck cancer. Br. J. Cancer 61:779-787, 1990

9. Wessels B.W., Harisiadis L. and Carabell S.C. Dosimetry and radiobiological efficacy of clinical radioimmunotherapy. J. Nucl. Med. 30: 827, 1989

10. Köhler G. and Milstein C. Continuous cultures of fused cells secreting antibody of predefined specificity. Nature 256: 495-497, 1975

11. Witzig T.E., White C.A., Wiseman G.A., Gordon L.I., Emmanouilides C., Raubitschek A., Janakiraman N., Gutheil J., Schilder R.J., Spies S., Silverman D.H., Parker E., Grillo-Lopez A.J. Phase I/II trial of IDEC-Y2B8 radioimmunotherapy for treatment of relapsed or refractory CD20⁺ B-cell non-Hodgkin's lymphoma. J. Clin. Oncol. 17: 3793-803, 1999

12. Knox S.J., Goris M.L., Trisler K., Negrin R., Davis T., Liles T.M., Grillo-Lopez A., Chinn P., Varns C., Ning S.C., Fowler S., Deb N., Becker M., Marquez C., Levy R. Yttrium-90-labeled anti-CD20 monoclonal antibody therapy of recurrent B-cell lymphoma. Clin. Cancer Res. 2: 457-70, 1996

13. Kaminski M.S., Zasadny K.R., Francis I.R., Fenner M.C., Ross C.W., Milik A.W., Estes J., Tuck M., Regan D., Fisher S., Glenn S.D., Wahl R.L. Iodine-131-anti-B1 radioimmunotherapy for B-cell lymphoma. J. Clin. Oncol. 14: 1974-1981, 1996

14. Press O.W., Eary J.F., Appelbaum F.R., Martin P.J., Nelp W.B., Glenn S., Fisher D.R., Porter B., Matthews D.C., Gooley T., et al. Phase II trial of 131I-B1 (anti-CD20) antibody therapy with autologous stem cell transplantation for relapsed B cell lymphomas. Lancet. 346: 336-40, 1995

15. De Bree R., Kuik D.J., Quak J.J., Roos J.C., Van den Brekel M.W.M., Castelijns J.A., Van Wagtendonk F.W., Greuter H., Snow G.B. and Van Dongen G.A.M.S. The impact of tumour volume and other characteristics on uptake of radiolabelled monoclonal antibodies in tumour tissue of head and neck cancer patients. Eur. J. Med. 25: 1562-1565, 1998

16. DeNardo G.L., O'Donnell R.T., Kroger L.A., Richman C.M., Goldstein D.S., Shen S., DeNardo S.J. Strategies for developing effective radioimmunotherapy for solid tumors. Clin. Cancer Res. 5(10): 3219- 3223, 1999

17. DeNardo S.J., O'Grady L.F., Richman C.M., Goldstein D.S., O'Donnell R.T., DeNardo D.A., Kroger L.D., Lamborn K.R., Hellstrom K.E., Hellstrom I. and DeNardo G.L. Radioimmunotherapy for advanced breast cancer using I-131-ChL6 antibody. Anticancer Res. 17: 1745-1751, 1997

18. Jacobs, A.J., Fer M., Su F.M., Breitz H., Thompson, J., Goodgold H., Cain J., Heaps J., Weiden P. A phase I trial of a rhenium 186-labeled monoclonal antibody administered intraperitoneally in ovarian carcinoma. Obstet. Gynecol. 82: 586-593, 1993

19. Crippa F., Bolis G., Seregni E., Gavoni N., Scarfone G., Ferraris C., Buraggi G.L. Bombardieri. Single-dose intraperitoneal radioimmunotherapy with the murine monoclonal antibody I-131 MOv18: clinical results in patients with minimal residual disease of ovarian cancer. E. Eur. J. Cancer 31A(5): 686-690 , 1995

20. Reynolds J.C., Del Vecchio S., Sakahara H., Lora M.E., Carrasquillo J.A., Neumann R.D., Larson S.M. Anti-murine response to mouse monoclonal antibodies: clinical findings and implications. Nucl. Med. Biol. 16: 121-125, 1989

21. Khazaeli M.B., Conry R.M. and LoBuglio A. Human immune response to monoclonal antibodies. J. Immunother. 15: 42-52 , 1994

22. Dillman R.O., Shawler D.L., McCallister T.J., Halpern S.E., Human anti-mouse antibody response in cancer patients following single low-dose injections of radiolabeled murine monoclonal antibodies. Cancer Biother. 9: 17-28, 1994

23. Juweid M., Sharkey R.M., Markowitz A., Behr T., Swayne L.C., Dunn R., Hansen H.J., Shevitz J., Leung S.O., Rubin A.D., Goldenberg D.M., Treatment of non-Hodgkin's lymphoma with radiolabeled murine, chimeric or humanized LL2, an anti-CD22 monoclonal antibody. Cancer Res. 55(suppl): 5899-5907, 1995

24. Jurcic J.G., Caron P.C., Nikula T.K., Papadapoulos E.B., Finn R.D., Gansow O.A., Miller W.H.J., Geerlings M.W., Warrell R.P.J., Larson S. Radiolabeled anti-CD33 monoclonal antibody M195 for myeloid leukemias. Cancer Res. 55 (suppl): 5908-5910, 1995

25. Baselga J., Tripathy D., Mendelsohn J., Baughman S., Benz C.C., Dontis L., Sklorin N.T., Seidman A.D., Hudis C.A., Moore J., Rosen P.P. Twaddell T., Henderson I.C., Norton L. Phase II study of weekly intravenous recombinant humanized anti-p185HER2 monoclonal antibody in patients with HER2/neu-overexpressing metastatic breast cancer. J. Clin. Oncol. 14: 737-744, 1996

26. Quak J.J., Van Dongen G.A.M.S., Balm A.J.M., Brakkee J.P.G., Scheper R.J., Snow G.B. and MeijerC.J.L.M. A 22-kDa surface antigen detected by monoclonal antibody E48 is exclusively expressed in stratified squamous and transitional epithelia. Am. J. Pathol. 136: 191-197, 1990

27. Quak J.J., Schrijvers A.H.G.J., Brakkee J.G.P., Davis H.D., Scheper R.J., Balm A.J.M., Meijer CJLM, Snow G.B. and Van Dongen G.A.M.S. Expression and characterization of two differentiation antigens in stratified squamous epithelia and carcinomas. Int. J. Cancer. 50: 507-513, 1992

516

28. Schrijvers A.H.G.J., Quak J.J., Uyterlinde A.M., Van Walsum M., Meijer C.J.L.M., Snow G.B. and Van Dongen G.A.M.S. MAb U36, a novel monoclonal antibody successful in immuno-targeting of squamous cell carcinoma of the head and neck. Cancer Res. 53: 4383-4390, 1993

29. Gerretsen M., Visser G.W.M., Van Walsum M., Meijer C.J.L.M., Snow G.B. and Van Dongen G.A.M.S. 186Re-labeled monoclonal antibody E48 immunoglobin G-mediated therapy of human head and neck squamous cell carcinoma xenografts. Cancer Res. 53: 3524-3529, 1993

30. Gerretsen M., Visser G.W.M., Brakenhoff R.H., Van Walsum M., Snow G.B. and Van Dongen G.A.M.S. Complete ablation of small squamous cell carcinoma xenografts with 186Re-labeled monoclonal antibody E48. Cell. Biophys. 24: 135-142, 1994

31. Van Gog F.B., Brakenhoff R.H., Stichter-Van Walsum M., Snow G.B. and Van Dongen G.A.M.S. Perspectives of combined radioimmunotherapy and anti-EGFR antibody therapy for the treatment of residual head and neck cancer. Int. J. Cancer. 77:13-18, 1998

32. Brakenhoff R.H., Gerretsen M., Knippels E.M.C., Van Dijk M., Van Essen H., Olde Weghuis D., Sinke R.J., Snow G.B. and Van Dongen G.AM.S. The human E48 Antigen, highly homologous to the murine Ly-6 antigen ThB, is a GPI-anchored molecule apparently involved in keratinocyte cell-cell adhesion. J. Cell. Biol. 129: 1677-1689, 1995

33. Schrijvers A.H.G.J., Gerretsen M., Fritz J., Van Walsum M., Quak J.J., Snow G.B., Van Dongen G.A.M.S. Evidence for a role of the monoclonal antibody E48 defined antigen in cell-cell adhesion in squamous epithelia and head and neck squamous cell carcinomas. Exp. Cell. Res. 196: 264-269, 1991

34. Van Hal N.L.W., Van Dongen G.A.M.S., Rood-Knippels E.M.S., Van der Valk P., Snow G.B. and Brakenhoff R.H. Monoclonal antibody U36, a suitable candidate for clinical immunotherapy of squamous cell carcinoma, recognizes a CD44 isoform. Int. J. Cancer. 69: 520-527, 1996

35. De Bree R., Roos J.C., Quak J.J., Den Hollander W., Van den Brekel M.W.M., Van der Wal J.E., Tobi H., Snow G.B. and Van Dongen G.A.M.S. Clinical imaging of head and neck cancer with technetium-99m-labeled monoclonal antibody E48 IgG and F(ab')₂. J. Nucl. Med. 35: 775-783, 1994

36. De Bree R., Roos J.C., Quak J.J., Den Hollander W., Wilhelm A.J., Van Lingen A., Snow G.B. and Van Dongen G.A.M.S. Biodistribution of radiolabeled monoclonal antibody E48 IgG and F(ab')₂ in patients with head and neck cancer. Clin. Cancer Res. 1: 277-286, 1995

37. De Bree R., Roos J.C., Quak J.J., Den Hollander W., Snow G.B. and Van Dongen G.A.M.S. Radioimmunoscintigraphy and biodistribution of monoclonal antibodyU36 in patients with head and neck cancer. Clin. Cancer Res. 1: 591-598, 1995

38. De Bree R., Roos J.C., Plaizier M.A.B.D., Quak J.J., Van Kamp G.J., Den Hollander W., Snow G.B. and Van Dongen G.A.M.S. Selection of monoclonal antibody E48 IgG or U36 IgG for adjuvant radioimmunotherapy in head and neck cancer patients. Brit. J. Cancer 75: 1049-1060, 1997

39. Heider K-H, Sproll M., Susani S., Patzelt E., Beaumier P., Ostermann E., Ahorn A., Adolf G.R. Characterization of a high affinity monoclonal antibody specific for CD44v6 as candidate for immunotherapy of squamous cell carcinomas. Cancer Immunol. Immunother. 43: 245-253, 1996

40. Heider K-H., Mulder J-W.R., Ostermann E., Susani S., Patzelt E., Pals S.T., Adolf G.R. Splice variants of the cell surface glycoprotein CD44 associated with metastatic tumour cells are expressed in normal tissues of humans and cynomolgus monkeys. Eur. J. Cancer. 31A: 2385-2391, 1995

41. Vaughan A.T.M., Keeling A., Yankuba S.C.S. the production and biological distribution of yttrium-90-labeled antibodies. Int. J. Appl. Radiat. Isot. 36: 803-806, 1985

42. Hird V., Stewart J.S., Snook D., Dhokia B., Coulter C., Lambert H.E., Mason W.P., Soutter W.P. and Epenetos A.A. Intraperetoneally administered 90Y-labelled monoclonal antibodies as a third line of treatment in ovarian cancer. A phase 1-2 trial: problems encountered and possible solutions. Br. J. Cancer. 10: 48-51, 1990

43. Wessels B.W. and Rogus R.D. Radionuclide selection and model absorbed dose calculations for radiolabeled tumor associated antibodies. Med. Phys. 11: 638-645, 1984

44. Breitz H.B., Weiden P.L., Vanderheyden J-L, Appelbaum J.W., Bjorn M.J., Fer M.F., Wolf S.B., Ratliff B.A., Seiler C.A., Foisie D.C., Fisher D.R., Schroff R.W., Fritzberg A.R., Abams P.G. Clinical experience with rhenium-186-labeled monoclonal antibodies for radioimmunotherapy: results of phase I trials. J. Nucl. Med. 33:1099-1112, 1992

45. Mausner L.F., Srivastava S.C., Selection of radionuclides for radioimmunotherapy. Med. Phys. 20: 503-509, 1993

46. Coursey B.M., Cessna J. and Garcia-Torano E. The standardization and decay scheme of rhenium-186. Int. J. Radiat. Appl. Instrum. Part A. 42: 865-869, 1991

47. O'Donoghue J.A., Bardies M. and Wheldon T.E. Relationships between tumor size and curability for uniformly targeted therapy with beta-emitting radionuclides. J. Nucl. Med. : 36: 1902-1909, 1995

48.   Visser G.W.M., Gerretsen M., Herscheid J., Snow G.B. and Van Dongen G.A.M.S. Labeling of monoclonal antibodies with 186Re using the MAG3 chelate for radioimmunotherapy of cancer: a technical protocol. J. Nucl. Med. 34: 1953-1963, 1993

49.   Colnot D.R., Quak J.J., Roos J.C., Van Lingen A., Wilhelm A.J., Van Kamp G.J., Huijgens P.C., Snow, G.B. and Van Dongen G.A.M.S. Phase I therapy study of 186Re-labeled chimeric monoclonal antibody U36 in patients with squamous cell carcinoma of the head and neck. J. Nucl. Med. 41: 1999-2010, 2000

50.   Colnot D.R., De Bree R., Quak J.J., Roos J.C., Huijgens P.C., Snow, G.B. and Van Dongen G.A.M.S. High-dose radioimmunotherapy using rhenium-186-labeled chimeric monoclonal antibody U36 with re-infusion of unprocessed, G-CSF-primed whole blood in head and neck cancer patients. Abstract, AACR San Francisco, April 2000

51.   Stroomer J.W.G., Roos J.C., Sproll M., Quak J.J., Heider K-H., Wilhelm B.J., Castelijns, J.A., Meyer R., Kwakkelstein M.O., Snow G.B. Adolf G.R. and Van Dongen G.A.M.S. Safety and biodistribution of ^{99m}Tc-labeled anti-CD44v6 monoclonal antibody BIWA 1 in head and cancer patients. Clin. Cancer. Res. 6: 3046-3055, 2000